INDEX OF BOXED NOTES

Hydrogen ion concentration (Ch 2)

Hyper/hyposecretion (Ch 10)

Hypersensitivity reactions (Ch 14)

Hypoglycemia (Ch 10)

Impotence (Ch 19)

In vitro fertilization (Ch 20)

Inguinal canal (Ch 19)

Insulin (Ch 10)

Interatrial septal defect (Ch 13)

Interferon (Ch 14)

Interleukin (Ch 14)

Internal jugular veins (Ch 13)

Isotonic/isometric contractions (Ch 7)

Ketone bodies (Ch 17)

Kidney stones (Ch 18)

Kwashiorkor (Ch 17)

Lactose intolerance (Ch 16)

Laryngitis (Ch 15)

Limbic system (Ch 8)

Lumbar puncture (Ch 8)

Lymph nodes (Ch 14)

Lysosomes (Ch 3)

Mastectomy (Ch 14)

Mastoid air cells (Ch 6)

Melanomas (Ch 5)

Melatonin (Ch 10)

Meningitis (Ch 8)

Mittelschmerz (Ch 19)

Morula (Ch 20)

Motion sickness (Ch 9)

Multiple ovulations (Ch 20)

Mumps (Ch 16)

Mutations (Ch 3)

Myocardial infarction (Ch 12)

Nephron number (Ch 18)

Nephroptosis (Ch 18)

Obstruction of lymph flow (Ch 14)

Odors (Ch 9)

Osteitis fibrosa cystica (Ch 10)

Osteoporosis (Ch 6)

Otitis media (Ch 9)

Otosclerosis (Ch 9)

Ovarian carcinoma (Ch 19)

Oxytocin (Ch 10, 20)

Papanicolaou smear (Ch 19)

Paranasal sinuses (Ch 6)

Parkinson's disease (Ch 8)

Perforated eardrum (Ch 9)

Pericarditis (Ch 12)

Peritonitis (Ch 4)

Pernicious anemia (Ch 11)

Peroxisomes (Ch 3)

Pharyngitis (Ch 15)

Placenta previa (Ch 20)

Pleurisy (Ch 15)

Pneumothorax (Ch 15)

Poisons (Ch 17)

Polycystic kidney disease (Ch 18)

Pott's fracture (Ch 6)

Preventing excessive bleeding (Ch 11)

Prolactin (Ch 10)

Prostaglandins (Ch 10)

Prostate cancer (Ch 19)

Protein-bound iodine (Ch 10)

Pupillary reflexes (Ch 9)

Quadriceps femoris (Ch 7)

Relationship of anatomy/physiology (Ch 1)

Renal diabetes (Ch 18)

Reticular formation (Ch 8)

Reticulocyte count (Ch 11)

Rhinitis (Ch 15)

Right and left brain (Ch 8)

Sarcomas (Ch 4)

Sensory adaptation (Ch 9)

Skin weight (Ch 5)

Spleen (Ch 14)

Sternum (Ch 6)

Stimulus for breathing (Ch 15)

Suction lipectomy (Ch 4)

Surfactant (Ch 15)

Taste blindness (Ch 9)

Taste receptors (Ch 9)

Tennis elbow (Ch 6)

Tetanus (Ch 7)

Tongue-tied (Ch 16)

Tonsils (Ch 14)

Torticollis (Ch 7)

Tracheostomy (Ch 15)

Tubal ligation (Ch 19)

Twins (Ch 20)

Umbilical cord stem cells (Ch 20)

Uremia (Ch 18)

Uremic frost (Ch 18)

Urinary incontinence (Ch 18)

Urinary tract infections (Ch 18)

Varicose veins (Ch 13)

Vasectomy (Ch 19)

Vitamin C (Ch 17)

Vitamin K (Ch 11)

Vitamin toxicity (Ch 17)

Vitamins (Ch 17)

Vomiting (Ch 16)

Water (Ch 2)

Weak pulse (Ch 13)

Wisdom teeth (Ch 16)

The Anatomy and Physiology Learning System

The
Anatomy
and
Physiology
Learning
Second Edition # System

Edith Applegate, MS

Professor of Science and Mathematics
Kettering College of Medical Arts
Kettering, Ohio

Illustrated by

Pat Thomas, CMI

W.B. SAUNDERS COMPANY
A Harcourt Health Sciences Company
Philadelphia   London   Toronto   Sydney

W.B. SAUNDERS COMPANY
A Harcourt Health Sciences Company

The Curtis Center
Independence Square West
Philadelphia, Pennsylvania 19106

Library of Congress Cataloging-in-Publication Data

Applegate, Edith J.
The anatomy and physiology learning system/Edith Applegate; illustrated by Pat Thomas—2nd ed.

p. cm.

Includes index.

ISBN 0–7216–8020–8

1. Human physiology.   2.Human anatomy.   I. Title.

QP34.5 .A67 2000   612—dc21   99–051568

THE ANATOMY AND PHYSIOLOGY LEARNING SYSTEM   ISBN 0–7216–8020–8

Printed in the United States of America

Last digit is the print number: 9   8   7   6   5   4   3

This book is dedicated to

FRIENDS

Colleagues who have encouraged me;

students who have challenged me;

editors who have stimulated me;

family who have loved me;

sons, **David** and **Douglas**,

who bring pride and joy to my life;

and my best friend for more than forty years,

my husband, **Stan**,

who makes life a joyous experience to be treasured.

Preface

The Anatomy and Physiology Learning System includes a textbook, a workbook, an instructor's manual, and overhead transparencies to help teachers present a quality educational experience for students preparing to enter one of the health related professions. It is designed for students enrolled in a one-semester course in human anatomy and physiology and is also a useful tool when reviewing for licensure examinations. The textbook presents fundamental information and concepts in a manner that encourages learning and understanding. The topics are consistent with those needed by students in the health related professions. Students with minimal science background, as well as those with greater preparation, will appreciate the clear and concise writing style that makes the book easy to read and understand. Numerous clinical applications add interest and provide a springboard for discussions or projects. The colorful illustrations in the textbook make it visually attractive and contribute reinforcement for comprehension. The textbook component is complete in the topics presented and can be used as a stand-alone item. The workbook provides an added dimension in the form of learning objectives, written exercises that correlate with the objectives, quizzes, and medical terminology exercises. These two components, used together, provide a package that facilitates learning, enhances understanding, relates information to medical applications, and enables the students to apply their knowledge to further study within their chosen health related professions.

EDITH APPLEGATE

Acknowledgments

This book, like all others, reflects the efforts of many people. From its inception to its completion, the editorial staff at W.B. Saunders has been a source of support and encouragement. The production staff kept the project on schedule even when I failed to meet deadlines. Designers and artists met the challenge of designing a book that is new, fresh, unique, and exciting in appearance. The copy editors and proofreaders were gracious and kind when correcting my errors. I greatly appreciate the work of these and many others I have not mentioned. Thank you to everyone who has had a part in the completion of *The Anatomy and Physiology Learning System, Second Edition*.

Note To Students

Dear Student,

You are starting on an adventure that is interesting, rewarding, exciting, and fascinating. It will also be rigorous, demanding, and require a significant portion of your time. Anatomy and physiology is fascinating because it is about you and your body. The human body is intricate, complex, and marvelous. Because of this, your adventure will be rigorous and demanding as you work through the intricacies of structure and function. It will be rewarding because you will learn more about yourself and it will help prepare you to serve in the health care professions. As you study, relate what you learn to your own body. It will make the study more relevant to you.

Anatomy and physiology forms the foundation for course work in the health related professions. Nearly every day, students tell me that what they learned in anatomy and physiology has helped them in some other course. Learn the subject well. You'll be glad you did.

I have written *The Anatomy and Physiology Learning System* with you in mind. It contains the topics that are most beneficial to students in health related professions. I have included study aids that my students find helpful. Pay attention to the **summary statements** within the text, answer the **QuickCheck** questions as you progress through the chapter (the answers are in the back of the book), and test yourself with the **chapter quizzes**. The **Learning System** includes a **workbook** to complement the textbook. Complete the **learning exercises** in the workbook, review with the **review questions**, test yourself with the workbook **chapter quizzes**, learn how to use the terminology with the **terminology exercises**, then relax and have a little fun with the **fun and games** pages. These study tools have been used successfully by hundreds of students.

On the first day of class, someone usually asks, "How do we study to get a good grade in this class?" My flippant response is, "Very hard and carefully!" Then I become more serious and give some study hints. I will share some of these study hints with you because, by using *The Anatomy and Physiology Learning System*, you become one of my students and I like to believe I may have some small part in your success. You must realize, however, that study methods are an individual thing. All methods do not work for all people and you have to select those that work best for you.

- Read the appropriate material in the textbook before the lecture. By doing this, the lecture is more meaningful because you are familiar with the terminology and ideas.
- Attend lectures faithfully, sit near the front if possible, and pay attention to the teacher.
- Take good lecture notes because these are your guide for further study.
- As soon as possible after class, while your learning curve is still

high and the subject is still fresh in your mind, review your lecture notes and fill in items you may have missed.
- Reread your textbook, with your notes, and highlight those topics your instructor considers to be important.
- Use the study aids available to you—the review questions at the end of the chapter, the learning exercises in the workbook, the objectives, the quizzes, the terminology exercises. Some people like to make flashcards. Using a variety of study methods adds interest and improves concentration.
- Study **every** day. Keep the material fresh in your mind.
- Keep current. Thoroughly understand one day's material before your next class appointment. The subject builds on previous material so if you haven't studied the previous material, the next lecture may not make much sense.
- Study for understanding rather than rote memory. Six-year-olds can recite a collection of words from memory but may not understand a word they are saying.
- If there is something you don't understand, make an appointment to see your teacher for further explanation. Make your teacher earn his or her paycheck!

It looks like my brief note to you has turned into a long letter and I know you are anxious to get started on your adventure. I hope you enjoy your study of the human body. I would like to hear from you and have your comments and suggestions about ways to improve *The Anatomy and Physiology Learning System*.

In closing, I offer my best wishes for success in this course, in your selected curriculum, and in your chosen career.

Sincerely,

Edith Applegate

EDITH APPLEGATE
Kettering College of Medical Arts
Department of Biological Science
3737 Southern Boulevard
Kettering, OH 45429-1299

CHAPTER 5

Integumentary System

Outline/Objectives

Structure of the Skin 77
- Describe the structure of the two layers of the skin.
- Name the supporting layer of the skin and describe its structure.

Skin Color 80
- Discuss three factors that influence skin color.

Epidermal Derivatives 80
- Describe the structure of hair and nails and their relationship to the skin.
- Discuss the characteristics and functions of the various glands associated with the skin.

Functions of the Skin 82
- Discuss four functions of the integumentary system.

Key Terms

Arrector pili
Ceruminous gland
Dermis
Epidermis
Keratinization
Melanin
Sebaceous gland
Subcutaneous layer
Sudoriferous gland

Building Vocabulary

WORD PART	MEANING
albin-	white
cer-	wax
cutane-	skin
derm-	skin
-ectomy	surgical excision
hidr-	sweat
ichthy-	scaly, dry
kerat-	hard, horny tissue
-lucid-	clear, light
melan-	black
onych-	nail
pachy-	thick
-plasty	surgical repair
rhytid-	wrinkles
seb-	oil
sud-	sweat

75

- **Clear and concise writing style** makes the book easy to read and understand.

- **Outlines and objectives** at the beginning of each chapter help the students organize their study material.

- ✳ **Building vocabulary** identifies prefixes, suffixes, and roots appropriate to each chapter to help students understand terminology.

- **Key terms** are identified at the beginning of each chapter.

TEXTBOOK FEATURES

Features designated by an asterisk are new to this edition.

✳ **Functional relationships** between the chapter topic system and the other body systems are highlighted with a full page illustration at the beginning of each system chapter. These reinforce the concept that all systems work together.

Functional Relationships of the
Integumentary System

Provides a barrier against hazardous materials and pathogens.

Skeletal

Muscular

Nervous

Endocrine

Cardiovascular

Lymphatic/Immune

Respiratory

Digestive

Urinary

Reproductive

76

- **Clinical terms** that relate to the topic are identified and defined. A guide for pronunciation is provided for each term.

- ✳ **Index of clinical terms** provides a chapter cross reference to make it easier to locate a given term in the book.

CLINICAL TERMS

Alopecia (al-oh-PEE-shee-ah) Absence of hair from skin areas where it normally grows; baldness; may be hereditary or due to disease, injury, or chemotherapy or may occur as part of aging
Basal cell carcinoma (BAY-sal SELL kar-sih-NOH-mah) Malignant tumor of the basal cell layer of the epidermis; most common form of skin cancer and usually grows slowly
Cellulitis (sell-yoo-LYE-tis) Infection of connective tissue with severe inflammation of the dermis and subcutaneous layer of the skin
Dermatitis (der-mah-TYE-tis) Inflammation of the skin
Eczema (ECK-zeh-mah) An inflammatory skin disease with red, itching, vesicular lesions that may crust over; common allergic reaction, but may occur without any obvious cause

Eschar (ESS-kar) A slough produced by a burn or gangrene
Hives (HYVZ) Eruption of itching and burning swellings on the skin; most commonly caused by infections, medications, food allergies, or emotional stress; also called urticaria
Impetigo (im-peh-TYE-go) Superficial skin infection caused by staphylococcal or streptococcal bacteria and characterized by vesicles, pustules, and crusted-over lesions; most common in children
Malignant melanoma (mah-LIG-nant mel-ah-NOH-mah) Cancerous growth composed of melanocytes; often arises in preexisting mole; an alarming increase in the incidence of malignant melanoma is attributed to excessive exposure to sunlight

Nevus (NEE-vus) An elevated, pigmented lesion on the skin; commonly called a mole; a dysplastic nevus is a mole that does not form properly and may progress to a type of skin cancer; plural, nevi
Pruritus (proo-RYE-tus) Severe itching; one of the most common problems in dermatology; arises as a result of stimulation of nerves in the skin by enzymes released in allergic reactions or by other irritating substances
Wart (WORT) Epidermal growth on the skin caused by a virus; plantar warts occur on the soles of the feet, juvenile warts occur on the hands and face of children, and venereal warts occur in the genital area

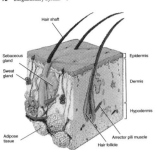

Hair shaft
Sebaceous gland
Sweat gland
Epidermis
Dermis
Hypodermis
Adipose tissue
Arrector pili muscle
Hair follicle

Figure 5-1 Structure of the skin. (From Jarvis C: Physical Examination and Health Assessment. Philadelphia, WB Saunders, 1992.)

cell changes shape. By the time the cells reach the surface, they are at or squamous and dead from lack of nutrients and are sloughed off. They are replaced by other cells that are pushed upward from below. As cells are pushed upward, away from the nutrient supply, and become keratinized, they take on different appearances and characteristics to form distinct regions. In thick skin, such as that on the soles of the feet and palms of the hand, the epidermis consists of ve regions, or strata, of cells (see Fig. 5–2). In the skin that covers the rest of the body, the regions are thinner and there are only four strata.

The epidermis is stratified squamous epithelium. In thick skin there are five distinct regions in the epidermis, but in thinner regions there are only four layers.

The bottom row of cells in the strati ed squamous epithelium that makes up the epidermis consists of actively dividing (mitotic) columnar cells. This layer is the **stratum basale** (BAY-sah-lee), the layer next to the basement membrane and closest to the blood supply (see Fig. 5–2). About one fourth of the cells in the stratum basale are **melanocytes** (meh-LAN-oh-sytes). These are specialized epithelial cells that produce a dark pigment called **melanin** (MEL-ah-nin). All individuals have the same number of melanocytes. However, melanocyte activity (the amount of melanin produced) differs according to genetic and environmental factors.

The bottom layer, or stratum basale, is closest to the blood supply and is actively mitotic. It also contains melanocytes.

Cancerous neoplasms composed of melanocytes, called malignant melanomas, account for 3 percent of all cancers, and the incidence is rising at a rate of 4.5 percent annually. Exposure to sunlight is the major risk factor for the development of malignant melanoma, and individuals with fair skin and light hair are at greatest risk. Melanomas often metastasize to the lung, liver, and brain.

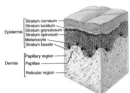

Stratum corneum
Stratum lucidum
Stratum granulosum
Stratum spinosum
Melanocyte
Stratum basale
Epidermis
Papillary region
Papillae
Reticular region
Dermis

Figure 5-2 Subdivisions of the epidermis and dermis.

• **Illustrations** are original, high quality, and colorful to add visual impact and reinforcement. They have been designed to correlate with the written material and help students visualize anatomical features and physiological processes.

• **Tables** within each chapter summarize information in a way that makes it easier to learn.

• **Summary statements** throughout each chapter provide reinforcement of key concepts.

• **Clinical applications** are highlighted in boxes throughout each chapter. These add interest and reinforce the relevance of the material.

✳ **Index of boxed notes** at the end of the book provide a chapter cross reference of the clinical applications notes to make it easier to locate a given clinical topic in the book.

• **Important words** are printed in bold type to highlight their significance.

• **Pronunciation guides** are given in parentheses after each scientific term when it appears the first time. This helps students verbalize the words correctly.

✳ **QuickCheck** questions throughout the chapter enable students to check their comprehension at various points within a chapter. Answers to these questions are in the back of the book.

• **Focus on aging** topics in each chapter describe some of the effects of aging on the body system discussed in that chapter.

• **Do you know this about . . . ?** box in each chapter provides additional information about a selected topic relevant to the chapter.

from the deeper tissues to the surface. However, if the skin becomes too cold, below 15°C (59°F), cutaneous blood vessels dilate to bring warm blood to the region so that the tissues are not damaged by the cold.

The skin helps to regulate body temperature through constriction and dilation of blood vessels, sweat gland activity, and the insulating effect of adipose tissue in the subcutaneous layer.

Synthesis of Vitamin D

Vitamin D is required for calcium and phosphorus absorption in the small intestine. The calcium and phosphorus are essential for normal bone metabolism and muscle function. Skin cells contain a precursor molecule that is converted to vitamin D when

the precursor is exposed to ultraviolet rays in sunlight. It takes only a small amount of ultraviolet light to stimulate vitamin D production, so this should not be used as an excuse to expose the skin to sun unnecessarily and to risk the damage that may result.

Vitamin D is synthesized in the skin when exposed to ultraviolet light.

☑ **QuickCheck**

• Why are infections and fluid loss of major concern for patients with severe burns?

• Jake is playing a vigorous game of volleyball on a warm summer day. Describe two ways the integument helps maintain internal body temperature in spite of the heat and exercise.

► FOCUS ON AGING

As the skin ages, the number of elastic fibers decreases and adipose tissue is lost from the dermis and subcutaneous layer. This causes the skin to wrinkle and sag. Loss of collagen fibers in the dermis makes the skin more fragile and makes it heal more slowly. Mitotic activity in the stratum basale slows so that the skin becomes thinner and appears more transparent. Reduced sebaceous gland activity causes dry, itchy skin. Loss of adipose tissue in the subcutaneous layer and reduced sweat gland activity lead to an intolerance of cold and susceptibility to heat. The ability of the skin to regulate temperature is reduced. There is a general reduction in melanocyte activity, which decreases protection from ultraviolet light, resulting in increased susceptibility to sunburn and skin cancer. Some melanocytes, however, may increase melanin production, resulting in "age spots."

Despite all the creams and "miracle" lotions, there is no known way to prevent skin from aging. Good nutrition and cleanliness may slow the aging process. Because skin that is exposed to sunlight ages more rapidly than unexposed skin, one of the best ways to slow the aging process is to avoid exposure by wearing protective clothing and by using sun blocks whenever possible.

DO YOU KNOW THIS ABOUT

Integument?

Burns

A burn is tissue damage that results from heat, certain chemicals, radiation, or electricity. The seriousness of burns is a result of their effect on the skin. The most serious threat to survival after a severe burn is uid loss because the waterproof protective covering, the skin, is destroyed. As uid seeps from the burned surfaces, electrolytes and proteins are also lost. The loss of uids, electrolytes, and proteins leads to osmotic imbalances, renal failure, and circulatory shock. Another problem is the imminent danger of massive infection. A large, severely burned region is bacteria heaven because there is easy access, ideal growing conditions, and no attack by the immune system. Bacteria have easy access to tissues because the protective barrier provided by the skin is absent. The protein-rich uid that seeps from burned areas is an ideal growth medium for bacteria, fungi, and other pathogens. Finally, the body s immune system, which normally ghts off threats of disease, becomes exhausted within 2 or 3 days after a severe burn injury.

Burns are classi ed as rst, second, or third degree according to their severity or depth. First-

REPRESENTATIVE DISORDERS OF THE INTEGUMENTARY SYSTEM

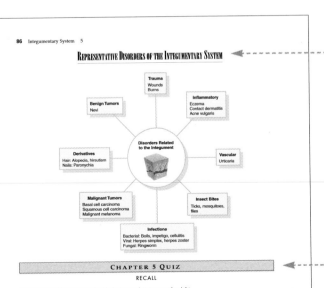

Trauma
Wounds
Burns

Inflammatory
Eczema
Contact dermatitis
Acne vulgaris

Benign Tumors
Nevi

Disorders Related to the Integument

Vascular
Urticaria

Derivatives
Hair: Alopecia, hirsutism
Nails: Paronychia

Malignant Tumors
Basal cell carcinoma
Squamous cell carcinoma
Malignant melanoma

Insect Bites
Ticks, mosquitoes, flies

Infections
Bacterial: Boils, impetigo, cellulitis
Viral: Herpes simplex, herpes zoster
Fungal: Ringworm

CHAPTER 5 QUIZ

RECALL

Match the definitions on the left with the appropriate term on the right.

1. Cells that produce a dark pigment

2. Outermost layer of the skin

3. Actively mitotic layer of the epidermis

4. Subcutaneous layer

A. Apocrine sweat glands
B. Arrector pili
C. Eponychium
D. Hair shaft

✳ **Representative disorders** of each body system are organized and presented in an illustration at the end of the chapter. The disorders are cross referenced and briefly described in a **glossary of disorders** at the end of the book.

• **Glossary** at the end of the book gives a pronunciation guide and definition for the scientific terms that appear throughout the textbook.

✳ **Chapter quizzes** at the conclusion of each chapter provide recall, thought, and application questions to check comprehension of the concepts within the chapter.

WORKBOOK FEATURES

✳ **Key concepts** are defined on the first page of each chapter in the workbook.

● **Chapter learning objectives** are organized according to textbook chapter outline headings. These objectives help students to focus on the important items presented in each chapter.

✳ **Chapter summary** is organized with the outline and objectives to provide a brief review of the chapter.

● **Learning exercises** are organized according to the chapter outlines and objectives. Five or more pages of exercises, including short answer, matching, and diagrams to label and color are provided for each chapter.

✳ **Chapter review** after the learning exercises provides questions for reinforcement and review of the concepts in the chapter.

● **Self-quizzes** give students an opportunity to check on their progress and understanding. There is a self quiz for each chapter.

● **Terminology exercises** gives students an opportunity to create and define words that relate to the topics presented in each chapter by using prefixes, suffixes, and word roots. This is excellent practice for their study in other courses relating to their chosen health related career.

● **Fun and games** is a lighter, more relaxed approach to the topics in each chapter. The final page of each workbook chapter is some type of word puzzle that incorporates words and concepts from the chapter. The workbook includes a variety of puzzles that provide reinforcement and show that learning can be fun.

ADDITIONAL MATERIAL FOR THE INSTRUCTOR

● **Instructor's Manual** is provided to adopters of **The Anatomy and Physiology Learning System**. This manual includes the answers to the review questions at the end of each chapter in the textbook and the answers for the learning exercises, quizzes, terminology exercises, and puzzles in the workbook. The manual also includes a collection of test questions with answers for each chapter.

● **Overhead Transparencies** are provided to adopters for use in lecture presentations. Fifty full-color illustrations from the textbook have been selected for this transparency set. They are certain to add interest and color to your lectures.

● **Computerized Test Bank** is provided to adopters for use in preparing tests and quizzes. This computer diskette package contains a minimum of 50 questions for each chapter to give a total of at least 1000 questions.

Contents

CHAPTER 1

Introduction to the Human Body   1

Anatomy and Physiology   2

Levels of Organization   2

Organ Systems   4

Life Processes   5

Homeostasis   9

    Negative and Positive Feedback   9

Anatomical Terms   10

    Anatomical Position   11

    Directions of the Body   11

    Planes and Sections of the Body   11

    Body Cavities   12

    Regions of the Body   14

CHAPTER 2

Chemistry, Matter, and Life   17

Elements   18

Structure of Atoms   18

Chemical Bonds   20

    Ionic Bonds   20

    Covalent Bonds   21

    Hydrogen Bonds   22

Compounds and Molecules   23

    Nature of Compounds   23

    Formulas   24

Chemical Reactions   24

    Chemical Equations   24

    Types of Chemical Reactions   25

    Reaction Rates   26

    Reversible Reactions   26

Mixtures, Solutions, and Suspensions   27

    Mixtures   27

Solutions   **27**

Suspensions   **27**

Electrolytes, Acids, Bases, and Buffers   **27**

Electrolytes   **28**

Acids   **28**

Bases   **28**

The pH Scale   **29**

Neutralization Reactions   **29**

Buffers   **30**

Organic Compounds   **30**

Carbohydrates   **30**

Proteins   **31**

Lipids   **32**

Nucleic Acids   **33**

Adenosine Triphosphate   **34**

CHAPTER **3**

Cell Structure and Function   39

Structure of the Generalized Cell   **40**

Plasma Membrane   **40**

Cytoplasm   **41**

Nucleus   **43**

Cytoplasmic Organelles   **43**

Filamentous Protein Organelles   **45**

Cell Functions   **45**

Movement of Substances Across the Cell Membrane   **45**

Cell Division   **50**

DNA Replication and Protein Synthesis   **52**

CHAPTER **4**

Tissues and Membranes   59

Body Tissues   **60**

Epithelial Tissue   **60**

Connective Tissue   **65**

Muscle Tissue   **68**

Nervous Tissue   **69**

Body Membranes   **70**

Mucous Membranes   **70**

Serous Membranes   **70**

Synovial Membranes   **71**

Meninges   **71**

CHAPTER **5**

Integumentary System   75

Structure of the Skin   **77**

Epidermis   **77**

Dermis   **79**

Subcutaneous Layer   **80**

Skin Color   **80**

Epidermal Derivatives   **80**

Hair and Hair Follicles   **80**

Nails   **81**

Glands   **82**

Functions of the Skin   **82**

Protection   **82**

Sensory Reception   **83**

Regulation of Body Temperature   **83**

Synthesis of Vitamin D   **84**

CHAPTER **6**

Skeletal System   89

Overview of the Skeletal System   **91**

Functions of the Skeletal System   **91**

Structure of Bone Tissue   **92**

Classification of Bones   **93**

General Features of a Long Bone   **93**

Bone Development and Growth   **94**

Division of the Skeleton   **97**

Bones of the Axial Skeleton   **97**

Skull   **97**

Hyoid Bone   **102**

Vertebral Column   **103**

Thoracic Cage   **105**

Bones of the Appendicular Skeleton   **106**

Pectoral Girdle   **106**

Upper Extremity   **107**

Pelvic Girdle   **109**

Lower Extremity   **111**

Articulations   **114**

Synarthroses   **114**

Amphiarthroses   **114**

Diarthroses   **114**

Spinal Nerves   **173**
Autonomic Nervous System   **174**

CHAPTER 7

Muscular System   **121**

Characteristics and Functions of the Muscular System   **123**
Structure of Skeletal Muscle   **123**
Whole Skeletal Muscle   **123**
Skeletal Muscle Attachments   **124**
Skeletal Muscle Fibers   **125**
Nerve and Blood Supply   **125**
Contraction of Skeletal Muscle   **126**
Stimulus for Contraction   **126**
Sarcomere Contraction   **127**
Contraction of a Whole Muscle   **127**
Energy Sources and Oxygen Debt   **129**
Movements   **133**
Skeletal Muscle Groups   **133**
Naming Muscles   **133**
Muscles of the Head and Neck   **133**
Muscles of the Trunk   **137**
Muscles of the Upper Extremity   **140**
Muscles of the Lower Extremity   **143**

CHAPTER 9

Sensory System   **183**

Receptors and Sensations   **184**
General Senses   **185**
Touch and Pressure   **185**
Proprioception   **186**
Temperature   **186**
Pain   **186**
Gustatory Sense   **186**
Olfactory Sense   **187**
Visual Sense   **188**
Protective Features and Accessory Structures of the Eye   **188**
Structure of the Eyeball   **190**
Pathway of Light and Refraction   **191**
Photoreceptors   **192**
Visual Pathway   **193**
Auditory Sense   **194**
Structure of the Ear   **194**
Physiology of Hearing   **196**
Sense of Equilibrium   **197**
Static Equilibrium   **197**
Dynamic Equilibrium   **198**

CHAPTER 8

Nervous System   **151**

Functions of the Nervous System   **153**
Organization of the Nervous System   **154**
Nerve Tissue   **155**
Neurons   **155**
Neuroglia   **156**
Nerve Impulses   **157**
Resting Membrane   **157**
Stimulation of a Neuron   **158**
Conducting Along a Neuron   **159**
Conduction Across a Synapse   **161**
Reflex Arcs   **162**
Central Nervous System   **163**
Meninges   **163**
Brain   **164**
Ventricles and Cerebrospinal Fluid   **169**
Spinal Cord   **170**
Peripheral Nervous System   **171**
Structure of a Nerve   **172**
Cranial Nerves   **172**

CHAPTER 10

Endocrine System   **203**

Introduction to the Endocrine System   **205**
Comparison of the Endocrine and Nervous Systems   **205**
Comparison of Exocrine and Endocrine Glands   **205**
Characteristics of Hormones   **205**
Chemical Nature of Hormones   **205**
Mechanism of Hormone Action   **205**
Control of Hormone Action   **206**
Endocrine Glands and Their Hormones   **207**
Pituitary Gland   **207**
Thyroid Gland   **212**
Parathyroid Glands   **213**
Adrenal (Suprarenal) Glands   **214**
Pancreas—Islets of Langerhans   **217**

Gonads (Testes and Ovaries)   218
Pineal Gland   219
Other Endocrine Glands   220
Prostaglandins   220

CHAPTER **11**

Blood   225

Functions and Characteristics of the Blood   226
Composition of the Blood   227
Plasma   227
Formed Elements   229
Hemostasis   233
Vascular Constriction   233
Platelet Plug Formation   233
Coagulation   234
Blood Typing and Transfusions   235
Agglutinogens and Agglutinins   235
ABO Blood Groups   235
RH Blood Groups   237

CHAPTER **12**

Heart   241

Overview of the Heart   243
Form, Size, and Location of the Heart   243
Coverings of the Heart   243
Structure of the Heart   244
Layers of the Heart Wall   244
Chambers of the Heart   245
Valves of the Heart   246
Pathway of Blood Through the Heart   247
Blood Supply to the Myocardium   248
Physiology of the Heart   249
Conduction System   249
Cardiac Cycle   251
Heart Sounds   251
Cardiac Output   252

CHAPTER **13**

Blood Vessels   259

Classification and Structure of Blood Vessels   260
Vessels   260

Arteries   260
Capillaries   261
Veins   262
Physiology of Circulation   263
Role of the Capillaries   263
Blood Flow   264
Pulse and Blood Pressure   266
Circulatory Pathways   269
Pulmonary Circuit   270
Systemic Circuit   270
Fetal Circulation   281

CHAPTER **14**

Lymphatic System and Body Defense   285

Functions of the Lymphatic System   287
Components of the Lymphatic System   287
Lymph   287
Lymphatic Vessels   288
Lymphatic Organs   289
Resistance to Disease   291
Nonspecific Defense Mechanisms   291
Specific Defense Mechanisms   293
Acquired Immunity   299

CHAPTER **15**

Respiratory System   305

Functions and Overview of Respiration   307
Ventilation   307
Conducting Passages   307
Mechanics of Ventilation   312
Respiratory Volumes and Capacities   314
Basic Gas Laws and Respiration   315
Properties of Gases   315
External Respiration   316
Internal Respiration   317
Transport of Gases   317
Oxygen Transport   317
Carbon Dioxide Transport   318
Regulation of Respiration   320
Respiratory Center   320

Factors That Influence Breathing   320

Nonrespiratory Air Movements   322

CHAPTER **16**

Digestive System   327

Functions of the Digestive System   329

General Structure of the Digestive Tract   330

Regions of the Digestive Tract   331

Mouth   331

Pharynx   334

Esophagus   335

Stomach   335

Small Intestine   338

Large Intestine   340

Accessory Organs of the Digestive System   341

Liver   341

Gallbladder   344

Pancreas   344

Chemical Digestion   345

Carbohydrate Digestion   345

Protein Digestion   346

Lipid Digestion   346

Absorption   346

CHAPTER **17**

Metabolism and Nutrition   353

Metabolism of Absorbed Nutrients   354

Anabolism   354

Catabolism   354

Energy From Foods   355

Carbohydrates   355

Uses for Energy   360

Basic Elements of Nutrition   361

Carbohydrates   362

Proteins   363

Lipids   364

Vitamins   365

Minerals   367

Water   367

Body Temperature   367

Heat Production   368

Heat Loss   368

Temperature Regulation   368

CHAPTER **18**

Urinary System and Body Fluids   373

Functions of the Urinary System   375

Components of the Urinary System   375

Kidneys   375

Ureters   379

Urinary Bladder   379

Urethra   380

Urine Formation   381

Glomerular Filtration   381

Tubular Reabsorption   381

Tubular Secretion   383

Regulation of Urine Concentration and Volume   384

Micturition   385

Characteristics of Urine   385

Physical Characteristics   385

Chemical Composition   385

Abnormal Constituents   385

Body Fluids   386

Fluid Compartments   386

Intake and Output of Fluid   387

Electrolyte Balance   387

Acid-Base Balance   388

CHAPTER **19**

Reproductive System   393

Male Reproductive System   395

Testes   395

Duct System   399

Accessory Glands   400

Penis   400

Male Sexual Response   401

Hormonal Control   402

Female Reproductive System   402

Ovaries   402

Genital Tract   406

External Genitalia   408

Female Sexual Response   408

Hormonal Control   409

Mammary Glands   412

CHAPTER 20

Development 419

Fertilization 420

Preembryonic Period 422

Cleavage 422

Implantation 423

Formation of Primary Germ Layers 424

Embryonic Development 424

Formation of Extraembryonic Membranes 424

Formation of the Placenta 425

Organogenesis 426

Fetal Development 427

Parturition and Lactation 428

Labor and Delivery 428

Adjustments of the Infant at Birth 429

Physiology of Lactation 429

Postnatal Development 430

Neonatal Period 431

Infancy 431

Childhood 431

Adolescence 432

Adulthood 432

Senescence 432

Answers for Quick Check Questions 436

Glossary of Disorders 439

Glossary of Word Parts 445

General Glossary 448

Index 475

CHAPTER 1

Introduction to the Human Body

Outline/Objectives

Anatomy and Physiology 2
- Define the terms *anatomy* and *physiology* and discuss the relationship between the two areas of study.

Levels of Organization 2
- List the six levels of organization within the human body.

Organ Systems 4
- Name the 11 organ systems of the body and briefly describe the major role of each system.

Life Processes 5
- List and define 10 life processes in the human body.
- List five physical environmental factors necessary for survival of the individual.

Homeostasis 9
- Discuss the concept of homeostasis.
- Distinguish between negative feedback mechanisms and positive feedback mechanisms.

Anatomical Terms 10
- Describe the four criteria that are used to describe the anatomic position.
- Use anatomical terms to describe body planes, body regions, and relative positions.
- Distinguish between the dorsal body cavity and the ventral body cavity, and list the subdivisions of each one.

Key Terms

Anatomical position
Anatomy
Differentiation
Homeostasis
Metabolism
Negative feedback
Physiology

Building Vocabulary

WORD PART	MEANING
al-	pertaining to
ana-	apart
cardi-	heart
dors-	back
epi-	upon, above
gastr-	stomach
homeo-	alike, same
integ-	a covering
-ism	process of
-itis	inflammation
-logy	study of, science of
metabol-	change
path-	disease
pelv-	basin
physi-	nature, function
proxim-	nearest
skelet-	a dried, hard body
-sta-	to control, staying
-tom-	to cut
vas-	vessel
viscer-	internal organs
-y	process, condition

he human body is an awesome masterpiece. Imagine billions of microscopic parts, each with its own identity, working together in an organized manner for the benefit of the total being. The human body is more complex than the greatest computer, yet it is very personal. The study of the human body is as old as history itself because people have always had an interest in how the body is put together, how it works, why it becomes defective (illness), and why it wears out (aging).

The study of the human body is essential for those planning a career in health sciences just as knowledge about automobiles is necessary for those planning to repair them. How can you fix an automobile if you do not know how it is put together or how it works? How can you help fix a human body if you do not know how it is put together or how it works?

Knowledge of the human body is also beneficial to the non-health care professional. Using this knowledge will help keep the body healthy. It will help you rate your activities as being beneficial or detrimental to your body, communicate with medical personnel, understand treatments that may be prescribed, and critically evaluate advertisements and reports in magazines. In addition to all this, the study of the human body is appealing. It lets us learn more about ourselves.

Anatomy and physiology are dynamic, applied sciences. New technology leads to new discoveries that may change the way certain aspects are viewed. For the student to keep up with the new discoveries and changes, it is necessary to have a strong foundation on which to build new knowledge. This book is an introduction designed to provide a basis for continuing study in the fascinating fields of anatomy and physiology.

Anatomy and Physiology

Anatomy (ah-NAT-oh-mee) is the scientific study of the structure or morphology of organisms and their parts. Human anatomy is the study of the shape and structure of the human body and its parts. It includes a wide range of study, including how structures develop, their microscopic organization, the relationship of one structure to another, and how structure and function are interrelated. Figure 1–1 depicts some of the subdivisions of the broad field of anatomy. **Gross human anatomy** deals with the large structures of the human body that can be seen through normal dissection. **Microscopic anatomy** deals with the smaller structures and fine detail that can be seen only with the aid of a microscope.

Physiology (fiz-ee-AHL-oh-jee) is the scientific study of the functions or processes of living things. It is the study of how the parts in anatomy work, what they do, and why. Some physiologists specialize in the study of a particular system such as the digestive system. Others deal with a single organ such as the stomach. Many people currently studying in the field of physiology deal with individual cells and how they work. This is called **cellular physiology.** Figure 1–1 shows some of the specialty areas within the study of physiology.

Anatomy and physiology are interrelated because structure and function are always closely associated. The function of an organ, or how it works, depends on how it is put together. Conversely, the anatomy or structure provides clues to understanding how it works. The structure of the hand, with its long, jointed fingers, is related to its function of grasping things. The heart is designed as a muscular pump that can contract to force blood into the blood vessels. By contrast, the lungs, whose function is the exchange of oxygen and carbon dioxide between the outside environment and the blood, are made of a very thin tissue. Imagine what would happen if the heart were made of thin tissue and the lungs were made of thick muscle. Structure and function are always related.

> Anatomy and physiology are interrelated because structure influences function and function affects structure.

> Often congenital anatomical abnormalities must be surgically repaired so that disruptions in physiology are corrected. For example a cleft palate (anatomy) is repaired so that food will enter (physiology) the pharynx instead of the nasal cavity. Broken bones (anatomy) are reset so that function (physiology) is restored.

Levels of Organization

One of the most outstanding features of the complex human body is its order and organization—how all the parts, from tiny atoms to visible structures, work together to make a functioning whole. There are six levels to the organizational scheme of the body (Fig. 1–2).

Starting with the simplest and proceeding to the most complex, the six levels of organization are chemical, cellular, tissue, organ, body system, and total organism. The structural and functional characteristics of all organisms are determined by their chemical makeup. The **chemical** level, discussed in Chapter 2, deals with the interactions of atoms (such as hydrogen and oxygen) and their combinations into molecules (such as water). Molecules contribute to the makeup of a cell, which is the basic unit of life. **Cells,** discussed in Chapter 3, are the basic living units of all organisms. Estimates indicate that

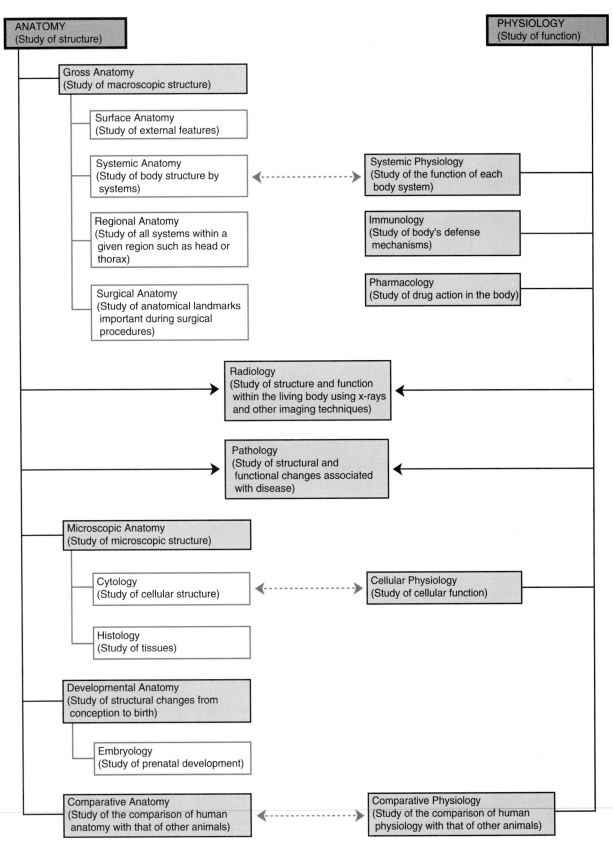

Figure 1–1 Examples of specialty areas of anatomy and physiology.

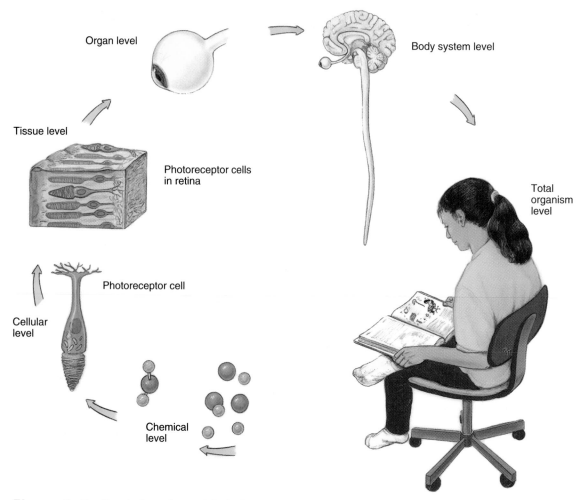

Figure 1–2   Organization scheme of the body.

there are about 100 trillion dynamic, living cells in the human body. These cells represent a variety of sizes, shapes, and structures and provide a vast array of functions. Cells with similar structure and function are grouped together as **tissues.** All of the tissues of the body are grouped into four main types: epithelial, connective, muscle, and nervous. The tissue level of organization is discussed in Chapter 4. Two or more tissue types that together form a more complex structure and work together to perform one or more functions make up **organs,** the next higher level of organization. Examples of organs include the skin, heart, ear, stomach, and liver. A body **system** consists of several organs that work together to accomplish a set of functions. Some examples of body systems include the nervous system, the digestive system, and the respiratory system. Finally, the most complex of all the levels is the **total organism,** which is made up of several systems that work together to maintain life. Beginning with Chapter 5, this book deals primarily with

the organs and organ systems that make up the total organism, the human body.

From the simplest to the most complex, the six levels of organization are chemical, cellular, tissue, organ, body system, and total organism.

✓ QuickCheck

- Would an immunologist be considered an anatomist or a physiologist? Why?

- Would an anatomist be more likely to study the structure or the function of the human body?

- On an organizational scale, are organs more complex or less complex than tissues?

Organ Systems

There are 11 major organ systems in the human body, each with specific functions, yet all are interrelated and working together to sustain life. Each system is described briefly here and then in more detail in later chapters. The organ systems are illustrated and summarized in Table 1–1.

Integumentary System. Integument means skin. The integumentary (in-teg-yoo-MEN-tar-ee) system consists of the skin and the various accessory organs associated with it. These accessories include hair, nails, sweat glands, and sebaceous (oil) glands. The components of the integumentary system protect the underlying tissues from injury, protect against water loss, contain sense receptors, help in temperature regulation, and synthesize chemicals to be used in other parts of the body.

Skeletal System. The skeletal (SKEL-eh-tull) system forms the framework of the body and protects underlying organs such as the brain, lungs, and heart. It consists of the bones and joints along with the ligaments and cartilages that bind the bones together. Bones serve as attachments for muscles and act with the muscles to produce movement. Tissues within bones produce blood cells and store inorganic salts containing calcium and phosphorus.

Muscular System. Muscles are the organs of the muscular (MUS-kyoo-lar) system. As muscles contract, they create the forces that produce movement and maintain posture. Muscles can store energy in the form of glycogen and are the primary source of heat within the body.

Nervous System. The nervous (NER-vus) system consists of the brain, spinal cord, and associated nerves. These organs work together to coordinate body activities. Nerve cells, or neurons, are specialized to transmit impulses (conductivity) from one point to another. In this way, body parts can communicate with each other and with the outside environment. Some nerve cells have special endings called sense receptors that detect changes in the environment (stimuli).

Endocrine System. The endocrine (EN-doh-krin) system includes all the glands that secrete chemicals called hormones that travel through the blood to act as messengers to regulate cellular activities. The endocrine and nervous systems act together to coordinate and regulate body activities to maintain a proper balance. The nervous system typically acts quickly, whereas the endocrine system acts slowly but with a more sustained effect. The endocrine system also regulates reproductive functions in both males and females.

Cardiovascular System. The cardiovascular (kar-dee-oh-VAS-kyoo-lar) system consists of the blood, heart, and blood vessels. The blood transports nutrients, hormones, and oxygen to tissue cells and removes waste products such as carbon dioxide. Certain cells within the blood defend the body against disease. The heart acts as a pump to create the forces necessary to maintain blood pressure and to circulate the blood. The blood vessels serve as pipes or channels for the flow of blood.

Lymphatic System. The lymphatic (lim-FAT-ik) system consists of a series of vessels that transport fluid (lymph) from the tissues back into the blood. The system includes lymph nodes and lymphoid organs like the tonsils, spleen, and thymus that filter the lymph to remove foreign particles as a protection against disease. Lymphoid organs also function in the body's defense mechanism by enhancing the activities of certain blood cells that produce immunity by inactivating specific pathogenic agents. The lymphatic system is sometimes considered to be a part of the cardiovascular system.

Digestive System. The organs of the digestive (dye-JES-tiv) system include the mouth, pharynx, esophagus, stomach, small intestine, and large intestine (colon), which make up the digestive tract, and the accessory organs, which consist of the teeth, tongue, salivary glands, liver, gallbladder, and pancreas. The functions of this system are to ingest food, process it into molecules that can be used by the body, and then eliminate the residue.

Respiratory System. The respiratory (reh-SPY-rah-tor-ee or res-per-ah-TOR-ee) system brings oxygen, in the form of air, into the lungs, removes the carbon dioxide, and provides a membrane for the exchange of the gases between the blood and lungs. The system consists of the nasal cavities, pharynx, larynx, trachea, bronchi, and lungs.

Urinary System. The kidneys, ureters, urinary bladder, and urethra make up the urinary (YOO-rin-air-ee) system. The kidneys remove various waste materials, especially nitrogenous wastes, from the blood and help to regulate the fluid level and chemical content of the body. The product of kidney function is urine, which is transported through the ureters and urethra. The urinary bladder serves as a reservoir or storage area for the urine.

Reproductive System. The reproductive (ree-pro-DUK-tiv) system is concerned with the production of new individuals. The system consists of the primary organs or gonads, ovaries in the female and testes in the male, that produce the reproductive cells, duct systems for transport, accessory glands, and supporting structures. In the female, the reproductive system produces ova or eggs, receives sperm from the male, and provides for the support and development of the embryo and fetus. The male reproductive system is concerned with the production and maintenance of sperm and the transfer of these cells to the female.

> The major organ systems of the body are the integumentary, skeletal, muscular, nervous, endocrine, cardiovascular, lymphatic, digestive, respiratory, urinary, and reproductive.

Life Processes

All living organisms have certain characteristics that distinguish them from nonliving forms. The basic processes of life include organization, metabolism, responsiveness, movement, and reproduction. In hu-

Table 1–1 Organ Systems of the Body

INTEGUMENTARY SYSTEM	SKELETAL SYSTEM	MUSCULAR SYSTEM
COMPONENTS: Skin, hair, nails, sweat and sebaceous glands FUNCTIONS: Covers and protects the body; regulates temperature	COMPONENTS: Bones, cartilage, ligaments FUNCTIONS: Provides body framework and support; protects; attaches muscles to bones; provides calcium storage	COMPONENTS: Muscles FUNCTIONS: Produces movement; maintains posture; provides heat
NERVOUS SYSTEM	**ENDOCRINE SYSTEM**	**CARDIOVASCULAR SYSTEM**
COMPONENTS: Brain, spinal cord, nerves, sense receptors FUNCTIONS: Coordinates body activities; receives and transmits stimuli	COMPONENTS: Pituitary, adrenal, thyroid, and other ductless glands FUNCTIONS: Regulates metabolic activities and body chemistry	COMPONENTS: Heart, blood vessels, and blood FUNCTIONS: Transports material from one part of the body to another; defends against disease

Table 1–1   Organ Systems of the Body *Continued*

LYMPHATIC SYSTEM	DIGESTIVE SYSTEM	RESPIRATORY SYSTEM

COMPONENTS: Lymph, lymph vessels, and lymphoid organs

FUNCTIONS: Returns tissue fluid to the blood; defends against disease

COMPONENTS: Mouth, esophagus, stomach, intestines, liver, and pancreas

FUNCTIONS: Ingests and digests food; absorbs nutrients into blood

COMPONENTS: Air passageways and lungs

FUNCTIONS: Exchanges gases between blood and external environment

URINARY SYSTEM	REPRODUCTIVE SYSTEM

COMPONENTS: Kidneys, ureter, urinary bladder, urethra

FUNCTIONS: Excretes metabolic wastes; regulates fluid balance and acid–base balance

COMPONENTS: Testes, ovaries, and accessory structures

FUNCTIONS: Forms new individuals to provide continuation of the human species mans, who represent the most complex form of life, there are additional requirements such as growth, differentiation, respiration, digestion, and excretion. All of these processes are interrelated. No part of the body, from the smallest cell to a complete body system, works in isolation. All function together, in fine-tuned balance, for the well-being of the individual and to maintain life. Disease and death represent a disruption of the balance in these processes. The following is a brief description of the life processes.

Organization. At all levels of the organizational scheme, there is a division of labor. Each component has its own job to perform in cooperation with others. Even a single cell, if it loses its integrity or organization, will die.

Metabolism. Metabolism (meh-TAB-oh-lizm) includes all the chemical reactions that occur in the body. One phase of metabolism is **catabolism** (kah-TAB-oh-lizm), in which complex substances are broken down into simpler building blocks and energy is released. **Anabolism** (ah-NAB-oh-lizm) is a building-up process in which complex substances are synthesized from simpler ones. This usually requires energy.

Responsiveness. Responsiveness or irritability is concerned with detecting changes in the internal or external environments and reacting to that change. It is the act of sensing a stimulus and responding to it. Conductivity is the ability to transmit a stimulus or information from one point to another.

Movement. There are many different types of movement within the body. On the cellular level, molecules move from one place to another. Blood moves from one part of the body to another. The diaphragm moves with every breath. The ability of muscle fibers to shorten and thus to produce movement is called contractility.

Reproduction. For most people, reproduction refers to the formation of a new person, the birth of a baby. In this way, life is transmitted from one generation to the next through reproduction of the organism. In a broader sense, reproduction also refers to the formation of new cells for the replacement and repair of old cells as well as for growth. This is cellular reproduction. Both are essential to the survival of the human race.

Growth. Growth refers to an increase in size either through an increase in the number of cells or through an increase in the size of each individual cell. For growth to occur, anabolic processes must occur at a faster rate than catabolic processes.

Differentiation. Differentiation (dif-er-en-she-AY-shun) is a developmental process by which unspecialized cells change into specialized cells with distinctive structural and functional characteristics. Through differentiation, cells develop into tissues and organs.

Respiration. Respiration refers to all the processes involved in the exchange of oxygen and carbon dioxide between the cells and the external environment. It includes ventilation, the diffusion of oxygen and carbon dioxide, and the transport of the gases in the blood. Cellular respiration deals with the cell's utilization of oxygen and release of carbon dioxide in its metabolism.

Digestion. Digestion is the process of breaking down complex ingested foods into simple molecules that can be absorbed into the blood and utilized by the body.

Excretion. Excretion is the process that removes the waste products of digestion and metabolism from the body. It gets rid of by-products that the body is unable to use, many of which are toxic and incompatible with life.

> Basic processes that distinguish human life from nonliving forms are organization, metabolism, responsiveness, movement, reproduction, growth, differentiation, respiration, digestion, and excretion.

The 10 life processes just described are not enough to ensure the survival of the individual. In addition to these processes, life depends on certain physical factors from the environment.

Water. Water is the most abundant substance in the body. About 60 percent of the body weight is attributed to water. It provides a medium in which chemical reactions occur, transports substances from one place to another within the body, and helps to regulate body temperature.

Oxygen. Oxygen is necessary for the metabolic reactions that provide energy.

Nutrients. Nutrients, such as carbohydrates, proteins, fats, vitamins, and minerals, come from the foods that we eat. They supply the chemicals that the body needs for energy and serve as raw materials for making new tissues for growth, replacement, and repair.

Heat. Heat, a form of energy, is necessary to keep the chemical reactions in the body proceeding at an appropriate rate. In general, the more heat there is, the faster the reaction, up to an optimum point. After that, the reaction rate decreases. Consequently the amount of heat in the body must be regulated. Temperature is a measure of the amount of heat that is present.

Pressure. Pressure is the application of a force. Atmospheric pressure is the force of the air acting on our bodies. This pressure plays an important role in breathing and in the exchange of gases between the lungs and the outside air. Hydrostatic pressure is the force applied by fluids. Blood pressure, a form of hydrostatic pressure, is essential for the circulation of blood.

> Physical factors from the environment that are essential to human life include water, oxygen, nutrients, heat, and pressure.

✓ Quick Check

- Which body system is responsible for the exchange of oxygen and carbon dioxide between the blood and the external environment?
- Which body system transports oxygen, carbon dioxide, and nutrients from one part of the body to another?
- What factors from the environment are necessary to sustain human life processes?

Homeostasis

Homeostasis (hoh-mee-oh-STAY-sis) refers to the constant internal environment that must be maintained for the cells of the body. The word is derived from two Greek words, "homeo," which means alike or the same, and "stasis," which means always or staying. Putting these together the word "homeostasis" means staying the same. When the body is healthy, the internal environment always stays the same. It remains stable within very limited normal ranges.

Everyone is familiar with aspects of the external environment—whether it is cold or hot, humid or dry, smoggy or clear. The internal environment is not quite as obvious. It refers to the tissue fluid that surrounds and bathes every cell of the body. Normal functional activities of the cell depend on the internal environment being maintained within very limited normal ranges. The chemical content, volume, temperature, and pressure of the fluid must stay the same (homeostasis), regardless of external conditions, so that the cell can function properly. If the conditions in the fluid deviate from normal, mechanisms respond that try to restore conditions to normal. If the mechanisms are unsuccessful, the cell malfunctions and dies. This leads to illness or disease and, if homeostasis is not restored, eventually to death of the individual.

■   A lack of homeostasis leads to illness or disease.

Negative and Positive Feedback

Any condition or stimulus that disrupts the homeostatic balance in the body is a **stressor.** When a stressor causes internal conditions to deviate from normal, all the body systems work to bring conditions back to the normal range. This is usually accomplished by a **negative feedback** mechanism that works much like a thermostat connected to a furnace and an air conditioner as illustrated in Figure 1–3A. When the temperature in the room decreases (stressor) below the thermostat setting (normal), the sensing device in the thermostat detects the change and causes the furnace to add heat to the room. When the room becomes too warm, the furnace stops and the air conditioner begins to cool. Negative feedback mechanisms do not prevent variation, but they keep variation within a normal range.

A

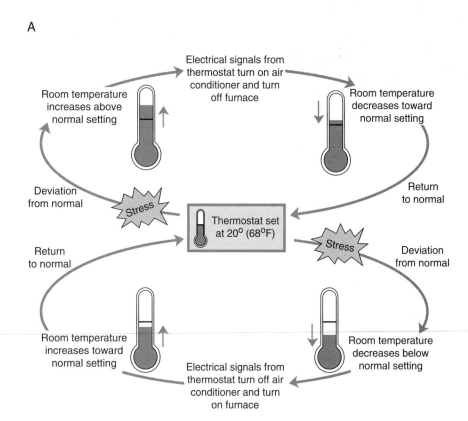

Figure 1–3   *A,* Negative feedback mechanism.

B

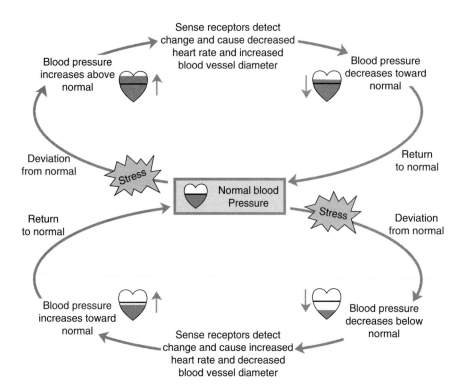

Figure 1–3 *Continued, B,* Physiologic example of negative feedback.

Homeostasis is usually maintained by negative feedback mechanisms.

An example of a physiologic homeostatic mechanism is illustrated in Figure 1–3B. When blood pressure decreases below normal, body sensors detect the deviation and initiate changes that bring the pressure back within the normal range. When the pressure increases above normal, changes occur to decrease the pressure to normal. Variations in blood pressure occur, but homeostatic mechanisms keep them within the limits of a normal range.

The nervous and endocrine systems work together to control homeostasis, but all the organ systems in the body help maintain the normal conditions of the internal environment. The brain contains centers that monitor temperature, pressure, volume, and the chemical conditions of body fluids. Endocrine glands secrete hormones in response to deviations from normal conditions, and these hormones affect other organs. The changes required to bring conditions back to the normal range are mediated by the various organ systems. Good health depends on homeostasis. Illness results when the negative feedback mechanisms that maintain homeostasis are disrupted. Medical therapy attempts to assist the negative feedback process to restore balance, or homeostasis.

All organ systems of the body, under direction from the nervous system, work together to maintain homeostasis.

Negative feedback mechanisms inhibit a change or deviation from normal. They create a response that is opposite to the deviation and that restores homeostasis. **Positive feedback mechanisms** stimulate or amplify changes. In the example of a thermostat, if there is an increase in temperature, a positive feedback mechanism brings about an even greater increase. Such responses tend toward instability because the variable, that is, the temperature, deviates farther and farther from the normal range. The process or change continues faster and faster until it comes to a quick conclusion. You may wonder why there is a need for positive feedback in physiology. There are times when positive feedback is beneficial because it quickly terminates a process that, if allowed to continue for a prolonged period, might be detrimental. The events in the birth of a baby and the formation of a blood clot are examples of positive feedback.

Positive feedback mechanisms are stimulatory. They are sometimes beneficial because they may bring a process to a rapid conclusion.

Anatomical Terms

Certain basic terms need to be understood to communicate effectively in the health care professions. In other words, you have to speak the language. This section deals with some basic terms that relate to the anatomy of the body. They are used to describe directions and regions of the body. This is the beginning of a new vocabulary that will expand as you progress through the book.

Anatomical Position

If directional terms are to be meaningful, there must be some knowledge of the beginning position. If you give a person directions to go somewhere, you must have a starting reference point. When using directions in anatomy and physiology, it is assumed that the body is in anatomical position. In this position, the body is standing erect, the face is forward, and the arms are at the sides with the palms and toes directed forward. Figure 1–4 illustrates the body in anatomical position.

> In anatomical position, the body is erect and facing forward with arms at the sides. The palms and toes are directed forward.

Directions in the Body

Directional terms are used to describe the relative position of one part to another. Note that in the following list of directional terms the two items in each pair of terms are opposites.

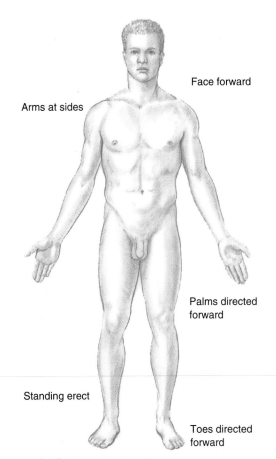

Arms at sides

Face forward

Palms directed forward

Standing erect

Toes directed forward

Figure 1–4 Anatomical position.

Superior (soo-PEER-ee-or) means that a part is above another portion, or closer to the head. The nose is superior to the mouth. **Inferior** (in-FEER-ee-or) means that a part is below another part, or closer to the feet. The heart is inferior to the neck.

Anterior (an-TEER-ee-or) (or ventral) means toward the front surface. The heart is anterior to the vertebral column. **Posterior** (pos-TEER-ee-or) (or dorsal) means that a part is toward the back. The heart is posterior to the sternum.

Medial (MEE-dee-al) means toward, or nearer, the midline of the body. The nose is medial to the ears. **Lateral** (LAT-er-al) means toward, or nearer, the side, away from the midline. The ears are lateral to the eyes.

Proximal (PRAHK-sih-mal) means that a part is closer to a point of attachment, or closer to the trunk of the body, than another part. The elbow is proximal to the wrist. The opposite of proximal is **distal** (DIS-tal), which means that a part is farther away from a point of attachment than is another part. The fingers are distal to the wrist.

Superficial (soo-per-FISH-al) means that a part is located on or near the surface. The superficial (or outermost) layer of the skin is the epidermis. The opposite of superficial is **deep,** which means that a part is away from the surface. Muscles are deep to the skin.

Visceral (VIS-er-al) pertains to internal organs or the covering of the organs. The visceral pericardium covers the heart. **Parietal** (pah-RYE-ih-tal) refers to the wall of a body cavity. The parietal peritoneum lines the wall of the abdominal cavity.

> Superior/inferior, anterior/posterior, medial/lateral, proximal/distal, superficial/deep, and visceral/parietal are six pairs of opposite terms used to describe the relative position of one body part to another.

Planes and Sections of the Body

To aid in visualizing the spatial relationships of internal body parts, anatomists use three imaginary planes, each of which is cut through the body in a different direction. Figure 1–5 illustrates these three planes.

A **sagittal** (SAJ-ih-tal) **plane** refers to a lengthwise cut that divides the body into right and left portions. This is sometimes called a longitudinal section. If the cut passes through the midline of the body it is called a **midsagittal plane,** and it divides the body into right and left halves.

A **transverse plane** or horizontal plane is perpendicular to the sagittal plane and cuts across the body horizontally to divide it into superior and inferior portions. Sections cut this way are sometimes called cross sections.

A **frontal plane** divides the body into anterior and posterior portions. It is perpendicular to both the sagittal plane and the transverse plane. This is sometimes called a **coronal** (ko-ROH-nal) **plane.**

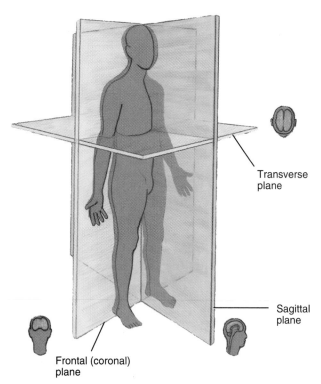

Figure 1–5   Transverse, sagittal, and frontal planes of the body.

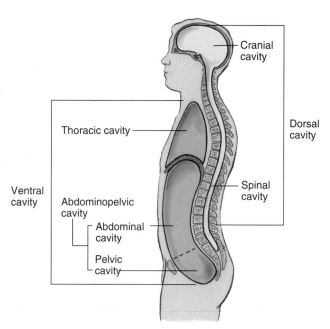

Figure 1–6   The two major cavities in the body.

> A sagittal plane divides the body into right and left parts; a transverse plane divides it into upper and lower regions; and a frontal or coronal plane divides it into front and back portions.

Body Cavities

The spaces within the body that contain the internal organs or viscera are called body cavities. The two main cavities are the **dorsal cavity** and the larger **ventral cavity,** which are illustrated in Figure 1–6. The dorsal cavity is divided into the **cranial** (KRAY-nee-al) **cavity,** which contains the brain, and the **spinal** (SPY-nal) **cavity,** which contains the spinal cord. The cranial and spinal cavities join with each other to form a continuous space.

> The dorsal body cavity consists of the cranial cavity, which contains the brain, and the spinal cavity, which contains the spinal cord.

The ventral cavity is much larger than the dorsal cavity and is subdivided into the **thoracic** (tho-RAS-ik) **cavity** and the **abdominopelvic** (ab-dahm-ih-noh-PEL-vik) **cavity.** The thoracic cavity is superior to the abdominopelvic cavity and contains the heart, lungs, esophagus, and trachea. It is separated from the abdominopelvic cavity by the muscular diaphragm. Although there is no clear-cut partition to divide it, the abdominopelvic cavity is separated

into the superior **abdominal** (ab-DAHM-ih-nal) **cavity** and the inferior **pelvic** (PEL-vik) **cavity.** The stomach, liver, gallbladder, spleen, and most of the intestines are in the abdominal cavity. The pelvic cavity contains portions of the small and large intestines, the rectum, the urinary bladder, and the internal reproductive organs.

> The ventral body cavity is subdivided into the thoracic cavity and the abdominopelvic cavity.

To help describe the location of body organs or pain, health care professionals frequently divide the abdominopelvic cavity into regions using imaginary lines. One such method uses the midsagittal plane and a transverse plane that passes through the umbilicus. This divides the abdominopelvic area into four quadrants, illustrated in Figure 1–7. Another system uses two sagittal planes and two transverse planes to divide the abdominopelvic area into the nine regions illustrated in Figure 1–8. The three central regions are, from superior to inferior, the **epigastric** (ep-ih-GAS-trik), **umbilical** (um-BIL-ih-kal), and **hypogastric** (hye-poh-GAS-trik) regions. Lateral to these, from superior to inferior, are the right and left **hypochondriac** (hye-poh-KAHN-dree-ak), right and left **lumbar,** and right and left **iliac** (ILL-ee-ak) or **inguinal** (ING-gwih-nal) regions.

> A convenient and commonly used system divides the abdominopelvic cavity into nine regions: epigastric, umbilical, hypogastric, right and left hypochondriac, right and left lumbar, and right and left iliac.

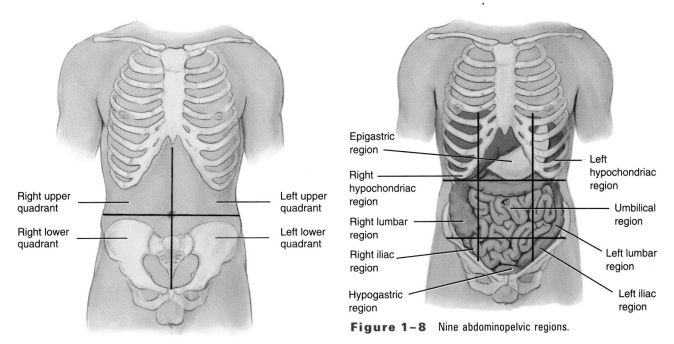

Figure 1-7   Abdominopelvic quadrants.

Right upper quadrant
Left upper quadrant
Right lower quadrant
Left lower quadrant

Epigastric region
Left hypochondriac region
Right hypochondriac region
Umbilical region
Right lumbar region
Left lumbar region
Right iliac region
Left iliac region
Hypogastric region

Figure 1-8   Nine abdominopelvic regions.

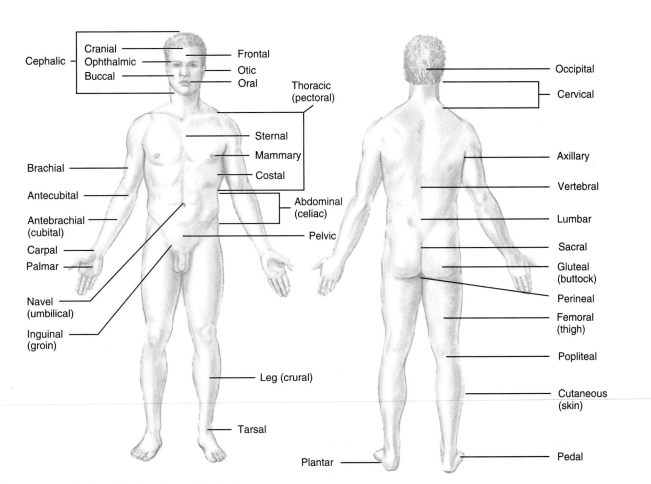

Cephalic
Cranial
Ophthalmic
Buccal
Frontal
Otic
Oral
Thoracic (pectoral)
Sternal
Mammary
Costal
Brachial
Antecubital
Abdominal (celiac)
Antebrachial (cubital)
Carpal
Pelvic
Palmar
Navel (umbilical)
Inguinal (groin)
Leg (crural)
Tarsal

Occipital
Cervical
Axillary
Vertebral
Lumbar
Sacral
Gluteal (buttock)
Perineal
Femoral (thigh)
Popliteal
Cutaneous (skin)
Plantar
Pedal

Figure 1-9   Terms for the regions of the body.

Regions of the Body

The body may be divided into the **axial** (AK-see-al) portion, which consists of the head, neck, and trunk, and the **appendicular** (ap-pen-DIK-yoo-lar) portion, which consists of the limbs. The trunk or **torso** includes the thorax, abdomen, and pelvis. In addition to these terms and the nine abdominopelvic regions identified in the previous section, there are numerous other terms that apply to specific body areas. Some of these are listed in the chart that follows this section and are identified in Figure 1–9.

> The axial portion of the body consists of the head, neck, and trunk. The limbs or appendages belong to the appendicular portion.

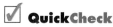 **QuickCheck**

- If the blood glucose level increases above normal, which is more likely to return it to normal, a positive feedback mechanism or a negative feedback mechanism?

- Which of the body planes would not intersect the hypochondriac and epigastric regions at the same time?

- Where would you expect the popliteal fossa to be located?

Body Area Terms

► Term	► Body Region	► Term	► Body Region
Abdominal (ab-DAHM-ih-nal)	Portion of the trunk below the diaphragm; between the thorax and pelvis	**Mammary** (MAM-ah-ree)	Breast
		Occipital (ahk-SIP-ih-tal)	Lower portion of the back of head
Antebrachial (an-te-BRAY-kee-al)	Region between the elbow and the wrist; forearm; cubital region	**Ophthalmic** (off-THAL-mik)	Eyes
		Oral (OH-ral or AW-ral)	Mouth
		Otic (OH-tik)	Ears
Antecubital (an-te-KYOO-bih-tal)	Space in front of the elbow	**Palmar** (PAWL-mar)	Palm of the hand
		Pectoral (PEK-toh-ral)	Chest region
Axillary (AK-sih-lair-ee)	Armpit area	**Pedal** (PED-al)	Foot
		Pelvic (PEL-vik)	Inferior region of the abdominopelvic cavity
Brachial (BRAY-kee-al)	Arm; proximal portion of the upper limb	**Perineal** (pair-ih-NEE-al)	Region between the anus and pubic symphysis; includes the region of the external reproductive organs
Buccal (BUK-al)	Region of the cheek		
Carpal (KAR-pal)	Wrist		
Celiac (SEE-lee-ak)	Abdomen		
Cephalic (seh-FAL-ik)	Head		
Cervical (SER-vih-kal)	Neck region	**Plantar** (PLAN-tar)	Sole of the foot
Costal (KAHS-tal)	Ribs	**Popliteal** (pop-LIT-ee-al or pop-lih-TEE-al)	Area behind the knee
Cranial (KRAY-nee-al)	Skull		
Cubital (KYOO-bih-tal)	Forearm; region between the elbow and wrist; antebrachial	**Sacral** (SAY-kral)	Posterior region between the hip bones
		Sternal (STIR-nal)	Anterior midline of the thorax
Cutaneous (kyoo-TAY-nee-us)	Skin	**Tarsal** (TAHR-sal)	Ankle and instep of the foot
Femoral (FEM-or-al)	Thigh; the part of the lower extremity between the hip and the knee	**Thoracic** (tho-RAS-ik)	Chest; part of the trunk inferior to the neck and superior to the diaphragm
Frontal (FRUN-tal)	Forehead		
Gluteal (GLOO-tee-al)	Buttock region	**Umbilical** (um-BIL-ih-kal)	Navel; middle region of the abdomen
Inguinal (IN-gwih-nal)	Depressed region between the abdomen and the thigh; groin	**Vertebral** (ver-TEE-bral or VER-teh-bral)	Pertaining to the spinal column; backbone
Leg (LEG)	Portion of the lower extremity between the knee and the foot; also called the crural region		
Lumbar (LUM-bar)	Region of the lower back and side between the lowest rib and the pelvis		

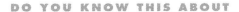

DO YOU KNOW THIS ABOUT

Medical Terminology?

Introduction to Terminology

Human anatomy and physiology, like any technical subject, has its own vocabulary. It is necessary to learn the language to understand the concepts. The sciences of medicine, anatomy, and physiology were born in the 18th century universities in which Greek and Latin were the languages used in lectures and in writing. As a result, the special vocabulary used in these sciences today consists of roots, prefixes, and suffixes based on Greek and Latin. These three principal parts are arranged in different combinations and sequences to make words. You need to be able to recognize, spell, pronounce, and use the roots, prefixes, and suffixes of these words to be an effective student in anatomy and physiology and in the medical sciences. Once you have learned the basic parts, you can recombine them to form or analyze new words. It is like having a mix and match wardrobe of words!

The **root** is the main part or subject of a word. It is the word's foundation and conveys the central meaning of the word. Sometimes two or more roots, connected by a combining vowel, are used in the same word. "Cardi" is the root meaning heart, "pulmon" refers to lung, and put together cardiopulmonary is a word that pertains to both the heart and lungs.

A **prefix** is a syllable, or group of syllables, placed before a root to alter or modify the meaning of the root. "Hyper" is a prefix that means over or above. Hypersensitive means overly sensitive. The root has been modified by the prefix before it.

A **suffix** is a syllable, or group of syllables, attached to the end of a root to modify the meaning of the root. The suffix "itis" means inflammation of, and "gastr" is a root that refers to the stomach. Thus, gastritis means inflammation of the stomach.

To make pronunciation easier, word parts are often linked together by a **combining vowel.** In the word cardiopulmonary, the vowel "o" is used to connect the two roots, "cardi" and "pulmon." The vowel "o" is also used to link the root "crani" with the suffix "tomy" to make the word craniotomy. The letter "o" is the most commonly used combining vowel.

The **plural form** of most English words is derived by adding "s" or "es" to the end of the word. In Greek and Latin, and consequently in medical terminology, the ending may be com-

pletely changed to designate the plural form (see Commonly Used Plural Endings).

Commonly Used Plural Endings

▶ Singular Ending	▶ Plural Ending
a as in aort**a**	**ae** as in aort**ae**
en as in foram**en**	**ina** as in foram**ina**
is as in test**is**	**es** as in test**es**
is as in ir**is**	**ides** as in ir**ides**
nx as in phala**nx**	**ges** as in phalan**ges**
on as in spermatozo**on**	**a** as in spermatozo**a**
um as in ov**um**	**a** as in ov**a**
us as in bronch**us**	**i** as in bronch**i**
x as in thora**x**	**ces** as in thora**ces**
y as in arter**y**	**ies** as in arter**ies**

Correct spelling is extremely important in medical terminology. When in doubt, look it up in the dictionary. Guessing has no place in medicine because one wrong letter may give the word an entirely new meaning.

Examples of Similarly Spelled Words that Have Very Different Meanings

▶ Term with letter difference	▶ Meaning of term
abduct	To lead **away** from midline
adduct	To lead **toward** the midline
arteritis	Inflammation of an **artery**
arthritis	Inflammation of a **joint**
ileum	Portion of **small intestine**
ilium	A **pelvic bone**

Medical and other scientific terms may look like they are hard to pronounce, especially if you have only read them and have not heard them. This text uses a phonetically spelled pronunciation guide, and you should practice saying each new word aloud to reinforce the pronunciation in your mind.

As you progress through this course, you will discover that medical terminology makes a lot of sense and is easy to understand. Practice it on your friends and family. You will find that once you learn the tricks of the trade it is easy and fun!

CHAPTER QUIZ

RECALL

Match the definitions on the left with the appropriate term on the right.

1. A part is closer to a point of attachment than another part

2. Stable internal environment

3. Divided body or part into anterior and posterior portions

4. Refers to skin

5. Complex substances are broken down into simpler building blocks and energy is released

6. Process by which unspecialized cells change into cells with distinctive structural and functional characteristics

7. Study of function and functional relationships

8. Contains the brain and spinal cord

9. Midline superior abdominal region

10. Space in front of the elbow

A. Antecubital

B. Catabolism

C. Cutaneous

D. Differentiation

E. Dorsal cavity

F. Epigastric

G. Frontal

H. Homeostasis

I. Physiology

J. Proximal

THOUGHT

1. Which of the following is more complex than tissues on the organizational scale?

   a. molecules

   b. organs

   c. cells

   d. organelles

2. Two body systems function to regulate and coordinate body activities. These systems are the

   a. cardiovascular and nervous

   b. lymphatic and endocrine

   c. nervous and reproductive

   d. endocrine and nervous

3. A student wants to separate a brain specimen into right and left halves. Along what plane should the student make the cut?

   a. transverse

   b. sagittal

   c. frontal

   d. midsagittal

4. Which of the following groups of organs is found in the abdominopelvic cavity?

   a. spinal cord, lungs, liver

   b. liver, stomach, heart

   c. brain, spinal cord, liver

   d. gallbladder, stomach, small intestine

5. Which body regions are inferior to the costal region?

   a. sternal and umbilical

   b. inguinal and pelvic

   c. inguinal and axillary

   d. buccal and brachial

APPLICATION

Ima Dock, MD, is able to visualize organ A of her patient in midsagittal, frontal, and transverse body planes. Which of the following is organ A?
a. kidney   b. spleen   c. gallbladder   d. urinary bladder

Chemistry, Matter, and Life

Outline/Objectives

Elements 18
- Define matter, element, and atom.
- Use chemical symbols to identify elements.

Structure of Atoms 18
- Illustrate the structure of an atom with a simple diagram showing the protons, neutrons, and electrons.
- Distinguish between atomic number and mass number of an element.
- Describe the electron arrangement that makes an atom most stable.

Chemical Bonds 20
- Describe the difference between ionic bonds, covalent bonds, and hydrogen bonds.

Compounds and Molecules 23
- Describe the relationship between atoms, molecules, and compounds and interpret molecular formulas for compounds.

Chemical Reactions 24
- Describe and write chemical equations for four types of chemical reactions and identify the reactants and products in each.
- Discuss five factors that influence the rate of chemical reactions.

Mixtures, Solutions, and Suspensions 27
- Distinguish between mixtures, solutions, and suspensions.

Electrolytes, Acids, Bases, and Buffers 27
- Differentiate between acids and bases and discuss how they relate to pH and buffers.

Organic Compounds 30
- Describe the five major groups of organic compounds that are important to the human body.

Key Terms

Acid

Atom

Base

Buffer

Carbohydrate

Compound

Covalent bond

Element

Ionic bond

Lipid

Molecule

Protein

Solute

Solvent

Building Vocabulary

WORD PART	MEANING
alkal-	basic
carb/o-	charcoal, coal, carbon
di-	two
end-	within, inner
erg-	work, energy
ex-	out of, away from
-genesis	to form, produce
hex-	six
hydro-	water
-ide	pertaining to
lact-	milk
lip/o-	fat
-lys	to take apart
mono-	one
-ose	sugar
oxy-	oxygen
pent-	five
poly-	many
sacchar-	sugar, sweet
tri-	three

hemistry is the science that deals with the composition of matter and the changes that may occur in that composition. Matter can be defined as anything that has mass and takes up space. For all practical purposes, mass is the same as weight, and thus these terms will be used interchangeably in this book. Technically, however, this is not correct. The mass of something remains the same throughout the universe. Weight varies with gravitational pull. An object that weighs 10 pounds on earth weighs less in space because there is less gravitational pull; however, its mass is the same wherever it is. Matter includes the solids, liquids, and gases that are in our bodies and in the environment around us. Because our bodies are composed of matter, an understanding of chemistry or the composition of matter is important to understanding the body, how it is put together, and how it works.

Elements

All matter, living and nonliving, is composed of elements. An element is the simplest form of matter; it cannot be broken down into a simpler form by ordinary chemical means. Examples of elements include gold, silver, oxygen, and hydrogen. There are about 90 naturally occurring elements and another 16 that are man-made in the laboratory. Of the 90 elements that occur naturally, only 20 are needed by living organisms. Four of the elements—carbon (C), oxygen (O), hydrogen (H), and nitrogen (N)—make up 95 percent of the human body by weight. Table 2–1 lists the principal elements found in the human body.

■ The simplest form of matter is an element.

Instead of writing out the complete name of an element, scientists use a shorthand method or chemical symbol to identify an element. The chemical symbol is usually the first one or two letters of the English or Latin name of the element. The chemical symbol for hydrogen is H, carbon is C, oxygen is O, Cl is chlorine, and Na is sodium (from *natrium*, the Latin word for sodium). The symbols for the elements in the human body are given in Table 2–1.

■ Chemical symbols are abbreviations used to identify elements.

Structure of Atoms

An element is composed of atoms that are all of the same kind. The element gold is made up entirely of gold atoms, and the element silver is made up entirely of silver atoms. An **atom** is the smallest particle of an element that still retains the properties of that element, and it is almost unbelievably small. It

Table 2–1 Elements Essential for Human Life

Element	Symbol	Atomic Number	Approximate Percent of Human Body by Weight	Importance
Oxygen	O	8	65.0%	Required for cellular metabolism; component of water; present in most organic compounds
Carbon	C	6	18.5%	Component of all organic compounds
Hydrogen	H	1	9.5%	Present in most organic compounds; component of water
Nitrogen	N	7	3.3%	Component of all proteins, phospholipids, nucleic acids
Calcium	Ca	20	1.5%	Component of bones and teeth; important in muscle contraction, nerve impulse conduction, blood clotting
Phosphorus	P	15	1.0%	Component of phospholipids, nucleic acids, and adenosine triphosphate; important in energy transfer
Potassium	K	19	0.4%	Principal cation inside cells; important in muscle contraction and nerve impulse conduction
Sulfur	S	16	0.3%	Component of most proteins
Sodium	Na	11	0.2%	Principal cation in fluid outside cells; important in muscle contraction and nerve impulse conduction
Chlorine	Cl	17	0.2%	Principal anion in fluid outside cells; important in fluid balance
Magnesium	Mg	12	0.1%	Part of many important enzymes; necessary for bones and teeth
Fluorine	F	9	Trace	Aids in development of teeth and bones
Chromium	Cr	24	Trace	Aids in carbohydrate metabolism
Manganese	Mn	25	Trace	Necessary for carbohydrate metabolism and bone formation
Iron	Fe	26	Trace	Component of hemoglobin; part of many enzymes
Cobalt	Co	27	Trace	Component of vitamin B_{12}
Copper	Cu	29	Trace	Necessary to maintain blood chemistry
Zinc	Zn	30	Trace	Necessary for growth, healing, and overall health
Selenium	Se	34	Trace	Aids vitamin E action and fat metabolism
Molybdenum	Mo	42	Trace	Component of enzymes necessary for metabolism
Iodine	I	53	Trace	Component of thyroid hormones

takes over 100 million average-sized atoms lined up side by side to make an inch, or 2.54 centimeters.

■ An atom is the smallest unit of an element.

Even though it is extremely small, an atom is made up of still smaller subunits or subatomic particles called **protons, neutrons,** and **electrons.** A dense region, called the nucleus, contains the protons and neutrons. Electrons are outside the nucleus. The number and nature of the subatomic particles present determine the physical and chemical characteristics of the atoms in an element. Protons, located in the nucleus, have a positive electrical charge, and each has a mass of one atomic mass unit (amu). An atomic mass unit is an arbitrarily assigned unit of mass based on a carbon atom. The number of protons in the nucleus is called the **atomic number.** The atomic number for each element is shown in the periodic table. All atoms of the same element have the same atomic number, or number of protons in the nucleus.

> The atomic number of an atom is the number of positively charged particles, protons, in the nucleus.

Neutrons, also found in the nucleus, have the same mass as protons but have no charge. Protons and neutrons together account for the mass of the atom and their number, collectively, is called the **mass number** of an atom. The element sodium is made up of sodium atoms, which have 11 protons and 12 neutrons in the nucleus. The atomic number of sodium is 11 (the number of protons), and the atomic mass number is 23 (the number of protons plus neutrons).

> Neutrons, also in the nucleus, have the same mass as protons but have no charge. The mass number of an atom equals the number of protons plus the number of neutrons.

Electrons are minute, negatively charged particles with almost no mass. They are located in the space surrounding the nucleus. The number of negatively charged electrons in an atom is always equal to the number of positively charged protons so that the atom is electrically neutral. The sodium atom, described in the previous paragraph, has 11 protons and 12 neutrons in the nucleus. Because the number of electrons equals the number of protons, there will be 11 electrons in the space surrounding the nucleus. It is impossible to know where a given electron will be at any given time, but it is possible to predict the region in which it will be located. Electrons are located in **energy levels,** or **shells,** around the nucleus. In general, electrons with higher energy levels are located in shells farther away from the nucleus than electrons with lower energy levels. The

shell closest to the nucleus has the lowest energy level and can hold two electrons. The next higher energy level can hold eight electrons. Higher energy levels can hold more than eight electrons, but an atom is most stable when there are eight electrons in the outermost shell, which has the highest energy level. Simplified diagrams of the atomic structure of some biologically important elements are shown in Figure 2–1.

> Electrons are negatively charged particles that are in constant motion outside the nucleus. The most stable atoms have eight electrons in their highest energy level.

✓ Quick**Check**

- The most abundant element in the body is abbreviated with the letter "O." What is this element?

- How many electrons, protons, and neutrons are in an element with an atomic number equal to 17 and a mass number equal to 35?

- How many energy levels or shells contain electrons in this element?

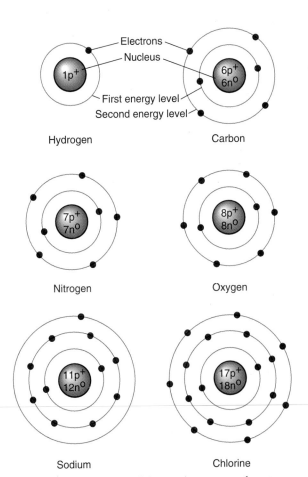

Figure 2–1 Diagrams of the atomic structure of some biologically important elements.

Chemical Bonds

An atom's chemical behavior, its chemical reactivity, is determined largely by the electrons in the outermost energy shell, which has the highest energy level. Atoms have a tendency to transfer or share electrons to achieve a stable configuration in the outermost energy shell. When electrons from the outermost energy level are transferred or shared between atoms, attractive forces called chemical bonds develop that "hold" the atoms together to form a molecule. There are two types of intramolecular chemical bonds: ionic bonds and covalent bonds. A third type of bond, the hydrogen bond, is intermolecular. It provides a weak bond between molecules.

| Chemical bonds are forces that hold atoms together.

Ionic Bonds

Ionic (eye-ON-ik) **bonds** are formed when one or more electrons are transferred from one atom to another. Because electrons have a negative charge, atoms are no longer neutral when they lose or gain electrons. The charged particles that result when atoms lose or gain electrons are called ions. The symbols for ions are symbols for the atoms from which they were derived with a superscripted plus ($^+$) or minus ($^-$) to indicate the charge. If more than one electron is lost or gained, then a number is used with the plus or minus sign. Table 2–2 lists some of the important ions in the human body.

| An ion is an atom that has lost or gained one or more electrons.

When an atom loses one or more electrons, it then has more protons than electrons, and it becomes a positively charged ion. Positively charged ions are called **cations** (KAT-eye-onz). A sodium (Na) atom has 11 protons in the nucleus and 11 electrons in the energy shells. It is electrically neu-

Table 2–2 Important Ions in the Body

Ion	Symbol	Importance
Calcium	Ca^{2+}	Component of bones and teeth; necessary for blood clotting and muscle contraction
Sodium	Na^+	Principal cation in fluid outside the cells; important in muscle contraction and nerve impulse conduction
Potassium	K^+	Principal cation in fluid inside the cells; important in muscle contraction and nerve impulse conduction
Hydrogen	H^+	Important in acid-base balance
Hydroxide	OH^-	Important in acid-base balance
Chloride	Cl^-	Principal anion in fluid outside the cells
Bicarbonate	HCO_3^-	Important in acid-base balance
Ammonium	NH_4^+	Important in acid-base balance; removes toxic ammonia from the body
Phosphate	PO_4^{3-}	Component of bones, teeth, and high-energy molecules; important in acid-base balance
Iron	Fe^{2+}	Important component of hemoglobin for oxygen transport

tral. When it loses an electron from its outermost shell, it still has 11 positively charged protons but only 10 negatively charged electrons. It has one more positive charge than it has negative charges so it becomes a positively charged sodium ion (Na^+). This is illustrated in Figure 2–2.

Atoms that gain or pick up one or more electrons and then have more electrons than they do protons become negatively charged ions. A negatively charged ion is called an **anion** (AN-eye-on). A chlorine atom has 17 protons and 17 electrons to make it electrically neutral. When it gains or picks up an electron, it still has 17 positively charged protons but now has 18 negatively charged electrons to

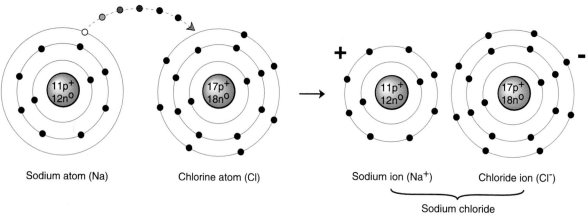

Sodium atom (Na)   Chlorine atom (Cl)   Sodium ion (Na^+)   Chloride ion (Cl^-)

Sodium chloride

Figure 2–2 Formation of ionic bonds.

make it a negatively charged chloride ion (Cl⁻) (see Fig. 2–2).

When an atom such as sodium loses or gives up an electron to another atom such as chlorine, two charged particles called ions are formed. One is a positively charged cation, the other is a negatively charged anion. Because of the opposite charges, the two ions are attracted to each other. The force of attraction between two oppositely charged ions is an ionic bond. Oppositely charged ions that are held together by ionic bonds are called **ionic compounds.** Sodium chloride (table salt), formed from sodium ions and chloride ions, is an example of an ionic compound.

Ionic bonds are the forces of attraction between cations and anions and form ionic compounds.

Covalent Bonds

Covalent (koh-VAY-lent) **bonds** are formed when two atoms share a pair of electrons. Two hydrogen atoms, for example, can share their electrons to form a molecule of hydrogen gas. Because only one pair of electrons is shared, a single covalent bond is formed (Fig. 2–3A). Carbon has four electrons in its outer shell that it can share with other atoms to

form covalent bonds. If it shares these electrons with four hydrogen atoms, then four single covalent bonds are formed and a molecule of methane gas results (Fig. 2–3B).

Covalent bonds result when atoms share electrons.

Some atoms may share more than one pair of electrons with another atom. For example, an oxygen atom shares two pairs of electrons with another oxygen atom to form a molecule of oxygen gas (Fig. 2–4A). This forms a double covalent bond. Carbon may share two electron pairs with each of two atoms of oxygen to form two double covalent bonds (Fig. 2–4B). A few atoms may share three pairs of electrons to form triple covalent bonds (Fig. 2–5).

A covalent bond formed by sharing a pair of electrons is sometimes indicated by drawing a straight line between the symbols for the two atoms. Two lines indicate a double covalent bond and three lines designate a triple covalent bond.

Atoms may share more than one pair of electrons, which results in double or triple covalent bonds.

There are times when the two electrons of a covalent bond are not shared equally between the two

A

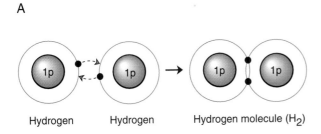

Hydrogen　　　Hydrogen　　　Hydrogen molecule (H₂)

B

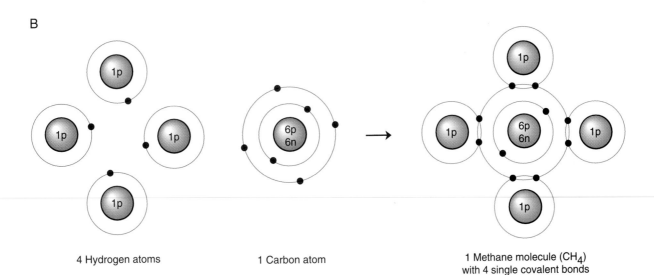

4 Hydrogen atoms　　　1 Carbon atom　　　1 Methane molecule (CH₄) with 4 single covalent bonds

Figure 2–3　*A,* Single covalent bonds in hydrogen gas. *B,* Single covalent bonds in methane.

A

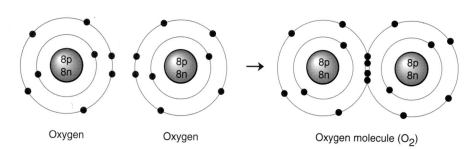

Oxygen   Oxygen   Oxygen molecule (O₂)

B

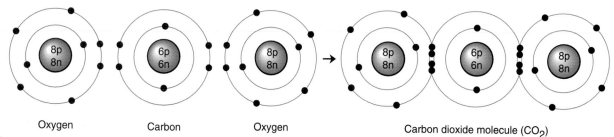

Oxygen   Carbon   Oxygen   Carbon dioxide molecule (CO₂)

Figure 2–4   *A,* Double covalent bonds in oxygen gas. *B,* Double covalent bonds in carbon dioxide.

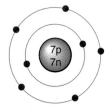

Nitrogen atom with 7 protons
and 7 neutrons in the nucleus
and 7 electrons in the electron
energy shell.

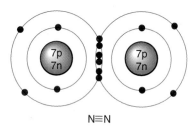

N≡N

A molecule of nitrogen gas.
The two nitrogen atoms share
three electron pairs to make a
triple covalent bond.

Figure 2–5   Triple covalent bonds.

atoms. Instead, the electrons tend to spend more time around the nucleus of one atom than the other. Another way of stating this is that the electrons are closer to the nucleus of one atom than the other. This unequal sharing of electrons is called a **polar covalent bond.** Water is a good example of this (Fig. 2–6). The shared pair of electrons spends more time with, or is closer to, the nucleus of the oxygen atom than the hydrogen atom. This results in a partial negative charge at the oxygen end of the molecule, and a partial positive charge on the hydrogen end, to form a polar molecule. The molecule as a whole is neutral; but because it has opposite partial charges, it is polar, and the bonds are polar covalent bonds. Molecules with polar covalent bonds have a weak attraction for ions or other covalent molecules. Polar covalent bonds are stronger than ionic bonds.

An unequal sharing of electrons results in polar covalent bonds.

Hydrogen Bonds

The ionic and covalent bonds just described hold atoms together within molecules. They are **intramolecular** bonds. The **hydrogen bond** is an **intermolec-**

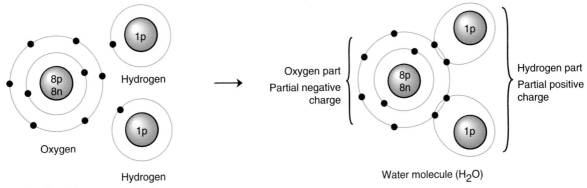

Figure 2-6 Polar covalent bonds.

ular bond or attraction between two molecules. The electropositive hydrogen end of a polar covalent molecule has a weak attraction for the negative portion of other polar covalent molecules or for negative ions. This weak attraction is called a hydrogen bond. Figure 2–7 illustrates how water molecules are held together by hydrogen bonds.

> The polar covalent molecules of water are attracted to each other to form hydrogen bonds.

✓ QuickCheck

- What type of chemical bond is formed when two elements share one or more pairs of electrons?

- Hydrogen bonds between covalent molecules of water are an example of what type of chemical bond?

Compounds and Molecules

Nature of Compounds

When two or more atoms chemically bond together, a **molecule** is formed. The atoms may be different, as they are in water when oxygen and hydrogen bond together, or they may be alike, as they are in oxygen gas when two atoms of oxygen combine. If the atoms are different, the new substance is a compound. The atoms in a molecule, whether they are alike or different, are held together by either ionic or covalent bonds.

> The atoms in a molecule are held together by chemical bonds.

A **compound** is formed when two or more different types of atoms chemically combine in a definite, or fixed, ratio to form a new substance that is different from any of the original atoms. Water is an example of a compound. It is formed from two atoms of hydrogen and one atom of oxygen that chemically combine. The ratio is always two hydrogen atoms to one oxygen atom, and the result of the chemical combination, water, is different from either hydrogen or oxygen. Carbon dioxide is another example. It is formed from one atom of carbon and two atoms of oxygen that chemically combine. Oxygen gas is formed from two atoms of oxygen, but it is not a compound because the two atoms are alike.

> Water is the most abundant compound in living organisms. It accounts for about two thirds of the weight of the adult human body. Water is physiologically important because it is a good solvent, it breaks down molecules by hydrolysis, it remains liquid over a broad temperature range, and it can absorb and transport relatively large quantities of heat without dramatic changes in its own temperature.

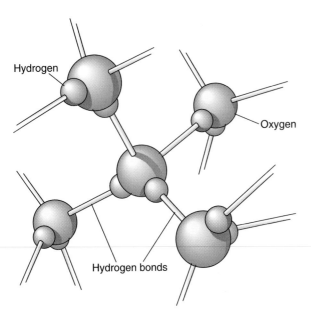

Figure 2-7 Hydrogen bonds in a water molecule.

A molecule is the smallest unit of a compound formed from two or more different atoms that still retains the properties of the compound. Molecules can be broken down into the atoms from which they were made, but then they will no longer have the properties of the compound. The principal particles of matter are summarized in Table 2–3.

> Atoms combine in definite ratios to form molecules, which are the smallest units of compounds.

Formulas

The **molecular formula** is a shorthand way to indicate the type and number of atoms in a molecule. The chemical symbols of the elements are used to indicate the types of atoms in the molecule, and a subscript number follows each symbol to show the number of atoms. If there is no subscript, the number 1 is implied. The molecular formula for water is H_2O. H is the symbol for hydrogen; the subscript 2 after the H indicates two atoms of hydrogen; O is the symbol for oxygen; and because there is no subscript the number 1 is implied, which indicates there is one atom of oxygen. The molecular formula for water, H_2O, indicates that one molecule of water is composed of two atoms of hydrogen and one atom of oxygen. A molecule of carbon dioxide, CO_2, is composed of one atom of carbon and two atoms of oxygen. The molecular formula for glucose, an important sugar in the body, is $C_6H_{12}O_6$, which indicates that there are 6 atoms of carbon, 12 atoms of hydrogen, and 6 atoms of oxygen in the molecule.

> Molecular formulas use chemical symbols to indicate the type of atoms and numerical subscripts to show how many of each atom are in a molecule of a compound.

Table 2–3 Principal Particles of Matter	
Particle	**Description**
Proton (p^+)	Relatively large particle; has a positive charge; found within nucleus of atoms; number of protons in nucleus equals atomic number
Neutron (n^0)	Relatively large particle; carries no charge; found within the nucleus of atoms
Electron (e^-)	Extremely small particle; has a negative charge; in constant motion around a nucleus
Atom	Smallest particle of an element that has the properties of that element; made up of protons, neutrons, and electrons
Ion	Atom that has lost or gained one or more electrons so that it is electrically charged
Molecule	Particle formed by the chemical union of two or more atoms; smallest particle of a compound

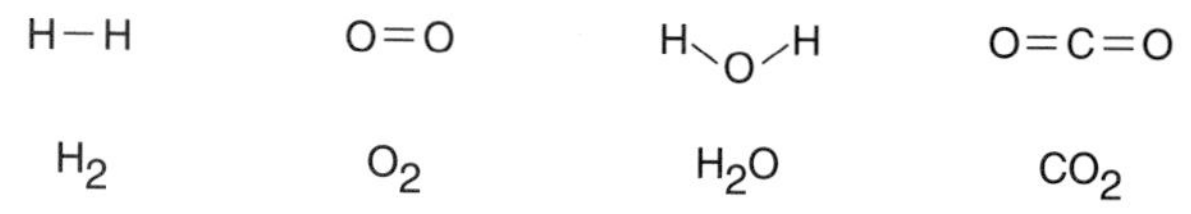

Figure 2–8 Structural formulas.

As mentioned earlier, covalent bonds are sometimes represented by straight lines between the symbols for the elements in the molecule. These representations show how atoms are arranged and joined together in a molecule. Illustrations of these bonding arrangements are called **structural formulas** (Fig. 2–8).

☑ Quick Check

● Identify the elements in a molecule of sodium bicarbonate: $NaHCO_3$.

● An atom is the smallest unit of an element. What is the smallest unit of a compound?

Chemical Reactions

A **chemical reaction** is the process by which atoms or molecules interact to form new chemical combinations. Bonds break and new ones form to create different molecules. The atoms and molecules present before the chemical reaction occurs are called the **reactants.** The new atoms and molecules that are created as a result of the reaction are called the **products.**

Chemical Equations

Reactions between molecules are represented by **chemical equations** that indicate the number and type of molecules involved in the reactions. The molecular formulas for the reactants are written on the left side of the equation, and the formulas for the products are written on the right. They are connected by an arrow that indicates the direction of the reaction, and the numeral before a molecular formula denotes the number of molecules of that particular substance involved. The following equation for the reaction between methane gas and oxygen provides a simple example.

$$CH_4 \;+\; 2O_2 \longrightarrow CO_2 \;+\; 2H_2O$$

methane   oxygen   carbon dioxide   water

This chemical equation indicates that 1 molecule of methane reacts with 2 molecules of oxygen to form 1 molecule of carbon dioxide and 2 molecules of water. The number of each *type of atom* must be the same in both the reactants and the products; that is, the equations must be balanced. In the above example, there is 1 carbon atom in the reactants and 1 carbon atom in the products. There are 4 hydrogen atoms and 4 oxygen atoms in the reactants and the same number in the products. Because changing a subscript in a formula indicates a different type of molecule, equations can be balanced only by adjusting the numerals before the molecular formulas.

The reaction between glucose and oxygen is an important one in the body. It provides much of the energy needed for body processes and daily activities.

$$C_6H_{12}O_6 + 6O_2 \longrightarrow 6CO_2 + 6H_2O$$

glucose   oxygen   carbon dioxide   water

This balanced chemical equation indicates that 1 molecule of glucose reacts with 6 molecules of oxygen to yield 6 molecules of carbon dioxide and 6 molecules of water. It is balanced because there are 6 carbon atoms, 12 hydrogen atoms, and 18 oxygen atoms on both the reactant and product sides of the equation.

▌ Chemical equations are an abbreviated method of showing the reactants and products in a chemical reaction.

Types of Chemical Reactions

Synthesis Reactions

When two or more simple reactants combine to form a new, more complex product, the reaction is called **synthesis, combination,** or **composition.** These are the anabolic reactions in the body. This is represented symbolically by the following equation.

$$A + B \longrightarrow AB$$

Oxygen and hydrogen combine to form water. Two simple molecules combine to form a more complex molecule. This is an example of a synthesis reaction.

$$2H_2 + O_2 \longrightarrow 2H_2O$$

When two simple molecules combine to form a more complex molecule by the removal of water, the reaction is called **dehydration synthesis.** Many anabolic reactions in the body, for example the conversion of glucose to glycogen for storage, are of this type.

▌ Synthesis reactions form a complex molecule from two or more simple molecules.

Decomposition Reactions

When the bonds in a complex reactant break to form new, simpler products, the reaction is **decomposition.** In the body, these are the catabolic reactions of metabolism. When water is used to break the bonds, the reaction is called **hydrolysis.** The digestion of food involves hydrolysis reactions. Decomposition reactions, represented symbolically by

the following equation, are the reverse of synthesis reactions.

$$AB \longrightarrow A + B$$

The bonds in water, the reactant, break to form oxygen gas and hydrogen gas, the products.

$$2H_2O \longrightarrow 2H_2 + O_2$$

▌ Decomposition reactions break down large molecules into simpler ones.

Single Replacement Reactions

Single replacement reactions, also called **single displacement reactions,** occur when one element in a compound is replaced by another. The general pattern for this type of reaction is represented symbolically as follows.

$$A + BC \longrightarrow AC + B$$

A single replacement reaction occurs when chlorine gas replaces bromine in a solution of sodium bromide to produce sodium chloride and a solution of bromine.

$$Cl_2 + 2NaBr \longrightarrow 2NaCl + Br_2$$

chlorine   sodium   sodium   bromine
           bromide   chloride

Double Replacement Reactions

Double replacement reactions (also called **double displacement** or **exchange** reactions) occur when substances in two different compounds replace each other. These reactions are partially decomposition and partially synthesis. The bonds in the original reactants must break (decomposition) before the new products can be formed (synthesis). The general equation pattern for a double replacement reaction is

$$AB + CD \longrightarrow AD + CB$$

where A has replaced C and C has replaced A from the original reactants. A and C have exchanged places. Certain double replacement reactions occur in the blood. One of these is the reaction between lactic acid and sodium bicarbonate.

$$H\text{-lactate} + NaHCO_3 \longrightarrow Na\text{-lactate} + H\text{-}HCO_3$$

lactic   sodium   sodium   carbonic
acid   bicarbonate   lactate   acid

▌ In single and double replacement reactions, the reactants exchange one or more parts to form new compounds.

Exergonic Reactions

Chemical reactions are important in the body because this is a way in which molecules can be produced when they are needed. The reactions are also important for the energy changes that occur when bonds break and form. Energy is stored in the chemical bonds of molecules. In **exergonic** (eks-er-GAHN-ik) reactions, there is more energy stored in the reactants than in the products. The extra energy is released. Some of the energy is released in the form of heat, which helps maintain body temperature. A common exergonic reaction that occurs in the body involves adenosine triphosphate (ATP), which breaks down to adenosine diphosphate (ADP) and a phosphate group, with the release of energy.

$$ATP \longrightarrow ADP + phosphate + energy$$

Endergonic Reactions

Endergonic (en-der-GAHN-ik) reactions have more energy stored in the products than in the reactants. An input of energy from exergonic reactions is needed to drive these reactions. The products of endergonic reactions store energy in their chemical bonds. In the human body, the large carbohydrate, lipid, and protein molecules are synthesized by endergonic reactions.

> Exergonic reactions release energy. Endergonic reactions require energy that is then stored in the chemical bonds.

Reaction Rates

Chemical reactions occur at different rates. Some are very slow, like the rusting of iron or the tarnishing of silver. Other reactions occur much faster, such as the setting of epoxy cement or the burning of paper. Some reactions occur so fast that they become explosive, like dynamite or the gasoline in a car. The rate at which chemical reactions occur is influenced by the nature of the reacting substances, temperature, concentration, catalysts, and surface area.

Certain substances are more reactive than others, depending on how readily bonds are broken and formed. Reactions involving ions are extremely fast because there are no bonds to break. Reactions in which covalently bonded molecules are involved require that bonds be broken and that new ones be formed. These occur more slowly. When hydrogen gas is mixed with oxygen gas, the reaction to produce water proceeds very slowly because the covalent bonds between the hydrogen atoms in the molecules of hydrogen gas and the covalent bonds between the oxygen atoms in the oxygen gas must first be broken. If a spark is introduced into this mixture of hydrogen and oxygen gas, the reaction occurs very rapidly because the spark supplies sufficient energy to break the covalent bonds.

As temperature increases, the speed of most chemical reactions also increases. In general, for every 10° C increase in temperature, the reaction rate nearly doubles. The opposite is also true. If temperature decreases, reaction rates decrease.

> When a person has a fever, reaction rates in the body increase. Some of this is manifested in an increased pulse and an increased respiratory rate. In certain types of surgery, the body is cooled so that metabolism is decreased during the procedure.

Within limits, the greater the concentration of the reactants, the faster will be the speed of the reaction. Because there are more molecules to react, the rate of reaction is increased. Under normal conditions, the concentration of oxygen molecules in body cells is sufficient to sustain the reactions that are necessary for life. If the concentration of oxygen decreases, the rate of the reactions decreases. This interferes with cell function and ultimately causes death.

A **catalyst** (KAT-ah-list) is a substance that changes the rate of a reaction without itself being chemically altered in the process. It increases the rate of a chemical reaction. In the body, organic catalysts called **enzymes** speed up the metabolic processes to a rate that is compatible with life. At normal body temperature, 37° C, most of the chemical reactions in the body would take place too slowly to sustain life if it were not for the enzymes. Enzymes are protein molecules that are very specific for the reactions they control. Each enzyme controls only one chemical reaction.

The rate of a chemical reaction also depends on the surface area of the reactants. Lumps of coal or charcoal briquettes burn quite slowly; however, coal dust is explosive and dangerous to coal miners. When a piece of coal is ground into coal dust, it greatly increases the total surface area of the particles. Many medications, such as antacids, are given as finely ground particles in a liquid so that they can react more rapidly.

> Reaction rates are affected by the nature of the reacting substances, temperature, concentration of the reactants, catalysts, and particle size.

Reversible Reactions

Many chemical reactions are **reversible.** This means that they can proceed from reactants into products or reverse the direction and proceed from products back into reactants. This is shown symbolically by using a double arrow with the points in opposite directions, as follows:

$$A + B \rightleftharpoons AB$$

Under certain conditions it is a synthesis reaction and proceeds from left to right. At other times, it is a decomposition reaction and proceeds from right to left. Whether a reversible reaction proceeds in one direction or the other depends on the relative proportions of the reactants and products, the energy necessary for the reaction, and the presence or absence of catalysts. At **equilibrium,** the reaction proceeds in both directions at the same rate. In other words, the rate of product formation is the same as the rate of reactant formation, and the amounts of products and reactants remain relatively constant.

The reaction between carbon dioxide and water to form hydrogen ions and bicarbonate ions is reversible.

$$CO_2 + H_2O \rightleftharpoons H^+ + HCO_3^-$$

If carbon dioxide is added to the system, the reaction proceeds to the right to produce more hydrogen and bicarbonate ions until equilibrium is reestablished. When hydrogen ions are added, the reaction proceeds to the left to produce more carbon dioxide and water until equilibrium is again reached. This reversible system is one mechanism that regulates the amount of hydrogen ions in the body, which is critical to normal functioning of metabolic processes.

> The body adjusts the hydrogen ion concentration in the blood by altering the breathing rate. If more hydrogen ions are needed in the body, the breathing rate decreases, which increases the amount of carbon dioxide in body fluids. This causes the reaction to proceed to the right and increases the hydrogen ions. If the hydrogen ion concentration is too high, the breathing rate increases, more carbon dioxide is exhaled and the reaction proceeds to the left to decrease the hydrogen ions.

| Some chemical reactions are reversible, and the direction in which they proceed depends on the existing conditions.

✓ QuickCheck

- During digestion, a molecule of sucrose forms the simpler molecules of glucose and fructose. This is an example of what type of reaction?

- Charcoal briquettes burn rather slowly, but coal dust can be explosive. Why?

Mixtures, Solutions, and Suspensions

Mixtures

A **mixture** is a combination of two or more substances, in varying proportions, that can be separated by ordinary physical means. The substances retain their original properties after they have been combined in a mixture. The components of a mixture may be elements (such as iron and sulfur), compounds (such as sugar and water), or elements and compounds (such as iodine and alcohol).

| A mixture consists of two or more substances that can be physically separated.

Solutions

Solutions are mixtures in which the component particles remain evenly distributed. All solutions consist of two parts: the **solute** and the **solvent.** The solute is the substance that is present in the smaller amount and that is being dissolved. It may be a gas, liquid, or solid. The solvent, usually a gas or liquid, is the component that is present in the larger amount and that does the dissolving. In a sugar solution, the sugar is the solute and the water is the solvent. Water is the most common solvent and is called the universal solvent. Alcohol and carbon tetrachloride are also commonly used solvents. When alcohol is the solvent, the solution is called a **tincture.** The composition of a solution is variable; that is, it may be weak or concentrated. In a sugar solution, whether there is a small amount of sugar or a large amount it is still a solution. Although a solution is always clear and the solute does not settle, the components may be separated by a physical means such as evaporation.

| Solutions consist of a solute that is being dissolved and a solvent that does the dissolving.

Suspensions

Some mixtures involving a liquid settle unless they are continually shaken. If sand is mixed with water, shaken, then allowed to settle, the particles of sand will fall to the bottom. This is a type of mixture called a **suspension.** A suspension is cloudy and its particles settle. Blood cells form a suspension in the plasma.

One type of mixture that is particularly important in the body is the **colloidal suspension.** The particles in a colloidal suspension are so small that they remain suspended in the liquid but they do not dissolve. Mayonnaise, although not of particular importance in the body, is a colloidal suspension. In this case, the vinegar is the suspending medium and the beaten egg provides the colloidal particles. More relevant, perhaps, is the fact that the fluid that fills the cells of the body, the cytoplasm, is a colloidal suspension.

| In most suspensions, the particles settle if left undisturbed. In colloidal suspensions, the particles are so small that they remain suspended but do not dissolve.

Electrolytes, Acids, Bases, and Buffers

Acids, bases, and salts belong to a large group of compounds called electrolytes. There are numerous electrolytes in the body, and their concentrations are an important aspect of health care.

Electrolytes

Electrolytes (ee-LEK-troh-lites) are substances that break up, or **dissociate,** in solution to form charged particles, or ions. These compounds are called *electrolytes* because the ions can conduct an electrical current. When an ionic compound such as sodium chloride, NaCl, is placed in water, the positively charged sodium ion is attracted to the negatively charged oxygen end of the water molecule. The negatively charged chloride ion is attracted to the hydrogens of the water molecule. Because the polar covalent bonds of the water are stronger than the ionic bonds of the sodium chloride, the sodium chloride breaks apart, or dissociates, into cations and anions in the water (Fig. 2–9).

> Electrolytes form cations and anions when they are placed in water.

> The electrocardiogram and electroencephalogram are graphic tracings of the electric currents created by the electrolytes in the heart and brain, respectively.

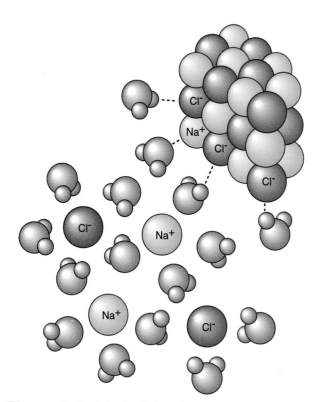

Figure 2–9 Behavior of electrolytes in water.

Acids

Everyone is familiar with acids of various types. Orange juice, lemon juice, vinegar, coffee, and aspirin all contain acids. Acids have a sour taste. An **acid** is defined as a **proton donor.** Now think about the structure of a hydrogen atom: it has one proton in the nucleus and one electron in the electron shell. When the hydrogen atom loses its one electron to become a hydrogen ion, its structure consists of the single proton in a nucleus. A hydrogen ion is a proton. Because an acid is a proton donor, any substance that releases hydrogen ions in water is a proton donor and an acid. Hydrochloric acid, the acid in the stomach, forms hydrogen ions (H^+) and chloride ions (Cl^-). Because it forms hydrogen ions, it is a proton donor.

$$HCl \longrightarrow H^+ + Cl^-$$

Carbonic acid also plays an important role in human physiology. When it dissociates or ionizes in water, it forms hydrogen ions and bicarbonate ions.

$$H_2CO_3 \longrightarrow H^+ + HCO_3^-$$

carbonic acid · · · · · · · · · hydrogen ion · · · · bicarbonate ion

The strength of an acid depends on the degree to which it dissociates in water. Hydrochloric acid is a strong acid because it dissociates readily to produce an abundance of hydrogen ions. There are very few hydrogen chloride molecules in the solution. On the other hand, carbonic acid is a relatively weak acid because most of the molecules remain intact in water and only a few dissociate into hydrogen ions and bicarbonate ions.

> Acids are proton donors.

Bases

Household ammonia, milk of magnesia, and egg white are just a few of the bases with which everyone is familiar. Bases feel slippery and taste bitter. A **base** is defined as a **proton acceptor.** A base accepts the protons that an acid donates. Sodium hydroxide (NaOH) is a common example of a base. When placed in water, it dissociates into sodium ions (Na^+) and hydroxide ions (OH^-).

$$NaOH \longrightarrow Na^+ + OH^-$$

It is a base because the hydroxide ions accept the protons or hydrogen ions from an acid to form water.

$$H^+ + OH^- \longrightarrow HOH (H_2O)$$

hydrogen ion · · · · · · hydroxide ion · · · · · · · · · · · water
proton donor · · · · · · proton acceptor

The degree of ionization or dissociation of a base determines its strength. A strong base is highly ionized in solution and at equilibrium will have more ions than molecules. Weak bases are poorly ionized, and at equilibrium their solutions have more molecules than ions.

■ Bases accept protons.

The pH Scale

The term **pH** is used to indicate the exact strength of an acid or base. The pH scale, illustrated in Figure 2–10, ranges from 0 to 14 and measures the hydrogen ion concentration of a solution. The greater the number of hydrogen ions, the more **acidic** the solution, and the lower the pH. Fewer hydrogen ions result in basic or **alkaline** solutions with a higher pH. A **neutral** solution has the same number of proton donors (hydrogen ions) as proton acceptors (hydroxide ions) and the pH is 7. Pure water is a neutral solution with a pH of 7. Solutions that are acidic have a pH of less than 7, and the lower the pH, the stronger the acid. Basic or alkaline

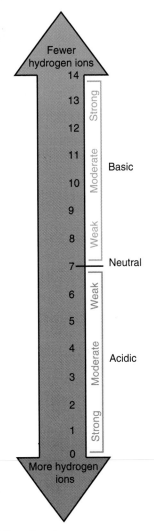

Figure 2–10 pH scale.

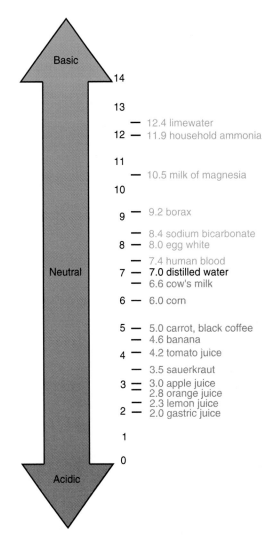

Figure 2–11 pH values of some common substances.

solutions have a pH greater than 7, and the higher the pH, the stronger it is. Because the scale is logarithmic, each unit on the pH scale represents a tenfold difference in the hydrogen ion concentration. For example, a solution with a pH of 6 has 10 times the hydrogen ion concentration as a solution with a pH of 7, and a solution with a pH of 5 has 10 times more than a solution with a pH of 6. A solution with a pH of 5 has 100 times the hydrogen ion concentration of a pH 7 solution. Figure 2–11 compares the pH values for some familiar acids and bases.

■ A pH value indicates the hydrogen ion concentration of a solution. A pH of 7 is neutral. Acids have a pH less than 7; bases have a pH greater than 7.

Neutralization Reactions

Neutralization is the reaction between an acid and a base. The hydrogen ion (H^+) from the acid reacts with the hydroxide ion (OH^-) from the base to form water. The acid removes or neutralizes the effect of the base and vice versa. The other product is called a **salt.** Salts are ionic compounds produced from neutralization reactions and consist of cations other than H^+ and anions other than OH^-. They are formed from the positive ion of the base and the negative ion of the acid.

$$HCl + NaOH \longrightarrow NaCl + H_2O$$

acid   base   salt   water

Neutralization reactions help maintain the proper pH of the blood. They also have many practical, everyday applications. One such application involves antacid medications. Antacids are basic in nature and are taken to neutralize excess acid in the stomach.

> Neutralization reactions occur between acids and bases to produce salts and water.

Buffers

If you add a few drops of a strong acid to some distilled water (pH = 7), the pH of the solution will decrease because hydrogen ions have been added. If a few drops of acid are placed in a buffer solution, the pH will change only slightly. A **buffer** is a solution that resists change in pH when either an acid or a base is added.

A buffer solution contains a weak acid and a salt of that same acid, which functions as a weak base. One of the most common buffering systems and one that is important in human physiology involves carbonic acid (H_2CO_3) and its salt, sodium bicarbonate ($NaHCO_3$). When hydrogen ions from a strong acid are added, they react with the salt to form a weaker acid and a neutral salt.

$$HCl + NaHCO_3 \longrightarrow H_2CO_3 + NaCl$$

strong acid   buffer salt   weak acid   neutral salt

In this way the hydrogen ions from the strong acid are incorporated into the weak acid and will have less effect on the pH. If a base such as NaOH is added to the buffer system, it will be neutralized by the acid to form water and a salt.

$$NaOH + H_2CO_3 \longrightarrow NaHCO_3 + H_2O$$

base   buffer acid   buffer salt   water

When either an acid or a base is added to a buffered solution, something neutral (water or salt) and a component of the buffer (weak acid or its salt) is formed. The pH doesn't change. Buffers are very important physiologically. Even a slight deviation from the normal pH range can cause pronounced changes in the rate of cellular chemical reactions and thus threaten survival. Buffers are one of the homeostatic control mechanisms that maintain normal pH.

> Buffers, which contain a weak aid and a salt of that same acid, resist pH changes by neutralizing the effects of stronger acids and bases.

In the human body, acid-base balance is regulated by chemical buffer systems, the lungs, and the kidneys.

✓ QuickCheck

● Black coffee is an acid. Is its pH greater or less than 7.0?

● Many of the foods we eat are acids, yet the pH of body fluids remains relatively constant. Why?

Organic Compounds

The term **organic chemistry** is inherited from the day when the science of chemistry was comparatively primitive. Compounds formed by living processes were termed organic. In the 19th century it was discovered that organic compounds can be created artificially in the laboratory from substances that do not arise from life processes. Since then, the field of organic chemistry has grown until today more than a million different organic compounds have been identified. By contrast, the inorganic compounds in the world number a mere 50,000!

Organic compounds are important because they are associated with all living matter in both plants and animals. Nearly all compounds related to living substances contain carbon; thus, organic compounds are carbon compounds. Carbohydrates, fats, proteins, hormones, vitamins, enzymes, and many drugs are organic compounds. Wool, silk, linen, cotton, nylon, and rayon all contain organic compounds. Add to this the perfumes, dyes, flavorings, soaps, gasoline, and oils and you see that the study of organic compounds is extensive.

The most important groups of organic compounds in the body are the carbohydrates, proteins, lipids, nucleic acids, and adenosine triphosphate.

> Organic compounds are associated with living matter and contain carbon.

Carbohydrates

Carbohydrate (kar-boh-HYE-drayt) molecules are composed of carbon, hydrogen, and oxygen in a ratio of 1C:2H:1O and range in size from small to very large. They are an important energy source in the body, contribute to the structure of some cellular components, and form a reserve supply of stored energy.

> Carbohydrates contain carbon, hydrogen, and oxygen. They are an important energy source.

The simplest carbohydrate molecules are the **monosaccharides** (mahn-oh-SAK-ah-rides) or simple sugars. The most important simple sugar is **glucose,** which has 6 carbon atoms, 12 hydrogen atoms, and 6 oxygen atoms, $C_6H_{12}O_6$. Because it has six carbon atoms, it is called a hexose. Glucose is also known as dextrose or grape sugar. It occurs normally in the blood and abnormally in the urine. Glucose requires no digestion; therefore, it can be given intravenously. Two other important hexoses are **fructose** and **galactose.** Even though they have the same molecular formula as glucose, $C_6H_{12}O_6$, their atoms are arranged differently, which gives them different structural formulas. Fructose is found in fruit juices and honey. It is called fruit sugar and is the sweetest of all sugars. Galactose is not found free in nature but is one of the components of lactose or milk sugar. When ingested, fructose and galactose are often converted to glucose in the liver.

Not all monosaccharides are hexoses. Some are **pentoses,** which contain five carbon atoms. **Ribose** and **deoxyribose** are important pentose monosaccharides in the body. They are components of nucleic acids, which are discussed later in this chapter.

| Glucose, fructose, and galactose are hexoses. Ribose and deoxyribose, components of nucleic acids, are pentoses.

When two hexose monosaccharides are linked together by a dehydration synthesis reaction, a **disaccharide** (die-SAK-ah-ride) or double sugar is formed. Disaccharides have the molecular formula $C_{12}H_{22}O_{11}$. Three common disaccharides are sucrose, maltose, and lactose. Sucrose is common, ordinary table sugar. It is formed from one glucose and one fructose. Maltose is malt sugar, found in germinating grain and in malt. The building blocks of maltose are two molecules of glucose. Lactose is milk sugar, the sugar found in milk. When lactose is digested or broken down by hydrolysis, it produces glucose and galactose. Certain bacteria produce enzymes that convert lactose to lactic acid, which sours the milk.

| Sucrose, maltose, and lactose are disaccharides or double sugars. They consist of two monosaccharides linked together.

Polysaccharides (pahl-ee-SAK-ah-rides) are long chains of monosaccharides linked together. Three important polysaccharides, all composed of glucose units, are starch, cellulose, and glycogen. Starch is the storage food of plants. It exists as small granules that are insoluble in water but if heated, the granules rupture and form a colloidal gel. Cellulose is the supporting tissue of plants. It is not affected by any enzymes in the human digestive system so it is not digestible and contributes to the "roughage" in

the diet. Glycogen, composed of many glucose units, is animal starch. It is the storage form of carbohydrates in the body and is found particularly in the liver and in muscle.

| Starch, cellulose, and glycogen are important polysaccharides. They consist of long chains of glucose molecules.

When blood sugar (glucose) levels decline, stored glycogen is broken down by hydrolysis into its component glucose units to restore blood glucose levels to normal.

Proteins

All **proteins** (PRO-teens) contain the elements carbon, hydrogen, oxygen, and nitrogen. Most of them

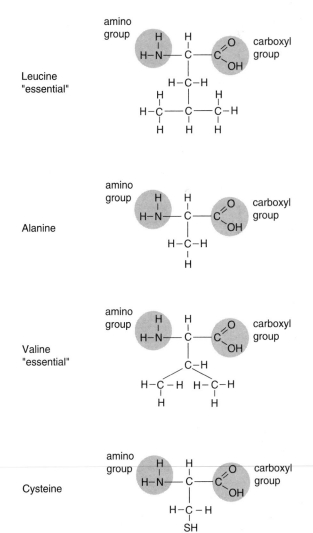

Figure 2-12 Structural formulas for some representative amino acids.

also contain sulfur and some include phosphorus. The building blocks of proteins are **amino acids,** molecules characterized by an amino group (—NH$_2$) and a carboxyl acid group (—COOH). Some amino acids are illustrated in Figure 2–12. There are about 20 different amino acids that occur commonly in proteins. Of these, humans can synthesize 10 from simple organic molecules, but the other 10 are "essential amino acids" and must be provided in the diet (Table 2–4). Amino acids are linked together by **peptide bonds,** produced by dehydration synthesis, to form chains that vary in length from less than 100 to more than 50,000 amino acids. The chains are then folded to form a three-dimensional protein molecule. The number, types, and sequence of amino acids, as well as the folding pattern, are unique for each specific protein.

> Proteins are formed from amino acids linked together by peptide bonds. They contain carbon, hydrogen, oxygen, nitrogen, usually sulfur, and often phosphorus.

Protein is the basic structural material of the body and performs many important functions. Some proteins are important structural components of cells and tissues whereas others act as antibodies in the fight against disease. Muscles contain specific proteins that are responsible for contraction. Other proteins provide identification marks and receptor sites on cell membranes. Enzymes and hormones have a critical role in all metabolic processes. Hemoglobin is a large protein molecule found inside red blood cells that has a specialized function to transport oxygen to body tissues. In addition to all of this, proteins provide a source of energy.

> Proteins are important to the health of an individual.

Table 2–5 Important Lipid Groups

Group	Components	Characteristics
Triglycerides	Glycerol and fatty acids	Most common lipid in the body, efficient energy storage; insulation
Phospholipids	Glycerol, fatty acids, phosphate and nitrogen groups	Component of cell membranes; also found in nerve tissue
Steroids	Complex carbon rings derived from lipids	Most common steroid is cholesterol; includes sex hormones, adrenocortical hormones, vitamin D

Lipids

Lipids represent a group of organic compounds that, like carbohydrates, are composed of carbon, hydrogen, and oxygen. They differ from carbohydrates in that they have a much lower oxygen content. This is illustrated by the molecular formula for the fat, glycerol tristearate, $C_{57}H_{110}O_6$. Lipids are insoluble in water but are generally soluble in nonpolar solvents such as alcohol, acetone, ether, and chloroform. Lipids include a variety of compounds such as fats, phospholipids, and steroids that have important functions in the body. These are summarized in Table 2–5.

> Lipids are insoluble in water but will dissolve in solvents such as alcohol and ether. They contain carbon, hydrogen, and oxygen.

The most common members of the lipid group are the fats or **triglycerides** (try-GLIS-ser-ides) that are the body's most highly concentrated source of energy and energy storage. They also provide protection, padding, and insulation. The building blocks of fats are **glycerol** and **fatty acids.** Glycerol is a three-carbon molecule that has a hydroxyl group (—OH) on each carbon (Fig. 2–13). Fatty acids are carbon chains with a carboxyl group (—COOH) at

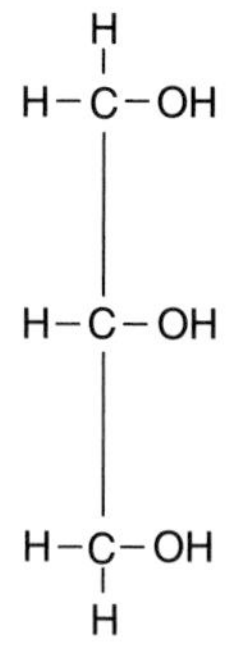

Table 2–4 Common Amino Acids

Name	Three-Letter	One-Letter	Name	Three-Letter	One-Letter
Alanine	Ala	A	Asparagine	Asn	N
Cysteine	Cys	C	Glutamine	Gln	Q
Glycine	Gly	G	**Isoleucine**	Ile	I
Leucine	Leu	L	**Methionine**	Met	M
Phenylalanine	Phe	F	Proline	Pro	P
Serine	Ser	S	**Threonine**	Thr	T
Tryptophan	Trp	W	Tyrosine	Tyr	Y
Valine	Val	V	Aspartic acid	Asp	D
Glutamic acid	Glu	E	**Arginine**	Arg	R
Histidine	His	H	**Lysine**	Lys	K

Essential amino acids are indicated in bold print.

```
          H
          |
     H — C — OH
          |
          |
     H — C — OH
          |
          |
     H — C — OH
          |
          H
```

Figure 2–13 Structural formula for glycerol.

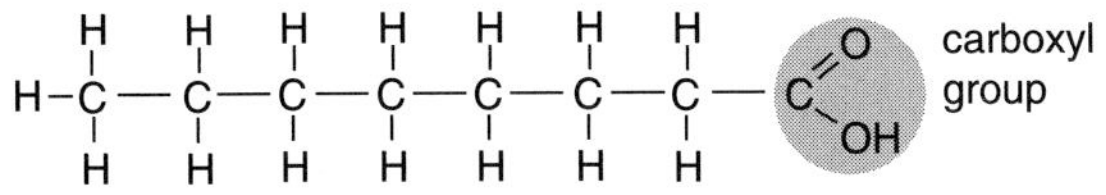

Figure 2-14 Structural formula for a representative fatty acid.

Table 2-6 Some Common Fatty Acids

Name	Number of Carbon Atoms	Formula	Saturated or Unsaturated
Butyric	4	C_3H_7COOH	Saturated
Caproic	6	$C_5H_{11}COOH$	Saturated
Caprylic	8	$C_7H_{15}COOH$	Saturated
Capric	10	$C_9H_{19}COOH$	Saturated
Lauric	12	$C_{11}H_{23}COOH$	Saturated
Myristic	14	$C_{13}H_{27}COOH$	Saturated
Palmitic	16	$C_{15}H_{31}COOH$	Saturated
Stearic	18	$C_{17}H_{35}COOH$	Saturated
Oleic	18	$C_{17}H_{33}COOH$	Unsaturated (1)
Linoleic	18	$C_{17}H_{31}COOH$	Unsaturated (2)
Linolenic	18	$C_{17}H_{29}COOH$	Unsaturated (3)
Arachidic	20	$C_{19}H_{39}COOH$	Saturated
Arachidonic	20	$C_{19}H_{31}COOH$	Unsaturated (4)

The numeral in parentheses by the unsaturated fatty acids indicates the number of double bonds.

one end (Fig. 2–14). The carbon chains in fatty acids vary in length but have an even number of carbon atoms. The carboxyl group gives it its acidic properties. If all the carbons in a fatty acid are joined together with single covalent bonds, then it is a **saturated fatty acid** (Fig. 2–15). It is saturated with hydrogen. If, however, there are double covalent bonds between some of the carbons in the chain, then it is an **unsaturated fatty acid** (Fig. 2–16). Table 2–6 lists some of the common fatty acids. Three fatty acids combine with one glycerol, by dehydration synthesis, to form a triglyceride or fat (Fig. 2–17). In natural fats, the fatty acids in the triglyceride are different. Triglycerides that contain only saturated fatty acids are called **saturated fats,** but if some of fatty acids are unsaturated, they are **unsaturated fats.** Saturated fats are typically animal fats and unsaturated fats are vegetable oils. Structurally animal fats and vegetable oils are similar except that the oils are synthesized from unsaturated fatty acids.

> The building blocks of triglycerides, commonly known as fats, are glycerol and fatty acids. Saturated fats contain only fatty acids that have single bonds between the carbon atoms.

Phospholipids, in addition to the glycerol and fatty acids, contain a phosphate group and a nitrogenous group. They are an important component of cell membranes in the body. They are particularly abundant in nerve and muscle cells.

> Phospholipids, which contain phosphates and nitrogen, are important components of cell membranes.

Steroids are compounds that are derivatives of lipids and have four interconnected rings of carbon atoms (Fig. 2–18). The most common steroid in the body is cholesterol, which is particularly abundant in the brain and nerve tissue. It is the chief component of gallstones. Sex hormones, steroid hormones

from the cortex of the adrenal gland, and vitamin D are all steroids and are derivatives of cholesterol.

> Steroids, which are derivatives of lipids, include cholesterol, certain hormones, and vitamin D.

Nucleic Acids

Nucleic acids are large, complex, organic compounds that contain carbon, hydrogen, oxygen, nitrogen, and phosphorus. The building blocks of nucleic acids are **nucleotides** (NOO-klee-oh-tides). A nucleotide consists of a five-carbon sugar or pentose, an organic nitrogenous base, and a phosphate group (Fig. 2–19). Nucleotides are joined together by dehydration synthesis into long chains to form the nucleic acid (Fig. 2–20). There are two classes of nucleic acids, deoxyribonucleic acid (DNA) and ribonucleic acid (RNA).

> Nucleotides are the building blocks of nucleic acids. They contain carbon, hydrogen, oxygen, nitrogen, and phosphorus.

Deoxyribonucleic acid (dee-ahk-see-rye-boh-noo-KLEE-ik AS-id), or **DNA,** is the genetic material of the cell. The sugar in DNA is deoxyribose and the

Figure 2-15 Structural formula for a representative saturated fatty acid showing the single bonds between carbon atoms.

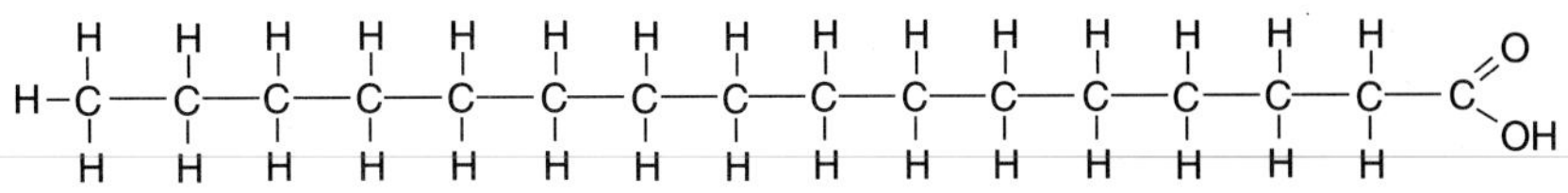

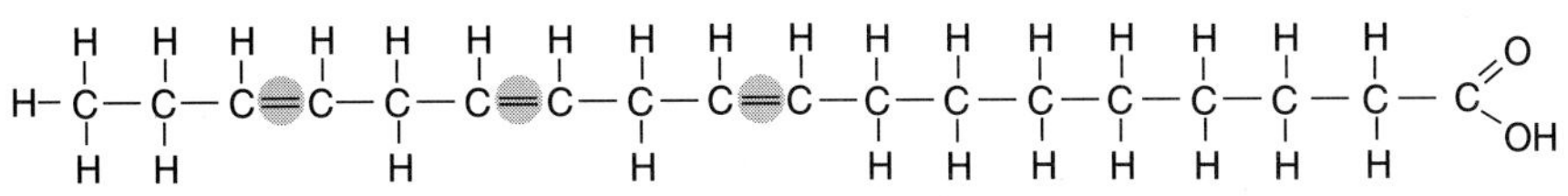

Figure 2-16 Structural formula for a representative unsaturated fatty acid showing double bonds between some carbon atoms.

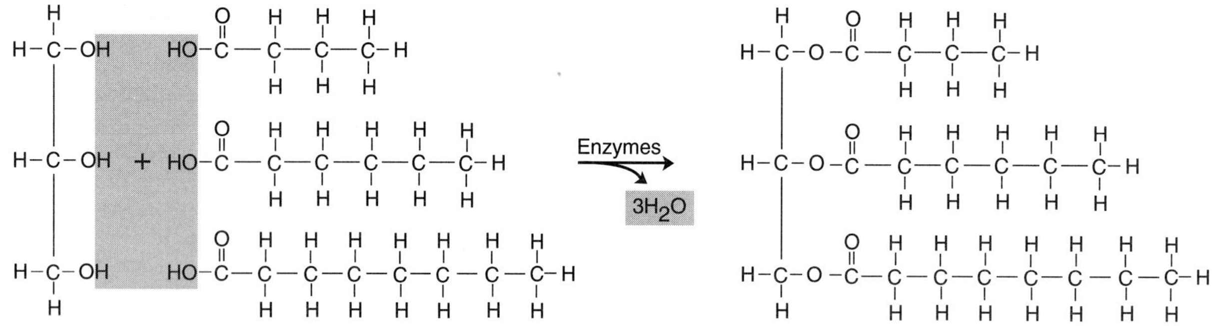

Figure 2-17 Structural formula for a representative triglyceride.

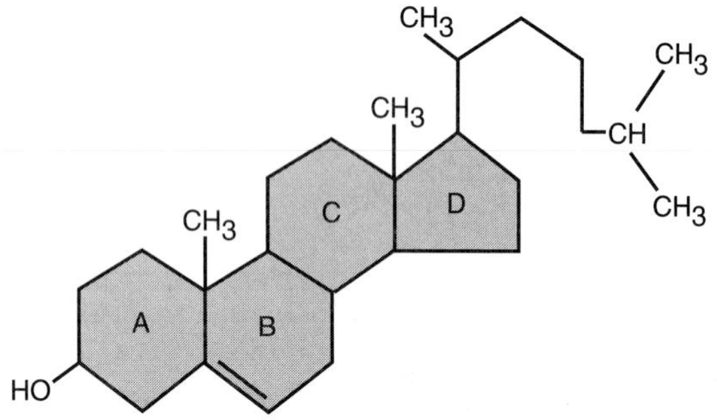

Figure 2-18 A common steroid, cholesterol.

| DNA is the genetic material of the cell, and RNA functions in the synthesis of proteins within the cell.

Adenosine Triphosphate

Adenosine triphosphate (ah-DEN-oh-sin trye-FOS-fate), or **ATP,** is a high-energy compound composed

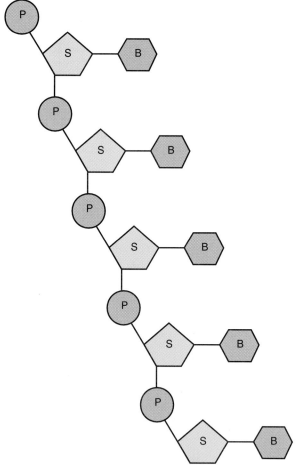

nitrogenous bases are adenine, thymine, cytosine, and guanine. The specific sequence of the nitrogenous bases constitutes the genetic code, which is all the genetic information of the cell in a code form. There are two chains of nucleotides in DNA that are loosely joined together by hydrogen bonds and then these two chains are twisted into a double helix (Fig. 2–21).

Ribonucleic acid (rye-boh-noo-KLEE-ik AS-id), or **RNA,** has several functions in the synthesis of proteins within the cell. RNA is a single chain of nucleotides in which the sugar is ribose and the nitrogenous bases are adenine, uracil, cytosine, and guanine. DNA, the genetic material, contains the instructions for making proteins but various types of RNA carry out the processes. DNA and RNA are compared in Table 2–7.

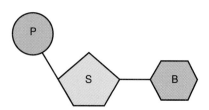

Figure 2-19 Components of a nucleotide. P = phosphate; S = sugar; B = base.

Figure 2-20 Components of a nucleic acid. P = phosphate; S = sugar; B = base.

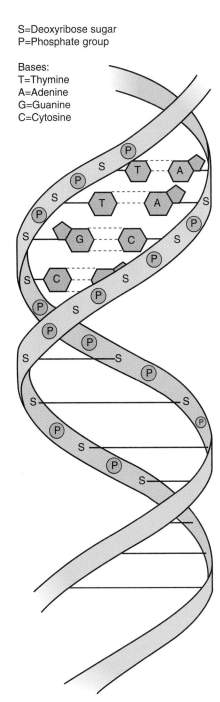

S=Deoxyribose sugar
P=Phosphate group

Bases:
T=Thymine
A=Adenine
G=Guanine
C=Cytosine

Figure 2–21   Deoxyribonucleic acid.

Feature	DNA	RNA
Sugar	Deoxyribose	Ribose
Bases	Adenine, thymine, guanine, cytosine	Adenine, uracil, guanine, cytosine
Strands	Two strands in double helix	Single strand

Table 2–7   Comparison of DNA and RNA

more energy and adenosine monophosphate. When energy is available, ATP can be resynthesized from ADP. The breakdown of nutrients releases energy that is used to synthesize ATP. In this way, the nutrient energy is converted to a form that is usable by the body through the high-energy bonds of ATP.

ATP is a high-energy compound that supplies energy in a from that is usable by body cells.

✓ QuickCheck

- Analysis of a given nucleic acid reveals cytosine, uracil, adenine, and guanine. Is this nucleic acid DNA or RNA?

- Analysis of an organic compound shows it contains only C, H, and a relatively small amount of O. Is this compound likely a carbohydrate, protein, lipid, or nucleic acid?

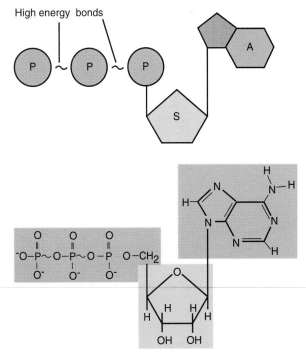

Figure 2–22   Components of adenosine triphosphate. P = phosphate; S = sugar; A = adenine.

of adenine (a nitrogenous base), ribose (a five-carbon sugar), and three phosphate groups (Fig. 2–22). The phosphate groups are linked together by high-energy chemical bonds that release chemical energy when they are broken. This chemical energy is usable by the body cells. When the phosphate group on the end is split off by hydrolysis, a molecule of adenosine diphosphate (ADP) remains.

$$ATP \longrightarrow ADP + phosphate + energy$$

Another phosphate can be split from ADP to release

Chemistry?

Radioactive Isotopes

All atoms of a given element have the same number of protons in the nucleus. This determines the atomic number. They also have the same number of electrons, equal to the number of protons, in the energy orbitals around the nucleus. The number and arrangement of the electrons determine how an atom reacts.

The number of neutrons in the nucleus may vary for different atoms of a given element, and this changes the atomic weight. For example, most hydrogen atoms have one proton and one electron, which gives an atomic weight of 1 amu. About 1.5 percent of the hydrogen atoms have a neutron with the proton in the nucleus and this gives them an atomic weight of 2 amu. A limited number have two neutrons in the nucleus and have an atomic weight of 3 amu. Atoms of a given element that have different numbers of neutrons, and consequently different atomic weights, are called **isotopes.** Deuterium is the isotope of hydrogen that has an atomic weight of 2 amu, and tritium is the isotope with an atomic weight of 3 amu.

Some of the isotopes of an element are stable, whereas others have unstable atomic nuclei that decompose, releasing energy or atomic particles. Unstable isotopes are called **radioactive isotopes,** and the energy or atomic particles they emit are called **atomic radiations.** These radiations include three common forms called alpha (α), beta (β), and gamma (γ). Alpha radiation consists of two protons and two neutrons from the atomic nuclei. This type of radiation travels relatively slowly and does not penetrate deeply. When alpha radiation is released within the body, it may cause severe tissue damage. Beta radiation is composed of electrons that travel more rapidly (almost the speed of light) and penetrate more deeply. Gamma radiation is electromagnetic energy and has the greatest penetrating power of the three forms. Although a given radioactive isotope may emit more than one form of radiation, the types and energies are specific for each isotope.

Each radioactive isotope loses its radioactivity at a particular rate. The **half-life** is the amount of time it takes for a given isotope to lose one half of its radioactivity. The times vary greatly from one isotope to another. For example, the half-life of cobalt 54 is 0.2 second, while for cobalt 60 it is 5.26 years. The half-life of iodine 131, commonly used to study thyroid function, is 8.1 days; that of strontium 85, used for diagnosis of bone diseases, is 64 days.

Because all isotopes of a given element, whether radioactive or nonradioactive, have the same number of electrons, they all react in the same way chemically. For example, each of the eight different isotopes of oxygen will function identically in metabolic reactions. This feature enables the medical profession to use radioactive isotopes in diagnosis and therapy.

In a simple form of diagnosis, a radioactive isotope called a **tracer** is injected intravenously, and a technician uses some form of radiation detector to monitor how the radiation is distributed. A good example of this is the use of iodine 131 to diagnose thyroid malfunction. The thyroid glands in the neck produce a hormone, called thyroxine, that contains iodine. When radioactive iodine 131 is injected into the bloodstream, the thyroid glands take it up and use it to make thyroxine just as they would nonradioactive iodine. A normally functioning thyroid absorbs about 12 percent of the administered iodine within a few hours. An overactive thyroid uses the iodine at a faster rate, and an underactive thyroid uses it at a slower rate. By counting the radiations emitted from the thyroid, one can determine the rate of uptake of iodine 131 and assess thyroid function. Other isotopes are used to study the functions of other organs in a similar manner.

Radioactive isotopes are used in therapy to destroy cancerous cells and tissues. Atomic radiations cause changes in the structure of cellular components and chemicals. This alters vital cellular processes and destroys both normal cells and cancerous cells. The idea, of course, is to kill cancerous cells but keep the normal cells intact. Because cancer cells, which divide rapidly, are more susceptible to radiation damage than normal cells, the cancer cells are destroyed more readily than the normal ones and damage to healthy tissues is minimized. Techniques are used that attempt to pinpoint the radiation to a localized area where the tumor is located. This also reduces the damage to normal tissue. The goal in radiation therapy is maximum destruction of diseased tissue with minimum damage to healthy cells.

CHAPTER 2 QUIZ

RECALL

Match the definitions on the left with the appropriate term on the right.

1. Positively charged particle in the nucleus of an atom

2. Atom that has lost or gained an electron

3. Substance being dissolved

4. Alcohol is the solvent

5. Positively charged ion

6. Has a pH less than 7

7. Bond between amino acids

8. Adenosine triphosphate

9. Building block of DNA

10. Smallest unit of a compound

A. Acid

B. ATP

C. Cation

D. Ion

E. Molecule

F. Nucleotide

G. Peptide

H. Proton

I. Solute

J. Tincture

THOUGHT

1. The symbol for sodium is
   a. Na
   b. So
   c. S
   d. N

2. The molecular formula for sodium bicarbonate is $NaHCO_3$. What is the total number of atoms in one molecule of sodium bicarbonate?
   a. 3
   b. 6
   c. 4
   d. 12

3. What type of reaction is represented by the following equation?

   $HgCl_2 + H_2S \longrightarrow HgS + 2HCl$

   a. synthesis
   b. decomposition
   c. single replacement
   d. double replacement

4. What type of organic molecule is represented by the formula $C_6H_{12}O_6$?
   a. carbohydrate
   b. protein
   c. lipid
   d. steroid

5. A nucleotide molecule consists of
   a. thymine, adenine, and guanine
   b. phosphate, adenine, and nitrogenous base
   c. pentose, phosphate group, nitrogenous base
   d. phosphate, adenosine, and ribose

APPLICATION

1. A chemical reaction is proceeding very slowly. Suggest four things you might try to speed up the reaction.
2. The following reaction is reversible.

$$CO_2 + H_2O \rightleftharpoons H^+ + HCO_3^-$$

As you breathe, you exhale CO_2, and remove it from the body. What effect does this have on the above reaction? Does the reaction proceed to the right or to the left as a result of exhaling CO_2?

CHAPTER 3

Cell Structure And Function

Outline/Objectives

Structure of the Generalized Cell 40

- Describe the cell membrane and list five functions of the proteins in the membrane.
- Describe the composition of the cytoplasm.
- Describe the components of the nucleus and state the function of each one.
- Identify and describe each of the cytoplasmic organelles and state the function of each one.

Cell Functions 45

- Explain how the cell membrane regulates the composition of the cytoplasm.
- Describe the various mechanisms that result in the transport of substances across the cell membrane.
- Name the phases of a typical cell cycle and describe the events that occur in each phase.
- Explain the difference between mitosis and meiosis.
- Summarize the process of protein synthesis, including the role of DNA and RNA.

Key Terms

Active transport
Cytokinesis
Diffusion
Meiosis
Mitosis
Osmosis
Passive transport
Phagocytosis
Pinocytosis

Building Vocabulary

WORD PART	MEANING
ana-	apart
cyt-	cell
-elle	little, small
extra-	outside, beyond
hyper-	excessive, above
hypo-	beneath, below
-ic-	pertaining to
intra-	within, inside
iso-	equal, same
-osis	condition of
-phag-	to eat, devour
-phil-	to love, have affinity for
-phob-	to hate, dislike
pino-	to drink
-plasm-	matter
-reti-	network, lattice
-som-	body
ton-	solute strength
-ul-, -ule	small, tiny
-um	presence of

39

Every individual begins life as a single cell, a fertilized egg. This single cell divides into 2 cells, then 4, 8, 16, and on and on, until the adult human body has an estimated 75 trillion cells. Cells are the structural and functional units of the human body. Homeostasis depends on the interaction between the cell and its environment.

Structure of the Generalized Cell

During development, cells become specialized in size, shape, characteristics, and function so that there is a large variety of cells in the body. It is impossible, in the scope of this book, to describe each different type of cell in detail. For descriptive purposes it is convenient to imagine a typical, generalized cell that contains the components of all the different cell types. Not all the components of a "generalized" cell are present in every cell type, but each component is present in some cells and has its particular function to maintain life. A generalized cell is illustrated in Figure 3–1, and the structure and functions of the cellular components are summarized in Table 3–1.

> There are many different types, sizes, and shapes of cells in the body. For descriptive purposes, the concept of a "generalized cell" is introduced. It includes features from all cell types.

Plasma Membrane

Every cell in the body is enclosed by a **plasma (cell) membrane.** The plasma membrane separates the material outside the cell (extracellular) from the material inside the cell (intracellular). It maintains the integrity of the cell. If the membrane ruptures, or is broken, the cell dies. The nature of the membrane determines what can go into, or out of, the cell. It is **selectively permeable,** which means that some substances can pass through the membrane but others cannot.

> A selectively permeable plasma membrane separates the extracellular material from the intracellular material.

The main structural components of the plasma membrane are **phospholipids** and **proteins.** Some carbohydrate and cholesterol molecules are present also. The phospholipid molecules are arranged in a double layer (bilayer) with the polar phosphate portions in contact with the outside and inside of the cell and the nonpolar lipid portions sandwiched between the phosphate layers (Fig. 3–2). You can visualize this as a cheese sandwich. The two slices of bread represent the phosphate layers, and the cheese is the lipid portion. The polar phosphate layers are **hydrophilic,** which means that they attract water and other polar molecules. These are the layers that are in contact with the intracellular and extracellular fluids. The middle nonpolar lipid portion is **hydrophobic,** which means that water will not mix with it. Nonpolar organic molecules such as ether and chloroform dissolve readily in the lipid layer and pass through the membrane.

> The plasma membrane is a double layer of phospholipid molecules.

Protein molecules are scattered throughout the phospholipid molecules. Some of the proteins contribute to the structural support of the membrane whereas others form channels that allow water and water-soluble substances to pass through the membrane. Although the lipid in the membrane is a barrier to these ions and molecules, some of the proteins selectively permit their passage. Other proteins

CLINICAL TERMS

Anaplasia (an-ah-PLAY-zee-ah) Loss of differentiation of cells; reversion to a more primitive cell type; characteristic of cancer

Atrophy (AT-roh-fee) Wasting away; a decrease in the size of a cell, tissue, organ, or part

Dysplasia (dis-PLAY-zee-ah) Abnormality in development; alteration in size, shape, and organization of cells

Hyperplasia (hye-per-PLAY-zee-ah) Abnormal increase in the number of cells due to an increase in the frequency of cell division

Hypertrophy (hye-PER-troh-fee) Enlargement of an organ due to an increase in the size of the individual constituent cells

Metaplasia (meh-tah-PLAY-zee-ah) Transformation of one cell type into another cell type

Metastasis (meh-TASS-tah-sis) Spread of a tumor to a secondary site

Necrosis (neh-KROH-sis) Death of cells or groups of cells

Neoplasm (NEE-oh-plazm) Any new and abnormal growth; a tumor

Carcinogen (kar-SIN-oh-jen) An agent that causes cancer; known carcinogens include chemicals and drugs, radiation, and viruses

Benign (bee-NYNE) Not malignant, not recurring

Malignant (mah-LIG-nant) Tending to become worse and result in death; refers to tumors having the characteristics of invasiveness, anaplasia, and metastasis

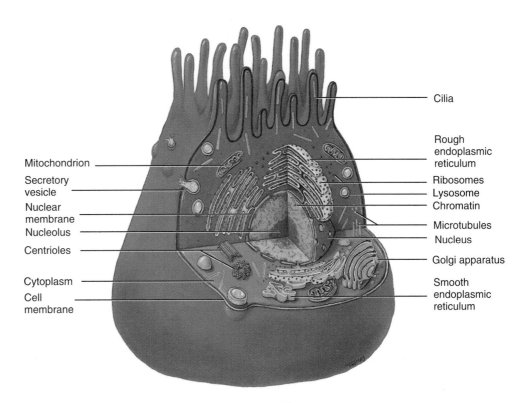

Figure 3–1
Generalized cell.

in the membrane act as receptor sites for hormones that affect the metabolic activity of the cell. Proteins also act as carrier molecules that combine with ions and molecules to transport them across the membrane. Proteins on the surface of the cell act as markers for identification. They are the "fingerprints" of the cell, such that the body recognizes and accepts its own cells but rejects those that are non-self or foreign. This is the basis of tissue and organ transplant rejection and defense mechanisms against disease. Autoimmune diseases result when the self-recognition process becomes faulty.

> Proteins in the cell membrane provide structural support, form channels for passage of materials, act as receptor sites, function as carrier molecules, and provide identification markers.

Cystic fibrosis is an inherited disorder that afflicts 1 in every 2,000 Caucasian live births. In cystic fibrosis the cell membrane proteins that function as channels for transporting chloride ions out of the cell are defective. Because chloride ion transport is altered, secretions such as mucus, sweat, and pancreatic juice are very salty and thick. Thick mucus in the lungs leads to impaired breathing and increased infections. The ducts in the pancreas become plugged, which stops the flow of digestive enzymes. Life expectancy, with therapy, is about 27 years.

Cytoplasm

The **cytoplasm** (SYE-toh-plazm) is the gel-like fluid inside the cell. When viewed with an ordinary light microscope, it appears homogeneous and empty. Electron microscopy reveals that the cytoplasm is highly organized, with numerous small structures, called **organelles,** suspended in it. These organelles (or-guh-NELZ), or "little organs," are the functional machinery of the cell and each organelle type has a specific role in the metabolic reactions that take place in the cytoplasm.

Chemically, the cytoplasm is primarily water, the **intracellular fluid.** About two thirds of the water in the body is in the cytoplasm of cells. The fluid contains dissolved electrolytes, metabolic waste products, and nutrients such as amino acids and simple sugars. Proteins suspended in the fluid give it colloidal properties and a gel-like consistency. Various **inclusions** may be suspended in the cytoplasm. These are bodies that are temporarily in the cell but that are not a part of the permanent metabolic machinery of the cell. Examples of inclusion bodies are membrane-enclosed (membrane-bound) fluid vacuoles, secretory products, glycogen granules, pigment granules, and lipid droplets.

> Cytoplasm, the gel-like fluid inside the cell, is largely water and has a variety of organelles suspended in it.

Table 3–1   Structure and Function of Cellular Components

Component	Structure	Function
Plasma membrane	Bilayer of phospholipid and protein molecules	Maintains integrity of cell; controls passage of materials into and out of the cell
Cytoplasm	Water; dissolved ions and nutrients; suspended colloids	Medium for chemical reactions; suspending medium for organelles
Nucleus	Spherical body near center of cell; enclosed in a membrane	Contains genetic material; regulates activities of the cell
Nuclear membrane	Double-layered membrane around nucleus; has pores	Separates cytoplasm from nucleoplasm; pores allow passage of material as necessary
Chromatin	Strands of DNA in the nucleus	Genetic material of the cell; becomes chromosomes during cell division
Nucleolus	Dense, nonmembranous body in the nucleus; composed of RNA and protein molecules	Forms ribosomes
Mitochondria	Rod-shaped bodies enclosed by a double-layered membrane in the cytoplasm; folds of inner membrane form cristae	Major site of ATP synthesis; converts energy from nutrients into a form that is usable by the body
Ribosomes	Granules of RNA in the cytoplasm	Protein synthesis
Endoplasmic reticulum	Interconnected membranous channels and sacs in the cytoplasm	Transports material through cytoplasm; rough endoplasmic reticulum aids in synthesis of protein; smooth endoplasmic reticulum involved in lipid synthesis
Golgi apparatus	Group of flattened membranous sacs usually near the nucleus	Packages products for secretion; forms lysosomes
Lysosomes	Membranous sacs of digestive enzymes in the cytoplasm	Digest material taken into the cell, debris from damaged cells, worn-out cell components
Cytoskeleton	Protein microfilaments and microtubules in cytoplasm	Provides support for cytoplasm; helps in movement of organelles
Centrioles	Pair of rod-shaped bodies composed of microtubules; located near the nucleus at right angles to each other	Distribute chromosomes to daughter cells during cell division
Cilia	Membrane-enclosed bundles of microtubules that extend outward from cell membrane; short and numerous	Move substances across surface of the cell
Flagella	Similar to cilia except usually long and single	Cell locomotion

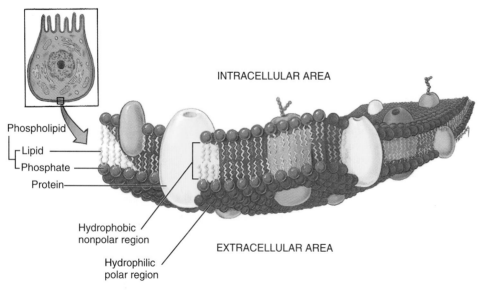

INTRACELLULAR AREA

Phospholipid
Lipid
Phosphate
Protein

Hydrophobic nonpolar region

Hydrophilic polar region

EXTRACELLULAR AREA

Figure 3–2   Structure of the cell membrane.

Nucleus

The **nucleus** (NOO-klee-us) is the control center that directs the metabolic activities of the cell. All cells have at least one nucleus at some time during their existence; some, however, such as red blood cells, lose their nucleus as they mature. Other cells, for example, skeletal muscle cells, have more than one nucleus.

The nucleus is a relatively large, spherical body that is usually located near the center of the cell (see Fig. 3–1). It is enclosed by a double-layered **nuclear membrane** that separates the cytoplasm of the cell from the **nucleoplasm,** the fluid portion inside the nucleus. At numerous points on the nuclear surface, the membrane becomes thin and is interrupted by pores that allow large molecules, such as ribonucleic acid (RNA), to pass from the nucleus into the cytoplasm. The nuclear membrane is more permeable than the cell membrane.

> The nucleus, formed by a nuclear membrane around a fluid nucleoplasm, is the control center of the cell.

The nucleus contains the genetic material of the cell. In the nondividing cell, the genetic material, deoxyribonucleic acid (DNA), is present as long, slender, filamentous threads called **chromatin** (see Fig. 3–1). When the cell starts to divide or replicate, the chromatin condenses and becomes tightly coiled to form short, rodlike **chromosomes.** Each chromosome, composed of DNA with some protein, contains several hundred genes arranged in a specific linear order. Human cells have 23 pairs of chromosomes that together contain all the information necessary to direct the synthesis of more than 100,000 different proteins.

> Threads of chromatin in the nucleus contain DNA, the genetic material of the cell.

The **nucleolus** (noo-KLEE-oh-lus) ("little nucleus") appears as a dark-staining, discrete, dense body within the nucleus (see Fig. 3–1). It has no enclosing membrane, and the number of nucleoli may vary from one to four in any given cell. The nucleolus has a high concentration of RNA and is the region of ribosome formation. In growing cells and others that are making large amounts of protein, the nucleoli are very large and distinct, reflecting the function of RNA in protein synthesis.

> The nucleolus is a dense region of RNA in the nucleus and is the site of ribosome formation.

Cytoplasmic Organelles

Cytoplasmic organelles are "little organs" that are suspended in the cytoplasm of the cell. Each type of organelle has a definite structure and a specific role in the function of the cell.

Mitochondria

Mitochondria (mye-toh-KON-dree-ah) are elongated, oval, fluid-filled sacs in the cytoplasm that contain their own DNA and can reproduce themselves (see Fig. 3–1). The membrane around a mitochondrion consists of two layers with a small space between the layers. The outer layer is smooth, but the inner layer has many invaginations that project like partitions into the interior matrix of the mitochondrion. These invaginations are called **cristae** (KRIS-tee) (Fig. 3–3). Enzymes necessary for the production of adenosine triphosphate (ATP) are located along the cristae. Mitochondria could be called the "power plant" of the cell because it is here that energy from nutrients is converted into a form that is usable by the cell. The enzymes in the mitochondria catalyze the reactions that form the high-energy bonds of ATP.

> Mitochondria are enclosed by a double membrane and function in the production of ATP.

Ribosomes

Ribosomes (RYE-boh-sohmz) are small granules of RNA in the cytoplasm. The RNA in the ribosomes is from the nucleolus, and when fully assembled, ribosomes function in protein synthesis. Some ribosomes are found free in the cytoplasm. These function in the synthesis of proteins for use within that same cell. Other ribosomes are attached to the membranes of the endoplasmic reticulum and function in the synthesis of proteins that are exported from the cell and used elsewhere. Ribosomes can attach to, or detach from, the endoplasmic reticulum, depending on the type of protein that is being produced.

> Ribosomes are granules of RNA that function in protein synthesis.

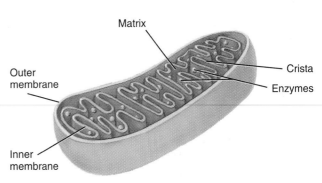

Figure 3–3 Mitochondrion.

Endoplasmic Reticulum

The **endoplasmic reticulum** (ER) (end-oh-PLAZ-mik reh-TICK-yoo-lum) is a complex series of membranous channels that extend throughout the cytoplasm. The interconnected membranes form fluid-filled flattened sacs and tubular canals. The membranes are connected to the outer layer of the nuclear membrane, to the inner layer of the cell membrane, and to certain other organelles. Endoplasmic reticulum provides a path to transport materials from one part of the cell to another.

Some of the membranes of the endoplasmic reticulum have granular ribosomes attached to the outer surface (see Fig. 3–1). This is called **rough endoplasmic reticulum** (RER) and, because of the ribosomes, it functions in the synthesis and transport of protein molecules. Other portions of the endoplasmic reticulum lack the ribosomes and appear smooth. This is the **smooth endoplasmic reticulum** (SER), which functions in the synthesis of certain lipid molecules such as steroids. There is also evidence that indicates that the SER is involved in the detoxification of drugs.

> The endoplasmic reticulum is a series of membranous channels that function in the transport of molecules. The RER transports proteins, and the SER transports certain lipids.

Golgi Apparatus

The **Golgi apparatus** (GOL-jee ap-ah-RAT-us) is a series of 4 to 6 flattened membranous sacs, usually located near the nucleus, and connected to the endoplasmic reticulum (see Fig. 3–1). It is the "packaging and shipping plant" of the cell.

Proteins from the RER and lipids from the SER are carried through the channels of the endoplasmic reticulum to the Golgi apparatus. Within the Golgi apparatus, the proteins may be modified or concentrated, or have a carbohydrate component added. Then they are surrounded by a piece of the Golgi membrane and are pinched off the end of the apparatus to become a **secretory vesicle,** a temporary inclusion in the cytoplasm (Fig. 3–4). The secretory vesicles move to the cell membrane and release their contents to the exterior of the cell.

The Golgi apparatus is especially abundant and well developed in glandular cells that secrete a product, but they also function in nonsecretory cells. In these cells they appear to package intracellular enzymes in the form of lysosomes. Because of the secretory vesicles pinching off the ends of the flattened membranous sacs, the Golgi apparatus is sometimes described as looking like a stack of pancakes with syrup dripping off the edge.

> The Golgi apparatus modifies substances produced in other parts of the cell and prepares these products for secretion.

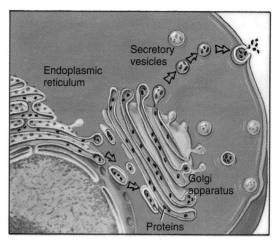

Figure 3–4   Golgi apparatus.

Lysosomes

Lysosomes (LYE-soh-sohmz) are membrane-enclosed sacs of various digestive enzymes that have been packaged by the Golgi apparatus. When cells are damaged, these enzymes destroy the cellular debris. They also function in the destruction of worn-out cell parts. The enzymes break down particles such as bacteria that have been taken into the cell. When a white blood cell phagocytizes or engulfs bacteria, the enzymes from the lysosomes destroy it. Lysosomal activity also seems to be responsible for decreasing the size of some body organs at certain periods. Atrophy of muscle due to lack of use, reduction in breast size after breast feeding, and decrease in the size of the uterus after parturition all seem to be due to lysosomal function.

> Lysosomes contain enzymes that break down substances taken in at the cell membrane. They also destroy cellular debris.

> Peroxisomes are organelles that are similar to lysosomes. They contain the enzymes peroxidase and catalase, which are important in the breakdown of hydrogen peroxide, a substance that is toxic to cells. Peroxisomes are often found in liver and kidney cells, where they function in the detoxification of harmful substances.

> Normally, the membrane around the lysosome is impermeable to the powerful digestive enzymes it contains. If the cell is injured or deprived of oxygen, the membrane becomes fragile and the contents escape. This results in self-digestion of the cell, a process called autolysis. This also happens normally when cells are destroyed as part of a reconfiguration process during embryologic development. It also occurs in white blood cells during inflammation.

Filamentous Protein Organelles

Several types of protein filaments are considered to be cellular organelles. The cytoskeleton and centrioles are in the cytoplasm, but the cilia and flagella project outward, away from the cell surface.

Cytoskeleton

The **cytoskeleton** helps to maintain the shape of the cell. At times it anchors certain organelles in position, but it may also move organelles from one position to another. Some parts of the cytoskeleton may move a portion of the cell membrane, whereas others may move the entire cell. The cytoskeleton also plays a role in muscle contraction.

The cytoskeleton is made up of protein **microfilaments** and **microtubules.** Microfilaments are long, slender rods of protein that support small projections of the cell membrane called **microvilli.** Microtubules are thin cylinders, larger than the microfilaments, and are composed of the protein **tubulin.** In addition to their role as part of the cytoskeleton, microtubules are also found in centrioles, cilia, and flagella.

> The cytoskeleton is formed from microfilaments and microtubules and helps to maintain the shape of the cell.

Centrioles

A dense area called the **centrosome** (SEN-troh-sohm), located near the nucleus, contains a pair of **centrioles** (SEN-tree-ohlz) (see Fig. 3–1). Each centriole is a nonmembranous rod-shaped structure composed of microtubules. The two members of the pair are at right angles to each other. Centrioles function in cell reproduction by aiding in the distribution of chromosomes to the new daughter cells.

> The centrosome contains a pair of centrioles that function in cell division.

Cilia

Cilia (SIL-ee-ah) are short, cylindrical, hairlike processes that project outward from the cell membrane. Each cilium consists of specialized microtubules surrounded by a membrane and anchored under the cell membrane. Cilia have an organized pattern of movement that creates a wavelike motion to move substances across the surface of the cell. They are found in large quantities on the surfaces of cells that line the respiratory tract, where their motion moves mucus, in which particles of dust are embedded, upward and away from the lungs.

> Cilia are short, hairlike projections that move substances across the surface of the cell.

Flagella

Similar in structure to cilia, **flagella** (fluh-JELL-ah) are much longer and fewer. In contrast to cilia, which move substances across the surface of the cell, flagella beat with a whiplike motion to move the cell itself. In the human, the tail of the spermatozoon, or sperm cell, is a single flagellum that causes the swimming motion of the cell.

> Flagella are long, threadlike projections that move the cell.

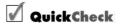 **QuickCheck**

● In which cellular organelle are proteins concentrated and prepared for secretion?

● What are the numerous short, hairlike processes that move mucus along the respiratory tract?

Cell Functions

The structural and functional characteristics of different types of cells are determined by the nature of the proteins present. Cells of various types have different functions because cell structure and function are closely related. It is apparent that a cell that is very thin is not well suited for a protective function. Bone cells do not have an appropriate structure for nerve impulse conduction. Just as there are many cell types, there are varied cell functions. The specific functions of cells will become more apparent as the tissues, organs, and systems are studied. This section deals with the more generalized cell functions, the functions that relate to the continued viability and continuation of the cell itself. These functions include movement of substances across the cell membrane, cell division to make new cells, and protein synthesis.

> The functions of specific cells are closely related to the structure of those cells.

Movement of Substances Across the Cell Membrane

The cell membrane provides a surface through which substances enter and leave the cell. The cell membrane controls the composition of the cell's cytoplasm by regulating the passage of substances through the membrane. If the membrane breaks, this control is removed and the cell dies. The survival of the cell depends on maintaining the difference between extracellular and intracellular material. Mechanisms of movement across the cell membrane include simple diffusion, osmosis, active transport, endocytosis, and exocytosis. These are summarized in Table 3–2.

> The cell membrane controls the composition of the cytoplasm by regulating movement of substances through the membrane.

Table 3–2 Summary of Membrane Transport Mechanisms

Mechanism	Description
Passive	
Simple diffusion	Molecular movement down a concentration gradient
Facilitated diffusion	Carrier molecules transport down a concentration gradient; requires membrane
Osmosis	Movement of solvent toward high solute (low solvent) concentration; requires membrane
Filtration	Movement of solvent using hydrostatic pressure; requires membrane filter
Active	
Active transport	Movement of ions/molecules against a concentration gradient; requires carrier molecule and ATP
Phagocytosis	Ingestion of solid particles by creating vesicles; requires ATP
Pinocytosis	Ingestion of fluid by creating vesicles; requires ATP
Exocytosis	Secretion of cellular products by creating vesicles, then liberating contents to outside of cell; requires ATP

ATP = adenosine triphosphate.

Diffusion

Simple diffusion (dif-YOO-zhun) is the movement of atoms, ions, or molecules from a region of high concentration to a region of low concentration. Odors permeate a room because the aromatic molecules diffuse through the air. A crystal of dye will color a whole beaker of water because the dye particles diffuse from the region of high concentration in the dye crystal to regions of low concentration in the water (Fig. 3–5).

Atoms, ions, and molecules are constantly moving at high speed. Each particle moves in a straight line until it collides with another particle or the edge of the container; then it changes directions until it hits another particle. Such random motion accounts for the mixing that occurs when two different substances are put together. Eventually the particles will be evenly distributed and **equilibrium** will exist. This does not mean that the particles cease their motion but as soon as a particle moves in one direction, others move in the opposite direction so that the concentration does not change.

If two solutions have different concentrations, then a **concentration gradient** exists between them. The gradient is the difference in the solute concentrations. When particles move from an area of high concentration to an area of low concentration they move down, or with, a concentration gradient. Generally, diffusion rates are faster if the gradients are steeper (there is a greater difference in concentrations). Anything that increases the speed of movement, such as heat or pressure, will also increase the rate of diffusion.

> Simple diffusion is the movement of particles (solutes) from a region of higher solute concentration to a region of lower solute concentration.

In the examples of diffusion cited, there has been no membrane involved. Diffusion can occur across a membrane as long as the membrane is permeable to the substances involved. Most physiologic examples involve a selectively permeable membrane. Many substances move through the extracellular and intracellular fluids of the body by diffusion. Because movement is down a concentration gradient and no cellular energy is involved, it is a form of passive transport or movement. Lipid-soluble substances and particles small enough to pass through protein membrane channels diffuse through the cell membrane. Oxygen and carbon dioxide are both lipid soluble so they are able to diffuse through the cell membrane. In this way, the gases are exchanged between the air and the blood in the lungs and between the blood and the cells of the various tissues (Fig. 3–6).

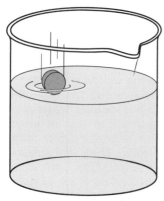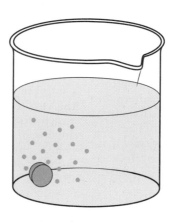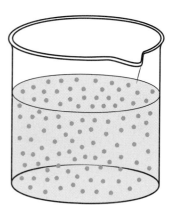

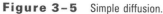

Figure 3–5 Simple diffusion.

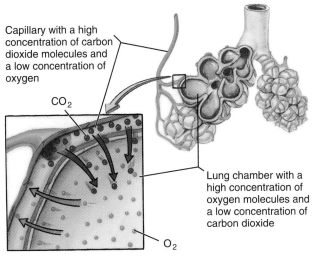

Capillary with a high concentration of carbon dioxide molecules and a low concentration of oxygen

CO_2

O_2

Lung chamber with a high concentration of oxygen molecules and a low concentration of carbon dioxide

Figure 3–6 Diffusion of oxygen and carbon dioxide in the lungs.

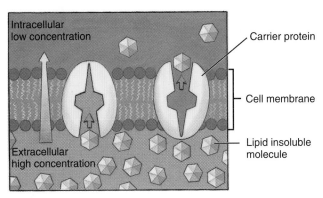

Intracellular low concentration

Carrier protein

Cell membrane

Lipid insoluble molecule

Extracellular high concentration

Figure 3–7 Facilitated diffusion.

Simple diffusion may take place through a selectively permeable membrane.

Normal functioning kidneys remove waste products from the blood. When the kidneys do not function properly, waste molecules can be removed from the blood artificially by a process called dialysis. Dialysis is a form of diffusion in which the size of the pores in a selectively permeable membrane separates smaller solute particles from larger solutes. In kidney dialysis small waste molecules pass through the membrane and are removed from the blood. The protein molecules, which are needed in the blood are too large to pass through the pores and thus are retained.

Facilitated diffusion is a special type of diffusion that involves a carrier molecule. The movement of glucose from the blood into cells is an example. Most sugar molecules, including glucose, are not soluble in lipids and are too large to pass through the membrane pores or channels. Yet they are able to diffuse across the membrane. A glucose molecule combines with a special protein carrier molecule in the cell membrane. This combination is soluble in lipid so it diffuses across the membrane. When it reaches the inside of the cell, the glucose portion is released and the protein carrier is free to pick up another glucose and "carry" it across the membrane (Fig. 3–7). Because the solute particles move down a concentration gradient and there is no expenditure of cellular energy, it is a process of diffusion, although it is "facilitated" by a carrier molecule. Facilitated diffusion is limited by the number of carrier molecules that are present.

Facilitated diffusion requires a special carrier molecule but still goes from a region of higher concentration to a region of lower concentration.

Osmosis

In the process of diffusion just discussed, any type of particles can move. Gases move through gases, gases move through liquids, solids dissolve and move through liquids, and liquids move through liquids. A membrane may or may not be involved in simple diffusion.

Osmosis (os-MOH-sis) involves the movement of **solvent** (water) molecules through a **selectively permeable** membrane from a region of higher concentration of water molecules (where the **solute** concentration is lower) to a region of lower concentration of water molecules (where the solute concentration is higher). Figure 3–8 illustrates osmosis. When equilibrium is reached, the solutions on both sides of the membrane have the same concentration but the solution that was more concentrated at the start (had more solute) will now have a greater volume. Water molecules continue to pass through the membrane after equilibrium, but because they move in both directions at the same rate there is no change in concentration or volume.

Osmosis is the diffusion of solvent or water molecules through a selectively permeable membrane.

If a red blood cell, which contains 5 percent glucose, is placed in a container of 5 percent glucose solution, water will move in both directions at the same rate because the glucose concentrations inside and outside the cell are the same. Solutions that have the same solute concentration are **isotonic** (Fig. 3–9A).

When a red blood cell is placed in a 10 percent glucose solution, water will leave the cell (where there are more water molecules) and enter the surrounding fluid (where there are fewer water molecules). When fluid leaves the cells, they will shrink or **crenate**. The 10 percent glucose solution is **hyper-**

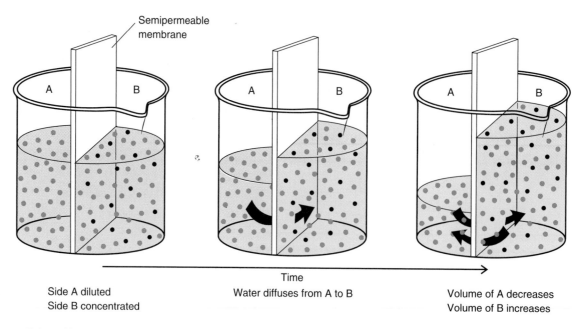

Semipermeable
membrane

Time

Side A diluted
Side B concentrated

Water diffuses from A to B

Volume of A decreases
Volume of B increases

● Solvent (water molecules)
● Solute

Figure 3–8   Osmosis.

tonic (greater solute concentration) to the cell (Fig. 3–9*B*).

Cells placed in a hypertonic solution will lose fluid because of osmosis and will shrink or crenate.

When a red blood cell is placed in distilled water, water will enter the cell because there are more water molecules outside the cell than inside. The distilled water is **hypotonic** (lower solute concentration) to the cell. As water enters the cell, it will swell, owing to the increased volume. If enough water goes into the cell, it may rupture. This is called **lysis.** When this happens to a red blood cell, it is called **hemolysis** (hee-MAHL-ih-sis) (Fig. 3–9*C*).

Cells placed in a hypotonic solution will take in water by osmosis and will swell, owing to the increased intracellular volume.

The terms *isotonic, hypotonic,* and *hypertonic* are relative. They are used to compare two solutions. A 5 percent glucose solution is hypertonic to distilled water but hypotonic to a 10 percent glucose solution.

Filtration

In diffusion and osmosis, particles, whether solute, solvent, or both, pass through a membrane by virtue of their own random movement, which is directed

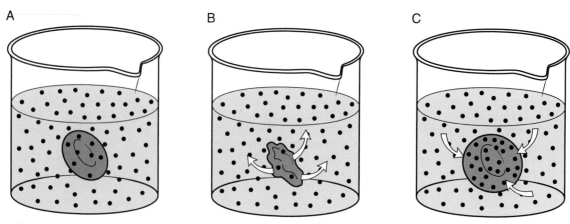

A   B   C

Figure 3–9   *A,* Isotonic solution. *B,* Hypertonic solution. *C,* Hypotonic solution.

by concentration gradients. In **filtration,** pressure pushes the particles through a membrane. Pressure gradients, rather than concentration gradients, direct the movement. Drip coffee makers use this principle. Water drips through the coffee and then the water and small particles pass through a filter. The large granules of coffee are too big to go through the pores in the filter. The size of the pores determines the size of the particles that can pass through the filter. The pressure is created by the weight of water on the paper. In the laboratory, filtration is often used to separate small solid particles from a liquid.

Contraction of the heart creates pressure in the blood. This fluid pressure or **hydrostatic pressure,** which is greater inside the blood vessels, pushes fluid, dissolved nutrients, and small ions through the capillary walls to form tissue fluid. The large protein molecules and blood cells are unable to pass through the pores in the capillary membrane. Blood is filtered through specialized membranes in the kidney as the initial step in urine formation. Water and small molecules and ions pass through the filtration membrane while blood cells and protein molecules remain in the blood.

> Filtration utilizes pressure to push substances through a membrane. The size of the pores in the membrane filter determines the size of particles that will pass through it.

Active Transport

In the transport mechanisms discussed thus far, no cellular energy has been involved and the molecules and/or ions moved from a region of high concentration to one of low concentration. **Active transport** differs from these processes in that it moves molecules and ions "uphill" against a concentration gradient and uses cellular energy in the form of ATP in the process. If ATP is not available, active transport ceases immediately. Active transport also uses a carrier molecule. Amino acids and glucose are transported from the small intestine into the blood by active transport, and all living cells show active transport of electrolytes.

As a result of active transport, some substances accumulate in significantly higher concentrations on one side of the cell membrane than on the other. Sodium ions are more concentrated outside the plasma membrane than inside the cell. Potassium is just the opposite; it is higher inside the cell. Normal passive transport, such as diffusion and osmosis, tends to equalize the concentrations on the two sides of the membrane. Active transport, in this case known as the sodium/potassium pump, moves sodium and potassium against concentration gradients so that sodium is pumped out of the cell and potassium is pumped into the cell. This keeps a high sodium concentration outside the cell and a high potassium concentration inside the cell. The process requires ATP and a protein carrier molecule.

> Active transport moves substances against a concentration gradient from a region of lower concentration to a region of higher concentration. It requires a carrier molecule and uses energy.

Endocytosis

Endocytosis (en-doh-sye-TOH-sis) refers to the formation of vesicles to transfer particles and droplets from outside to inside the cell. In this case, the material is too large to enter the cell by diffusion or active transport. The cell membrane surrounds the particle or droplet, and then that portion of the membrane pinches off to form a vesicle in the cytoplasm. The process requires energy in the form of ATP. **Phagocytosis** (fag-oh-sye-TOH-sis), which means "cell eating," involves solid material (Fig. 3–10). The cell membrane engulfs a particle to form a vesicle in the cytoplasm. Lysosomes fuse with the vesicle and the enzymes digest the particle. Certain white blood cells are called phagocytes because they engulf and destroy bacteria in this manner. Another form of endocytosis is **pinocytosis** (pin-oh-sye-TOH-sis) or "cell drinking." It differs from phagocytosis in that the vesicles that are formed are much smaller and their contents are fluids. Pinocytosis is important in cells that function in absorption.

> Phagocytosis (solids) and pinocytosis (liquids) are types of endocytosis.

Exocytosis

In certain cells, secretory products are packaged into vesicles by the Golgi apparatus and are then released from the cell by a process of **exocytosis** (eck-soh-sye-TOH-sis). The secretory vesicle moves to the cell membrane, where the vesicle membrane fuses with the cell membrane and the contents are discharged to the outside of the cell (Fig. 3–11). Secretion of digestive enzymes from the pancreas and secretion of milk from the mammary glands are examples of exocytosis. Exocytosis and endocytosis are similar except they work in opposite directions. They are both active processes that require cellular

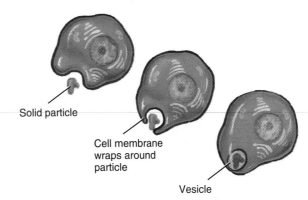

Solid particle

Cell membrane wraps around particle

Vesicle

Figure 3–10 Phagocytosis.

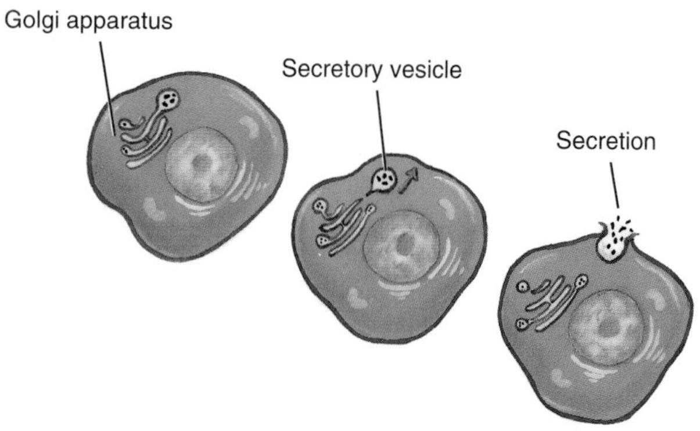

Golgi apparatus

Secretory vesicle

Secretion

Figure 3–11 Exocytosis.

energy (ATP). Exocytosis releases substances to the outside of the cell, and endocytosis brings substances to the inside of the cell.

Secretory vesicles are moved from the inside to the outside of the cell by exocytosis.

Cell Division

Cell division is the process by which new cells are formed for growth, repair, and replacement in the body. This process includes division of the nuclear material and division of the cytoplasm. Periods of growth and repair are special periods in the life of an individual when it is obvious that new cells are needed either to increase the number of cells or to repair tissues after an injury. General maintenance and replacement needs of the body may not be quite as obvious. More than 2 million red blood cells are worn out and replaced in the body every

second of every day. Skin cells are continually sloughed off the body's surface and must be replaced. The lining of the stomach is replaced every few days. All cells in the body (somatic cells), except those that give rise to the eggs and sperm (gametes), reproduce by **mitosis** (mye-TOH-sis). Egg and sperm cells are produced by a special type of nuclear division called **meiosis** (mye-OH-sis) in which the number of chromosomes is halved. Division of the cytoplasm is called **cytokinesis.**

New cells are continually needed for growth, repair, and replacement.

Mitosis

All somatic cells reproduce by mitosis, in which a single cell divides to form two new "daughter cells," each identical to the parent cell. Humans have 23 pairs of, or 46, chromosomes in their cells. Each new cell that forms must also have 23 pairs or 46 chromosomes. For this to occur, events must proceed in an organized manner, chromosome material must replicate exactly, and then the chromosomes must separate precisely so that each new cell gets a set that is a carbon copy of the parent cell's. For descriptive purposes it is convenient to divide the events of mitosis into stages, as illustrated in Figure 3–12. It is important to remember that the process is a continual one and that there are no starting and stopping points along the way.

Somatic cells reproduce by mitosis, which results in two cells identical to the one parent cell.

The period between active cell divisions is called **interphase.** This is a time of growth and metabolism

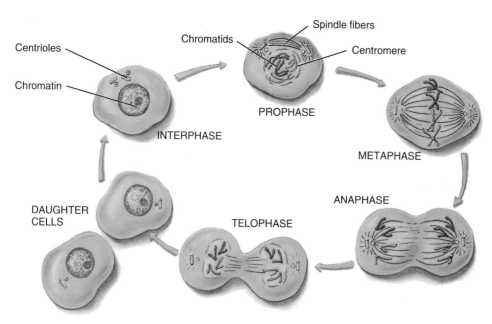

Centrioles

Chromatin

Chromatids

Spindle fibers

Centromere

INTERPHASE

PROPHASE

METAPHASE

ANAPHASE

TELOPHASE

DAUGHTER CELLS

Figure 3–12 Mitosis.

and is usually the longest period of the cell cycle. In cells that are rapidly dividing it may last for as little as a few hours, but in other cells it may take days, weeks, or even months. Some highly specialized cells, such as nerve and muscle, may never divide and spend their whole life in interphase.

During interphase, the cell increases in size and synthesizes an exact copy of the DNA in its nucleus so that when the cell begins to divide it has identical sets of genetic information. Also just before division, the cell synthesizes an additional pair of centrioles and some new mitochondria. In addition to these synthetic activities that are a preparation for division, normal cellular function takes place during interphase.

> Interphase is the period between successive cell divisions. It is the longest part of the cell cycle.

After interphase, the cell begins mitosis. The first stage of mitosis is **prophase.** During prophase, the chromatin shortens, thickens, and becomes tightly coiled to form chromosomes. As a result of the replication in interphase, each chromosome has two identical parts, called **chromatids,** that are joined by a special region on each called the **centromere.** The two pairs of centrioles separate and go to opposite ends of the cytoplasm. Microtubules called **spindle fibers** form and extend from the centromeres to the centrioles. The nucleolus and nuclear membrane disappear during the latter part of prophase.

Prophase ends when the nuclear membrane disintegrates, and this signals the beginning of the next stage, **metaphase.** The chromosomes align themselves along the center of the cell during metaphase. This is the time when the chromosomes are most clearly visible and distinguishable.

The third stage of mitosis is **anaphase.** After the chromosomes are aligned along the center of the cell, the centromeres separate so that each chromatid now becomes a chromosome. At this time, there are actually two sets of chromosomes in the cell. The two chromatids (now chromosomes) from each pair migrate to the centrioles at opposite ends of the cell. The microtubules that are attached to the centrioles and centromeres shorten and pull the chromosomes toward the centrioles. At the end of anaphase, the cytoplasm begins to divide.

The final stage of mitosis is **telophase.** This stage is almost the reverse of prophase. After the chromosomes reach the centrioles at the ends of the cell, a new nuclear membrane forms around them. The spindle fibers disappear. The chromosomes start to uncoil to become long, slender strands of chromatin, and nucleoli appear in the newly formed nucleus. During this time, the cell membrane constricts in the middle to divide the cytoplasm and organelles into two parts that are approximately equal. Division of the cytoplasm is called **cytokinesis** (sye-toh-kih-NEE-sis). Except for size, the two newly formed daughter cells are exact copies of the parent cell.

Table 3–3	Summary of Mitotic Events
Stage	**Events**
Interphase	DNA, mitochondria, and centrioles replicate
Prophase	Chromatin shortens and thickens to become chromosomes; centrioles move to opposite ends of the cell; spindle fibers form; nucleolus and nuclear membrane disappear
Metaphase	Chromosomes align along center of cell
Anaphase	Centromeres separate and spindle fibers shorten to pull chromatids (chromosomes) toward centrioles at opposite ends of cell
Telophase	Chromosomes uncoil to become long filaments of chromatin; nuclear membrane and nucleolus reappear; cytokinesis occurs; daughter cells form and enter interphase

The two daughter cells now become interphase cells to carry out designated cellular functions and to undergo mitosis as necessary. The events of mitosis are summarized in Table 3–3.

> The successive stages of mitosis are prophase, metaphase, anaphase, and telophase. Cytokinesis, division of the cytoplasm, occurs during telophase.

Meiosis

Meiosis is a special type of cell division that occurs in the production of the gametes, or eggs and sperm. These cells have only 23 chromosomes, one-half the number found in somatic cells, so that when fertilization takes place, the resulting cell will again have 46 chromosomes, 23 from the egg and 23 from the sperm. Meiosis is discussed in greater detail in Chapter 19. In brief, meiosis consists of two divisions but DNA is replicated only once. The result is four cells, but each one has only 23 chromosomes. Table 3–4 and Figure 3–13 compare mitosis and meiosis.

Table 3–4	Comparison of Mitosis and Meiosis	
Feature	**Mitosis**	**Meiosis**
Type of cell where it occurs	Somatic cells	Reproductive cells
Chromosomes in parent cell	46 (23 pairs)	46 (23 pairs)
Chromosome replication	Yes—once	Yes—once
Number of cytoplasmic divisions	1	2
Number of cells formed	2	4
Number of chromosomes in each new cell formed	46 (23 pairs)	23

MITOSIS   MEIOSIS

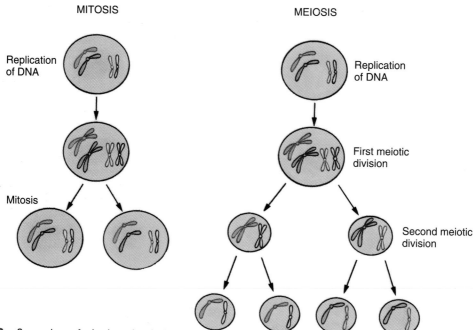

Replication of DNA

Replication of DNA

First meiotic division

Mitosis

Second meiotic division

Figure 3–13 Comparison of mitosis and meiosis.

Eggs and sperm are produced by meiosis. In this process, a single cell produces four cells, each with one-half the number of chromosomes as the parent cell.

DNA Replication and Protein Synthesis

Proteins that are synthesized in the cytoplasm function as structural materials, enzymes that regulate chemical reactions, hormones, and other vital substances. Because DNA in the nucleus directs the synthesis of the proteins in the cytoplasm, it ultimately determines the structural and functional characteristics of an individual. Whether a person has blue or brown eyes, brown or blond hair, or light or dark skin is determined by the types of proteins synthesized in response to the genetic information contained in the DNA in the nucleus. The portion of a DNA molecule that contains the genetic information for making one particular protein molecule is called a **gene.** If a cell produced for replacement or repair is to function exactly as its predecessor, then it must have the same genes, a carbon copy of the DNA. This is the purpose of DNA replication in cell division.

DNA in the nucleus directs protein synthesis in the cytoplasm. A gene is the portion of a DNA molecule that controls the synthesis of one specific protein molecule.

DNA Replication

As described in Chapter 2, DNA consists of two long chains of nucleotides that are loosely held to-

gether by hydrogen bonds and then are twisted to form a double helix. Each nucleotide in the chains has a phosphate, a sugar called deoxyribose, and a nitrogenous base. The bases are adenine, thymine, cytosine, and guanine. Uncoiled, the DNA looks something like a ladder. The sugar and phosphate alternate to form the uprights of the ladder. The bases from each chain project toward each other and are held together by hydrogen bonds to form the crossbars or rungs of the ladder (Fig. 3–14). There is a specific pattern to the combination of bases. Adenine is always opposite thymine, and cytosine always pairs with guanine.

When DNA replicates during interphase before starting mitosis, the DNA molecule uncoils, the hydrogen bonds between the complementary base pairs break, and the two strands separate. Enzymes then catalyze the formation of new complementary strands from nucleotides that are present in the nucleoplasm. Because adenine always pairs with thymine, and guanine always pairs with cytosine, the new complementary strands are identical to the previous ones (Fig. 3–15). As a result of this process, two identical molecules of DNA are produced, each with one strand from the old molecule and one new strand. The cell is now ready to begin mitosis.

The specific pairing of nitrogenous bases in DNA results in the formation of new but identical complementary strands during DNA replication.

Role of DNA and RNA in Protein Synthesis

The genetic information, contained in the DNA, that controls protein synthesis is located in the nucleus.

S=Deoxyribose sugar
P=Phosphate group

Bases:
T=Thymine
A=Adenine
G=Guanine
C=Cytosine

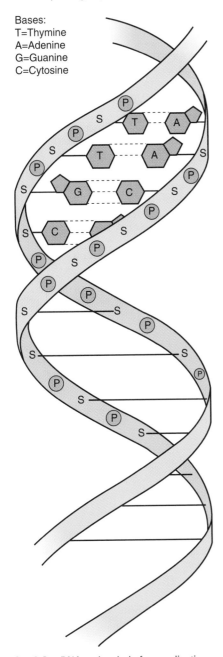

Figure 3–14 DNA molecule before replication.

Messenger RNA carries the genetic information from the DNA in the nucleus to the sites of protein synthesis in the cytoplasm.

The first step in protein synthesis is to transfer the genetic information from DNA to mRNA. This process is called **transcription** and is illustrated in Figure 3–16. First, the DNA strands uncoil and separate; then the RNA nucleotides pair with the complementary DNA nucleotides on the coding strand of DNA. Because there is no thymine in RNA, adenine on DNA will pair with uracil on RNA. Enzymes catalyze the formation of chemical bonds between the RNA nucleotides to form a molecule of mRNA. The sequence of bases on the mRNA is determined by the sequence on DNA because of the complementary base pairing. If the sequence on the

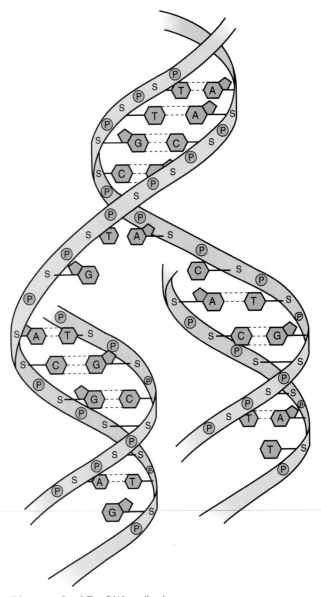

Figure 3–15 DNA replication.

The process of protein synthesis takes place in the cytoplasm outside the nucleus. Because the DNA is unable to leave the nucleus there must be a "messenger" molecule that can take the information from the DNA to the cytoplasm. This molecule is **messenger RNA** (mRNA). The structure of RNA is discussed in Chapter 2. Briefly, RNA is a single chain of nucleotides, the sugar is ribose, and uracil is substituted for thymine in the bases.

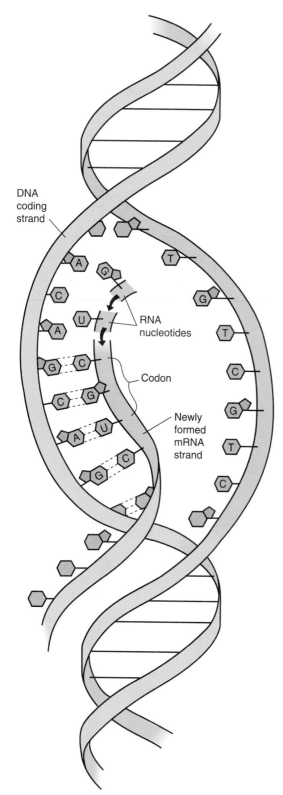

DNA coding strand

RNA nucleotides

Codon

Newly formed mRNA strand

Figure 3–16   Synthesis of mRNA—transcription.

come associated with ribosomes in the cytoplasm and to act as templates for protein synthesis. The genetic information is carried in groups of three nucleotides called **codons.** Each codon, a sequence of three bases, on mRNA codes for a specific amino acid. The three codons in the above example are GAA, UGG, and GCA. These code for glutamic acid, tryptophan, and alanine, respectively. There are also instruction codons that indicate where protein synthesis is to start and where it is to stop. Some examples of mRNA codons are listed in Table 3–5.

> During the process of transcription, the genetic code is transferred from DNA to mRNA. A sequence of three nucleotide bases on mRNA represents a codon that codes for a specific amino acid.

There are two additional types of RNA in the cytoplasm, **ribosomal RNA** (rRNA) and **transfer RNA** (tRNA). These are also produced in the nucleus and then move to the cytoplasm. The rRNA, as its name implies, is part of the ribosomes. One portion of tRNA consists of three nucleotides, called an **anticodon.** Another portion attaches to an amino acid. There are specific tRNA nucleotide base sequences for each of the 20 amino acids (see Table 3–5).

> Anticodons on tRNA have nitrogenous bases that are complementary to the codons on mRNA.

In the cytoplasm, a ribosome, which coordinates the activities of the codons and anticodons, attaches to mRNA near a codon. A tRNA with an anticodon complementary to the mRNA codon brings its specific amino acid into place. The ribosome moves along the mRNA, codon by codon, which allows complementary tRNA anti-codons to put their respective amino acids in place. Enzymes catalyze the formation of peptide bonds between the amino acids. Once a tRNA has released its amino acid, it is free to pick up another amino acid of the same kind and "transfer" it to the amino acid chain. The process is repeated again and again, until the amino acid sequence for the protein is completed. The process of creating a protein in response to the codons on mRNA is called **translation,** which is illustrated in Figure 3–17.

> Each tRNA carries a specific amino acid to the developing molecule. The amino acid sequence is determined by the complementary base pairs on the mRNA and tRNA. This process of creating a protein in response to mRNA codons is called translation.

coding strand of DNA is CTTACCCGT, then the sequence on mRNA will be GAAUGGGCA. After it is formed, the mRNA molecules leave the nucleus through the pores in the nuclear membrane to be-

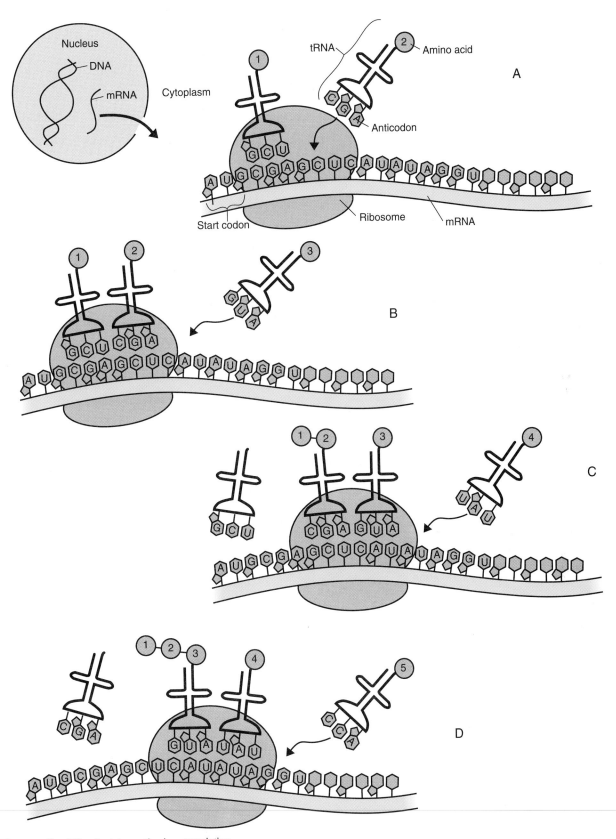

Figure 3-17   Protein synthesis—translation.

Table 3–5 Examples of Nucleotide Sequences of the Genetic Code			
Amino Acid	**DNA Triplet**	**mRNA Codon**	**tRNA Anticodon**
Alanine	CGA, CGG, CGT, CGC	GCU, GCC, GCA, GCG	CGA, CGG, CGU, CGC
Cysteine	ACA, ACG	UGU, UGC	ACA, ACG
Glutamic acid	CTT, CTC	GAA, GAG	CUU, CUC
Histidine	GTA, GTG	CAU, CAC	GUA, GUG
Lysine	TTT, TTC	AAA, AAG	UUU, UUC
Tryptophan	ACC	UGG	ACC
Stop synthesis	ATT, ATC, ACT	UAA, UAG, UGA	AUU, AUC, ACU

☑ QuickCheck

● What happens to cells when they are placed in a hypertonic solution?

● Phagocytic cells are likely to have a large quantity of which organelle?

● During which stage of mitosis does cytokinesis occur?

Genetic disorders are pathologic conditions caused by mistakes, or mutations, in a cell's genetic code. Mutations may occur naturally, or they may be induced by mutagens such as radiation and certain chemicals. If the mutations occur in the gametes, the faulty code is passed from one generation to the next. Errors in the genes (DNA) cause the production of abnormal proteins, which result in abnormal cellular function. For example, in sickle cell anemia, a genetic blood disorder, red blood cells have abnormal hemoglobin because there is an "error" in the gene that directs hemoglobin synthesis.

● FOCUS ON AGING

Many of the cellular effects of aging are attributed to damage to DNA. Normal cells have built-in mechanisms to repair minor DNA damage, but this ability appears to diminish in aging cells. Because DNA directs protein synthesis, DNA damage is reflected in changes in the membranes and enzymes that are made by the cell. The cell membrane exhibits changes in its transport of ions and nutrients. Membrane-bound organelles, such as mitochondria and lysosomes, are present in reduced numbers. In addition, they are less effective, presumably because of changes in their membranes and in the enzymes that regulate their reactions.

Cells?

Abnormal Cell Division—Cancer

The word **cancer** brings emotions of fear and despair, along with visions of pain and death, to almost everyone. Nearly one third of all Americans will develop some form of cancer in their lifetime. It may occur in any body tissue and at any age, although it is found most frequently in older people. Treatment is expensive and contributes to the overall rising cost of health care in this country. Although half of all patients who develop cancer are cured of their disease, at least temporarily, it currently accounts for one fifth of all deaths in the United States.

Normally, body cells divide at a rate required to replace the dying ones. Normal cells are subject to control mechanisms that prevent overpopulation and competition for nutrients and space. Occasionally, a series of events occurs that alters some cells so they lack the control mechanisms that tell them when to stop dividing. When the cells do not stop reproducing, they form an abnormal growth called a **tumor,** or **neoplasm.**

Neoplasms are classified as either benign or malignant. A **benign neoplasm** consists of highly organized cells that closely resemble normal tissue. It grows slowly, is often encapsulated, and does not infiltrate surrounding tissue or spread beyond its original site. Benign neoplasms seldom kill their hosts, but they may be surgically removed if they interfere with normal body function. In contrast, a **malignant neoplasm,** or cancer, consists of unorganized and immature cells that are incapable of normal function. The malignant cells tend to multiply rapidly and invade the surrounding tissues. Cancerous cells from a malignant neoplasm may detach themselves from the tumor site, travel in the bloodstream or lymphatic system to another site, and establish a new tumor. This secondary growth is called a **metastasis.** This is probably the most devastating property of malignant cells.

Before cancer can start, a precise sequence of events must occur that transforms a normal cell into a cancerous one. The process is not completely understood, but the key to malignant transformation lies in the genetic material (DNA) of the cell. Certain chemicals and radiation can be **carcinogenic** (cancer-causing) and serve as triggers. Examples of chemical carcinogens include hydrocarbons found in cigarette tar and radon gas from the earth. Radiation and some viruses also have been implicated in the development of cancer.

Most chemical carcinogens never gain entry into our cells because of alert defense mechanisms that destroy invaders. Those that do enter the cells are usually inactivated by lysosomes and peroxisomes. Even with these protective mechanisms, some of the carcinogens may still enter the nucleus and bind with DNA. Cancer is still unlikely, however, because the body has a built-in DNA repair system. This system detects the altered DNA, removes it in a type of molecular surgery, and prompts the synthesis of a new normal DNA segment. If the repair is faulty or if mitosis occurs before DNA is repaired, the altered segment of DNA is copied abnormally and the daughter cells receive a mutated gene.

In most cases the mutated gene destroys only a single cell and cancer still does not develop. When the mutation involves a critical region of DNA, one that removes or disables the cell's control over mitosis, the first step toward cancer initiation is completed. The body still attempts to destroy these abnormal cells, but in some cases, the abnormal cells reproduce more rapidly than they can be destroyed and cancer develops.

With radiation and viruses, the sequence of events before interaction with DNA is slightly different, but the effect is the same—altered DNA. Whether cancer develops depends on the body's ability to "detoxify" the cancer-causing agent and repair the DNA damage.

Exposure to ultraviolet radiation in sunlight is implicated in certain types of skin cancer. Moderation in sun exposure and the use of sunscreening products are advisable, especially in people with light hair and fair complexion. Sensible dietary guidelines to reduce cancer risk include decreasing the amount of fat and increasing the amount of fiber in the diet, avoiding extreme obesity, and avoiding excessive alcohol ingestion. Worldwide, one third of all cancers result from the use of cigarettes and other tobacco products. In the United States, recent estimates implicate cigarette smoking as a cause of 85 percent of all lung cancers and 30 percent of all cancer deaths. Data indicate that the single most effective way to prevent cancer and to decrease cancer mortality is to avoid tobacco products.

CHAPTER QUIZ

RECALL

Match the definitions on the left with the appropriate term on the right.

1. Attracts water

2. Inside the cell

3. Small granules of RNA in cytoplasm

4. Cellular ingestion of solid particles

5. Diffusion of water through a selectively permeable membrane

6. Greater solute concentration

7. Division of cytoplasm

8. Transfer of genetic information from DNA to mRNA

9. Sequence of three bases on mRNA

10. Results in eggs and sperm

A. Codon

B. Cytokinesis

C. Hydrophilic

D. Hypertonic

E. Intracellular

F. Meiosis

G. Osmosis

H. Phagocytosis

I. Ribosomes

J. Transcription

THOUGHT

1. The plasma membrane is composed primarily of
   a. phospholipid and cholesterol
   b. cholesterol and glycoprotein
   c. phospholipid and protein
   d. protein and carbohydrate

2. Which of the following organelles functions in the production of ATP?
   a. Golgi apparatus
   b. endoplasmic reticulum
   c. centrioles
   d. mitochondria

3. A cell is placed in a hypotonic solution. What will happen?
   a. water will enter the cell
   b. the cell will shrink

   c. nothing, because the plasma membrane is impermeable to water
   d. solute particles will leave the cell

4. The stage of mitosis in which cytokinesis occurs is
   a. prophase
   b. telophase
   c. anaphase
   d. metaphase

5. In DNA replication
   a. adenine pairs with guanine
   b. cytosine pairs with thymine
   c. cytosine pairs with guanine
   d. adenine pairs with uracil

APPLICATION

A given cell is active in the synthesis of secretory proteins. Name three organelles that are likely to be abundant in this cell.

Tissues and Membranes

Outline/Objectives

Body Tissues 60

- List the four main types of tissues found in the body.
- Describe the various types of epithelial tissues in terms of structure, location, and function.
- Describe the classification of glandular epithelium according to structure and method of secretion; give an example of each type.
- Describe the general characteristics of connective tissues.
- Name three types of connective tissue cells and state the function of each one.
- Describe the features and location of the various types of connective tissue.
- Distinguish between skeletal muscle, smooth muscle, and cardiac muscle in terms of structure, location, and control.
- Name two categories of cells in nerve tissue and state their general functions.

Body Membranes 70

- Describe four types of membranes and specify the location and function of each.

Key Terms

Chondrocyte
Collagenous fibers
Elastic fibers
Fibroblast
Histology
Macrophage
Mast cell
Neuroglia
Neuron
Osteocyte
Tissue

Building Vocabulary

WORD PART	MEANING
a-	without, lacking
aden-	gland
adip-	fat
-blast	to form, sprout
chrondr-	cartilage
erythr-	red
fibro-	fiber
glia-	glue
hist-	tissue
leuk-	white
macro-	large
multi-	many
neur-	nerve
-oma	tumor, swelling, mass
os-	bone
pseudo-	false
squam-	flattened, scale
strat-	layer
thromb-	clot
vas-	vessel

tissue is a group of cells that have similar structure and that function together as a unit. The microscopic study of tissues is called **histology** (hiss-TAHL-oh-jee). A nonliving material, called the intercellular matrix, fills the spaces between the cells. This may be abundant in some tissues and minimal in others. The intercellular matrix may contain special substances such as salts and fibers that are unique to a specific tissue and give that tissue distinctive characteristics.

Body Tissues

There are four main tissue types in the body: epithelial, connective, muscle, and nervous. Each is designed for specific functions.

> A tissue is a group of similar cells collected together by an intercellular matrix.

Epithelial Tissue

Epithelial (ep-ih-THEE-lee-al) **tissues** are widespread throughout the body. They form the covering of all body surfaces, line body cavities and hollow organs, and are the major tissue in glands. They perform a variety of functions that include protection, secretion, absorption, excretion, filtration, diffusion, and sensory reception.

> Epithelial tissues function in protection, secretion, absorption, excretion, filtration, diffusion, and sensory reception.

The cells in epithelial tissue are tightly packed with very little intercellular matrix. Because the tissues form coverings and linings, the cells have one free surface that is not in contact with other cells. Opposite the free surface, the cells are attached to underlying connective tissue by a noncellular **basement membrane.** This membrane is a mixture of carbohydrates and proteins secreted by the epithelial and connective tissue cells. Because epithelial tissues are typically **avascular,** they must receive their nutrients and oxygen supply by diffusion from the blood vessels in the underlying tissues. Another characteristic of epithelial tissues is that they regenerate, or reproduce, quickly. For example, the cells of the skin and stomach are continually damaged and replaced and skin abrasions heal quite rapidly.

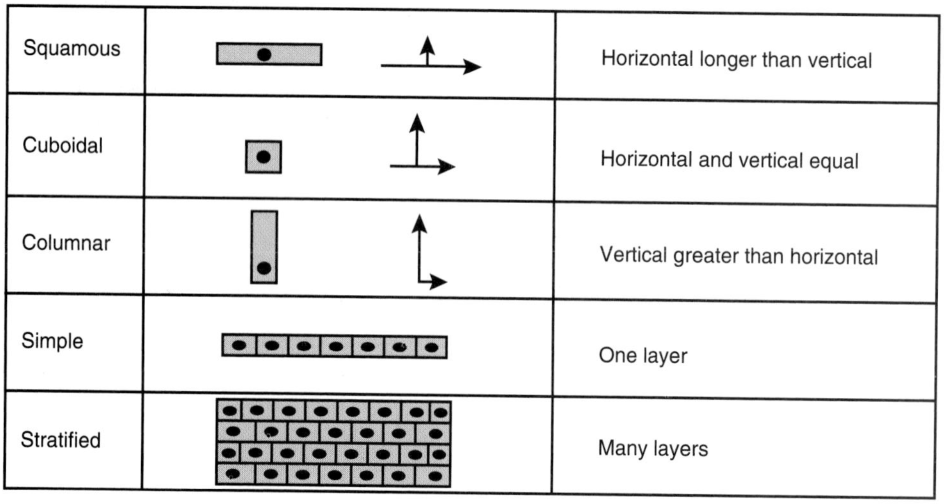

Squamous		Horizontal longer than vertical
Cuboidal		Horizontal and vertical equal
Columnar		Vertical greater than horizontal
Simple		One layer
Stratified		Many layers

Figure 4–1 Classification of epithelium.

CLINICAL TERMS

Adhesion (add-HEE-shun) Abnormal joining of tissues by fibrous scar tissue
Biopsy (BYE-ahp-see) Removal and microscopic examination of body tissue
Carcinoma (kar-sih-NOH-mah) A malignant growth derived from epithelial cells
Histology (hiss-TAHL-oh-jee) Branch of microscopic anatomy that studies tissues

Marfan's syndrome (mahr-FAHNZ SIN-drohm) A congenital disorder of connective tissue characterized by abnormal length of the extremities and cardiovascular abnormalities
Pathology (pah-THAHL-oh-jee) Branch of medicine that studies the essential nature of disease, especially the structural and functional changes in tissues

Sarcoma (sar-KOH-mah) A malignant growth derived from connective tissue cells
Scurvy (SKUR-vee) A condition caused by a deficiency of vitamin C in the diet, which results in abnormal collagen synthesis

Table 4-1   Summary of Epithelial Tissues

Type	Description	Location
Simple squamous	Single layer of thin, flat cells	Alveoli of the lungs, capillary walls, kidneys
Simple cuboidal	Single layer of cuboidal cells	Ovary, thyroid gland, kidney tubules, pancreas, salivary glands
Simple columnar	Single layer of tall cells; often contains goblet cells	Stomach, intestines
Pseudostratified columnar	Single layer of uneven columnar cells; often contains cilia and goblet cells	Respiratory tract, tubes of reproductive system
Stratified squamous	Several layers with flat cells at the free surface	Skin, mouth, vagina, anus
Transitional	Specialized for stretching; several layers that decrease in number and cells that become thinner when distended	Urinary bladder

> Epithelial tissues consist of tightly packed cells with little intercellular matrix, have one free surface, are avascular, and reproduce readily.

> Epithelial cells may be squamous, cuboidal, or columnar in shape and may be arranged in single or multiple layers.

> Carcinomas are solid cancerous tumors that are derived from epithelial tissue. Approximately 85 percent of all malignant neoplasms are carcinomas.

Epithelia are classified according to cell shape and the number of layers in the tissue (Fig. 4–1). Classified according to shape, the cells are squamous, cuboidal, or columnar, and the shape of the nucleus corresponds to the cell shape. **Squamous** cells are flat and the nuclei are usually broad and thin. **Cuboidal** cells are cubelike, as tall as they are wide, and the nuclei are spherical and centrally located. **Columnar** cells are tall and narrow like columns, and the nuclei are usually in the lower portion of the cell near the basement membrane. According to the number of layers, epithelia are **simple** if they have only one layer of cells and **stratified** if they have multiple layers. Stratified epithelia are named according to the type of cells at the free surface of the tissue. Epithelial tissues are summarized in Table 4–1.

Simple Squamous Epithelium

Simple squamous epithelium (Fig. 4–2) consists of a single layer of thin, flat cells that fit closely together with very little intercellular matrix. Because it is so thin, simple squamous epithelium is well suited for areas in which diffusion and filtration take place. The alveoli or air sacs of the lungs, where diffusion of oxygen and carbon dioxide gases occurs, are made of simple squamous epithelium. This tissue is also found in the kidney, where the blood is filtered. Capillary walls, where oxygen and carbon dioxide diffuse between the blood and tissues, are made of simple squamous epithelium. Because it is so thin and delicate, this tissue is damaged easily and offers very little protective function.

> The single layer of flat cells in simple squamous epithelium makes it well suited for diffusion and filtration.

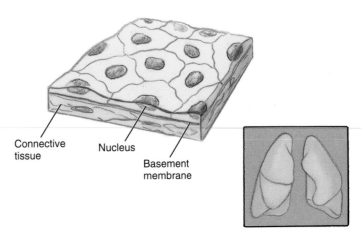

Connective tissue   Nucleus   Basement membrane

Figure 4-2   Simple squamous epithelium.

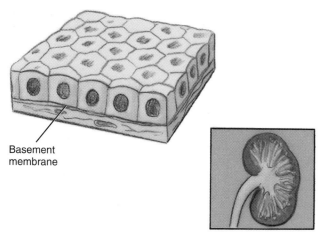

Basement
membrane

Figure 4-3 Simple cuboidal epithelium.

Simple Cuboidal Epithelium

Simple cuboidal epithelium (Fig. 4–3) consists of a single layer of cube-shaped cells. These cells have more volume than squamous cells and also have more organelles. Simple cuboidal epithelium is found as a covering of the ovary, lining the kidney tubules, and in many glands such as the thyroid, pancreas, and salivary glands. In the kidney tubules, the tissue functions in absorption and secretion. In glands, simple cuboidal cells form the secretory portions and the ducts that deliver the products to their destination.

> Simple cuboidal epithelium is found in glandular tissue and in the kidney tubules.

Simple Columnar Epithelium

A single layer of cells that are taller than they are wide makes up **simple columnar epithelium** (Fig. 4–4). The nuclei are in the bottom portion of the cell near the basement membrane. Simple columnar epi-

thelium is found lining the stomach and intestines, where it secretes digestive enzymes and absorbs nutrients. Because the cells are taller (or thicker) than either squamous or cuboidal cells, this tissue offers some protection to underlying tissues.

> Simple columnar epithelium lines the stomach and intestines.

In regions where absorption is of primary importance, such as in parts of the digestive tract, the cell membrane on the free surface has numerous small projections called **microvilli.** Microvilli increase the surface area that is available for absorption of nutrients. **Goblet cells** are frequently interspersed among the simple columnar cells. Goblet cells are flask- or goblet-shaped cells that secrete mucus onto the free surface of the tissue. **Cilia** may be present to move secretions along the surface.

> Microvilli, goblet cells, and cilia are frequently found in simple columnar epithelium.

Pseudostratified Columnar Epithelium

Pseudostratified columnar epithelium (Fig. 4–5) appears to have multiple layers (stratified) but it really does not. This is because the cells are not all the same height. Some cells are short and some are tall, and the nuclei are at different levels. Close examination reveals that all the cells are attached to the basement membrane but that not all cells reach the free surface of the tissue. Cilia and goblet cells are often associated with pseudostratified columnar epithelium. This tissue lines portions of the respiratory tract in which the mucus, produced by the goblet cells, traps dust particles and is then moved upward by the cilia. Pseudostratified columnar epithelium also lines some of the tubes of the male reproductive system. Here the cilia help propel the sperm from one region to another.

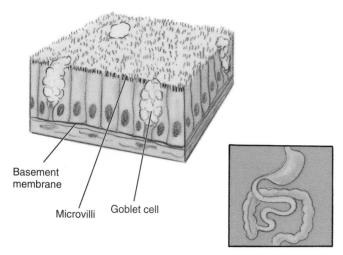

Basement
membrane

Microvilli Goblet cell

Figure 4-4 Simple columnar epithelium.

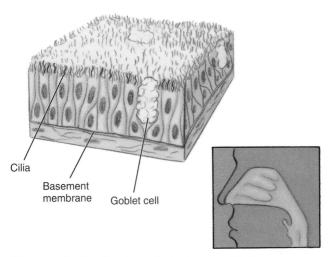

Figure 4–5 Pseudostratified columnar epithelium.

> Pseudostratified columnar epithelium lines portions of the respiratory tract and some of the tubes of the male reproductive tract. It usually has cilia and/or goblet cells.

Stratified Squamous Epithelium

Stratified squamous epithelium, the most widespread stratified epithelium, is thick because it consists of many layers of cells (Fig. 4–6). Because stratified epithelia are named according to the shape of the surface cells, it follows that the cells on the surface are flat. The cells on the bottom layer, next to the basement membrane, are usually cuboidal or columnar, and these are the cells that undergo mitosis. As the cells are pushed toward the surface, they become thinner, so the surface cells are squamous.

As the cells are pushed farther away from the basement membrane, it is more difficult for them to receive oxygen and nutrients from underlying connective tissue and the cells die. As cells on the surface are damaged and die, they are sloughed off and replaced by cells from the deeper layers. Because this tissue is thick, it is found in areas in which protection is a primary function. Stratified squamous epithelium forms the outer layer of the skin and extends a short distance into every body opening that is continuous with the skin.

> Protection is the primary function of stratified squamous epithelium because it is thicker than other epithelial tissues.

Transitional Epithelium

Transitional epithelium (Fig. 4–7) is a specialized type of tissue that has several layers but can be stretched in response to tension. The lining of the urinary bladder is a good example of this type of tissue. When the bladder is empty and contracted, the epithelial lining has several layers of cuboidal cells. As the bladder fills and is distended or stretched, the cells become thinner and the number of layers decreases.

> Transitional epithelium can be distended or stretched. The cells change shape when they are stretched, so this epithelium is called transitional.

Glandular Epithelium

Glandular epithelium consists of cells that are specialized to produce and secrete substances. It normally lies deep to the epithelia that cover and line parts of the body. If the gland secretes its product onto a free surface via a duct, it is called an **exocrine gland.** If the gland secretes its product directly

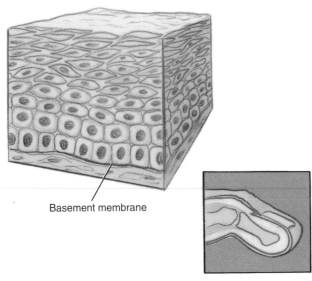

Figure 4–6 Stratified squamous epithelium.

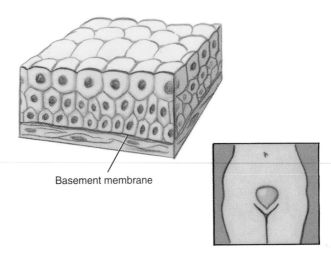

Figure 4–7 Transitional epithelium.

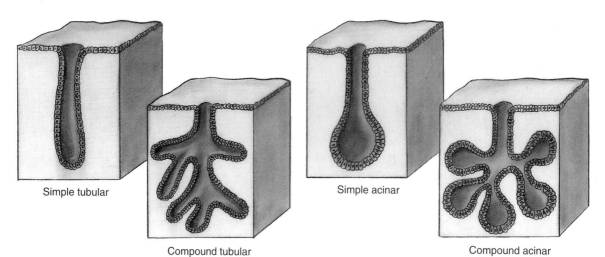

Simple tubular

Compound tubular

Simple acinar

Compound acinar

Figure 4–8 Structural classification of exocrine glands.

into the blood, it is a ductless, or **endocrine, gland.** Endocrine glands are discussed in Chapter 10.

> Glandular epithelium is specialized to produce and secrete substances. Glands may be exocrine or endocrine.

> A benign tumor of glandular epithelial cells is called an adenoma. An adenocarcinoma is a cancerous tumor arising from glandular cells.

Exocrine glands that consist of only one cell are called **unicellular** glands. Goblet cells, which produce mucus in the lining of the digestive, respiratory, urinary, and reproductive tracts, are examples of unicellular glands. Most glands are **multicellular** because they consist of many cells. These glands have a secretory portion and a duct derived from epithelium. Multicellular glands are classified according to their structure and to the type of secretion they produce.

> Goblet cells are unicellular exocrine glands. Other exocrine glands are multicellular.

A gland is **simple** if its duct has no branches. If the duct branches, then the gland is **compound.** The glands are **tubular** if the gland and duct merge with no change in diameter. Glands in which the distal part of the duct expands to form a saclike structure are called **acinar** (AS-ih-nur) or **alveolar** (al-VEE-oh-lar). The structural classification of exocrine glands is illustrated in Figure 4–8.

> Structurally, multicellular glands may be classified as simple or compound, tubular or alveolar.

Glands are also classified according to their mode of secretion (Fig. 4–9). **Merocrine** (MER-oh-krin)

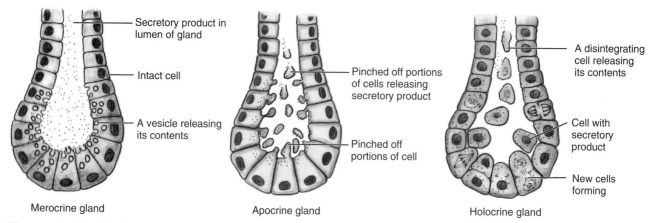

Secretory product in lumen of gland

Intact cell

A vesicle releasing its contents

Merocrine gland

Pinched off portions of cells releasing secretory product

Pinched off portions of cell

Apocrine gland

A disintegrating cell releasing its contents

Cell with secretory product

New cells forming

Holocrine gland

Figure 4–9 Classification of glands according to mode of secretion.

Table 4–2   Summary of Glandular Modes of Secretion

Secretion Mode	Description	Examples
Merocrine	Fluid released through cell membrane; no cytoplasm lost	Salivary glands, pancreatic glands, certain sweat glands
Apocrine	Portion of cell is pinched off with the secretion	Mammary glands and certain sweat glands
Holocrine	Entire cell discharged with secretion	Sebaceous glands

glands secrete a fluid that is released through the cell membrane by exocytosis with no loss of cytoplasm. Most glandular cells are of this type. Salivary glands, pancreatic glands, and certain sweat glands are merocrine glands. The cells of merocrine glands may be either **serous** cells or **mucous** cells. Serous cells secrete a thin, watery serous fluid that often contains enzymes. Mucous cells secrete a thick fluid called mucus that contains the glycoprotein mucin. In **apocrine** (AP-oh-krin) glands, the secretory product accumulates in one region of the cell and then that portion pinches off so that a small portion of the cell is lost with the secretion. The cell repairs itself and repeats the process. Examples of apocrine glands include certain sweat glands and mammary glands. In **holocrine** (HOH-loh-krin) glands, the cells become filled with the secretory product and then rupture, releasing their products. The cells have to be replaced. Sebaceous (oil) glands are holocrine glands. Modes of glandular secretion are summarized in Table 4–2.

Glands are also classified according to the amount of cytoplasm that is secreted with the product. This classification scheme divides the glands into merocrine, apocrine, and holocrine.

Connective Tissue

Connective tissues bind structures together, form a framework and support for organs and the body as a whole, store fat, transport substances, protect against disease, and help repair tissue damage. They occur throughout the body. Connective tissues are characterized by an abundance of intercellular matrix with relatively few cells. Connective tissue cells are able to reproduce but not as rapidly as epithelial cells. Most connective tissues have a good blood supply but some do not. The various types of connective tissue are summarized in Table 4–3.

Connective tissues have an abundance of intercellular matrix with relatively few cells.

Table 4–3   Summary of Connective Tissues

Type	Description	Functions/Locations
Loose (areolar)	Collagenous and elastic fibers produced by fibroblasts are embedded in a gel-like matrix	Binds organs together/beneath the skin, between muscles
Adipose	Cells are filled with fat droplets so that nucleus and cytoplasm are pushed to the periphery; little intercellular matrix	Cushions, insulates, stores energy/beneath the skin, around the kidneys, heart, eyeballs
Dense fibrous	Matrix filled with parallel bundles of collagenous fibers	Binds structures together/tendons and ligaments
Osseous (bone)	Hard matrix with mineral salts; matrix arranged in lamellae around haversian canal; osteocytes in lacunae	Protects, supports, provides framework/bones of the skeleton
Blood	Liquid matrix called plasma with erythrocytes, leukocytes, and platelets suspended in it	Transports oxygen, protects against disease, functions in the clotting mechanism/blood vessels and heart
Elastic	Matrix filled with yellow elastic fibers	Elasticity/vocal cords and ligaments between adjacent vertebrae
Cartilage		
Hyaline	Solid matrix with fibers and scattered cells; chondrocytes located in lacunae	Supports, protects, provides a framework/ends of long bones, connects ribs to sternum, tracheal rings, fetal skeleton
Fibrocartilage	Numerous collagenous fibers in matrix	Cushions and protects/intervertebral disks, pads in knee joint, pad between two pubic bones
Elastic	Numerous elastic fibers in matrix	Supports and provides framework/external ear, epiglottis, auditory tubes

Sarcomas are cancerous tumors that are derived from connective tissue. These account for approximately 10 percent of all malignant neoplasms.

The intercellular matrix in connective tissue has a gel-like base of water, nonfibrous protein, and other molecules. Various mineral salts in the matrix of some connective tissues, such as bone, make them hard. Two types of fibers, collagenous (koh-LAJ-eh-nus) and elastic, are frequently embedded in the matrix. **Collagenous fibers,** composed of the protein collagen, are strong and flexible but are only slightly elastic. They are able to withstand considerable pulling force and are found in areas in which this is important, such as in tendons and ligaments. When collagenous fibers are grouped together in parallel bundles, the tissue appears white so they are sometimes called white fibers. **Elastic fibers,** composed of the protein elastin, are not very strong, but they are elastic. They can be stretched and will return to their original shape and length when released. Elastic fibers, also called yellow fibers, are located where structures are stretched and released, such as the vocal cords.

Collagenous fibers are strong and flexible, but not very elastic. Elastic fibers are not very strong but return to their natural shape and length after being stretched.

Collagen turns into a soft gelatin when it is boiled. Meat that has a lot of collagenous fibers is tough, but it becomes more tender when it is boiled or simmered because the collagen softens.

Numerous cell types are found in connective tissue. Three of the most common are the **fibroblast, macrophage,** and **mast cell.** As the name implies, fibroblasts produce the fibers that are in the intercellular matrix. Macrophages are large phagocytic cells that are able to move about and clean up cellular debris and foreign particles from the tissues. Mast cells contain heparin, an anticoagulant, and histamine, a substance that promotes inflammation and that is active in allergies.

Fibroblasts, macrophages, and mast cells are three of the most common connective tissue cells.

Loose Connective Tissue

Loose connective tissue, also called **areolar** (ah-REE-oh-lar) **connective tissue,** is one of the most widely distributed tissues in the body. It is the packing material in the body. It attaches the skin to the underlying tissues and fills the spaces between muscles. Most epithelial tissue is anchored to this tissue by the basement membrane, and the blood vessels

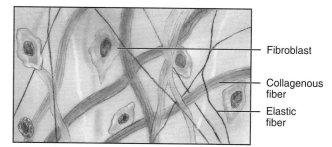

Figure 4–10 Loose (areolar) connective tissue.

in the loose connective tissue supply nutrients to the epithelium above. The matrix is characterized by a loose network of collagenous and elastic fibers. The predominant cell is the fibroblast, but other connective tissue cells are also present (Fig. 4–10).

Loose (areolar) connective tissue fills spaces in the body and binds structures together.

Adipose Tissue

Commonly called fat, **adipose** (ADD-ih-pose) **tissue** is really a specialized form of loose connective tissue in which there is very little intercellular matrix. Some of the cells accumulate liquid triglyceride, or fat, droplets. When this happens, the cytoplasm and nucleus are pushed off to one side, and the cells swell and become closely packed together (Fig. 4–11). Fat cells have the ability to take up fat and then release it at a later time. Adipose tissue forms a protective cushion around the kidneys, heart, eyeballs, and various joints. It also accumulates under the skin where it provides insulation for heat. Adipose tissue is an efficient energy storage material for excess calories.

Adipose tissue, commonly called fat, forms a protective cushion around certain organs, provides insulation, and is an efficient energy storage material.

Suction lipectomy is a cosmetic surgical procedure in which adipose tissue is suctioned from fatty areas of the body.

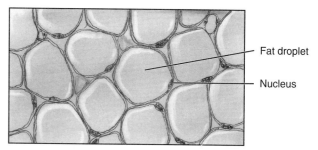

Figure 4–11 Adipose tissue.

Dense Fibrous Connective Tissue

Dense fibrous connective tissue is characterized by closely packed parallel bundles of collagenous fibers in the intercellular matrix (Fig. 4–12). There are relatively few cells and the ones that are present are fibroblasts to produce the collagenous fibers. This is the tissue that makes up **tendons,** which connect muscles to bones, and **ligaments,** which connect one bone to another. Dense fibrous connective tissue has a poor blood supply and this, along with the relatively few cells, accounts for the slow healing of this tissue.

> Tendons and ligaments are formed from dense fibrous connective tissue.

Elastic Connective Tissue

Elastic connective tissue has closely packed elastic fibers in the intercellular matrix. This type of tissue yields easily to a pulling force and then returns to its original length as soon as the force is released. The vocal cords and the ligaments that connect adjacent vertebrae are composed of elastic connective tissue.

Cartilage

Cartilage has an abundant matrix that is solid, yet flexible, with fibers embedded in it. The matrix contains the protein **chondrin** (KON-drihn). Cartilage cells, or **chondrocytes** (KON-droh-sytes), are located in spaces called **lacunae** (lah-KOO-nee) that are scattered throughout the matrix. Typically, cartilage is surrounded by a dense fibrous connective tissue covering called the **perichondrium**. There are blood vessels in the perichondrium, but they do not penetrate the cartilage itself; and the cells obtain their nutrients by diffusion through the solid matrix. Cartilage heals slowly because there is no direct blood supply, and this also contributes to slow cellular reproduction. Cartilage protects underlying tissues, supports other structures, and provides a framework for attachments.

> Blood vessels do not penetrate cartilage so cellular reproduction and healing occur slowly.

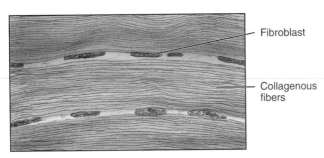

Figure 4–12 Fibrous connective tissue.

— Fibroblast

— Collagenous fibers

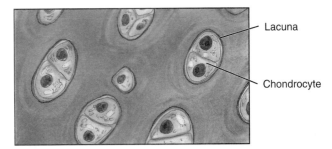

Figure 4–13 Hyaline cartilage.

— Lacuna

— Chondrocyte

Hyaline cartilage (Fig. 4–13) is the most common type of cartilage. It has fine collagenous fibers in the matrix and a shiny, white, opaque appearance. It is found at the ends of long bones, in the costal cartilages that connect the ribs to the sternum, and in the supporting rings of the trachea. Most of the fetal skeleton is formed of hyaline cartilage before it is replaced by bone.

Fibrocartilage has an abundance of strong collagenous fibers embedded in the matrix. This allows it to withstand compression, act as a shock absorber, and resist pulling forces. It is found in the pads between the vertebrae, or intervertebral disks; in the symphysis pubis, or the pad between the two pubic bones; and between the bones in the knee joint.

Elastic cartilage has numerous yellow elastic fibers embedded in the matrix, which makes it more flexible than hyaline cartilage or fibrocartilage. It is found in the framework of the external ear, the epiglottis, and the auditory tubes.

> The three types of cartilage are hyaline cartilage, fibrocartilage, and elastic cartilage.

Bone

Osseous tissue or **bone** is the most rigid of all the connective tissues. Collagenous fibers in the matrix give strength to bone, and its hardness is derived from the mineral salts, particularly calcium, that are deposited around the fibers. Bones form the framework for the body and help protect underlying tissues. They serve as attachments for muscles and act as mechanical levers in producing movement. Bone also contributes to the formation of blood cells and functions as a storage area for mineral salts.

> Bone is a rigid connective tissue. The matrix is strengthened and hardened by mineral salts.

Cylindrical structural units, called **osteons** or **haversian** (hah-VER-shun) **systems,** are packed together to form the substance of compact bone (Fig. 4–14). The center or hub of the osteon is a tubular **osteonic** or **haversian** canal that contains a blood vessel. The matrix is deposited in concentric rings called **lamellae** (lah-MEL-ee) around the canal. **Osteocytes,** or

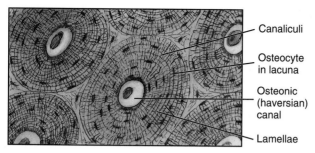

Canaliculi

Osteocyte
in lacuna

Osteonic
(haversian)
canal

Lamellae

Figure 4–14   Compact bone (osseous tissue).

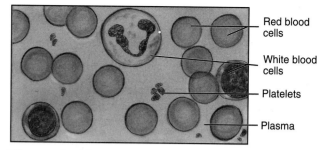

Red blood
cells

White blood
cells

Platelets

Plasma

Figure 4–15   Blood.

bone cells, are located in lacunae between the lamellae so that they are also arranged in concentric rings. Slender processes from the bone cells extend, through tiny tubes in the matrix called **canaliculi** (kan-ah-LIK-yoo-lye), to other cells or to the osteonic canals. This provides a readily available blood supply for the bone cells, which allows a faster repair process for bone than for cartilage.

> The haversian system, or osteon, is the structural unit of bone.

Blood

Blood is a unique connective tissue because it is the only one that has a liquid matrix. It is a vehicle for transport of substances throughout the body. **Erythrocytes,** or red blood cells, and **leukocytes,** or white blood cells, are suspended in a liquid matrix called **plasma** (Fig. 4–15). The red blood cells transport oxygen from the lungs to the tissues. White blood cells are important in fighting disease. Another formed element in the blood is the **platelet,** or **thrombocyte,** which is not actually a cell but a fragment of a giant cell in the bone marrow. Platelets are important in initiating the blood clotting process. Blood is discussed in more detail in Chapter 11.

> Blood is a connective tissue that has a liquid matrix called plasma. The cells are the erythrocytes, leukocytes, and thrombocytes.

Muscle Tissue

Muscle tissue is composed of cells that have the special ability to shorten or contract in order to produce movement of body parts. The tissue is highly cellular and is well supplied with blood vessels. The cells are long and slender so they are sometimes called muscle fibers, and these are usually arranged in bundles or layers that are surrounded by connective tissue. The contractile proteins **actin** and **myosin** form microfilaments in the cytoplasm and are responsible for contraction. There are three types of muscle tissue: skeletal muscle, smooth muscle, and cardiac muscle. Features of muscle tissues are summarized in Table 4–4.

> Actin and myosin are, contractile proteins in muscle tissue.

Skeletal Muscle

Skeletal muscle tissue (Fig. 4–16) is what is commonly thought of as "muscle." It is the meat of animals. and it constitutes about 40 percent of an individual's body weight. Skeletal muscle cells (fibers) are long and cylindrical with many nuclei (multinucleated) peripherally located next to the cell membrane. The cells have alternating light and dark bands that are perpendicular to the long axis of the cell. These bands are due to the organized arrangement of the contractile proteins in the cytoplasm

Table 4–4 Summary of Muscle Tissues			
Feature	Skeletal	Smooth	Cardiac
Location	Attached to bones	Walls of internal organs and blood vessels	Heart
Function	Produces body movement	Contracts viscera and blood vessels	Pumps blood through the heart and blood vessels
Cell shape	Cylindrical	Spindle shaped, tapered ends	Cylindrical, branching, intercalated disks join cells together end to end
Number of nuclei	Many; peripherally located	One; centrally located	One; centrally located
Striations	Present	Absent	Present
Speed of contraction	Fastest	Slowest	Intermediate
Length of contraction	Least	Greatest	Intermediate
Type of control	Voluntary	Involuntary	Involuntary

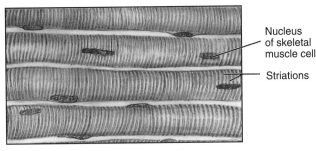

Figure 4-16 Skeletal muscle.

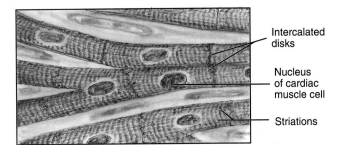

Figure 4-18 Cardiac muscle.

and give the cell a **striated** appearance. Skeletal muscle fibers are collected into bundles and wrapped in connective tissue to form the muscles, which are attached to the skeleton and which cause body movements when they contract in response to nerve stimulation. Skeletal muscle action is under conscious or voluntary control. Chapter 7 describes skeletal muscles in more detail.

> Skeletal muscle fibers are cylindrical, multinucleated, striated, and under voluntary control.

Smooth Muscle

Smooth muscle tissue (Fig. 4–17) is found in the walls of hollow body organs such as the stomach, intestines, urinary bladder, uterus, and blood vessels. It normally acts to propel substances through the organ by contracting and relaxing. It is called smooth muscle because it lacks the striations evident in skeletal muscle. Because it is found in the viscera or body organs, it is sometimes called **visceral muscle.** Smooth muscle cells are shorter than skeletal muscle cells, are spindle shaped and tapered at the ends, and have a single, centrally located nucleus. Smooth muscle usually cannot be stimulated to contract by conscious or voluntary effort, so it is called involuntary muscle.

> Smooth muscle cells are spindle shaped, have a single, centrally located nucleus, and lack striations. They are called involuntary muscles.

Cardiac Muscle

Cardiac muscle tissue (Fig. 4–18) is found only in the wall of the heart. The cardiac muscle cells are cylindrical and appear striated like the skeletal muscle cells. Cardiac muscle cells are shorter than skeletal muscle cells and have only one nucleus per cell. The cells branch and interconnect to form complex networks. At the point where one cell attaches to another, there is a specialized intercellular connection called an intercalated (in-TER-kuh-lay-ted) disk. Cardiac muscle appears striated like skeletal muscle but its contraction is involuntary. It is responsible for pumping the blood through the heart and into the blood vessels.

> Cardiac muscle has branching fibers, one nucleus per cell, striations, and intercalated disks. Its contraction is not under voluntary control.

Nervous Tissue

Nervous tissue is found in the brain, spinal cord, and nerves. It is responsible for coordinating and controlling many body activities. It stimulates muscle contraction, creates an awareness of the environment, and plays a major role in emotions, memory, and reasoning. To do all of these things, cells in nervous tissue need to be able to communicate with each other by way of electrical nerve impulses.

The cells in nervous tissue that generate and conduct impulses are called **neurons** (NOO-rons) or

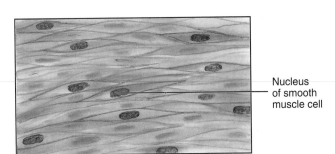

Figure 4-17 Smooth muscle.

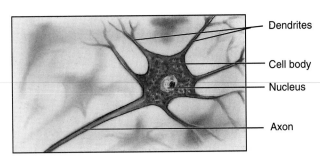

Figure 4-19 Neuron (nervous tissue).

nerve cells. These cells have three principal parts: the dendrites, the cell body, and one axon (Fig. 4–19). The main part of the cell, the part that carries on the general functions, is the **cell body. Dendrites** are extensions, or processes, of the cytoplasm that carry impulses to the cell body. An extension or process called an **axon** carries impulses away from the cell body.

> Neurons are the conducting cells of nervous tissue. They have a cell body with processes called axons and dendrites.

Nervous tissue also includes cells that do not transmit impulses but instead support the activities of the neurons. These are the **glial** (GLEE-al) **cells** (or neuroglial cells), together termed the **neuroglia** (noo-ROG-lee-ah). Supporting, or glial, cells bind neurons together and insulate the neurons. Some are phagocytic and protect against bacterial invasion, whereas others provide nutrients by binding blood vessels to the neurons. Further detail on nerve tissue is presented in Chapter 8.

> The neuroglia, composed of the glial cells, is the supporting structure of nervous tissue. Glial cells do not conduct nerve impulses.

✓ QuickCheck

- Which of the four types of tissues forms the coverings and linings of the body?

- Cartilage, bone, and blood are what type of tissue?

- One type of muscle tissue has branching fibers, striations, and intercalated disks. Where in the body is this muscle tissue located?

Body Membranes

Body membranes are thin sheets of tissue that cover the body, line body cavities, cover organs within the cavities, and line the cavities in hollow organs. By this definition, the skin is a membrane because it covers the body, and indeed, the skin, or integument, is sometimes called the **cutaneous membrane.** This membrane is discussed in Chapter 5. This section deals with two epithelial membranes and two connective tissue membranes. Epithelial membranes consist of epithelial tissue and the connective tissue to which it is attached. The two main types of epithelial membranes are the mucous membranes and serous membranes. Connective tissue membranes contain only connective tissue. Synovial membranes and meninges belong to this category.

> Mucous and serous membranes are epithelial membranes. Synovial membranes and the meninges are connective tissue membranes.

Mucous Membranes

Mucous membranes are epithelial membranes that consist of epithelial tissue that is attached to an underlying loose connective tissue. These membranes, sometimes called **mucosae,** line the body cavities that open to the outside. The entire digestive tract is lined with mucous membranes. Other examples include the respiratory, excretory, and reproductive tracts. The type of epithelium varies depending on its function. In the mouth, the epithelium is stratified squamous for its protection function, but the stomach and intestines are lined with simple columnar epithelium for absorption and secretion. The mucosa of the urinary bladder is transitional epithelium so that it can expand. Mucous membranes get their name from the fact that the epithelial cells secrete mucus for lubrication and protection.

> Mucous membranes secrete mucus and line body cavities that open to the exterior.

Serous Membranes

Serous membranes line body cavities that do not open directly to the outside, and they cover the organs located in those cavities. A serous membrane, or **serosa,** consists of a thin layer of loose connective tissue covered by a layer of simple squamous epithelium called **mesothelium.** These membranes always have two parts. The part that lines a cavity wall is the **parietal** layer and the part that covers the organs in the cavity is the **visceral** layer (Fig. 4–20). Serous membranes are covered by a thin layer

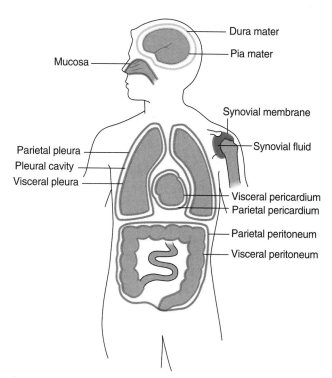

Dura mater
Pia mater
Mucosa
Synovial membrane
Synovial fluid
Parietal pleura
Pleural cavity
Visceral pleura
Visceral pericardium
Parietal pericardium
Parietal peritoneum
Visceral peritoneum

Figure 4–20 Body membranes.

of **serous fluid** that is secreted by the epithelium. Serous fluid lubricates the membrane and reduces friction and abrasion when organs in the thoracic or abdominopelvic cavity move against each other or the cavity wall.

> Serous membranes line the closed body cavities and cover the organs within those cavities. These membranes secrete a serous fluid between the parietal and visceral layers.

Serous membranes have special names given according to their location. The serous membrane that lines the thoracic cavity and covers the lungs is the **pleura,** with the parietal pleura lining the cavity and the visceral pleura covering the lungs. The **pericardium** (pair-ih-KAR-deeum) lines the pericardial cavity and covers the heart. The serous membrane in the abdominopelvic cavity is the **peritoneum** (pair-ih-toh-NEE-um).

> The pleura, pericardium, and peritoneum are serous membranes.

An inflammation of the serous membranes in the abdominal cavity is called peritonitis. This is sometimes a serious complication of an infected appendix.

Synovial Membranes

Synovial (sih-NOH-vee-al) **membranes** are connective tissue membranes that line the cavities of the freely movable joints such as the shoulder, elbow, and knee. Like serous membranes, they line cavities that do not open to the outside. Unlike serous membranes, they do not have a layer of epithelium. Synovial membranes secrete **synovial fluid** into the joint cavity, and this lubricates the cartilage on the ends of the bones so that they can move freely and without friction. In certain types of arthritis, these membranes become inflamed and the fluid becomes viscous. This reduces lubrication and increases friction, and movement becomes difficult and painful.

> Synovial membranes are connective tissue membranes that line joint cavities. They secrete synovial fluid for lubrication.

Meninges

The connective tissue coverings around the brain and spinal cord, within the dorsal cavity, are called **meninges** (meh-NIN-jeez). They provide protection for these vital structures. The outermost layer of the meninges is the toughest and is called the **dura mater** (DOO-rah MAY-ter). The middle layer, the **arachnoid** (ah-RAK-noyd), is quite fragile. The **pia mater** (PEE-ah MAY-ter), the innermost layer, is very delicate and closely adherent to the surface of the brain and spinal cord. Inflammation of the meninges is **meningitis.** Further discussion of the meninges appears in Chapter 8.

> The dura mater, arachnoid, and pia mater are connective tissue membranes around the brain and spinal cord.

 QuickCheck

- The pericardium and peritoneum are examples of which type of epithelial membrane?
- What is the name of the connective tissue membrane that lines joint cavities?

 FOCUS ON AGING

Because tissues consist of cells, cellular aging alters the tissues formed by those cells. There is a general loss of fluid in the tissues. Most of this dehydration is from intracellular fluid, but there is also a reduction in extracellular fluid. Elastic tissues lose some of their elasticity. Changes that occur in connective tissues exaggerate the normal curvatures of the spinal column and cause changes in the joints, in the arches of the foot, and in the intervertebral disks. These changes are manifested in a loss of height. Most organs show a loss of mass with aging because of tissue atrophy.

Tissues?

Inflammation and Tissue Repair

Inflammation is a nonspecific defense mechanism that attempts to localize or contain tissue injury and to prepare the area for healing. It is a normal mechanism that is manifested by redness, swelling, heat, and pain.

Damaged tissues release chemicals that cause blood vessels in the area to dilate and become more permeable. Blood vessel dilation increases blood flow to the area, which accounts for the redness and the increased temperature. Increased blood vessel permeability permits fluid and phagocytic white blood cells to leave the blood vessels and to infiltrate the surrounding tissue spaces. Phagocytic white blood cells engulf invading bacteria and debris from the damaged cells. The increased fluid in the tissue spaces accounts for the swelling associated with inflammation, and swelling puts pressure on the nerves, causing pain. The fluid dilutes toxins and cleanses the area. It also contains clotting proteins that construct a clot to stop the loss of blood, to hold the edges of the wound together, and to isolate or "wall off" the area to prevent bacteria and toxins from spreading to surrounding tissues. If the wound is in the skin, the portion of the clot that is exposed to air dehydrates and hardens to form a scab that forms a temporary covering over the break in the skin. Even though inflammation may be painful, it is a beneficial process that cleanses the damaged area and sets the stage for repair and restoration.

There are two types of tissue repair: regeneration and fibrosis, or scar formation. The type that occurs depends on the characteristics of the tissue and the severity of the damage. Usually both types are involved in the repair process. Because nearly everyone has experienced a skin wound, it is used to illustrate the process of repair.

Regeneration is the replacement of destroyed tissue by the proliferation of cells that are identical to the original cells. This occurs in superficial skin abrasions when mitosis of healthy and undamaged cells restores the skin to its original thickness. Regeneration occurs only in tissues that have mitotic capability. Skeletal muscle, cardiac muscle, and nerve tissue in the brain and spinal cord cannot regenerate. These damaged tissues have to be replaced by fibrous scar tissue, which may interfere with the normal function of the organ involved.

Fibrosis is the replacement of destroyed tissue by the generation of fibrous connective tissue. This is the formation of scar tissue. Fibroblasts proliferate in the region of the wound and produce collagen fibers that form the basis of the scar. These fibers help draw the edges of the wound together and strengthen the area. This new, immature scar tissue is called **granulation tissue.** While the collagen fibers are forming, undamaged capillaries in the region develop buds that grow into the area of the wound to form new capillaries. The abundance of new capillaries, necessary to bring nutrients to the active cells, makes the immature scar tissue appear pink.

While the granulation tissue is forming, the surface epithelium regenerates and grows over the surface between the scab and the granulation tissue. When the epithelium is complete, the scab detaches. As the granulation tissue matures, it contracts, and the capillaries regress when the extra blood supply is no longer needed. The regenerating epithelium thickens until it matches the surrounding epithelium. The result is a fully regenerated layer of epithelium over an underlying area of fibrosis or scar tissue. The scar may or may not be evident, depending on the severity of the wound. Figure 4–21 illustrates tissue repair in a skin laceration.

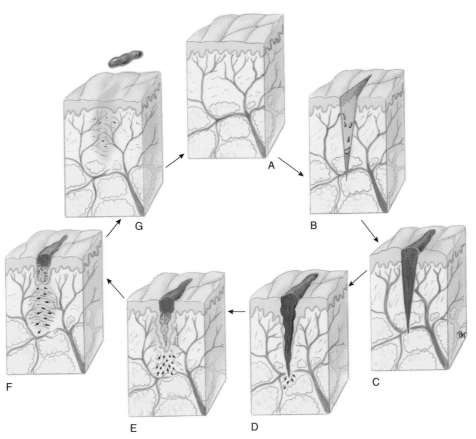

Figure 4–21 Steps in tissue regeneration and repair: *A*, Normal skin. *B*, Wound with bleeding. *C*, Clot forms. *D*, Fibroblasts migrate to the area. *E*, Fibroblasts proliferate and begin forming fibers of collagen. Scab forms. *F*, Surface epithelium regenerates and grows between scab and granulation tissue. *G*, Formation of granulation tissue (scar) is complete and scab detaches.

CHAPTER 4 QUIZ

RECALL

Match the definitions on the left with the appropriate term on the right.

1. Flat cells

2. More than one layer of cells

3. Unicellular glands that produce mucus

4. Entire cell discharged with secretion

5. Strong, flexible connective tissue fibers

6. Large, phagocytic cell

7. Fat tissue

8. Bone cell

9. Nerve cell

10. Contractile protein in muscle

A. Adipose

B. Collagenous

C. Goblet cell

D. Holocrine

E. Macrophage

F. Myosin

G. Neuron

H. Osteocyte

I. Squamous

J. Stratified

THOUGHT

1. A tissue is composed of a single layer of flat cells, closely packed together. This tissue is likely to be found

   a. covering the outside of the body

   b. forming the alveoli or air sacs of the lungs

   c. lining the intestines

   d. as packing between neurons in the brain

2. A gland in which a portion of the secretory cell is pinched off and released with the secretion

   a. is a merocrine gland

   b. is a sebaceous gland

   c. is an apocrine gland

   d. is a goblet cell

3. Tendons and ligaments are formed from

   a. dense fibrous connective tissue

   b. osseous tissue

   c. hyaline cartilage

   d. extensions of muscle tissue

4. Muscle tissue that is spindle shaped with tapered ends and no apparent striations is

   a. found in the heart wall

   b. called skeletal muscle

   c. found in the wall of the stomach

   d. usually attached to bones

5. Meninges are membranes that

   a. secrete a serous fluid

   b. line joint cavities

   c. line the respiratory tract

   d. cover the brain and spinal cord

APPLICATION

Approximately 85% of all cancers are carcinomas, meaning that they arise from epithelial tissue. Why do you think there are so many more carcinomas than sarcomas that arise from connective tissue?

Integumentary System

Outline/Objectives

Structure of the Skin 77
- Describe the structure of the two layers of the skin.
- Name the supporting layer of the skin and describe its structure.

Skin Color 80
- Discuss three factors that influence skin color.

Epidermal Derivatives 80
- Describe the structure of hair and nails and their relationship to the skin.
- Discuss the characteristics and functions of the various glands associated with the skin.

Functions of the Skin 82
- Discuss four functions of the integumentary system.

Key Terms

Arrector pili
Ceruminous gland
Dermis
Epidermis
Keratinization
Melanin
Sebaceous gland
Subcutaneous layer
Sudoriferous gland

Building Vocabulary

WORD PART	MEANING
albin-	white
cer-	wax
cutane-	skin
derm-	skin
-ectomy	surgical excision
hidr-	sweat
ichthy-	scaly, dry
kerat-	hard, horny tissue
-lucid-	clear, light
melan-	black
onych-	nail
pachy-	thick
-plasty	surgical repair
rhytid-	wrinkles
seb-	oil
sud-	sweat

Functional Relationships of the
Integumentary System

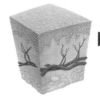

Provides a barrier against hazardous materials and pathogens.

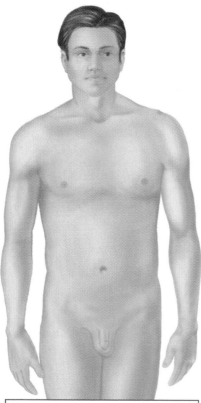

Skeletal
Provides structural support.

Synthesizes vitamin D needed for calcium absorption and metabolism for bone growth and maintenance.

Muscular
Generates heat to warm the skin; muscle contraction pulls on skin to produce facial expressions.

Synthesizes vitamin D needed for absorption and metabolism of calcium essential for muscle contraction.

Nervous
Controls diameter of cutaneous blood vessels and sweat gland activity for temperature regulation.

Dermis contains receptors that detect stimuli related to touch, pressure, pain, and temperature.

Endocrine
Sex hormones influence hair growth, sebaceous gland activity, and distribution of subcutaneous adipose.

Synthesizes vitamin D needed for the absorption and metabolism of calcium, which acts as a messenger in some hormone actions.

Cardiovascular
Transports gases, nutrients, wastes, and hormones to and from the skin; hemoglobin provides color.

Prevents fluid loss from the blood; vasoconstriction of dermal vessels diverts blood flow to other organs.

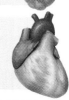

Lymphatic/Immune
Prevents loss of interstitial fluid from skin, protects against skin infection, and promotes tissue repair.

Prevents pathogen entry; connective tissue cells in the skin activate the immune response.

Respiratory
Furnishes oxygen and removes carbon dioxide by gaseous exchange with blood.

Hairs of nasal cavity filter particles that may damage the upper respiratory tract.

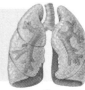

Digestive
Provides nutrients needed for skin growth, maintenance, and repair.

Provides vitamin D for intestinal absorption of calcium.

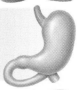

Urinary
Eliminates metabolic wastes and maintains normal body fluid composition.

Alternative excretory route for some salts and nitrogenous wastes; limits fluid loss.

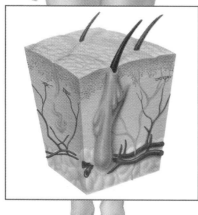

Reproductive
Gonads provide hormones that promote growth, maturation, and maintenance of skin.

Skin forms scrotum that protects testes; tactile receptors in skin provide sensations associated with sexual behaviors.

The skin and the glands, hair, nails, and other structures that are derived from it make up the **integumentary** (in-teg-yoo-MEN-tar-ee) **system.** Because it is on the outside of the body, this is the organ system with which we are most familiar. This is our contact with the external environment. It is the part that is, at least partially, exposed so others can see it. There is probably no other system that receives as much personal attention. We spend millions of dollars each year in attempts to "beautify" the integumentary system through creams, lotions, oils, color, rinses, conditioners, permanents, manicures, pedicures, polishes, and more. The list goes on and on. Yet because it is on the outside of the body, this system is subjected to continual abuse in the form of bumps, abrasions, cuts, scrapes, toxic chemicals, pollutants, wind, and sun. However, the skin is resilient and versatile. Generally, it quickly repairs itself and continues to perform its many functions year after year.

The integumentary system includes the skin and its derivatives.

For an "average" person, the skin weighs about 5 kilograms, has a surface area of approximately 2 square meters, and varies in thickness from 0.05 to 0.4 centimeter.

Structure of the Skin

The skin, sometimes called the **cutaneous** (kyoo-TAY-nee-us) **membrane,** consists of two distinct layers of tissues. The outer layer is the **epidermis,** and the inner layer is the **dermis.** These are anchored to underlying structures by a third layer, the **subcutaneous tissue.**

The structure of the skin is illustrated in Figures 5-1 and 5-2.

The skin has an outer epidermis and an inner dermis anchored to underlying structures by subcutaneous tissue.

Epidermis

The outer layer of the skin is the **epidermis.** This layer is stratified squamous epithelium (see Fig. 5-1). Because the epidermis is epithelium, there are no blood vessels present and the cells receive their nutrients, by diffusion, from vessels in the underlying tissue. The cells on the bottom, near the basement membrane, receive adequate nutrients and actively grow and divide. As cells are pushed upward toward the surface by the growing cells next to the basement membrane, they receive fewer nutrients. They also undergo a process called **keratinization** (ker-ah-tin-ih-ZAY-shun). During keratinization, a protein called keratin is deposited in the cell, the chemical composition of the cell changes, and the

CLINICAL TERMS

Alopecia (al-oh-PEE-shee-ah) Absence of hair from skin areas where it normally grows; baldness; may be hereditary or due to disease, injury, or chemotherapy or may occur as part of aging

Basal cell carcinoma (BAY-sal SELL kar-sih-NOH-mah) Malignant tumor of the basal cell layer of the epidermis; most common form of skin cancer and usually grows slowly

Cellulitis (sell-yoo-LYE-tis) Infection of connective tissue with severe inflammation of the dermis and subcutaneous layer of the skin

Dermatitis (der-mah-TYE-tis) Inflammation of the skin

Eczema (ECK-zeh-mah) An inflammatory skin disease with red, itching, vesicular lesions that may crust over; common allergic reaction, but may occur without any obvious cause

Eschar (ESS-kar) A slough produced by a burn or gangrene

Hives (HYVZ) Eruption of itching and burning swellings on the skin; most commonly caused by infections, medications, food allergies, or emotional stress; also called urticaria

Impetigo (im-peh-TYE-go) Superficial skin infection caused by staphylococcal or streptococcal bacteria and characterized by vesicles, pustules, and crusted-over lesions; most common in children

Malignant melanoma (mah-LIG-nant mel-ah-NOH-mah) Cancerous growth composed of melanocytes; often arises in preexisting mole; an alarming increase in the incidence of malignant melanoma is attributed to excessive exposure to sunlight

Nevus (NEE-vus) An elevated, pigmented lesion on the skin; commonly called a mole; a dysplastic nevus is a mole that does not form properly and may progress to a type of skin cancer; plural, nevi

Pruritus (proo-RYE-tus) Severe itching; one of the most common problems in dermatology; arises as a result of stimulation of nerves in the skin by enzymes released in allergic reactions or by other irritating substances

Wart (WORT) Epidermal growth on the skin caused by a virus; plantar warts occur on the soles of the feet, juvenile warts occur on the hands and face of children, and venereal warts occur in the genital area

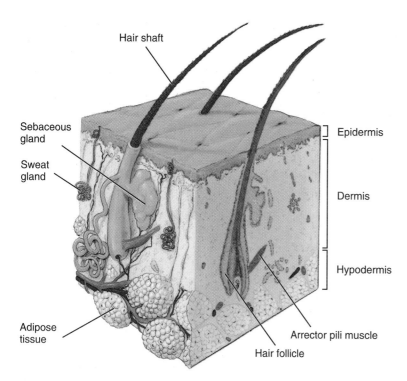

Hair shaft

Sebaceous gland

Sweat gland

Adipose tissue

Hair follicle

Arrector pili muscle

Epidermis

Dermis

Hypodermis

Figure 5–1 Structure of the skin. (From Jarvis C: Physical Examination and Health Assessment. Philadelphia, WB Saunders, 1992.)

cell changes shape. By the time the cells reach the surface, they are flat or squamous and dead from lack of nutrients and are sloughed off. They are replaced by other cells that are pushed upward from below. As cells are pushed upward, away from the nutrient supply, and become keratinized, they take on different appearances and characteristics to form distinct regions. In thick skin, such as that on the soles of the feet and palms of the hand, the epidermis consists of five regions, or strata, of cells (see Fig. 5–2). In the skin that covers the rest of the body, the regions are thinner and there are only four strata.

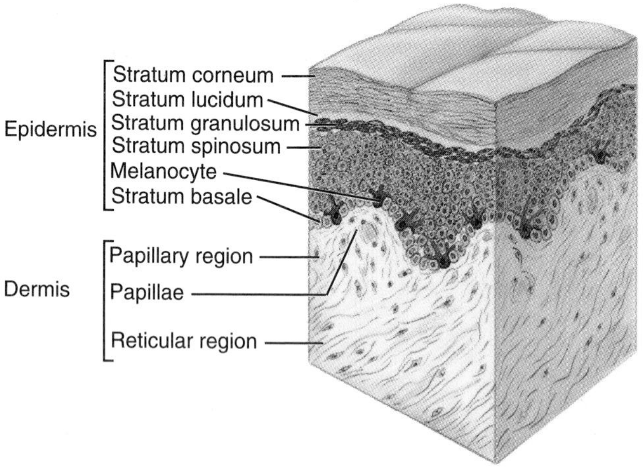

The epidermis is stratified squamous epithelium. In thick skin there are five distinct regions in the epidermis, but in thinner regions there are only four layers.

The bottom row of cells in the stratified squamous epithelium that makes up the epidermis consists of actively dividing (mitotic) columnar cells. This layer is the **stratum basale** (BAY-sah-lee), the layer next to the basement membrane and closest to the blood supply (see Fig. 5–2). About one fourth of the cells in the stratum basale are **melanocytes** (meh-LAN-oh-sytes). These are specialized epithelial cells that produce a dark pigment called **melanin** (MEL-ah-nin). All individuals have the same number of melanocytes. However, melanocyte activity (the amount of melanin produced) differs according to genetic and environmental factors.

The bottom layer, or stratum basale, is closest to the blood supply and is actively mitotic. It also contains melanocytes.

Epidermis

Stratum corneum
Stratum lucidum
Stratum granulosum
Stratum spinosum
Melanocyte
Stratum basale

Dermis

Papillary region
Papillae
Reticular region

Figure 5–2 Subdivisions of the epidermis and dermis.

Cancerous neoplasms composed of melanocytes, called malignant melanomas, account for 3 percent of all cancers, and the incidence is rising at a rate of 4.5 percent annually. Exposure to sunlight is the major risk factor for the development of malignant melanoma, and individuals with fair skin and light hair are at greatest risk. Melanomas often metastasize to the lung, liver, and brain.

The **stratum spinosum** (spy-NOH-sum) consists of several layers of cells immediately above the stratum basale (see Fig. 5–2). These cells have slender projections, or spiny processes, that connect them with other cells. When a cell in the stratum basale undergoes mitosis and divides into two cells, one of the daughter cells remains in the stratum basale and the other one is pushed upward into the stratum spinosum. Because the cells in the stratum spinosum show limited mitotic ability, this layer combined with the stratum basale is called the **stratum germinativum** (JER-mih-nah-tiv-um).

> Cells in the stratum spinosum are derived from mitosis of stratum basale cells.

The **stratum granulosum** (gran-yoo-LOH-sum) is a very thin region consisting of two or three layers of flattened cells (see Fig. 5–2). Keratinization begins in this layer. The cells appear granular, which gives this layer its name.

> Keratinization begins in the stratum granulosum.

The **stratum lucidum** (LOO-sih-dum) appears as a translucent band just above the stratum granulosum (see Fig. 5–2). It consists of a few layers of flattened, anucleate cells. The stratum lucidum is present only in thick skin.

> The stratum lucidum is a translucent band that is present only in thick skin.

The **stratum corneum** (KOR-nee-um) is the outermost or surface region of the epidermis and constitutes about three fourths of the epidermal thickness. It consists of 20 to 30 layers of flattened, dead, completely keratinized cells (see Fig. 5–2). The cells in the stratum corneum are continually shed and replaced. About 5 weeks after a cell has been produced in the stratum basale, it is sloughed off the surface of the stratum corneum. The keratin that is present is a tough, water-repellent protein, and its inclusion in the stratum corneum provides protection against water loss from the body.

> The stratum corneum is the outermost layer of the epidermis. Its dead keratinized cells are continually sloughed off and replaced by cells from deeper layers.

Dermis

The **dermis,** or **stratum corium** (KOR-ee-um), is dense connective tissue that is deeper and usually thicker than the epidermis (see Fig. 5–1). Hair, nails, and certain glands, although derived from the stratum basale of the epidermis, are embedded in the dermis. The dermis contains both collagenous and elastic fibers to give it strength and elasticity. If the skin is overstretched, the dermis may be damaged, leaving white scars called **striae** (STRY-ee), commonly called "stretch marks." Fibers also form a framework for the numerous blood vessels and nerves that are present in the dermis but generally absent in the epidermis. Many of the nerves in the dermis have specialized endings called **sensory receptors** that detect changes in the environment such as heat, cold, pain, pressure, and touch. Because there are no nerves in the epidermis, these receptors are the body's contact with the environment.

> The dermis, thicker than the epidermis, is connective tissue with hairs, nails, glands, fibers, sense receptors, blood vessels, and nerves embedded in it.

The dermis is the portion of an animal's skin that is used to make leather because the collagen in the dermis becomes very tough when treated with tannic acid.

The dermis is divided into two indistinct layers. The upper **papillary** (PAP-ih-lair-ee) **layer** derives its name from the numerous **papillae,** or projections, that extend into the epidermis (see Fig. 5–2). Blood vessels, nerve endings, and sensory receptors extend into the papillae to bring them into closer proximity to the epidermis and the surface. On the palms, fingertips, and the soles of the feet, the papillae form distinct patterns or ridges that provide friction for grasping objects. The patterns are genetically determined and are unique for each individual. These are the basis of fingerprints and footprints.

> The papillary layer of the dermis is the basis of fingerprints and footprints.

The **reticular** (reh-TICK-yoo-lar) **layer** of the dermis is deeper and thicker than the papillary layer (see Fig. 5–2). Bundles of connective tissue fibers run in many different directions to provide the strength and resilience needed to stretch in many planes. More bundles usually run in one direction than in the others, and this produces **cleavage lines.** Incisions across cleavage lines tend to gape more and produce more scar tissue than those that are parallel to the cleavage lines.

> The reticular layer is the deeper region of the dermis that provides strength to the skin.

A blister is a fluid-filled pocket between the dermis and the epidermis. When the skin is burned or irritated some plasma escapes from the blood vessels in the dermis and accumulates between the two layers, where it forms the blister.

Subcutaneous Layer

The **subcutaneous layer** (see Fig. 5–1) is not actually a part of the skin, but it loosely anchors the skin to underlying organs. Because it is beneath the dermis, it is sometimes called the **hypodermis.** It is also referred to as **superficial fascia.** The subcutaneous layer consists largely of loose connective tissue and adipose tissue. The fibers in the loose connective tissue are continuous with those in the dermis and, as a result, there is no distinct boundary between the dermis and the subcutaneous tissue.

> The hypodermis, or subcutaneous layer, anchors the skin to underlying organs.

The adipose tissue in the subcutaneous layer cushions the underlying organs from mechanical shock and acts as a heat insulator in temperature regulation. Fat in the adipose tissue can be mobilized and used for energy when necessary. The distribution of subcutaneous adipose is largely responsible for the differences in body contours between men and women.

> Subcutaneous adipose tissue acts as a cushion and as a heat insulator and can be used as an energy source.

Skin Color

Skin color is due to many factors: some genetic, some physiologic, and some environmental. Basic skin color is due to the dark pigment **melanin** produced by the melanocytes in the stratum basale of the epidermis. Melanocytes have long slender processes by which they transfer the melanin to surrounding cells in the skin and in hair. Everyone has about the same number of melanocytes. The activity of the melanocytes, however, is genetically controlled. A large number of melanin granules results in dark skin; fewer granules result in lighter skin. Although many genes are responsible for skin color, a single mutation can result in an inability to produce melanin. This results in a condition called **albinism** (AL-bih-nizm) in which individuals have very light skin, white hair, and unpigmented irises in the eyes.

Some people have the yellowish pigment **carotene** (KAIR-oh-teen) in addition to melanin. This gives a yellow tint to the skin. A pinkish tint in the skin is due to the blood in the vessels in the dermis. Ultraviolet light increases melanocyte activity so that more melanin is produced and the skin becomes darker or tanned.

> Basic skin color is due to the amount of melanin produced in the basal layer of the epidermis. Other pigments and blood flow are also factors in skin color.

In people with light skin, when dermal blood vessels dilate and blood flow increases (e.g., during blushing and increased temperature), the skin may be quite red. If the vessels constrict and blood flow decreases, the individual is pale or "white as a sheet."

 Quick Check

- The epidermis is constantly sloughed off and replaced. What layer of the epidermis is the source of replacement cells?

- Sensory receptors and blood vessels are embedded in which layer of the skin?

- Melanin is the basic dark pigment responsible for skin color. Where in the skin is this produced?

Epidermal Derivatives

Accessory structures of the skin include hair, nails, sweat glands, and sebaceous glands. They are derived from the stratum basale of the epidermis and are embedded in the reticular layer of the dermis. Figure 5–1 illustrates some of the accessory structures associated with the skin.

> Hair, nails, sweat glands, and sebaceous glands are derived from the epidermis and are embedded in the dermis.

Hair and Hair Follicles

Hair is found on nearly all body surfaces. It is absent on the palms of the hands, soles of the feet, lips, nipples, certain external genitalia, and distal segments of the fingers and toes. All hair has essentially the same structure. It consists of a shaft and a root that are composed of dead, keratinized epithelial cells. The root is enclosed in a hair follicle that extends through the epidermis and is embedded in the dermis. The structure of hair and hair follicles is illustrated in Figure 5–3.

The **shaft** of a hair is that portion that extends beyond the surface of the epidermis. It is the part that you can see. Because it contains no nerves, it can be cut with no sensation of pain. The **root** is the portion of the hair that is below the surface of the skin. It is surrounded by a hair follicle. The shaft and root are continuous and together make up the hair, which is produced by the hair follicle. The central core of a hair is the **medulla.** This is surrounded by several layers of cells called the **cortex.** The outermost covering is a single layer of overlapping, keratinized cells called the **cuticle.** On the shaft of the hair, the cuticle is exposed to the environment and subjected to abrasion. It tends to wear away at the tip of the shaft. When this happens, the keratin fibers in the cells of the cortex and medulla

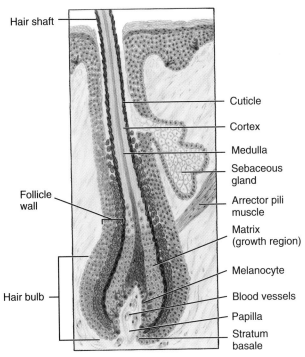

Hair shaft

Cuticle

Cortex

Medulla

Sebaceous gland

Arrector pili muscle

Follicle wall

Matrix (growth region)

Melanocyte

Blood vessels

Hair bulb

Papilla

Stratum basale

Figure 5–3   Structure of hair and hair follicles.

project from the tip of the shaft, resulting in "split ends."

> The central core of hair is the medulla, which is surrounded by the cortex and the cuticle. Hair is divided into the shaft, which is visible, and the root, which is embedded in the skin and surrounded by the hair follicle.

The root of a hair is enclosed in a tubular **hair follicle.** At the end deep in the dermis, the follicle expands to form a **hair bulb.** A **papilla** of dermis with a cluster of blood vessels projects into the center of the bulb. This provides the blood supply for the epithelial cells. As the follicle nears the hair bulb, the follicle becomes thinner so that only a single layer of stratum basale cells covers the papilla. The stratum basale cells, like those in the skin, provide the mitotic cells that divide and undergo keratinization to produce the hair. The stratum basale cells of the hair follicle can, if necessary, grow onto the surface of the skin to repair wounds there.

> The distal end of the hair follicle expands to form a bulb around a central papilla. Stratum basale cells in the bulb undergo mitosis to form hair.

Hair color is determined by the type of melanin produced by the melanocytes in the stratum basale. Yellow, brown, and black pigments are present in varying proportions to produce different hair colors. With age, the melanocytes become less active. Hair

in which melanin is replaced with air bubbles is white.

> Hair color is determined by melanocytes in the stratum basale.

The shape of the hair shaft determines whether hair is straight or curly. If the shaft is round, the hair is straight. If it is oval, the hair is wavy. If it is flat, the hair is curly or kinky. A permanent flattens the hair to make it curly.

A bundle of smooth muscle cells, called the **arrector pili** (ah-REK-tor PY-lee) muscle, is associated with each hair follicle. Most hair follicles are at a slight angle to the surface of the skin. The arrector pili muscles are attached to the hair follicles in such a way that contraction pulls the hair follicles into an upright position or causes the hair to "stand on end." Contraction of the arrector pili muscles also causes raised areas on the skin, or "goose bumps." Action of the arrector pili muscles is controlled by the nervous system in response to cold and fright.

> Arrector pili muscles, smooth muscles associated with hair, contract in response to cold and fear.

Nails

Nails are thin plates of dead stratum corneum that contain a very hard type of keratin and cover the dorsal surfaces of the distal ends of the fingers and toes (Fig. 5–4). Each nail has a **free edge;** a **nail body,** which is the visible portion; and a **nail root,** which is covered with skin. The **eponychium** (eh-poh-NICK-ee-um) or **cuticle** is a fold of stratum corneum that grows onto the proximal portion of the

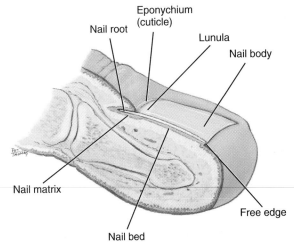

Eponychium (cuticle)

Nail root

Lunula

Nail body

Nail matrix

Free edge

Nail bed

Figure 5–4   Structure of nails. (From Jarvis C: Physical Examination and Health Assessment. Philadelphia, WB Saunders, 1992.)

nail body. Stratum basale from the epidermis grows under the nail body to form the **nail bed.** This is thickened at the proximal end to form the **nail matrix,** which is responsible for nail growth. As cells are produced by the matrix, they become keratinized and slide over the nail bed. The portion of the body over the matrix appears as a whitish, crescent-shaped area called the **lunula** (LOO-nyoo-lah). Nails appear pink because of the rich supply of blood vessels in the underlying dermis.

> Nails are thin plates of keratinized stratum corneum. They are derived from the stratum basale in the nail bed.

Glands

The two major glands associated with the skin are the **sebaceous** (see-BAY-shus) **glands** and the **sweat glands.** A third type, the **ceruminous** (see-ROOM-ih-nus) **glands,** are modified sweat glands.

Sebaceous Glands

Generally, sebaceous glands are associated with hair follicles and are found in all areas of the body that have hair (see Figs. 5–1 and 5–3). Those not associated with hair follicles open directly onto the surface of the skin. Functionally, they are holocrine glands, which means that the glandular cells are destroyed and released along with the secretory product. The oily secretion, called **sebum,** is transported by a duct into a hair follicle, and from there it reaches the surface of the skin. Sebum functions to keep hair and skin soft and pliable. It also inhibits growth of bacteria on the skin and helps to prevent water loss. Secretory activity of the sebaceous glands is stimulated by sex hormones so that the glands are relatively inactive in childhood, become highly active during puberty, and decrease in activity during old age. Decreased sebum, in part, accounts for the dry skin and brittle hair that are common in older people.

> Sebaceous glands are oil glands and are associated with hair follicles. They secrete sebum to keep hair and skin soft and pliable. Sebum also helps prevent fluid loss.

Acne is a problem that plagues many teenagers. Increased hormone activity at puberty causes an increase in sebaceous gland activity. Sebum and dead cells may block the hair follicle and form blackheads. Bacteria infect the blocked follicle, and the sebum/dead cell mixture accumulates until the follicle ruptures. This initiates an inflammatory response that soon appears on the surface as a pus-filled pimple.

Sweat (Sudoriferous) Glands

Sweat glands, also called **sudoriferous** (soo-door-IF-er-us) **glands,** are widely distributed over the body, except for the lips, nipples, and parts of the external genitalia. They are most numerous in the palms and soles. It is estimated that an individual has more than 2.5 million sweat glands.

Merocrine sweat glands are the more numerous and more widely distributed of the two types of sweat glands. The glandular portion is a coiled tube that is embedded in the dermis of the skin, and the duct opens onto the surface of the skin through a **sweat pore** (see Fig. 5–1). The secretion of these glands is primarily water with a few salts. When temperature increases, the glands are stimulated to produce sweat, which evaporates and has a cooling effect. Sweat, or **perspiration,** is also produced in response to nerve stimulation as a result of emotional stress.

> Merocrine sweat glands open to the surface of the skin through sweat pores.

Apocrine sweat glands are larger than the merocrine glands, and their distribution is limited to the axillae and external genitalia. Their ducts open into the hair follicles in these regions. The secretion consists of water and salts and also contains organic compounds such as fatty acids and proteins. These glands become active at puberty and are stimulated by the nervous system in response to pain, emotional stress, and sexual arousal. The secretion is odorless when released but is quickly broken down by bacteria to cause what is known as body odor.

> Apocrine sweat glands, limited to the axillae and external genitalia, open into hair follicles.

Ceruminous Glands

Ceruminous glands are modified sweat glands that are found in the external auditory (ear) canal. They secrete an oily, sticky substance called **cerumen** (see-ROOM-men), or earwax, that is thought to repel insects and trap foreign material.

 QuickCheck

- Hair and nails are derived from which layer of the epidermis?

- Which type of sweat gland is most widely distributed?

Functions of the Skin

Protection

The skin forms a protective covering over the entire body. The keratin in the cells waterproofs the cells and helps prevent fluid loss from the body. This waterproofing also prevents too much water from entering the body during swimming and bathing. Unbroken skin forms the first line of defense against bacteria and other invading organisms. The oily secretions of the sebaceous glands are acidic and inhibit bacterial growth on the skin. Melanin pigment absorbs light and helps protect underlying tissues from the damaging effects of ultraviolet light. Skin also protects underlying tissues from mechanical, chemical, and thermal injury.

> The skin protects against water loss, ultraviolet light, invading organisms, and other injuries.

Sensory Reception

The dermis contains numerous sense receptors for heat, cold, pain, touch, and pressure. Even though hair itself has no sense receptors, the movement of hair can be detected by receptors clustered around a hair follicle. The sense receptors in the dermis relay information about the environment to the brain so that changes can be made to prevent or minimize injury. The sense receptors are also a means of communication between individuals.

> Sense receptors in the skin detect information about the environment and also serve as a means of communication between individuals.

Regulation of Body Temperature

Normally, body temperature is maintained at 37°C (98.6°F). It is important that body temperature be regulated because changes in temperature alter the speed of chemical reactions in the body. About 40 percent of the energy in a glucose molecule is stored in the bonds of adenosine triphosphate (ATP) to be used by the cells. The remaining 60 percent of the energy is heat to maintain body temperature. Often this amount is more than is necessary to maintain body temperature, and the excess heat must be removed from the body. The skin has two ways that it helps to regulate body temperature: by dilation and constriction of blood vessels, and by activity or inactivity of the sweat glands. Both of these mechanisms are examples of negative feedback in maintaining homeostasis. The role of the skin in temperature regulation is summarized in Figure 5–5. The adipose tissue in the subcutaneous layer also helps by acting as an insulator.

> People who lose weight rapidly may feel cold because they have reduced their adipose insulation.

When there is excess heat in the body, and body temperature rises above normal, the small arteries in the dermis dilate to increase blood flow through the skin. This brings the heat from the deeper tissues to the surface so that it can escape into the surrounding air. Sweat glands become active in response to increased temperature. Moisture, in the form of sweat, accumulates on the surface of the skin and then evaporates to provide cooling.

If body temperature falls below normal, the sweat glands are inactive and the blood vessels in the skin constrict to reduce blood flow. Constriction of the blood vessels reduces the amount of heat transferred

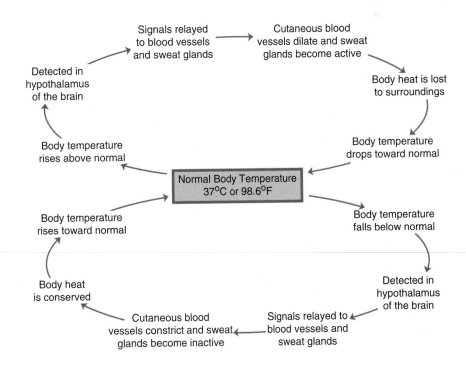

Figure 5-5 Role of skin in temperature regulation.

from the deeper tissues to the surface. However, if the skin becomes too cold, below 15°C (59°F), cutaneous blood vessels dilate to bring warm blood to the region so that the tissues are not damaged by the cold.

> The skin helps to regulate body temperature through constriction and dilation of blood vessels, sweat gland activity, and the insulating effect of adipose tissue in the subcutaneous layer.

Synthesis of Vitamin D

Vitamin D is required for calcium and phosphorus absorption in the small intestine. The calcium and phosphorus are essential for normal bone metabolism and muscle function. Skin cells contain a precursor molecule that is converted to vitamin D when

the precursor is exposed to ultraviolet rays in sunlight. It takes only a small amount of ultraviolet light to stimulate vitamin D production, so this should not be used as an excuse to expose the skin to sun unnecessarily and to risk the damage that may result.

> Vitamin D is synthesized in the skin when exposed to ultraviolet light.

 QuickCheck

- Why are infections and fluid loss of major concern for patients with severe burns?

- Jake is playing a vigorous game of volleyball on a warm summer day. Describe two ways the integument helps maintain internal body temperature in spite of the heat and exercise.

 ## FOCUS ON AGING

As the skin ages, the number of elastic fibers decreases and adipose tissue is lost from the dermis and subcutaneous layer. This causes the skin to wrinkle and sag. Loss of collagen fibers in the dermis makes the skin more fragile and makes it heal more slowly. Mitotic activity in the stratum basale slows so that the skin becomes thinner and appears more transparent. Reduced sebaceous gland activity causes dry, itchy skin. Loss of adipose tissue in the subcutaneous layer and reduced sweat gland activity lead to an intolerance of cold and susceptibility to heat. The ability of the skin to regulate temperature is reduced. There is a general reduction in melanocyte activity, which decreases pro-

tection from ultraviolet light, resulting in increased susceptibility to sunburn and skin cancer. Some melanocytes, however, may increase melanin production, resulting in "age spots."

Despite all the creams and "miracle" lotions, there is no known way to prevent skin from aging. Good nutrition and cleanliness may slow the aging process. Because skin that is exposed to sunlight ages more rapidly than unexposed skin, one of the best ways to slow the aging process is to avoid exposure by wearing protective clothing and by using sun blocks whenever possible.

DO YOU KNOW THIS ABOUT

Integument?

Burns

A burn is tissue damage that results from heat, certain chemicals, radiation, or electricity. The seriousness of burns is a result of their effect on the skin. The most serious threat to survival after a severe burn is fluid loss because the waterproof protective covering, the skin, is destroyed. As fluid seeps from the burned surfaces, electrolytes and proteins are also lost. The loss of fluids, electrolytes, and proteins leads to osmotic imbalances, renal failure, and circulatory shock. Another problem is the imminent danger of massive infection. A large, severely burned region is bac-

teria "heaven" because there is easy access, ideal growing conditions, and no attack by the immune system. Bacteria have easy access to tissues because the protective barrier provided by the skin is absent. The protein-rich fluid that seeps from burned areas is an ideal growth medium for bacteria, fungi, and other pathogens. Finally, the body's immune system, which normally fights off threats of disease, becomes exhausted within 2 or 3 days after a severe burn injury.

Burns are classified as first, second, or third degree according to their severity or depth. **First-**

degree burns damage only the epidermis. They appear red, there may be some swelling, and they are somewhat painful. Some portion of the stratum basale remains intact, and regeneration occurs within a few days. A sunburn is usually a first-degree burn.

Second-degree burns involve damage to the epidermis and a portion of the dermis. These also appear red, with some swelling, and are painful. In addition, excessive fluid accumulates between the dermis and the epidermis to form blisters. If the burn extends only to the upper portion of the dermis, scar tissue is not likely to form in the healing process. If the burn reaches the lower region of the dermis, scar tissue is likely to develop. In second-degree burns, the epithelium regenerates from the edges of the wound and from the stratum basale in the hair follicles. Both first- and second-degree burns are sometimes referred to as partial-thickness burns.

Third-degree burns are full-thickness burns. The epidermis and dermis are destroyed, and the burn extends into the subcutaneous tissue or below. The area appears white or charred and there is little or no edema. Because the nerve endings in the dermis are destroyed, there is no pain. However, the surrounding area, which probably has received first- and second-degree burns, may be painful. Third-degree burns are serious and require skilled medical treatment because of the problems associated with fluid loss and infection. Skin grafts are necessary to protect the area while healing takes place. Repair involves the formation of scar tissue. The epithelium may regenerate from the stratum basale at the edges of the wound, but this is a slow process, especially if the injury is extensive.

The treatment of burns depends on their severity and on the amount of surface area that is damaged. For this reason, it is helpful to be able to estimate quickly the amount of surface area that is burned. One easy method for making a quick estimate is called the **rule of nines.** In this method (Fig. 5–6), each body region constitutes a percentage of the total that is some multiple of nine. Each upper extremity is 9 percent of the total body surface area; each lower limb is 18 percent; the anterior and posterior trunk regions are each 18 percent; the head and neck together make up 9 percent; and the perineum has the final 1 percent.

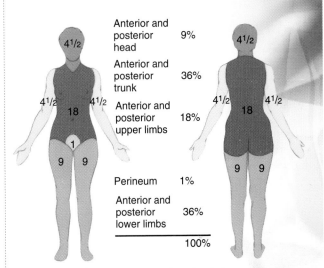

Anterior and posterior head	9%
Anterior and posterior trunk	36%
Anterior and posterior upper limbs	18%
Perineum	1%
Anterior and posterior lower limbs	36%
	100%

Figure 5–6 Illustration of the rule of nines.

Representative Disorders of the Integumentary System

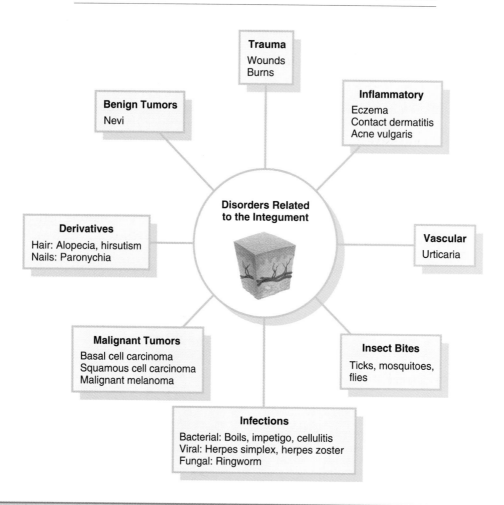

Trauma
Wounds
Burns

Inflammatory
Eczema
Contact dermatitis
Acne vulgaris

Benign Tumors
Nevi

Derivatives
Hair: Alopecia, hirsutism
Nails: Paronychia

**Disorders Related
to the Integument**

Vascular
Urticaria

Malignant Tumors
Basal cell carcinoma
Squamous cell carcinoma
Malignant melanoma

Insect Bites
Ticks, mosquitoes,
flies

Infections
Bacterial: Boils, impetigo, cellulitis
Viral: Herpes simplex, herpes zoster
Fungal: Ringworm

CHAPTER 5 QUIZ

RECALL

Match the definitions on the left with the appropriate term on the right.

1. Cells that produce a dark pigment

2. Outermost layer of the skin

3. Actively mitotic layer of the epidermis

4. Subcutaneous layer

5. Visible portion of hair

6. Cuticle of fingernail

7. Glands that open into hair follicles

8. Muscle attached to hair follicles

9. Tough, water repellant protein in epidermis

10. Upper layer of the dermis

A. Apocrine sweat
   glands

B. Arrector pili

C. Eponychium

D. Hair shaft

E. Hypodermis

F. Keratin

G. Melanocytes

H. Papillary layer

I. Stratum basale

J. Stratum corneum

THOUGHT

1. Sandy Shore was walking barefoot along the beach when she stepped on a broken shell and cut her foot. The sequence in which the shell penetrated her foot was

   a. stratum corneum, stratum lucidum, stratum granulosum, stratum spinosum, stratum basale, stratum corium

   b. stratum corium, stratum corneum, stratum basale, stratum granulosum, stratum spinosum, stratum lucidum

   c. stratum corium, stratum granulosum, stratum lucidum, stratum spinosum, stratum basale, stratum corneum

   d. stratum corneum, stratum granulosum, stratum spinosum, stratum lucidum, stratum basale, stratum corium

2. The layer of skin that is responsible for fingerprints and footprints is the

   a. stratum corneum

   b. stratum granulosum

   c. reticular layer of dermis

   d. papillary layer of dermis

3. Receptors for the sensation of touch are located in the

   a. stratum corneum

   b. stratum basale

   c. dermis

   d. hypodermis

4. In response to warm temperature,

   a. cutaneous blood vessels dilate and sweat glands become active

   b. cutaneous blood vessels dilate and sweat glands become inactive

   c. cutaneous blood vessels constrict and sweat glands become active

   d. cutaneous blood vessels constrict and sweat glands become inactive

5. Why are infants and the elderly more susceptible to temperature changes than other people?

   a. they have fewer sweat glands to carry away heat

   b. they have less adipose in the subcutaneous tissue for insulation

   c. they have fewer sebaceous glands to form sebum for insulation

   d. their blood vessels don't dilate and constrict as readily

APPLICATION

Joyce is scheduled for surgery and is concerned about the scar that may result. Her surgeon explains that scarring will be minimal because the incision will be parallel to cleavage lines. Explain this so she will understand.

CHAPTER 6

Skeletal System

Outline/Objectives

Overview of the Skeletal System 91
- Discuss five functions of the skeletal system.
- Distinguish between compact and spongy bone on the basis of structural features.
- Classify bones according to size and shape, and identify the general features of a long bone.
- Discuss the processes by which bones develop and grow.
- Distinguish between the axial and appendicular skeletons, and state the number of bones in each.

Bones of the Axial Skeleton 97
- Identify the bones of the skull and their important surface markings.
- Identify the general structural features of vertebrae and compare cervical, thoracic, lumbar, sacral, and coccygeal vertebrae; state the number of each type.
- Identify the structural features of the ribs and sternum.

Bones of the Appendicular Skeleton 106
- Identify the features of the pectoral girdle and upper extremity.
- Identify the features of the pelvic girdle and lower extremity.

Articulations 114
- Compare the structure and function of three types of joints.

Key Terms

Amphiarthrosis

Diaphysis

Diarthrosis

Endochondral ossification

Epiphyseal plate

Epiphysis

Intramembranous ossification

Osteoblast

Osteoclast

Osteocyte

Osteon

Synarthrosis

Building Vocabulary

WORD PART	MEANING
acetabul-	little cup
appendicul-	little attachment
artic-	joint
arthr-	joint
-blast	to form, sprout
burs-	pouch
-clast-	to break
corac-	beak
cribr-	sieve
crist-	crest, ridge
ethm-	sieve
-fic-	make
kyph-	hump
odont-	tooth
-oid	like, resembling
oste-, oss-	bone
-poie-	making
syn-	together
sphen-	wedge
-tion	act or process of

Functional Relationships of the
Skeletal System

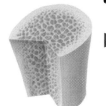

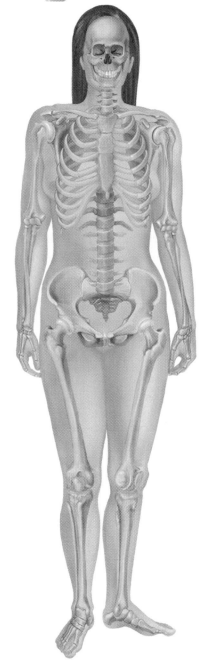

▶ Provides mechanical support.

Integument
◀ Provides barrier against harmful substances; synthesis of vitamin D for absorption of calcium necessary for bone growth, maintenance, and repair.

▶ Bones close to surface give shape to skin.

Muscular
◀ Stabilizes position of bones; tension from muscle contraction influences bone shape and size.

▶ Provides attachment sites for muscles; bones act as levers for muscle action; stores calcium necessary for muscle contraction.

Nervous
◀ Interprets impulses relating to pain and position from receptors in bones and joints.

▶ Surrounds brain and spinal cord for protection; stores calcium necessary for neural function.

Endocrine
◀ Hormones from the pituitary, thyroid, and gonads influence bone growth; calcitonin and parathyroid hormone regulate calcium uptake and release from bones.

▶ Protects glands in the head, thorax, and pelvis.

Cardiovascular
◀ Supplies oxygen and nutrients for bone tissue metabolism and removes metabolic wastes from bone.

▶ Produces blood cells in bone marrow and supplies calcium necessary for cardiac muscle contraction and blood clotting.

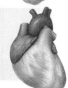

Lymphatic/Immune
◀ Maintains interstitial fluid balance in bone tissue; assists in defense against pathogens and repair of bone tissue following trauma.

▶ Cells of immune response are produced and stored in bone marrow.

Respiratory
◀ Supplies oxygen for bone tissue metabolism and removes carbon dioxide.

▶ Encases the lungs for protection; provides passageways for air through nasal cavity.

Digestive
◀ Absorbs nutrients, including calcium, for bone growth, maintenance, and repair.

▶ Provides protection for portions of the digestive tract and liver.

Urinary
◀ Eliminates metabolic wastes; conserves calcium and phosphate ions for bone growth, maintenance, and repair.

▶ Supports and protects organs of the urinary system.

Reproductive
◀ Gonads produce hormones that influence bone growth, maintenance, and closure of epiphyseal plates.

▶ Provides protection for reproductive organs in the pelvis.

The skeletal system consists of the bones and the cartilages, ligaments, and tendons associated with the bones. It accounts for about 20 percent of the body weight. Bones are rigid structures that form the framework for the body. People often think of bones as dead, dry, inert pipes and plates because that is how they are seen in the laboratory. In reality, the living bones in our bodies contain active tissues that consume nutrients, require a blood supply, use oxygen and give off waste products in metabolism, and change shape or remodel in response to variations in mechanical stress. The skeletal system is strong but lightweight. It is well adapted for the functions it must perform. It is a masterpiece of design.

▌ Bones are living, dynamic tissue.

Overview of the Skeletal System

Functions of the Skeletal System

The skeletal system gives form and shape to the body. Without the skeletal components, we would appear as big "blobs" inefficiently "oozing" around on the ground. Besides contributing to shape and form, our bones perform several other functions and play an important role in homeostasis.

Support

Bones provide a rigid framework that supports the soft organs of the body. Bones support the body against the pull of gravity, and the large bones of the lower limbs support the trunk when standing.

Protection

The skeleton protects the soft body parts. The fused bones of the cranium surround the brain to make it less vulnerable to injury. The vertebrae surround and protect the spinal cord. The bones of the rib cage help protect the heart and lungs in the thorax.

Movement

Bones provide sites for muscle attachment. Bones and muscles work together as simple mechanical lever systems to produce body movement. A mechanical lever system has four components: (1) a rigid bar, (2) a pivot or fulcrum, (3) an object or weight that is moved, and (4) a force that supplies the mechanical energy for the movement. In the body, bones are the rigid bars, the joints between the bones are the pivots, the body or a part of it is the weight that is moved, and the muscles supply the force.

CLINICAL TERMS

Arthritis (ahr-THRYE-tis) Inflammation of a joint

Bunion (BUN-yun) Abnormal swelling of the joint between the big toe and the first metatarsal bone, resulting from a buildup of soft tissues and bone caused by chronic irritation from ill-fitting shoes

Carpal tunnel syndrome (KAHR-pull TUH-nul SIN-drohm) Condition characterized by pain and burning sensations in the fingers and hand, caused by compression of the median nerve as it passes between a wrist ligament and the bones and tendons of the wrist

Dislocation (dis-loh-KAY-shun) Displacement of a bone from its joint with tearing of ligaments, tendons, and articular capsule; also called luxation

Gout (GOWT) A form of acute arthritis in which uric acid crystals develop within a joint and irritate the cartilage, causing acute inflammation, swelling, and pain; most commonly occurs in middle-aged and older men

Lyme disease (LYME dih-ZEEZ) A bacterial disease transmitted to humans by deer ticks; characterized by joint stiffness, headache, fever and chills, nausea, and back pain; complications include severe arthritis and cardiac problems; early stages of the disease respond well to antibiotics

Osteomalacia (ahs-tee-oh-mah-LAY-shee-ah) Softening of bone because of inadequate amounts of calcium and phosphorus; bones bend easily and become deformed; in childhood this is called rickets

Osteomyelitis (ahs-tee-oh-my-eh-LYE-tis) Inflammation of the bone marrow caused by bacteria

Osteoporosis (ahs-tee-oh-por-OH-sis) Decrease in bone density and mass; commonly occurs in postmenopausal women as a result of increased osteoclast activity due to diminished estrogen; bones fracture easily

Osteosarcoma (ahs-tee-oh-sahr-KOH-mah) Malignant tumor derived from bone; also called osteogenic sarcoma; osteoblasts multiply without control and form large tumors in bone

Sprain (SPRAYN) Twisting of a joint with pain, swelling, and injury to ligaments, tendons, muscles, blood vessels, and nerves; most often occurs in the ankle; more serious than a strain, which is the overstretching of the muscles associated with a joint

Talipes (TAL-ih-peez) Congenital deformity of the foot in which the patient cannot stand with the sole of the foot flat on the ground; clubfoot

Storage

The intercellular matrix of bone contains large amounts of calcium salts, the most important being calcium phosphate. Calcium is necessary for vital metabolic processes. When blood calcium levels decrease below normal, calcium is released from the bones so that there will be an adequate supply for metabolic needs. When blood calcium levels are increased, the excess calcium is stored in the bone matrix. Storage and release are dynamic processes that go on almost continually.

Bone tissue contains lesser amounts of other inorganic ions such as sodium, magnesium, potassium, and carbonate. Fat is stored in the yellow bone marrow.

Blood Cell Formation

Blood cell formation, called **hematopoiesis** (hee-mat-oh-poy-EE-sis), takes place mostly in the red marrow of bones. Red marrow is found in the cavities of most bones in an infant. With age, it is largely replaced by yellow marrow for fat storage. In the adult, red marrow is limited to the spongy bone in the skull, ribs, sternum, clavicles, vertebrae, and pelvis. Red marrow functions in the formation of red blood cells, white blood cells, and blood platelets.

> Functions of bones include support, protection, movement, mineral storage, and formation of blood cells.

Structure of Bone Tissue

There are two types of bone tissue: compact and spongy. The names imply that the two types differ in density, or how tightly the tissue is packed together. There are three types of cells that contribute to bone homeostasis. Osteoblasts are bone-forming cells, osteoclasts resorb or break down bone, and osteocytes are mature bone cells. An equilibrium between osteoblasts and osteoclasts maintains bone tissue.

Compact Bone

The microscopic unit of compact bone, the osteon (haversian system), was described in Chapter 4. Briefly, the osteon consists of a central canal called the osteonic (haversian) canal that is surrounded by concentric rings (lamellae) of matrix. Between the rings of matrix, the bone cells (osteocytes) are located in spaces called lacunae. Small channels (canaliculi) radiate from the lacunae to the osteonic (haversian) canal to provide passageways through the hard matrix. In compact bone the haversian systems are packed tightly together to form what appears to be a solid mass. The osteonic canals contain blood vessels that are parallel to the long axis of the bone. These blood vessels interconnect, by way of perforating (Volkmann's) canals, with vessels on the surface of the bone. The microscopic structure of compact bone is illustrated in Figure 6–1.

> Compact bone consists of closely packed osteons, or haversian systems.

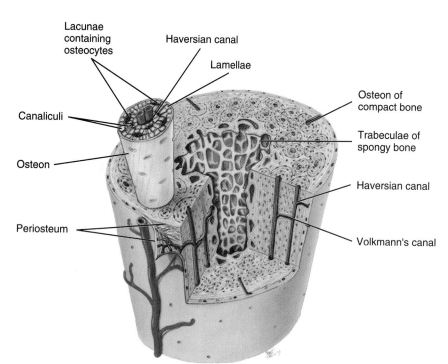

Figure 6–1 Structure of compact and spongy bone.

Spongy (Cancellous) Bone

Spongy (cancellous) bone is lighter and less dense than compact bone (see Fig. 6–1). Spongy bone consists of plates and bars of bone adjacent to small, irregular cavities that contain red bone marrow. The plates of bone are called **trabeculae** (trah-BEK-yoo-lee). The canaliculi, instead of connecting to a central haversian canal, connect to the adjacent cavities to receive their blood supply. It may appear that the trabeculae are arranged in a haphazard manner, but they are organized to provide maximum strength much as braces are used to support a building. The trabeculae of spongy bone follow the lines of stress and can realign if the direction of stress changes.

> Spongy bone consists of plates of bone, called trabeculae, around irregular spaces that contain red bone marrow.

Classification of Bones

Bones come in a variety of sizes and shapes. Bones that are longer than they are wide are called long bones. They consist of a long shaft with two bulky ends or extremities. They are primarily compact bone but may have a large amount of spongy bone at the ends. Examples of long bones are those in the thigh, leg, arm, and forearm.

Short bones are roughly cube shaped with vertical and horizontal dimensions approximately equal. They consist primarily of spongy bone, which is covered by a thin layer of compact bone. Examples of short bones include the bones of the wrist and ankle.

Flat bones are thin, flattened, and usually curved. They are usually made like a sandwich with a middle layer of spongy bone called the **diploë** (DIP-loh-ee). The diploë is covered on each side by a layer of compact bone; these layers are called the **inner** and **outer tables.** Most of the bones of the cranium are flat bones.

Bones that are not in any of the above three categories are classified as irregular bones. They are primarily spongy bone that is covered with a thin layer of compact bone. The vertebrae and some of the bones in the skull are irregular bones.

> Bones may be classified as long, short, flat, or irregular.

General Features of a Long Bone

Most long bones have the same general features, which are illustrated in Figure 6–2.

The shaft of a long bone is called the **diaphysis** (dye-AF-ih-sis). It is formed from relatively thick compact bone that surrounds a hollow space called the **medullary** (MED-yoo-lair-ee) **cavity.** In adults, the medullary cavity contains yellow bone marrow so it is sometimes called the yellow marrow cavity.

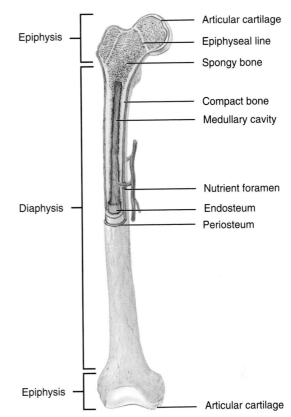

Figure 6–2   General features of long bones.

At each end of the diaphysis, there is an expanded portion called the **epiphysis** (ee-PIF-ih-sis). The epiphysis is spongy bone covered by a thin layer of compact bone. The end of the epiphysis, where it meets another bone, is covered by hyaline cartilage, called the **articular cartilage.** This provides smooth surfaces for movement in the joints. In growing bones, there is an **epiphyseal** (ep-ih-FIZ-ee-al) **plate** of hyaline cartilage between the diaphysis and epiphysis. Bones grow in length at the epiphyseal plate. Growth ceases when the cartilaginous epiphyseal plate is replaced by a bony **epiphyseal line.** Except in the region of the articular cartilage, the outer surface of long bones is covered by a tough, fibrous connective tissue membrane called the **periosteum.** The periosteum is richly supplied with nerve fibers, lymphatic vessels, blood vessels, and osteoblasts. The blood vessels enter the diaphysis of the bone through small openings called **nutrient foramina.** The surface of the medullary cavity is lined with a thinner connective tissue membrane, the **endosteum,** which contains osteoclasts.

> The diaphysis of a long bone is the central shaft. There is an epiphysis at each end of the diaphysis.

In addition to the general features that are present in most long bones, all bones have surface markings and characteristics that make a specific bone unique. There are holes, depressions, smooth facets, lines, projections, and other markings. These usually represent passageways for vessels and nerves, points of articulation with other bones, or points of attachment for tendons and ligaments. Some of the bony markings are described in Table 6–1.

Bone Development and Growth

The terms **osteogenesis** and **ossification** are often used synonymously to indicate the process of bone formation. Parts of the skeleton form during the first few weeks after conception. By the end of the eighth week after conception, the skeletal pattern is formed in cartilage and connective tissue membranes, and ossification begins. Bone development continues throughout adulthood. Even after adult stature is attained, bone development continues for repair of fractures and for remodeling to meet changing lifestyles. Three types of cells are involved in the devel-

opment, growth, and remodeling of bones. **Osteoblasts** are bone-forming cells; **osteocytes** are mature bone cells; and **osteoclasts** break down and reabsorb bone.

> Osteoporosis is a common bone disorder due to decreased osteoblast activity. It is characterized by loss of the organic matrix, collagenous fibers, and minerals in the bone tissue. People with osteoporosis are susceptible to deformities of the vertebral column and fractures because the bones are not strong enough to support the weight of the body. Osteoporosis occurs most frequently in postmenopausal Caucasian women. Factors that influence its occurrence are aging, malnutrition, lack of exercise, and hormone imbalance. Supplemental estrogen after menopause may be of benefit, and exercise is always important in maintaining bone strength.

Table 6–1 Terms Related to Bone Markings

Term	Description	Examples
Projections for Articulation		
Condyle (KON-dial)	Smooth, rounded articular surface	Occipital condyle on the occipital bone; lateral and medial condyles on the femur
Facet (FASS-et)	Smooth, nearly flat articular surface	Facets on thoracic vertebrae for articulation with ribs
Head (HED)	Enlarged, often rounded, end of bone	Head of the humerus; head of the femur
Projections for Muscle Attachment		
Crest (KREST)	Narrow ridge of bone	Iliac crest on the ilium
Epicondyle (ep-ih-KON-dial)	Bony bulge adjacent to or above a condyle	Lateral and medial epicondyles of the femur
Process (PRAH-sess)	Any projection on a bone; often pointed and sharp	Styloid process on the temporal bone
Spine (SPYN)	Sharp, slender projection	Spine of the scapula
Trochanter (tro-KAN-turr)	Large, blunt, irregularly shaped projection	Greater and lesser trochanters on the femur
Tubercle (TOO-burr-kul)	Small, rounded, knoblike projection	Greater tubercle of the humerus
Tuberosity (too-burr-AHS-ih-tee)	Similar to a tubercle, but usually larger	Tibial tuberosity on the tibia
Depressions, Openings, and Cavities		
Fissure (FISH-ur)	Narrow cleft or slit; usually for passage of blood vessels and nerves	Superior orbital fissure
Foramen (foh-RAY-men)	Opening through a bone; usually for passage of blood vessels and nerves	Foramen magnum in the occipital bone
Fossa (FAW-sah)	A smooth, shallow depression	Mandibular fossa on the temporal bone; olecranon fossa on the humerus
Fovea (FOH-vee-ah)	A small pit or depression	Fovea capitis femoris on the head of the femur
Meatus (canal) (mee-ATE-us)	A tubelike passageway; tunnel	External auditory meatus in the temporal bone
Sinus (SYE-nus)	A cavity or hollow space in a bone	Frontal sinus in the frontal bone

Osteogenesis is the process of bone formation. Three types of cells, osteoblasts, osteocytes, and osteoclasts, are involved in bone formation and remodeling.

Intramembranous Ossification

Intramembranous ossification (in-tra-MEM-bran-us ah-sih-fih-KAY-shun) involves the replacement of sheetlike connective tissue membranes with bony tissue. Bones formed in this manner are called **intramembranous bones.** They include certain flat bones of the skull and some of the irregular bones. The future bones are first formed as connective tissue membranes. Osteoblasts migrate to the membranes and deposit bony matrix around themselves. When the osteoblasts are surrounded by matrix they are called osteocytes.

In intramembranous ossification, connective tissue membranes are replaced by bone. This process occurs in the flat bones of the skull.

Endochondral Ossification

Endochondral ossification (en-doh-KON-dral ah-sih-fih-KAY-shun) involves the replacement of hyaline cartilage with bony tissue. Most of the bones of the skeleton are formed in this manner and are called **endochondral bones.** In this process, illustrated in Figure 6–3, the future bones are first formed as hyaline cartilage models. During the third month after conception, the perichondrium that surrounds the hyaline cartilage "models" becomes infiltrated with blood vessels and osteoblasts and changes into a periosteum. The osteoblasts form a collar of compact bone around the diaphysis. At the same time,

the cartilage in the center of the diaphysis begins to disintegrate. Osteoblasts penetrate the disintegrating cartilage and replace it with spongy bone. This forms a **primary ossification center.** Ossification continues from this center toward the ends of the bones. After spongy bone is formed in the diaphysis, osteoclasts break down the newly formed bone to open up the medullary cavity.

The cartilage in the epiphyses continues to grow so the developing bone increases in length. Later, usually after birth, **secondary ossification centers** form in the epiphyses. Ossification in the epiphyses is similar to that in the diaphysis except that the spongy bone is retained instead of being broken down to form a medullary cavity. When secondary ossification is complete, the hyaline cartilage is totally replaced by bone except in two areas. A region of hyaline cartilage remains over the surface of the epiphysis as the **articular cartilage.** Another area of cartilage remains between the epiphysis and diaphysis. This is the **epiphyseal plate** or growth region.

In endochondral ossification, bone tissue replaces hyaline cartilage models. Most bones are formed in this manner.

Bone Growth

Bones grow in length at the epiphyseal plate by a process that is similar, in many ways, to endochondral ossification. The cartilage in the region of the epiphyseal plate next to the epiphysis continues to grow by mitosis. The chondrocytes in the region next to the diaphysis age and degenerate. Osteoblasts move in and ossify the matrix to form bone. This process continues throughout childhood and the adolescent years until the cartilage growth slows

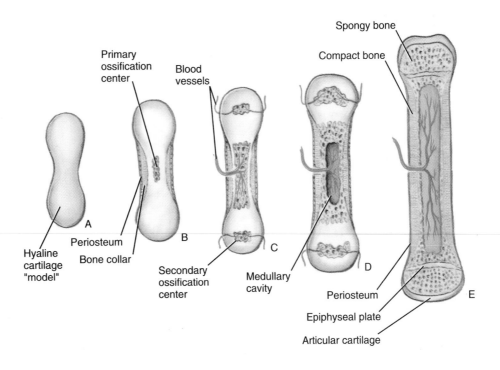

Figure 6–3 Events in endochondral ossification.

and finally stops. When cartilage growth ceases, usually in the early 20s, the epiphyseal plate completely ossifies so that only a thin **epiphyseal line** remains and the bones can no longer grow in length. Bone growth is under the influence of growth hormone from the anterior pituitary gland and sex hormones from the ovaries and testes.

> Bones grow in length at the epiphyseal plate between the diaphysis and the epiphysis. When the epiphyseal plate completely ossifies, bones no longer increase in length.

> The epiphyseal plates of specific long bones ossify at predictable times. Radiologists frequently can determine a young person's age by examining the epiphyseal plates to see whether they have ossified. A difference between bone age and chronologic age may indicate some type of metabolic dysfunction.

Even though bones stop growing in length in early adulthood, they can continue to increase in thickness or diameter throughout life in response to stress from increased muscle activity or to weight. The increase in diameter is called **appositional (ap-poh-ZISH-un-al) growth.** Osteoblasts in the periosteum form compact bone around the external bone surface. At the same time, osteoclasts in the endosteum break down bone on the internal bone surface, around the medullary cavity. These two processes together increase the diameter of the bone and, at the same time, keep the bone from becoming excessively heavy and bulky.

> Osteoblasts and osteoclasts work together to increase the diameter of bones. This is called appositional growth.

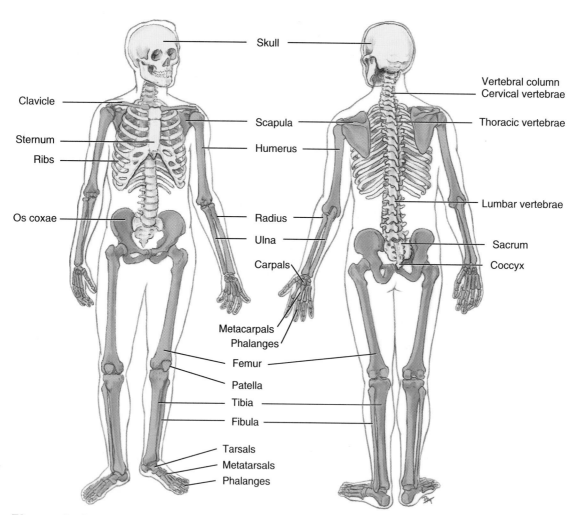

Figure 6–4 Divisions of the skeleton with major bones identified.

✓ QuickCheck

- What type of bone tissue is predominant in the diaphysis of a long bone?
- How does appositional growth differ from growth at the epiphyseal plate?

Divisions of the Skeleton

The adult human skeleton usually consists of 206 named bones. In addition to the named bones, there are two other types that vary in number from one individual to another and do not have specific names. **Wormian** (WER-mee-an) **bones** or **sutural** (SOO-cher-ahl) **bones** are small bones in the joints between certain cranial bones. **Sesamoid** (SEH-sah-moyd) **bones** are small bones that grow in certain tendons in which there is considerable pressure. The **patella**, or kneecap, is an example of a sesamoid bone that is named, but other sesamoid bones are not named.

For convenience, the bones of the skeleton are grouped in two divisions, as illustrated in Figure 6–4. The 80 bones of the **axial skeleton** form the vertical axis of the body. They include the bones of the head, vertebral column, ribs, and breastbone or sternum. The **appendicular skeleton** consists of 126 bones and includes the free appendages and their attachments to the axial skeleton. The free appendages are the upper and lower extremities, or limbs, and their attachments are called girdles. The named bones of the body are listed by category in Table 6–2.

> There are 206 named bones in the adult human skeleton. The axial skeleton, with 80 bones, forms the axis of the body and consists of the head, vertebrae, ribs, and sternum. The appendicular skeleton, with 126 bones, consists of the appendages and their attachments.

Bones of the Axial Skeleton

The axial skeleton, with 80 bones, is divided into the skull, hyoid, vertebral column, and rib cage.

> An articulation, or joint, is the place of junction between two or more bones of the skeleton.

Skull

There are 28 bones in the skull, illustrated in Figures 6–5 through 6–9. Eight of these form the cranium, which houses the brain. The anterior aspect of the skull, the face, consists of 14 bones. The remaining six bones are the auditory ossicles, tiny bones in the middle ear cavity. With the exception of the lower jaw, or mandible, and the auditory ossicles, the

Table 6–2 Named Bones of the Body Listed by Category

Bones	Number
Axial Skeleton (80 bones)	
Skull (28 bones)	
Cranial bones	8
Parietal (2)	
Temporal (2)	
Frontal (1)	
Occipital (1)	
Ethmoid (1)	
Sphenoid (1)	
Facial bones	14
Maxilla (2)	
Zygomatic (2)	
Mandible (1)	
Nasal (2)	
Palatine (2)	
Inferior nasal concha (2)	
Lacrimal (2)	
Vomer (1)	
Auditory ossicles	6
Malleus (2)	
Incus (2)	
Stapes (2)	
Hyoid	1
Vertebral column	26
Cervical vertebrae (7)	
Thoracic vertebrae (12)	
Lumbar vertebrae (5)	
Sacrum (1)	
Coccyx (1)	
Thoracic cage	25
Sternum (1)	
Ribs (24)	
Appendicular Skeleton (126 bones)	
Pectoral girdles	4
Clavicle (2)	
Scapula (2)	
Upper extremity	60
Humerus (2)	
Radius (2)	
Ulna (2)	
Carpals (16)	
Metacarpals (10)	
Phalanges (28)	
Pelvic girdle	2
Coxal, innominate, or hip bones (2)	
Lower extremity	60
Femur (2)	
Tibia (2)	
Fibula (2)	
Patella (2)	
Tarsals (14)	
Metatarsals (10)	
Phalanges (28)	

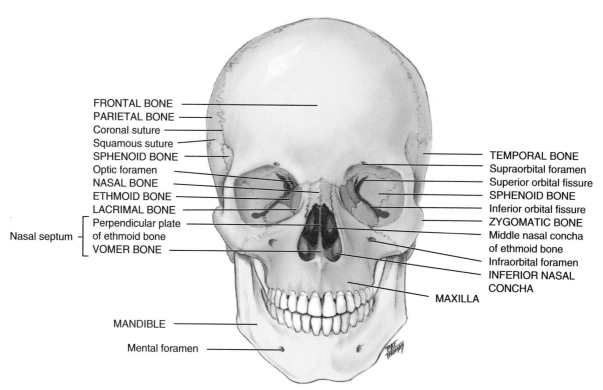

FRONTAL BONE
PARIETAL BONE
Coronal suture
Squamous suture
SPHENOID BONE
Optic foramen
NASAL BONE
ETHMOID BONE
LACRIMAL BONE
Perpendicular plate
of ethmoid bone
VOMER BONE
Nasal septum
MANDIBLE
Mental foramen

TEMPORAL BONE
Supraorbital foramen
Superior orbital fissure
SPHENOID BONE
Inferior orbital fissure
ZYGOMATIC BONE
Middle nasal concha
of ethmoid bone
Infraorbital foramen
INFERIOR NASAL
CONCHA
MAXILLA

Figure 6-5 Skull, anterior view.

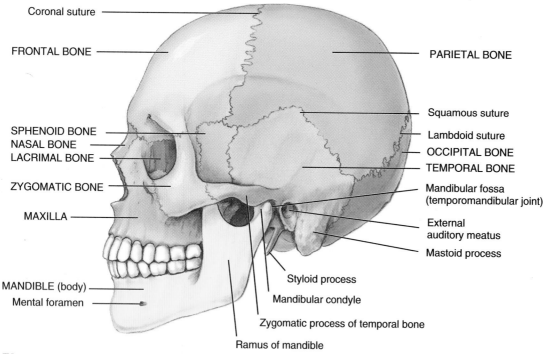

Coronal suture

FRONTAL BONE

SPHENOID BONE
NASAL BONE
LACRIMAL BONE

ZYGOMATIC BONE

MAXILLA

MANDIBLE (body)
Mental foramen

PARIETAL BONE

Squamous suture

Lambdoid suture
OCCIPITAL BONE
TEMPORAL BONE

Mandibular fossa
(temporomandibular joint)

External
auditory meatus
Mastoid process

Styloid process

Mandibular condyle

Zygomatic process of temporal bone

Ramus of mandible

Figure 6-6 Skull, lateral view.

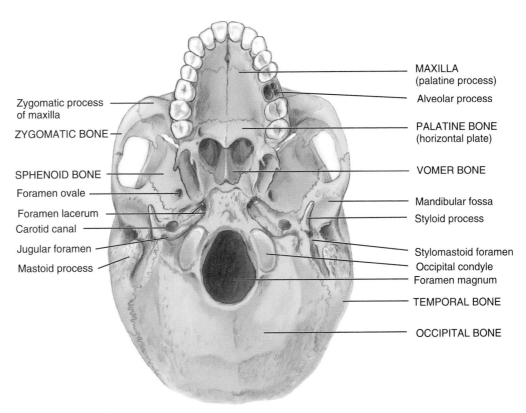

MAXILLA
(palatine process)

Alveolar process

Zygomatic process
of maxilla

ZYGOMATIC BONE

PALATINE BONE
(horizontal plate)

SPHENOID BONE

VOMER BONE

Foramen ovale

Mandibular fossa

Foramen lacerum

Styloid process

Carotid canal

Jugular foramen

Stylomastoid foramen

Mastoid process

Occipital condyle

Foramen magnum

TEMPORAL BONE

OCCIPITAL BONE

Figure 6–7   Skull, inferior view.

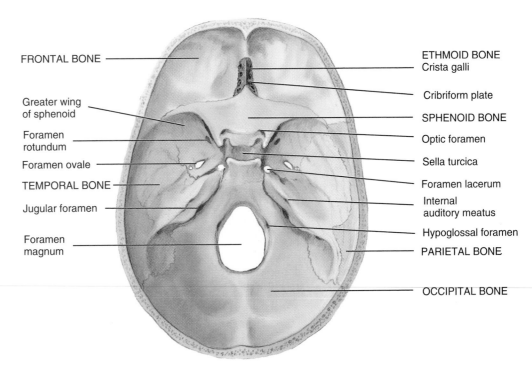

FRONTAL BONE

ETHMOID BONE
Crista galli

Cribriform plate

Greater wing
of sphenoid

SPHENOID BONE

Foramen
rotundum

Optic foramen

Foramen ovale

Sella turcica

TEMPORAL BONE

Foramen lacerum

Jugular foramen

Internal
auditory meatus

Foramen
magnum

Hypoglossal foramen

PARIETAL BONE

OCCIPITAL BONE

Figure 6–8   Skull, cranial floor viewed from above.

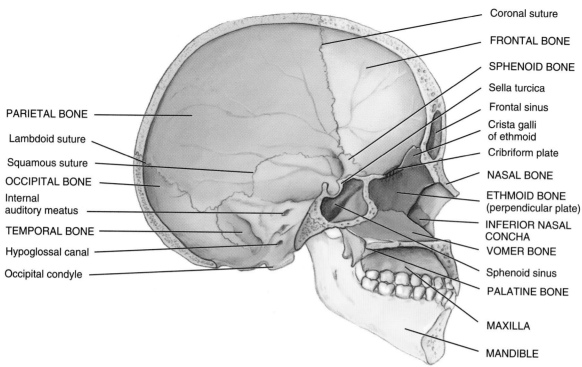

Coronal suture

FRONTAL BONE

SPHENOID BONE

Sella turcica

Frontal sinus

Crista galli
of ethmoid

Cribriform plate

NASAL BONE

ETHMOID BONE
(perpendicular plate)

INFERIOR NASAL
CONCHA

VOMER BONE

Sphenoid sinus

PALATINE BONE

MAXILLA

MANDIBLE

PARIETAL BONE

Lambdoid suture

Squamous suture

OCCIPITAL BONE

Internal
auditory meatus

TEMPORAL BONE

Hypoglossal canal

Occipital condyle

Figure 6–9   Skull, midsagittal section.

bones in the skull are tightly interlocked along irregular lines called **sutures.** Some of the bones in the skull contain **sinuses.** These are air-filled cavities that are lined with mucous membranes. The sinuses help to reduce the weight of the skull. The paranasal sinuses are arranged around the nasal cavity and drain into it.

The bones with paranasal sinuses are the frontal sphenoid ethmoid and the two maxillae. The sinuses are lined with mucous membranes that are continuous with the nasal cavity. Allergies and infections cause inflammation of the membranes, which results in sinusitis. The swollen membranes may reduce drainage from the sinuses so that pressure within the cavities increases, resulting in sinus headaches.

There are numerous openings, or **foramina,** in the bones of the skull to allow for passage of blood vessels and nerves. Major foramina of the skull are listed in Table 6–3 and illustrated in Figures 6–5 through 6–9.

The 28 bones in the skull include 8 bones in the cranium, 14 facial bones, and 6 auditory ossicles.

Cranium

The eight bones of the cranium are interlocked together to enclose the brain (see Figs. 6–5 through 6–9).

Frontal Bone. The frontal bone forms the anterior portion of the skull above the eyes (forehead), a portion of the nose, and the superior portion of the orbit (eye socket). On the superior margin of each orbit, there is a **supraorbital foramen** (or supraorbital notch in some skulls) through which blood vessels and nerves pass to the tissues of the forehead. On either side of the midline, just above the eyes, there is a cavity in the frontal bone. These are the paranasal **frontal sinuses.**

Parietal Bones. The two parietal (pah-RYE-eh-tal) bones form most of the superolateral aspects of the skull. The are joined to each other in the midline by the **sagittal suture** and to the frontal bone by the **coronal suture.**

Occipital Bone. The single occipital (ahk-SIP-ih-tal) bone forms most of the dorsal part of the skull and the base of the cranium. It is joined to the parietal bones by the **lambdoid** (lamm-DOYD) **suture.** Wormian bones are frequently found in the lambdoid suture. The **foramen magnum** is a large opening on the lower surface of the occipital bone. The spinal cord passes through this opening. **Occipital condyles** are rounded processes on each side of the foramen magnum. They articulate with the first cervical vertebra.

Table 6–3   Major Foramina of the Skull

Foramen	Location	Structures Transmitted
Carotid canal	Temporal bone	Internal carotid artery
Hypoglossal	Occipital bone	Hypoglossal nerve
Inferior orbital (fissure)	Floor of orbit	Maxillary branch of trigeminal nerve and infraorbital vessels
Infraorbital	Maxilla bone	Infraorbital vessels and nerves
Internal auditory (meatus)	Temporal bone	Vestibulocochlear nerve
Jugular	Temporal bone	Internal jugular vein; vagus, glossopharyngeal, and spinal accessory nerves
Magnum	Occipital bone	Medulla oblongata / spinal cord; accessory nerves; vertebral and spinal arteries
Mental	Mandible	Mental nerve and vessels
Nasolacrimal canal	Lacrimal bone	Nasolacrimal (tear) duct
Olfactory	Ethmoid bone	Olfactory nerves
Optic	Sphenoid bone	Optic nerve
Ovale	Sphenoid bone	Mandibular branch of trigeminal nerve
Rotundum	Sphenoid bone	Maxillary branch of trigeminal nerve
Stylomastoid	Temporal bone	Facial nerve
Superior orbital (fissure)	Orbit of the eye	Oculomotor (III), trochlear (IV), ophthalmic branch of trigeminal (V), and abducens (VI) nerves
Supraorbital	Frontal bone	Supraorbital artery and nerve

Temporal Bones. The two temporal bones, one on each side of the head, form parts of the sides and base of the cranium. On each side, a temporal bone meets the parietal bone at the **squamous** (SKWAY-mus) **suture.** Near the inferior margin of the temporal bone, there is an opening, the **external auditory meatus,** which is a canal that leads to the middle ear. Just anterior to the external auditory meatus, there is a shallow depression, the **mandibular** (man-DIB-yoo-lar) **fossa,** that articulates with the mandible. Posterior and inferior to each external auditory meatus, there is a rough protuberance, the **mastoid process.** The mastoid process contains air cells that drain into the middle ear cavity. The **styloid process** is a long, pointed projection inferior to the external auditory meatus. A **zygomatic** (zye-goh-MAT-ik) **process** projects anteriorly from the temporal bone and helps form the prominence of the cheek.

The mastoid air cells are separated from the cranial cavity by only a thin partition of bone. A middle ear infection that spreads to the mastoid air cells (mastoiditis) is serious because there is danger that the infection will spread from the air cells to the membranes around the brain.

Sphenoid Bone. The sphenoid (SFEE-noyd) bone is an irregularly shaped bone that spans the entire width of the cranial floor. It is wedged between other bones in the anterior portion of the cranium. This bone helps form the sides of the skull, the base of the cranium, and the lateral and inferior portions of each orbit. Within the cranial cavity, there is a saddle-shaped central portion, called the **sella turcica** (SELL-ah TUR-sih-kah), with a depression for the pituitary gland. Anterior to the sella turcica are two openings, one on each side, called the **optic foramina,** for the passage of the optic nerve. The **greater wings** extend laterally from the region of the sella turcica and are the portions of the sphenoid seen in the orbits and external wall of the skull. The sphenoid bone also contains paranasal **sphenoid sinuses.**

Ethmoid Bone. The ethmoid (ETH-moyd) bone is located anterior to the sphenoid bone and forms most of the bony area between the nasal cavity and the orbits. In the anterior portion of the cranial cavity, the **crista galli** (KRIS-tah GAL-lee) is seen as a triangular process that projects upward. It is an attachment for the membranes that surround the brain. On each side of the crista galli there is a small, flat **cribriform** (KRIB-rih-form) **plate** that is full of tiny holes. The holes are the **olfactory foramina.** Nerve fibers from the sense receptors for smell in the nasal cavity pass through the olfactory foramina. The **perpendicular plate** of the ethmoid projects downward in the middle of the nasal cavity to form the superior part of the nasal septum. Delicate, scroll-like projections, called the **superior and middle nasal conchae** (KONG-kee) or **turbinates,** form ledges along the lateral walls of the nasal cavity. The conchae are lined with mucous membranes to warm and moisten inhaled air. The ethmoid bone contains many small, paranasal **ethmoidal sinuses.**

The bones in the skull of a newborn are not completely joined together but are separated by fibrous membranes. There are six large areas of membranes called **fontanels,** or soft spots. The anterior fontanel is on the top of the head, at the junction of the frontal and parietal bones. The posterior fontanel is at the junction of the occipital and parietal bones. On each side of the head there is a mastoid (posterolateral) fontanel near the mastoid region of the temporal bone and a sphenoid (anterolateral) fontanel just superior to the sphenoid bone.

Facial Bones

The facial skeleton consists of 14 bones. Thirteen of these are interlocked together, and there is one movable mandible, the lower jawbone. These bones form the basic framework and shape of the face. They also provide attachments for the muscles that control facial expression and move the jaw for chewing. All the bones except the vomer and mandible are paired. Facial bones are illustrated in Figures 6–5 through 6–9.

Maxillary Bones. The maxillary bones, or **maxillae** (maks-ILL-ee), form the upper jaw. Additionally, they form the lateral walls of the nose, floor of the orbits, and the anterior part of the roof of the mouth. The portion in the hard palate, or roof of the mouth, is the **palatine process.** The inferior border of each maxilla projects downward to form the **alveolar** (al-VEE-oh-lar) **process,** which contains the teeth. Each maxilla has a large paranasal **maxillary sinus.** These are the largest of all the paranasal sinuses.

Palatine Bones. The palatine (PAL-ah-tyne) bones are behind, or posterior to, the maxillae. Each one is roughly L-shaped. The **horizontal plates** form the posterior portion of the hard palate. The vertical portions help form the lateral walls of the nasal cavity.

Nasal Bones. The two nasal bones are small rectangular bones that form the bridge of the nose.

Lacrimal Bones. The small, thin, lacrimal (LACK-rih-mal) bones are located in the medial walls of the orbits, between the ethmoid bone and the maxilla. Each one has a small **lacrimal groove** that is a pathway for a tube that carries tears from the eyes to the nasal cavity.

Zygomatic Bones. The zygomatic (zye-goh-MAT-ik) bones, also called **malar** bones, form the prominences of the cheeks and a portion of the lateral walls of the orbits. Each one has a **temporal process** that projects toward the zygomatic process of the temporal bone to form the **zygomatic arch.**

Inferior Nasal Conchae. The inferior nasal conchae (KONG-kee) are thin, curved bones that are attached to the lateral walls of the nasal cavity. They project into the nasal cavity just below the middle conchae of the ethmoid bone.

Vomer. The thin, flat vomer (VOH-mer) is in the inferior portion of the midline in the nasal cavity. It joins with the perpendicular plate of the ethmoid bone to form the **nasal septum.**

Mandible. The mandible (MAN-dih-bul) is the lower jaw. It has a horseshoe-shaped **body** that forms the chin and a flat portion, the **ramus,** that projects upward at each end. On the superior portion of the ramus, there is a knoblike process, the **mandibular condyle,** that fits into the mandibular fossa of the temporal bone to form the **temporomandibular** (tem-por-oh-man-DIB-yoo-lar) **joint.** The superior border of the mandible projects upward to form the **alveolar process** that contains the teeth.

Auditory Ossicles

There are three tiny bones that form a chain in each middle ear cavity in the temporal bone. These are the **malleus, incus,** and **stapes.** These bones transmit sound waves from the tympanic membrane, or eardrum, to the inner ear where the sound receptors are located.

Hyoid Bone

The hyoid bone is not really part of the skull, so it is listed separately. It is a U-shaped bone in the neck, between the mandible and the larynx, or voice box. Figure 6–10 illustrates the position and shape of the hyoid bone. It is unique because it is the only bone in the body that does not articulate directly with another bone. Instead it is suspended under the mandible and anchored by ligaments to the styloid processes of the temporal bones. It functions as a base for the tongue and as an attachment for several muscles associated with swallowing.

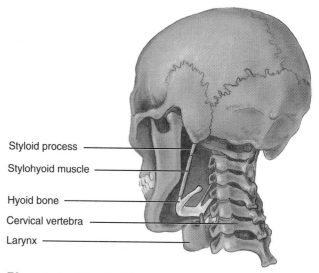

Styloid process

Stylohyoid muscle

Hyoid bone

Cervical vertebra

Larynx

Figure 6–10 Hyoid bone.

The hyoid bone, a U-shaped bone in the neck, does not articulate directly with any other bone.

Vertebral Column

The vertebral column extends from the skull to the pelvis and contains 26 bones called **vertebrae** (singular, vertebra). The bones are separated by pads of fibrocartilage called **intervertebral disks.** The disks act as shock absorbers and allow the column to bend. Normally there are four curvatures, illustrated in Figure 6–11, that increase the strength and resilience of the column. They are named according to the region in which they are located. The **thoracic** and **sacral curvatures** are concave anteriorly and are present at birth. The **cervical curvature** develops when an infant begins to hold its head erect. The **lumbar curvature** develops when an infant begins to stand and walk. Both the cervical and lumbar curvatures are convex anteriorly.

The vertebral column consists of 26 vertebrae separated by intervertebral disks. Four curvatures add strength and resilience to the column.

An abnormally exaggerated lumbar curvature is called lordosis, or swayback. This is often seen in pregnant women as they adjust to their changing center of gravity. An increased roundness of the thoracic curvature is kyphosis, or hunchback. This is frequently seen in elderly people. Abnormal side-to-side curvature is scoliosis. Abnormal curvatures may interfere with breathing and other vital functions.

General Structure of Vertebrae

All vertebrae have a common structural pattern, illustrated in Figure 6–12, although there are variations between them. The thick anterior, weight-bearing portion is the **body** or **centrum.** The posterior curved portion is the **vertebral arch.** The vertebral arch and body surround a central large opening, the **vertebral foramen.** When all the vertebrae are stacked together in a column, the vertebral foramina make a canal that contains the spinal cord. **Transverse processes** project laterally from the vertebral arch, and in the posterior midline there is a **spinous process.** These processes are places for muscle attachment. The spinous processes can be felt as bony projections along the midline of the back.

Although all vertebrae have similar general features, there are regional variations that distinguish one type of vertebra from another. These are illustrated in Figure 6–13.

Cervical Vertebrae

There are seven **cervical vertebrae,** designated C1 through C7. In general, the cervical vertebrae, shown in Figure 6–13C, can be distinguished from

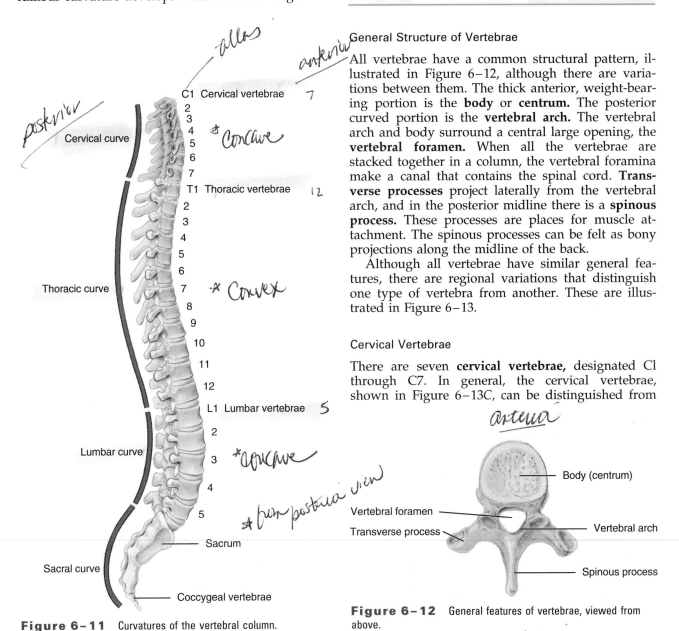

C1 Cervical vertebrae   7
2
3
4
5
6
7
T1 Thoracic vertebrae   12
2
3
4
5
6
7
8
9
10
11
12
L1 Lumbar vertebrae   5
2
3
4
5

Cervical curve

Thoracic curve

Lumbar curve

Sacral curve

Sacrum

Coccygeal vertebrae

Figure 6–11   Curvatures of the vertebral column.

Body (centrum)

Vertebral foramen

Transverse process

Vertebral arch

Spinous process

Figure 6–12   General features of vertebrae, viewed from above.

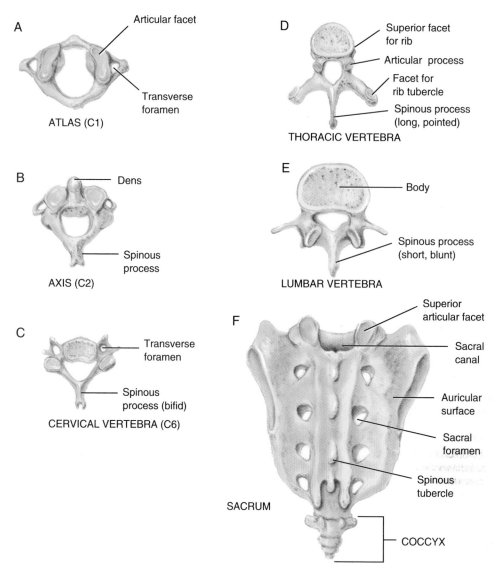

A ATLAS (C1)
- Articular facet
- Transverse foramen

B AXIS (C2)
- Dens
- Spinous process

C CERVICAL VERTEBRA (C6)
- Transverse foramen
- Spinous process (bifid)

D THORACIC VERTEBRA
- Superior facet for rib
- Articular process
- Facet for rib tubercle
- Spinous process (long, pointed)

E LUMBAR VERTEBRA
- Body
- Spinous process (short, blunt)

F SACRUM
- Superior articular facet
- Sacral canal
- Auricular surface
- Sacral foramen
- Spinous tubercle

COCCYX

Figure 6–13 Regional differences in vertebrae.

other vertebrae because the cervicals have **transverse foramina** in the transverse processes and the spinous processes are forked, or **bifid.** The first two cervical vertebrae are greatly modified and there is no disk between them. The **atlas** (C1), illustrated in Figure 6–13A, has no body, no spinous process, and short transverse processes. It is essentially a ring with large facets that articulate with the occipital condyles on the occipital bone. The **axis** (C2), shown in Figure 6–13B, has a **dens,** or **odontoid** (oh-DON-toyd) **process** that projects upward from the vertebral body like a tooth. The odontoid process acts as a pivot for rotation of the atlas.

The atlas holds up the skull and permits you to nod "yes." The axis allows you to rotate your head from side to side to indicate "no."

Thoracic Vertebrae

There are 12 **thoracic vertebrae,** designated T1 through T12. These can be distinguished from other vertebrae by the facets, located on the bodies and transverse processes, for articulation with the ribs. They also have long, pointed spinous processes. These features are illustrated in Figure 6–13D.

Lumbar Vertebrae

There are five **lumbar vertebrae,** designated L1 through L5, that make up the part of the vertebral column in the small of the back. The lumbar vertebrae, shown in Figure 6–13E, have large, heavy bodies because they support most of the body weight and have many back muscles attached to them. They also have short, blunt, spinous processes.

Sacrum

The **sacrum,** shown in Figure 6–13F, is a triangular bone just below the lumbar vertebrae. In the child there are five separate bones, but these fuse to form a single bone in the adult. The sacrum articulates with the pelvic girdle laterally, at the **sacroiliac** (say-kro-ILL-ee-ak) **joint,** and forms the posterior wall of the pelvic cavity.

Coccyx

The **coccyx** (KOK-siks), or tailbone, is the last part of the vertebral column (see Figs. 6–11 and 6–13F). There are four (the number varies from three to five) separate small bones in the child but these fuse to form a single bone in the adult. Several muscles have some point of attachment on the coccyx.

> The seven cervical vertebrae are characterized by transverse foramina and bifid spinous processes; 12 thoracic vertebrae are identified by articular facets for the ribs; five lumbar vertebrae have large bodies; five sacral vertebrae fuse into one sacrum; and three to five coccygeal vertebrae fuse into one coccyx.

Thoracic Cage

The thoracic cage, or bony thorax, protects the heart, lungs, and great vessels. It also supports the bones of the shoulder girdle and plays a role in breathing. The components of the thoracic cage are the thoracic vertebrae dorsally, the ribs laterally, and the sternum and costal cartilages anteriorly.

Sternum

The **sternum,** or breastbone, is in the anterior midline (Fig. 6–14). It consists of three parts: the superior, triangular **manubrium** (mah-NOO-bree-um); the middle, slender **body;** and the inferior, small **xiphoid** (ZYE-foyd) **process.** The xiphoid process, for muscle attachment, is composed of hyaline cartilage in the child, but it ossifies in the adult. An important anatomical landmark, the **jugular (suprasternal) notch** is an easily palpable, central indentation in the superior margin of the manubrium. The manubrium articulates with the clavicles and the first two pairs of ribs. The manubrium and body of the sternum meet at a slight angle that can be felt as a horizontal ridge below the jugular notch. This is the **sternal angle,** and it is a convenient way to locate the second rib (see Fig. 6–14). The body of the sternum has notches along the sides where it attaches to the cartilages of the third through seventh ribs.

> The sternum forms the anterior portion of the thoracic cage. It consists of the manubrium, body, and xiphoid.

The sternum is frequently used for a red marrow biopsy because it is accessible. The sample for biopsy is obtained by performing a sternal puncture, in which a large needle is inserted into the sternum to remove a sample of red bone marrow.

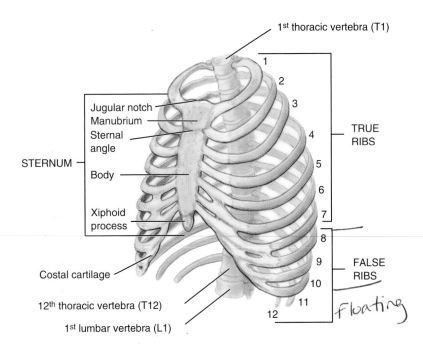

1ˢᵗ thoracic vertebra (T1)

1
2
3
4
5
6
7
8
9
10
11
12

TRUE RIBS

FALSE RIBS

Floating

Jugular notch
Manubrium
Sternal angle
STERNUM
Body
Xiphoid process

Costal cartilage

12ᵗʰ thoracic vertebra (T12)
1ˢᵗ lumbar vertebra (L1)

Figure 6–14 Thoracic cage.

Ribs

Twelve pairs of **ribs,** illustrated in Figure 6–14, form the curved, lateral margins of the thoracic cage. One pair is attached to each of the 12 thoracic vertebrae. The upper seven pairs of ribs are called **true,** or **vertebrosternal** (ver-TEE-broh-stir-nal), **ribs,** because they attach to the sternum directly by their individual **costal cartilages.** The lower five pairs of ribs are called **false ribs** because their costal cartilages do not reach the sternum directly. The first three pairs of false ribs reach the sternum indirectly by joining with the cartilages of the ribs above. These are called **vertebrochondral** (ver-TEE-broh-kahn-dral) **ribs.** The bottom two rib pairs have no anterior attachment and are called **vertebral ribs,** or **floating ribs.**

> There are seven pairs of vertebrosternal ribs, three pairs of vertebrochondral ribs, and two pairs of vertebral, or floating, ribs.

☑ **Quick**Check

- What bones contain paranasal sinuses?
- What bones are involved if there is a fracture of the nasal septum?
- What is the posterior attachment of all ribs?

Bones of the Appendicular Skeleton

The 126 bones of the appendicular skeleton are suspended from two yokes or girdles that are anchored to the axial skeleton. They are additions or appendages to the axis of the body. The appendicular skeleton is designed for movement. If a portion is immobilized for a period of time, we realize how awkward life can be without appendicular movement.

Pectoral Girdle

Each half of the **pectoral girdle,** or **shoulder girdle,** consists of two bones: an anterior **clavicle** (KLAV-ih-kul) and a posterior **scapula** (SKAP-yoo-lah). The term "girdle" implies something that encircles or a complete ring. The pectoral girdle, however, is an incomplete ring. Anteriorly, the bones are separated by the sternum. Posteriorly, there is a gap between the two scapulae because they do not articulate with each other or with the vertebral column. The bones of the pectoral girdle, illustrated in Figure 6–15, form the connection between the upper extremities and the axial skeleton. The clavicles and scapulae, with their associated muscles, also form the shoulder.

The **clavicle** is commonly called the **collarbone.** It is an elongated S-shaped bone that articulates proximally with the manubrium of the sternum. The other end articulates with the scapula.

> The clavicle is the most frequently fractured bone in the body because it transmits forces from the arm to the trunk. The force from falling on the shoulder or outstretched arm is often sufficient to fracture the clavicle.

The **scapula,** commonly called the **shoulder blade,** is a thin, flat, triangular bone on the posterior surface of the thoracic wall. It articulates with the clavicle and the humerus. The scapula has points of

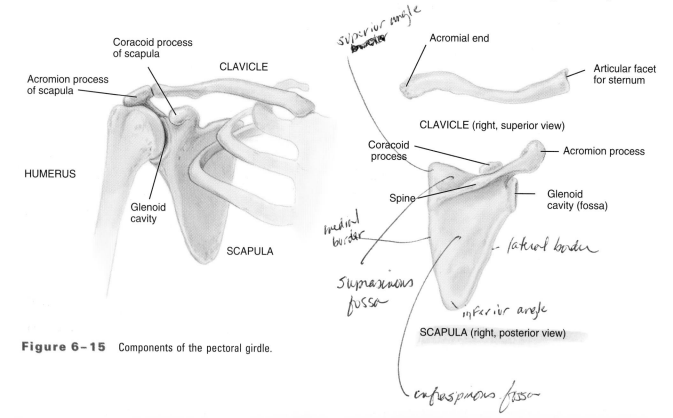

Figure 6–15 Components of the pectoral girdle.

attachment for numerous muscles that are involved in movement of the shoulder and arm. A bony ridge called the **spine** divides the dorsal surface into two unequal portions. The lateral end of the spine broadens to form the **acromion** (ah-KRO-mee-on) **process,** which articulates with the clavicle and is a site of muscle attachment. It forms the point of the shoulder. Another process, the **coracoid** (KOR-ah-koyd) **process,** forms a hook that projects forward, under the clavicle. It also serves as a place for muscle attachments. Between the two processes there is a shallow depression, the **glenoid cavity** (fossa), where the head of the humerus connects to the scapula.

> The two clavicles, or collarbones, and two scapulae, or shoulder blades, make up the pectoral girdle.

Upper Extremity

The upper extremity (limb) consists of the bones of the arm, forearm, and hand.

Arm

The arm, or **brachium,** is the region between the shoulder and the elbow. It contains a single long bone, the **humerus,** illustrated in Figure 6–16. The **head** is the large, smooth, rounded end that fits into the scapula. Lateral to the head, there are two blunt projections for muscle attachment. These are the **greater** and **lesser tubercles,** and the shallow groove between them is the **intertubercular groove.** The **deltoid tuberosity** is an elongated rough area along the shaft. The deltoid muscle attaches to the humerus along this region. The **lateral** and **medial epicondyles,** for the attachment of forearm muscles, project from the sides of the humerus at the distal end, near the elbow region. On the posterior surface, between the two epicondyles, there is a depression, the **olecranon fossa,** where the ulna fits with the humerus to form the hinged elbow joint. On the anterior surface is a shallow depression, the **coronoid fossa,** also for the ulna. Two smooth, rounded projections are evident on the distal end of the humerus. The **capitulum** is on the lateral side and articulates with the radius of the forearm. The **trochlea** is on the medial side and articulates with the ulna of the forearm. Table 6–4 describes important anatomical features on the humerus.

> Tennis elbow is an inflammation of the tissues surrounding the lateral epicondyle of the humerus. Six muscles that control movement of the hand attach in this region, and repeated contraction of these muscles irritates the attachments. The medical term for tennis elbow is *lateral epicondylitis.*

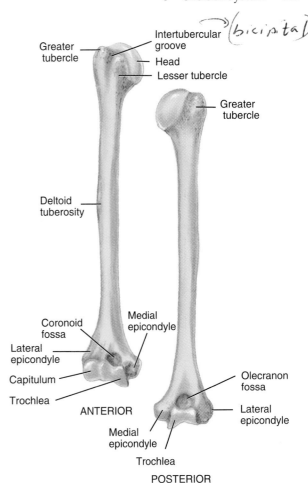

Figure 6–16   Humerus.

Forearm

The forearm is the region between the elbow and wrist. It is formed by the **radius** on the lateral side and the **ulna** on the medial side when the forearm is in anatomical position. When the hand is turned so the palm faces backward, the radius crosses over the ulna. The radius and ulna are illustrated in Figure 6–17.

The radius has a circular disklike **head** on the proximal end. This articulates with the capitulum of the humerus. Just inferior to the head and on the medial side of the bone, there is a small rough region called the **radial tuberosity,** which is an attachment for the biceps brachii muscle. On the distal end, the prominent markings of the radius are the **styloid process,** a pointed projection on the lateral side, and the **ulnar notch,** a smooth region on the medial side.

The proximal end of the ulna has a wrenchlike shape, with the opening of the wrench being the **trochlear notch,** or semilunar notch. The projection at the upper end of the notch is the **olecranon process,** which fits into the olecranon fossa of the hu-

Table 6–4	Important Markings on the Humerus	
Marking	**Description**	**Purpose**
Head	Large, smooth, rounded surface on the proximal end	Fits into the glenoid cavity of the scapula
Greater and lesser tubercles	Blunt projections, lateral to the head, on the proximal end	Attachment for muscles that move the shoulder and arm
Intertubercular groove	Shallow groove between the two tubercles	Holds tendon for the biceps brachii muscle
Deltoid tuberosity	Rough area along shaft	Attachment for deltoid muscle
Lateral and medial epicondyles	Lateral projections from the distal end	Attachment for muscles of the forearm
Olecranon fossa	Depression on the posterior distal end	Space for the olecranon process of the ulna when the elbow is extended
Coronoid fossa	Shallow depression on the anterior distal end	Space for the coronoid process of the ulna when the elbow is flexed
Capitulum	Smooth, rounded condyle on the lateral side of the distal end	Articulates with the head of the radius of the forearm
Trochlea	Smooth, pulley-shaped condyle on the medial side of the distal end	Articulates with the ulna of the forearm

merus and forms the bony point of the elbow. The projection at the lower end of the notch is the **coronoid process,** which fits into the coronoid fossa of the humerus. The **radial notch,** a smooth region on the lateral side of the coronoid process, is where the head of the radius fits. The **head** is at the distal end, and on the medial side of the head the pointed **styloid process** serves as an attachment point for ligaments of the wrist. The important features of the radius and ulna are described in Table 6–5.

Hand

The hand, illustrated in Figure 6–18, is composed of the wrist, palm, and five fingers. The wrist, or **carpus,** contains 8 small **carpal bones,** tightly bound by ligaments and arranged in two rows of 4 bones each. The carpal bones are identified in Figure 6–18. The palm of the hand, or **metacarpus,** contains 5 **metacarpal bones,** one in line with each finger. These bones are not named but are numbered 1 to 5

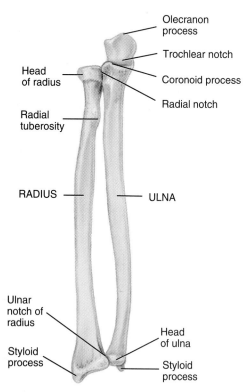

Figure 6–17 Radius and ulna.

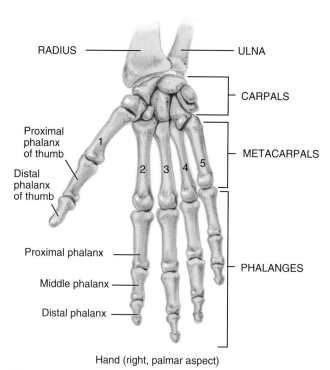

Hand (right, palmar aspect)

Figure 6–18 Hand.

Table 6–5   Important Markings on the Radius and Ulna

Marking	Description	Purpose
Radius		
Head	Circular disklike proximal end	Articulates with the capitulum of the humerus and fits into the radial notch of the ulna
Radial tuberosity	Small rough process on the medial side, near the head	Attachment for the biceps brachii muscle
Styloid process	Pointed process on the lateral side of the distal end	Attachments for ligaments of the wrist
Ulnar notch	Small, smooth facet on the medial side of the distal end	Articulates with the head of the ulna
Ulna		
Trochlear notch (semilunar notch)	Wrench-shaped opening or cavity at the proximal end	Articulates with the trochlea of the humerus
Olecranon process	Projection at the upper end of the trochlear notch	Articulates with the olecranon fossa of the humerus when the elbow is extended; provides attachment for muscles
Coronoid process	Projection at the lower end of the trochlear notch	Articulates with the coronoid fossa of the humerus when the elbow is flexed; provides attachment for muscles
Radial notch	Smooth facet on the lateral side of the coronoid process	Articulates with the head of the radius
Head	Knoblike process at the distal end	Articulates with the ulnar notch of the radius
Styloid process	Pointed process on the medial side of the distal end	Attachments for ligaments of the wrist

starting on the thumb side. The 14 bones of the fingers are called **phalanges** (fah-LAN-jeez). Some people refer to these as digits. There are three phalanges in each finger (a proximal, middle, and distal phalanx) except the thumb, or pollex, which has two. The thumb lacks a middle phalanx. The proximal phalanges articulate with the metacarpals.

> Each upper extremity includes the humerus in the arm, the radius (lateral) and ulna (medial) in the forearm, eight carpals in the wrist, five metacarpals in the palm of the hand, and 14 phalanges in the fingers.

Pelvic Girdle

The **pelvic girdle,** or **hip girdle,** attaches the lower extremities to the axial skeleton and provides a strong support for the weight of the body. It also provides support and protection for the urinary bladder, a portion of the large intestine, and the internal reproductive organs, which are located in the pelvic cavity.

The pelvic girdle consists of two **coxal** (hip) **bones,** illustrated in Figure 6–19, and their important features are described in Table 6–6. The coxal bones are also called the **ossa coxae,** or **innominate bones.** Anteriorly, the two bones articulate with each other at the **symphysis pubis;** posteriorly, they articulate with the sacrum at the **iliosacral joints.** During childhood, each coxal bone consists of three separate parts: the **ilium,** the **ischium,** and the **pubis.** In the adult, these bones are firmly fused to form a single bone. Where the three bones meet, there is a large depression, the **acetabulum** (as-seh-TAB-yoo-lum), which holds the head of the femur. The **obturator foramen** is a large opening between the pubis and ischium that functions as a passageway for blood vessels, nerves, and muscle tendons.

The major portion of the coxal bone is formed by the ilium, which has a large, flared region called the **ala,** or wing. The concavity on the medial surface of the ala is the **iliac fossa.** The superior margin of the ala is the **iliac crest,** which ends anteriorly as a blunt projection, the **anterior superior iliac spine.** Just inferior to this is another blunt projection, the **anterior inferior iliac spine.** Posteriorly, the crest ends in the **posterior superior iliac spine** and just inferior to this there is a **posterior inferior iliac spine.** The **greater sciatic notch** forms a deep indentation in the posterior region. The sciatic nerve passes through this notch. The **auricular surface** is the rough region on the posterior part of the ilium, where it meets the sacrum to form the iliosacral (sacroiliac) joint. The **iliopectineal line,** a sharp line at the inferior margin of the iliac fossa, marks the pelvic brim.

The lower, posterior portion of the coxal bone is

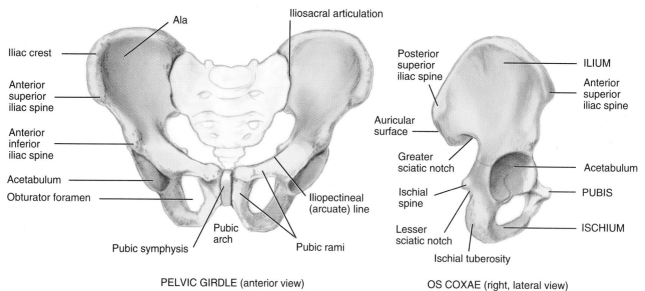

Figure 6-19 Bones of the pelvic girdle.

In the figure:

PELVIC GIRDLE (anterior view) — labels: Iliac crest, Ala, Iliosacral articulation, Anterior superior iliac spine, Anterior inferior iliac spine, Acetabulum, Obturator foramen, Pubic symphysis, Pubic arch, Pubic rami, Iliopectineal (arcuate) line

OS COXAE (right, lateral view) — labels: Posterior superior iliac spine, ILIUM, Anterior superior iliac spine, Auricular surface, Greater sciatic notch, Acetabulum, Ischial spine, PUBIS, Lesser sciatic notch, ISCHIUM, Ischial tuberosity

Table 6–6	Important Markings on the Coxal Bones	
Marking	**Description**	**Purpose**
Acetabulum	Deep depression on lateral surface of coxal bone	Socket for articulation with head of femur (thigh bone)
Obturator foramen	Large opening between the pubis and ischium	Passageway for blood vessels, nerves, muscle tendons; largest foramen in the body
Ilium	Large flaring region that forms the major portion of the coxal bone	
Alae (wings)	Large flared portions of the ilium	Large area for numerous muscle attachments; form false pelvis
Iliac crest	Thickened superior margin of the ilium	Muscle attachment; forms prominence of hips
Anterior superior iliac spine	Blunt projection at anterior end of the iliac crest	Attachment for muscles of trunk, hip, thigh; can be easily palpated
Posterior superior iliac spine	Blunt projection at posterior end of the iliac crest	Attachment for muscles of trunk, hip, thigh
Anterior inferior iliac spine	Projection on ilium inferior to the anterior superior iliac spine	Attachment for muscles of trunk, hip, thigh
Posterior inferior iliac spine	Projection on ilium inferior to the posterior superior iliac spine	Attachment for muscles of trunk, hip, thigh
Greater sciatic notch	Deep indentation inferior to the posterior inferior iliac spine	Passageway for sciatic nerve and some muscle tendons
Iliac fossa	Slight concavity on medial surface of alae	Attachment for iliacus muscle
Auricular surface	Large, rough region at posterior margin of iliac fossa	Articulates with sacrum to form the iliosacral (sacroiliac) joint
Iliopectineal (arcuate) line	Sharp curved line at inferior margin of iliac fossa	Attachment for muscles; marks the pelvic brim
Ischium	Lower, posterior portion of the coxal bone	
Ischial spine	Projection near junction of ilium and ischium; projects into pelvic cavity	Attachment for a major ligament; distance between the two spines tells the size of the pelvic cavity
Ischial tuberosity	Large rough inferior portion of ischium	Muscle attachment; portion on which we sit; strongest part of coxal bones
Lesser sciatic notch	Indentation below the ischial spine	Passageway for blood vessels and nerves
Pubis	Most anterior part of coxal bone	
Pubic symphysis	Anterior midline where two pubic bones meet	
Pubic rami	Armlike portions that project from the pubic symphysis	Form margins of the obturator foramen
Pubic arch	V-shaped arch inferior to the pubic symphysis and formed by the inferior pubic rami	Broadens or narrows the dimensions of the true pelvis

the ischium. The **ischial tuberosity** is the large, rough, inferior portion of the ischium. Near the junction of the ilium and ischium, the **ischial spine** forms a pointed projection. The indentation inferior to the spine is the **lesser sciatic notch.**

The most anterior portion of the coxal bone is the pubis. The two pubic bones meet at the pubic symphysis and extend laterally and inferiorly from this point. The armlike extensions are the **pubic rami.** Inferiorly the pubic rami form a V-shaped arch called the **pubic arch.**

> Two ossa coxae, or innominate bones, form the pelvic girdle. Each os coxa is formed by the ilium, ischium, and pubis, which meet and fuse in the acetabulum. The two ossa coxae meet anteriorly at the symphysis pubis.

Together, the sacrum, coccyx, and pelvic girdle form the basin-shaped pelvis. The **false pelvis** (greater pelvis) is surrounded by the flared portions of the ilium bones and the lumbar vertebrae. The **true pelvis** (lesser pelvis) is smaller and inferior to the false pelvis. It is the region below the **pelvic brim,** or **pelvic inlet,** and it is encircled by bone. The large opening at the bottom of this region is the **pelvic outlet.** The dimensions of the true pelvis are especially important in childbirth. Differences between the male and female pelvis, described in Table 6–7, reflect the modifications of the female pelvis for childbearing.

> The false pelvis is the region between the flared portions of the ilium bones. The true pelvis is the region below the pelvic brim.

The female pelvis is shaped to accommodate childbearing. Because the fetus must pass through the pelvic outlet, the physician carefully measures this opening to make sure there is enough room. The distance between the two ischial spines is a good indication of the size of the pelvic outlet. If the opening is too small, a cesarean delivery is indicated.

Lower Extremity

The lower extremity (limb) consists of the bones of the thigh, leg, foot, and patella, or kneecap. The lower extremities support the entire weight of the body when we are erect and they are exposed to tremendous forces when we walk, run, and jump. With this in mind, it is not surprising that the bones of the lower extremity are larger and stronger than those in the upper extremity.

Thigh

The **thigh** is the region from the hip to the knee. It contains a single long bone, the **femur,** illustrated in Figure 6–20. It is the largest, longest, and strongest bone in the body.

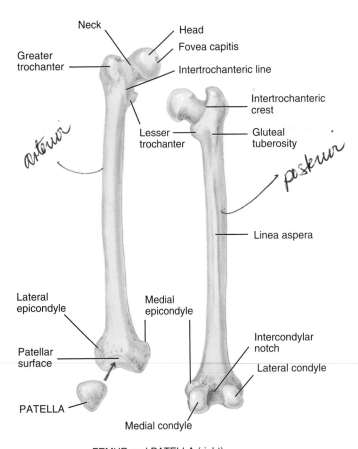

FEMUR and PATELLA (right)

Figure 6–20   Femur.

Table 6–7	Differences Between Male and Female Pelvis
Characteristic	**Description of Difference**
Bone thickness	In the female, the bones are lighter, thinner, and smoother than in the male; markings are more prominent in the male
Pelvic cavity	In the female, the pelvic cavity is broad, oval, and shallow; in the male, it is narrow, deep, and funnel shaped
Pubic arch/angle	Less than 90° in male; 90° or more in the female
Ilium	Bones are more flared in the female than in the male; therefore, the female has broader hips
Ischial spines	Farther apart in the female
Ischial tuberosities	Farther apart in the female
Acetabulum	Smaller and farther apart in the female
Pelvic inlet	Wider and more oval in the female; narrow, almost heart shaped in the male

The large, smooth, ball-like **head** of the femur has a small depression called the **fovea capitis.** A ligament attaches here. Prominent projections at the proximal end, the **greater** and **lesser trochanters,** are major sites for muscle attachment. The **intertrochanteric crest** on the posterior side and the **intertrochanteric line** on the anterior side are between the trochanters and are also for muscle attachment. The **neck** is between the head and the trochanters. On the posterior surface, a rough area, the **gluteal tuberosity,** continues inferiorly as the **linea aspera.** Both of these are regions of muscle attachment. The distal end is marked by two large, rounded surfaces, the **lateral** and **medial condyles.** These form joints with the bones of the leg. The **intercondylar notch** is a depression between the condyles that contains ligaments associated with the knee joint. Two small projections superior to the condyles are the **epicondyles.** On the anterior surface, between the condyles, a smooth **patellar surface** marks the area for the kneecap. Table 6–8 describes important anatomical features on the femur.

Elderly people, particularly those with osteoporosis, are susceptible to "breaking a hip." The femur is a weight-bearing bone, and when it is weakened, it cannot support the weight of the body and the neck of the femur fractures under the stress. Instead of saying, "Grandma fell and broke her hip," often it is more appropriate to say, "Grandma broke her hip, then fell."

Leg

The **leg** is the region between the knee and the ankle. It is formed by the slender **fibula** (FIB-yoo-lah) on the lateral side and the larger, weight-bearing **tibia** (TIB-ee-ah), or shin bone, on the medial side. The tibia articulates with the femur to form the knee joint and with the **talus** (one of the foot bones) to allow flexion and extension at the ankle.

The proximal end of the fibula is the **head** and the projection at the distal end is the **lateral malleolus,** which forms the lateral bulge of the ankle. The superior surface of the tibia is flattened and smooth, with two slightly concave regions called the **lateral** and **medial condyles.** The condyles of the femur fit into these regions. Just below the condyles, the **tibial tuberosity** forms a rough area for the attachment of ligaments associated with the knee. The **anterior crest** is a sharp ridge on the anterior surface and forms the shin. On the medial side of the distal end, the **medial malleolus** forms the medial bulge of the ankle. Figure 6–21 illustrates the tibia and fibula, and their important features are summarized in Table 6–9.

Skiers frequently fracture the distal part of the fibula as a result of a twisting, or shearing, force near the ankle. This is called Pott's fracture. Sometimes, the force is sufficient to fracture the medial malleolus at the same time.

Table 6–8	Important Markings on the Femur	
Marking	**Description**	**Purpose**
Head	Large, ball-like proximal end	Fits into the acetabulum of the coxal bone
Fovea capitis	Small depression on head of femur	Attachment for ligamentum teres femoris
Greater trochanter	Prominent projection from proximal part of the shaft	Attachment for gluteus maximus muscle
Lesser trochanter	Smaller projection inferior and medial to greater trochanter	Site of attachment for buttock and hip muscles
Intertrochanteric crest	Between the trochanters on the posterior side	Muscle attachment
Neck	Between the head and the trochanters	Muscle attachment; offsets thigh from hip joint for ease in movement
Intertrochanteric line	Between the trochanters of the anterior side	Muscle attachment
Gluteal tuberosity	Rough area below the trochanters on the posterior surface	Attachment for gluteal muscles
Linea aspera	Sharp ridge that is a continuation of gluteal tuberosity	Muscle attachment
Lateral and medial condyles	Large rounded surfaces on distal end of femur	Articulate with the tibia
Lateral and medial epicondyles	Small projections just above the condyles	Muscle attachment
Patellar surface	Smooth area between the condyles on the anterior surface	Articulates with the patella
Intercondylar notch	Large U-shaped depression between the condyles on the posterior surface	Contains ligaments associated with the knee joint

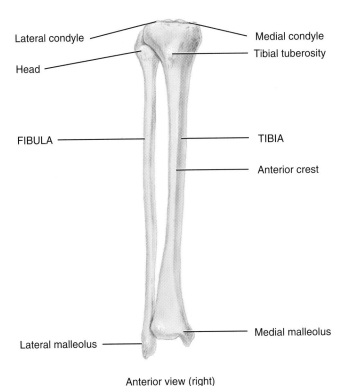

Lateral condyle

Head

FIBULA

Lateral malleolus

Medial condyle

Tibial tuberosity

TIBIA

Anterior crest

Medial malleolus

Anterior view (right)

Figure 6–21 Tibia and fibula.

Foot

The **foot,** illustrated in Figure 6–22, is composed of the ankle, instep, and five toes. The ankle, or **tarsus,** contains seven **tarsal bones.** These correspond to the carpals in the wrist. The largest tarsal bone is the **calcaneus** (kal-KAY-nee-us), or heel bone. The **talus,** another tarsal bone, rests on top of the calcaneus and articulates with the tibia. The tarsal bones are identified in Figure 6–22. The instep of the foot, or **metatarsus,** contains five **metatarsal bones,** one in line with each toe. The distal ends of these bones form the ball of the foot. These bones are not

named, but are numbered one through five starting on the medial side. The tarsals and metatarsals, together with strong tendons and ligaments, form the arches of the foot. The 14 bones of the toes are called **phalanges.** There are three phalanges in each toe (a proximal, middle, and distal phalanx), except in the great (or big) toe, or hallux, which has only two. The great toe lacks a middle phalanx. The proximal phalanges articulate with the metatarsals.

Poorly fitted shoes may compress the toes so that there is a lateral deviation of the big toe toward the second toe. When this occurs, a bursa and callus form at the joint between the first metatarsal and proximal phalanx. This creates a bunion.

Patella

The **patella,** or **kneecap,** is a flat, triangular sesamoid bone enclosed within the major tendon that anchors the anterior thigh muscle to the tibia. It provides a smooth surface for the tendon as it turns the corner between the thigh and leg when the knee is flexed. It also protects the knee joint anteriorly.

Each lower extremity includes the femur in the thigh, the tibia (medial) and fibula (lateral) in the leg, seven tarsal bones in the ankle, five metatarsal bones in the instep of the foot, 14 phalanges in the toes, and one patella.

✓ QuickCheck

● What bone is involved if there is a fracture on the lateral side of the forearm?

● What is the purpose of the acetabulum?

● Sally developed some bone spurs on her heel. What bone was involved?

Table 6–9	Important Markings on the Tibia and Fibula	
Marking	**Description**	**Purpose**
Tibia		
Medial and lateral condyles	Slightly concave, smooth surfaces on proximal end of tibia	Articulate with condyles of femur
Tibial tuberosity	Large rough area on anterior surface just below the condyles	Attachment of patellar ligament
Anterior crest	Sharp ridge on the anterior surface of the shaft	Forms the shin
Medial malleolus	Medial, rounded process at the distal end	Forms the medial bulge of the ankle; attachment for ligaments
Fibula		
Head	Proximal end	Articulates with the tibia
Lateral malleolus	Projection at distal end	Forms the lateral bulge of the ankle; attachment for ligaments

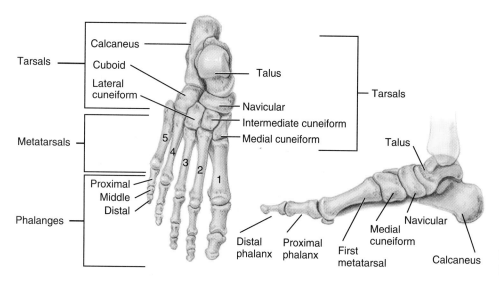

Figure 6-22 Bones of the foot.

Articulations

An **articulation** (ahr-tik-yoo-LAY-shun), or joint, is where two bones come together. In terms of the amount of movement they allow, there are three types of joints: immovable, slightly movable, and freely movable.

Synarthroses

Synarthroses (sin-ahr-THROH-seez) are immovable joints. The singular form is synarthrosis. In these joints, the bones come in very close contact and are separated only by a thin layer of fibrous connective tissue. The **sutures** in the skull are examples of immovable joints.

Amphiarthroses

Slightly movable joints are called **amphiarthroses** (am-fee-ahr-THROH-seez). The singular form is amphiarthrosis. In this type of joint, the bones are connected by hyaline cartilage or fibrocartilage. The ribs connected to the sternum by costal cartilages are slightly movable joints connected by hyaline cartilage. The symphysis pubis is a slightly movable joint in which there is a fibrocartilage pad between the two bones. The joints between the vertebrae, the intervertebral disks, are also of this type.

> Immovable joints, such as sutures in the skull, are classified as synarthroses; slightly movable joints, such as intervertebral disks and the symphysis pubis, are amphiarthroses.

Diarthroses

Most joints in the adult body are **diarthroses** (dye-ahr-THROH-seez), or freely movable joints. The singular form is diarthrosis. In this type of joint, the ends of the opposing bones are covered with hyaline cartilage, the **articular cartilage,** and they are separated by a space called the **joint cavity.** The components of the joints are enclosed in a dense fibrous **joint capsule** (Fig. 6-23). The outer layer of the capsule consists of the ligaments that hold the bones together. The inner layer is the **synovial membrane** that secretes **synovial fluid** into the joint cavity for lubrication. Because all of these joints have a synovial membrane, they are sometimes called **synovial joints.**

> Gout was commonly known as the disease of the kings because it was believed that it was caused by a rich diet and fine wines. The disease is no respecter of persons, however, and occurs across the entire population. A rich diet and fine wines may contribute to the disease, but they are not the definitive cause. Gout is caused by the excessive accumulation of uric acid that forms needlelike crystals within the joint, producing pain and inflammation. The great toe is the most commonly affected joint. The disorder is diagnosed by aspirating joint fluid and observing the crystals under the microscope. There is no cure for gout, but it can be effectively controlled with anti-inflammatory drugs and diet.

> Joints classified as diarthroses are freely movable. They have a joint capsule lined with synovial membrane, so they are also called synovial joints.

Some diarthroses have pads and cushions associated with them. The knee has fibrocartilaginous pads, called **semilunar cartilages** or the **lateral meniscus** (meh-NIS-kus) and **medial meniscus,** which rest on the lateral and medial condyles of the tibia. The pads help stabilize the joint and act as shock

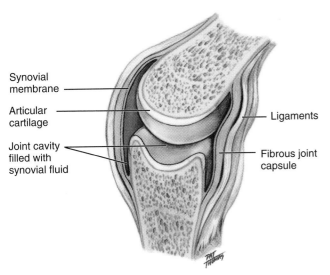

Figure 6-23 Generalized structure of a synovial joint.

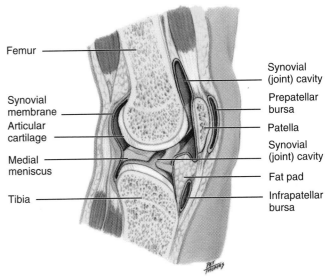

Figure 6-24 Sagittal section of the knee joint illustrating bursae and menisci.

absorbers. **Bursae** are fluid-filled sacs that act as cushions and help reduce friction. Bursae are lined with a synovial membrane that secretes synovial fluid into the sac. They are commonly located between the skin and underlying bone or between tendons and ligaments. Inflammation of a bursa is called **bursitis**. Figure 6–24 illustrates some menisci and bursae associated with the knee joint.

> Menisci and bursae are special structures that act as protective cushions in some synovial joints.

There are six types of diarthrotic or freely movable joints based on the shapes of their parts and the types of movement they allow. These are described in Table 6–10.

✓ QuickCheck

● An athlete is diagnosed as having a torn meniscus. Which joint is affected and what type of joint is it?

● Which type of joint is the only one with a joint cavity?

The term *torn cartilage* refers to a damaged meniscus, usually the medial, in the knee. Frequently this can be repaired with relatively minor arthroscopic surgery. A torn ligament in the knee involves one of the cruciate ligaments. The surgical procedure to repair this damage is quite involved, and recovery of function may require months of rehabilitative therapy.

Table 6-10 Types of Freely Movable Joints

Type	Shape of Joint Surfaces	Range of Movement	Examples
Ball-and-socket	Ball-shaped end of one bone fits into cup-shaped socket of another	Permits widest range of movement in all planes, including rotation	Shoulder, hip
Condyloid	Oval-shaped condyle fits into elliptical cavity of another	Angular motion but not rotation	Occipital condyles with atlas; metacarpals and metatarsals with phalanges
Saddle	Articulating surfaces of both bones have concave and convex regions; shapes of the two bones complementary to each other	Permits wide range of movement	Carpometacarpal joint of the thumb is only saddle joint in the body
Pivot	Rounded or conical surface of one bone fits into a ring of bone or tendon	Rotation	Joint between the atlas and axis; proximal radioulnar joint
Hinge	Convex projection of one bone fits into concave depression in another	Permits flexion and extension only	Elbow and knee joints
Gliding	Flat or slightly curved surfaces are moving against each other	Sliding or twisting without circular movement	Between the carpals in the wrist and between the tarsals in the ankle

FOCUS ON AGING

The major age-related change in the skeletal system is the loss of calcium from the bones. Calcium loss occurs in both men and women, but it starts at an earlier age and is more severe in women. The exact reasons for the loss are unknown and possibly involve a combination of several factors. These may include an imbalance between osteoblast and osteoclast activity, imbalance between calcitonin and parathormone levels, reduced absorption of calcium and/or vitamin D from the digestive tract, poor diet, and lack of exercise. Whatever the cause, there is no sure way of preventing the loss, but adequate calcium and vitamin D in the diet may help reduce the effects. Estrogen replacement therapy after menopause may help in women.

Another change with age is a decrease in the rate of collagen synthesis. This means that the bones have less strength and are more brittle. Bones fracture more readily in elderly individuals and the healing process may be slow or incomplete. Tendons and ligaments become less flexible because of the changes in collagen.

The articular cartilage at the ends of bones tends to become thinner and deteriorates with age. This causes joint disorders that are commonly found in older individuals. People also appear to get shorter as they get older. This is partially due to loss of bone mass and partially due to compression of the intervertebral disks.

Age-related changes in the skeletal system cannot be prevented. An active and healthy lifestyle with appropriate exercise and an adequate diet help reduce the effect of the changes in the skeletal system.

DO YOU KNOW THIS ABOUT THE

Skeleton?

Fractures and Fracture Repair

A bone fracture is any break in the continuity of a bone. Traumatic injury is the most common cause of fractures, although metabolic disorders and aging may weaken bones to the point at which they can withstand very little stress and they fracture spontaneously. Fractures occur more frequently in children than in adults because children have slender bones and are more active. Fortunately for the children, their bones tend to heal more quickly than adults because of greater osteoblast activity in young people.

Bone fractures may be classified in several ways. The following list defines some of the more commonly used terms for describing fractures.

Complete—The break extends across the entire section of bone.

Incomplete—The fracture still has pieces of the bone partially joined together.

Open—The broken end of the bone protrudes through the surrounding tissues and skin, which presents an open pathway for infection; also called a compound fracture.

Closed—The fractured bone does not extend through the skin so that there is less chance of bacterial invasion; also called a simple fracture.

Transverse—The bone is broken at right angles to the long axis of the bone.

Linear—The fracture is parallel to the long axis of the bone.

Spiral—The bone is broken by twisting.

Oblique—The bone is broken on a slant.

Comminuted—The bone is crushed into small pieces.

Greenstick—An incomplete fracture occurs in which one side of the bone is broken and the other side bends; occurs in children.

Displaced—The pieces of bone are not in correct alignment.

Usually, the pieces of bone in a displaced fracture can be brought into normal position by physical manipulation without surgery. This is called a **closed reduction.** In some cases, surgery is necessary to expose the fractured bone fragments and bring them into normal alignment. This process is called **open reduction.**

After the reduction of a fracture, a complex series of events occurs that usually results in satisfactory healing. Anyone who has ever had a fracture knows firsthand that the healing process is slow. Several factors contribute to this. The blood vessels to the bone are damaged by the break and whenever vascular supply is reduced, there is a corresponding reduction in cellular metabolism and mitosis. The physical trauma of the break tears and destroys tissues in the region and a lack of blood supply further damages tissues. This dead and damaged tissue inhibits repair. A third factor that makes bone repair slow is the fact that the bone cells reproduce slowly. An infection slows the process even further.

When a bone fracture occurs, the periosteum and numerous blood vessels that cross the fracture line are torn. The blood from the torn vessels forms a clot, or **fracture hematoma,** which plugs the gap between the ends of the bones. The fracture hematoma, usually formed within a few hours after the injury, stops blood circulation in the region so that cells in the area, including periosteal and bone cells, die. This dead tissue and reduced vascular supply in the traumatized area seem to initiate the healing process.

After the fracture hematoma forms, blood capillaries start to grow into the hematoma and organize it into a **procallus.** These new vessels bring phagocytic cells, such as neutrophils and macrophages, to start cleaning up the dead debris. The cleanup is an ongoing process that takes several weeks. While cleanup is in progress, fibroblasts from neighboring healthy tissue migrate to the fracture area and produce collagen fibers within the procallus. The fibers help tie the ends of the bones together. Chondroblasts, which develop from bone cells that do not receive enough blood, produce fibrocartilage that transforms the procallus into a **fibrocartilaginous callus.** This lasts about 3 weeks.

Osteoblasts from neighboring healthy bone tissue start to produce trabeculae of spongy bone. As the trabeculae grow, they infiltrate the fibrocartilaginous callus to make a **bony callus.** This bony callus, consisting of spongy bone, lasts for 3 to 4 months before it is remodeled into bone that is very similar to the original. **Remodeling** is the final step in the repair process. Osteoblasts lay down new compact bone around the periphery whereas osteoclasts reabsorb spongy bone from the inside and form a new medullary cavity. Successful healing results in a repaired bone that is so similar in structure to the original that the fracture line may not be visible on a radiograph, although the bone may be slightly thicker in that region. If healing is complete, original bone strength is also restored.

Sometimes bones do not heal properly or are very slow to heal. In some cases surgery is indicated to remove dead or infected tissue and to cleanse the area or to stabilize the broken pieces of bone. Some cases may be helped by using electrotherapy. This technique uses a weak electrical current, called **pulsating electromagnetic fields,** to stimulate osteoblast activity, vascularization, and calcification.

REPRESENTATIVE DISORDERS OF THE SKELETAL SYSTEM

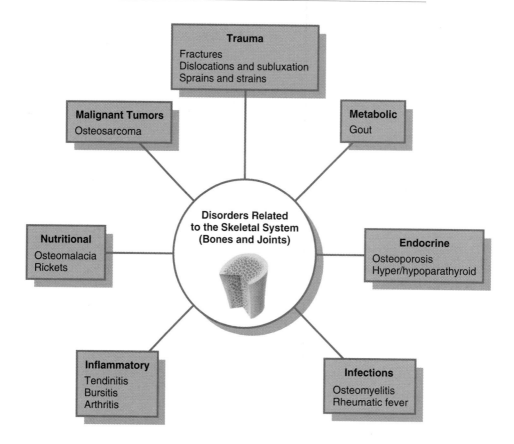

Trauma
Fractures
Dislocations and subluxation
Sprains and strains

Malignant Tumors
Osteosarcoma

Metabolic
Gout

Nutritional
Osteomalacia
Rickets

**Disorders Related
to the Skeletal System
(Bones and Joints)**

Endocrine
Osteoporosis
Hyper/hypoparathyroid

Inflammatory
Tendinitis
Bursitis
Arthritis

Infections
Osteomyelitis
Rheumatic fever

CHAPTER QUIZ

RECALL

Match the definitions on the left with the appropriate term on the right.

1. Blood cell formation

2. Shaft of a long bone

3. Opening in bone for blood vessels and nerves

4. Bone cells

5. Connective tissue is replaced by bone

6. Increase in bone diameter

7. Slightly movable joints

8. Inflammation of fluid-filled sacs related to joints

9. Narrow cleft or slit

10. Location of red bone marrow

A. Amphiarthroses

B. Appositional
growth

C. Bursitis

D. Diaphysis

E. Fissure

F. Foramen

G. Hematopoiesis

H. Intramembranous
ossification

I. Osteocytes

J. Spongy bone

THOUGHT

1. Intramembranous ossification occurs in the

   a. femur

   b. parietal bone

   c. radius

   d. carpals

2. Which of the following does not belong to the appendicular skeleton?

   a. clavicle

   b. scapula

   c. sternum

   d. patella

3. The bone on the lateral side of the forearm is the

   a. humerus

   b. ulna

   c. fibula

   d. radius

4. The bones that form the pectoral girdle are the

   a. scapula and sternum

   b. sternum and clavicle

   c. scapula and clavicle

   d. humerus and scapula

5. An example of a diarthrosis is the

   a. coronal suture

   b. elbow

   c. symphysis pubis

   d. joints between two vertebrae

APPLICATION

Why do you think lumbar vertebrae have large, thick bodies and thick intervertebral disks instead of small ones like the cervical vertebrae?

CHAPTER 7

Muscular System

Outline/Objectives

Characteristics and Functions of the Muscular System 123
- List the characteristics and functions of muscle tissue.

Structure of Skeletal Muscle 123
- Describe the structure of a skeletal muscle, including its connective tissue coverings.
- Identify the bands and lines that make up the striations on myofibers of skeletal muscle and relate these striations to actin and myosin.

Contraction of Skeletal Muscle 126
- Describe the sequence of events involved in the contraction of a skeletal muscle fiber.
- Compare the different types of muscle contractions.
- Describe how energy is provided for muscle contraction and how oxygen debt occurs.
- Describe and illustrate movements accomplished by the contraction of skeletal muscles.

Skeletal Muscle Groups 133
- Locate, identify, and describe the actions of the major muscles of the axial skeleton.
- Locate, identify, and describe the actions of the major muscles of the appendicular skeleton.

Key Terms

Actin

All-or-none principle

Antagonist

Insertion

Motor unit

Myosin

Neuromuscular junction

Origin

Prime mover

Sarcomere

Synergist

Building Vocabulary

WORD PART	MEANING
a-	without, lacking
act-	motion
bi-	two
cep-	head
delt-	triangle
dia-	through
duct-	movement
flex-	bend
-in	neutral substance
iso-	same, alike
lemm-	peel, rind
masset-	chew
metr-	measure
myo-, mys-	muscle
phragm-	fence, partition
sarco-	flesh, muscle
syn-	together
tetan-	stiff
ton-	tone, tension
troph-	nourish, develop

Functional Relationships of the
Muscular System

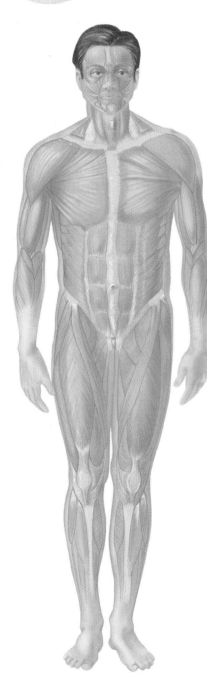

► Generates heat to maintain body temperature.

Integument

◄ Covers muscles and provides barrier against harmful substances; synthesis of vitamin D for absorption of calcium necessary for bone growth, maintenance, and repair; radiates excess heat generated by muscle contraction.

► Facial muscles contract and pull on the skin to provide facial expressions.

Skeletal

◄ Provides attachment sites for muscles; bones act as levers for muscle action; stores calcium necessary for muscle contraction.

► Stabilizes position of bones; supplies forces for movement; tension from muscle contraction influences bone shape and size and maintains bone mass.

Nervous

◄ Coordinates muscle contraction; adjusts cardiovascular and respiratory systems to maintain cardiac output and oxygen for muscle contraction.

► Muscles carry out motor commands originating in the nervous system, give expression to emotions and thoughts.

Endocrine

◄ Hormones influence muscle metabolism, mass, and strength; epinephrine and norepinephrine influence cardiac and smooth muscle activity.

► Provides protection for some endocrine glands.

Cardiovascular

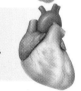

◄ Delivers oxygen and nutrients to muscle tissue and removes waste products and heat.

► Skeletal muscle contraction aids venous return, contributes to growth of new blood vessels, promotes cardiac strength; smooth and cardiac muscle contraction contributes to vessel and heart function.

Lymphatic/Immune

◄ Maintains interstitial fluid balance in muscle tissue; assists in defense against pathogens and repair of muscle tissue following trauma.

► Skeletal muscle contraction aids in the flow of lymph; protects superficial lymph nodes.

Respiratory

◄ Supplies oxygen for muscle metabolism and contraction; removes carbon dioxide.

► Muscle contractions control airflow through respiratory passages and create pressure changes necessary for ventilation.

Digestive

◄ Absorbs nutrients for muscle growth, maintenance, and repair; liver metabolizes lactic acid from muscle contraction.

► Provides support and protection for digestive system organs; muscular sphincters control openings in the GI tract; function in chewing and swallowing; aids in defecation.

Urinary

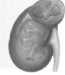

◄ Eliminates metabolic wastes from muscle metabolism; conserves calcium ions for muscle contraction.

► Supports and protects organs of the urinary system; sphincters control voluntary urination.

Reproductive

◄ Gonads produce hormones that influence muscle development and size.

► Provides support for reproductive organs in the pelvis; muscle contractions contribute to orgasm in both sexes; aid in childbirth.

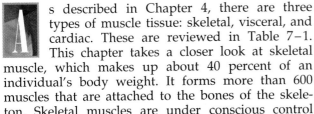s described in Chapter 4, there are three types of muscle tissue: skeletal, visceral, and cardiac. These are reviewed in Table 7–1. This chapter takes a closer look at skeletal muscle, which makes up about 40 percent of an individual's body weight. It forms more than 600 muscles that are attached to the bones of the skeleton. Skeletal muscles are under conscious control and when they contract they move the bones. Skeletal muscles also allow us to smile, frown, pout, show surprise, and exhibit other forms of facial expression.

Characteristics and Functions of the Muscular System

Skeletal muscle has four primary characteristics that relate to its functions:

Excitability—Excitability (eks-eye-tah-BILL-ih-tee) is the ability to receive and respond to a stimulus. To function properly, muscles have to respond to a stimulus from the nervous system.

Contractility—Contractility (kon-track-TILL-ih-tee) is the ability to shorten or contract. When a muscle responds to a stimulus, it shortens to produce movement.

Extensibility—Extensibility (eks-ten-sih-BILL-ih-tee) means that a muscle can be stretched or extended. Skeletal muscles are often arranged in opposing pairs. When one muscle contracts, the other muscle is relaxed and is stretched.

Elasticity—Elasticity (ee-lass-TISS-ih-tee) is the capacity to recoil or return to the original shape and length after contraction or extension.

> Four characteristics of skeletal muscle tissue are excitability, contractility, extensibility, and elasticity.

Muscle contraction fulfills four important functions in the body:

- Movement
- Posture
- Joint stability
- Heat production

Nearly all **movement** in the body is the result of muscle contraction. Exceptions to this are the action of cilia, the flagellum on sperm cells, and ameboid movement of some white blood cells. The integrated action of joints, bones, and skeletal muscles produces obvious movements such as walking and running. Skeletal muscles also produce more subtle movements that result in various facial expressions, eye movements, and respiration. **Posture,** such as sitting and standing, is maintained as a result of muscle contraction. The skeletal muscles are continually making fine adjustments that hold the body in stationary positions. Skeletal muscles contribute to **joint stability.** The tendons of many muscles extend over joints and in this way contribute to joint stability. This is particularly evident in the knee and shoulder joints, where muscle tendons are a major factor in stabilizing the joint. **Heat production,** to maintain body temperature, is an important byproduct of muscle metabolism. Nearly 85 percent of the heat produced in the body is the result of muscle contraction.

> Four functions of muscle contraction are movement, posture, joint stability, and heat production.

Structure of Skeletal Muscle

A whole skeletal muscle is considered an organ of the muscular system. Each organ or muscle consists of skeletal muscle tissue, connective tissue, nerve tissue, and blood or vascular tissue.

Whole Skeletal Muscle

An individual skeletal muscle may be made up of hundreds, or even thousands, of muscle fibers bun-

---

CLINICAL TERMS

Cramp (KRAMP) Painful involuntary muscle spasm; often caused by myositis but can be a symptom of any irritation or ion imbalance

Electromyography (ee-lek-troh-mye-AHG-rah-fee) The process of recording the strength of muscle contraction as a result of electrical stimulation

Muscle biopsy (MUSS-uhl BYE-ahp-see) Removal of muscle tissue for microscopic examination

Muscular dystrophy (MUSS-kyoo-lar DIS-troh-fee) An inherited, chronic, progressive wasting and weakening of muscles without involvement of the nervous system

Myasthenia gravis (mye-as-THEE-nee-ah GRAY-vis) An autoimmune disease, more common in females, that is characterized by weakness of skeletal muscles caused by an abnormality at the neuromuscular junction

Myopathy (mye-AHP-ah-thee) Muscle disease

Myositis (mye-oh-SYE-tis) Inflammation of muscle tissue

Tic (TICK) A spasmodic involuntary twitching of a muscle that is normally under voluntary control

Table 7–1 Summary of Muscle Tissue

Feature	Skeletal	Visceral	Cardiac
Location	Attached to bones	Walls of internal organs and blood vessels	Heart
Function	Produce body movement	Contraction of viscera and blood vessels	Pump blood through the heart and blood vessels
Cell shape	Cylindrical	Spindle shaped, tapered ends	Cylindrical, branching
Number of nuclei	Many	One	One
Striations	Present	Absent	Present
Type of control	Voluntary	Involuntary	Involuntary

dled together and wrapped in a connective tissue covering. Each muscle is surrounded by a connective tissue sheath called the **epimysium** (ep-ih-MYE-see-um). Fascia, connective tissue outside the epimysium, surrounds and separates the muscles. Portions of the epimysium project inward to divide the muscle into compartments. Each compartment contains a bundle of muscle fibers. Each bundle of muscle fibers is called a **fasciculus** (fah-SIK-yoo-lus) and is surrounded by a layer of connective tissue called the **perimysium** (pair-ih-MYE-see-um). Within the fasciculus, each individual muscle cell, called a muscle fiber, is surrounded by connective tissue called the **endomysium** (end-oh-MYE-see-um). Connective tissue fibers of the endomysium are continuous with those in the perimysium, which, in turn, are continuous with the epimysium. Skeletal muscle cells (fibers), like other body cells, are soft and fragile. The connective tissue coverings furnish support and protection for the delicate cells and allow them to withstand the forces of contraction. The coverings also provide pathways for the passage of blood vessels and nerves. The organization and connective tissue wrappings of skeletal muscle fibers are illustrated in Figure 7–1.

> Each muscle fiber is surrounded by endomysium. The fibers are collected into bundles covered by perimysium. Many bundles, or fasciculi, are wrapped together by the epimysium to form a whole muscle.

Skeletal Muscle Attachments

In some instances, fibers of the epimysium fuse directly with the periosteum of a bone to form a **direct** attachment. More commonly, the epimysium, perimysium, and endomysium extend beyond the fleshy part of the muscle, the **belly** or **gaster,** to form a thick ropelike **tendon** or a broad, flat, sheetlike **aponeurosis** (ah-pah-noo-ROE-sis). The tendon and aponeurosis form **indirect** attachments from muscles to the periosteum of bones or to the connective tissue of other muscles. Typically, a muscle spans a joint and is attached to bones by tendons at both ends. One of the bones remains relatively fixed

or stable while the other end moves as a result of muscle contraction. The fixed or stable end is called the **origin** of the muscle, and the more movable attachment is called the **insertion.**

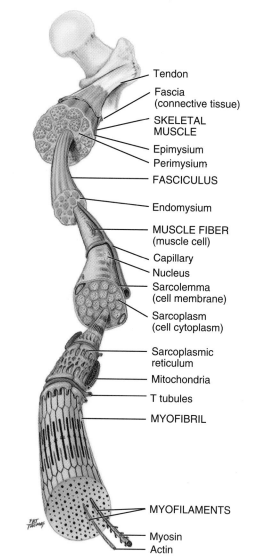

Tendon
Fascia (connective tissue)
SKELETAL MUSCLE
Epimysium
Perimysium
FASCICULUS
Endomysium
MUSCLE FIBER (muscle cell)
Capillary
Nucleus
Sarcolemma (cell membrane)
Sarcoplasm (cell cytoplasm)
Sarcoplasmic reticulum
Mitochondria
T tubules
MYOFIBRIL
MYOFILAMENTS
Myosin
Actin

Figure 7–1 Organization and connective tissue components of skeletal muscle.

Muscles are attached to bones by tendons. The more stable attachment of a muscle is the origin; the more movable end is the insertion.

Skeletal Muscle Fibers

Each skeletal muscle fiber is a single cylindrical muscle cell. The cell membrane is called the **sarcolemma** (sar-koh-LEM-mah), the cytoplasm is the **sarcoplasm** (SAR-koh-plazm), and a specialized form of smooth endoplasmic reticulum that stores calcium ions is the **sarcoplasmic reticulum** (sar-koh-PLAZ-mik reh-TIK-yoo-lum). There are multiple nuclei next to the sarcolemma at the periphery of the cell. Because the muscle cell needs energy for contraction, there are numerous mitochondria. The sarcolemma has multiple inward extensions, or invaginations, called transverse tubules or **T tubules.**

A skeletal muscle fiber is a muscle cell with typical cellular organelles.

Microscopic examination of a skeletal muscle fiber reveals alternating light **I** (isotropic) **bands** and dark **A** (anisotropic) **bands.** These are the striations visible in a light microscope. Closer inspection shows that the sarcoplasm is packed with filamentous **myofibrils** (mye-oh-FYE-brills) that have the same characteristic banding as the muscle fiber. The myofibrils consist of still smaller protein threads called **myofilaments** (mye-oh-FILL-ah-ments). Thick filaments are formed by the protein **myosin,** whereas thin filaments are formed primarily from the protein **actin.** The overlapping arrangement of actin and myosin, illustrated in Figure 7–2, accounts for the bands and lines observed on the myofibrils and muscle fibers.

The sarcoplasm of muscle cells is packed with myofibrils composed of actin and myosin myofilaments.

The **I band** is the region where there are only thin (actin) filaments. A dark **Z line** bisects the I band. The Z line is actually a protein disk that serves as a point of attachment for the actin mole-

cules. **A bands,** alternating with the I bands, extend the full length of the thick (myosin) filaments. Each A band is subdivided into three regions. The **zone of overlap** is at the ends of the A band where the actin overlaps the myosin. The central region of the A band where the actin does not overlap and where there are only myosin filaments is the **H zone** or **H band.** An **M line,** where thick filaments interconnect, bisects the H band. Refer to Figure 7–2 to identify these regions.

The arrangement of the actin and myosin myofilaments accounts for the A, I, and H bands. The Z and M lines are points of myofilament connections.

A **sarcomere** (SAR-koh-meer), the functional unit of a myofibril, extends from one Z line to the next. The typical myofibril consists of 10,000 or more **sarcomeres** that are strung together in long chains. When a muscle cell contracts, all the sarcomeres in all the myofibrils of that cell shorten at the same time.

Nerve and Blood Supply

Skeletal muscles have an abundant supply of blood vessels and nerves. This is directly related to the primary function of skeletal muscle—contraction. Before a skeletal muscle fiber can contract, it has to receive an impulse from a nerve cell. Muscle contraction requires adenosine triphosphate (ATP), and blood vessels deliver the necessary nutrients and oxygen to produce it. Blood vessels also remove the waste products that are produced as a result of muscle contraction.

In general, an artery and at least one vein accompany each nerve that penetrates the epimysium of a skeletal muscle. Branches of the nerve and blood vessels follow the connective tissue components of the muscle so that each muscle fiber is in contact with a branch of a nerve cell and with one or more minute blood vessels called capillaries.

Skeletal muscles have an abundant blood and nerve supply.

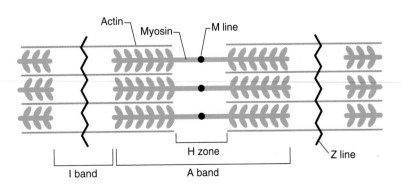

Figure 7–2 Arrangement of myofilaments in skeletal muscle.

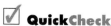

✓ QuickCheck

● When dissecting a muscle, what is the outermost connective tissue wrapping that is encountered?

● What band of striation has only thin (actin) myofilaments?

Contraction of Skeletal Muscle

Skeletal muscle contraction is the result of a complex series of events, based on chemical reactions, at the cellular (muscle fiber) level. This chain of reactions begins with stimulation by a nerve cell and ends when the muscle fiber is again relaxed. Contraction of a whole muscle is the result of the simultaneous contraction of many muscle fibers.

> Skeletal muscle contraction is produced by simultaneous and synchronized contraction of many muscle fibers.

Stimulus for Contraction

Skeletal muscles are stimulated to contract by special nerve cells called **motor neurons.** As the axon of the motor neuron penetrates the muscle, the axon branches, so there is an axon terminal for each muscle fiber. A single motor neuron and all the muscle fibers it stimulates is called a **motor unit.** Some motor units include several hundred individual fibers; others contain less than 10. Because all the muscle fibers in a motor unit receive a nerve impulse at the same time, all the fibers contract at the same time.

The region in which an axon terminal meets a muscle fiber is called a **neuromuscular,** or myoneural, **junction,** which is illustrated in Figure 7–3. The axon terminal does not actually touch the sarcolemma of the muscle cell but fits into a shallow depression in the cell membrane. The fluid-filled space between the terminal and sarcolemma is called a **synaptic cleft** (gap). **Acetylcholine (ACh)** (ah-see-till-KOH-leen), a neurotransmitter, is contained within synaptic vesicles in the axon terminal. Receptor sites for the acetylcholine are located on the sarcolemma.

> A neuromuscular junction is the region in which an axon terminal is closely associated with a muscle fiber.

When a nerve impulse reaches the axon terminal, acetylcholine is released. The acetylcholine diffuses across the synaptic cleft and binds with the receptor sites on the sarcolemma. This reaction is the stimulus for contraction. A stimulus is a change in the cellular environment that alters the cell membrane and causes a response. In this case, the response is a muscle impulse, similar to a nerve impulse, that travels in all directions on the sarcolemma. From the sarcolemma, it travels into the T tubules, where it initiates physiologic activity within the muscle cell that results in contraction.

> Acetylcholine is the neurotransmitter that diffuses across the synaptic cleft to stimulate the sarcolemma.

Meanwhile, back at the synaptic cleft, the acetylcholine that was released is rapidly inactivated by the enzyme **acetylcholinesterase** (ah-see-till-koh-lin-ES-ter-ase). This ensures that one nerve impulse will result in only one muscle impulse and only one contraction of the muscle fiber. Anything that interferes with the production, release, or inactivation of acetylcholine, or its ability to bind with the receptor sites on the sarcolemma, will have an effect on muscle contraction. Muscle relaxant drugs work in this manner.

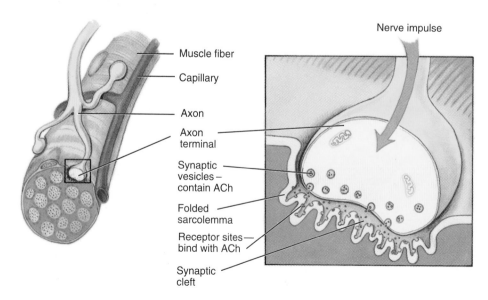

Figure 7–3 Neuromuscular junction.

Anything that interferes with the action of acetylcholine will have an effect on muscle contraction.

Sarcomere Contraction

In a relaxed muscle fiber, myosin receptor sites on the actin thin filaments are covered or inactivated. Heads or cross-bridges on the myosin are also inactivated and are bound to ATP. Calcium is stored in the sarcoplasmic reticulum and has a low concentration in the sarcoplasm.

When an impulse travels from an axon to the sarcolemma and down the T tubule, calcium ions are released from the sarcoplasmic reticulum. This rapid influx of calcium ions into the sarcoplasm causes a change in the configuration of the troponin on the actin filaments and exposes the myosin binding sites. Simultaneously, the ATP on the myosin heads is broken down to adenosine diphosphate (ADP) so that the myosin is energized and interacts with the actin. The energized myosin heads that are now bound to actin to form cross-bridges rotate in a "power stroke" to pull the actin toward the center of the myosin. Because actin is firmly anchored to the Z line, the Z lines move closer together and the sarcomere shortens. The length of each myofilament remains the same. The actin just slides over the myosin to decrease the length of the sarcomere. When new ATP binds with the myosin, the cross-bridges detach, and the cycle is repeated with another binding site. These events are illustrated in Figure 7–4. Because the actin "slides" over the myosin, this is known as the **sliding filament theory** of muscle contraction.

Calcium and ATP change the configuration of actin and myosin so that actin "slides" toward the center of myosin. This action shortens the length of a sarcomere.

The term *rigor mortis* means the "stiffness of death." Within a short time of death, the ATP in muscles breaks down so there is no ATP available to detach the cross-bridges between myosin and actin. The myofilaments remain locked in a contracted position and the body becomes rigid. A day or so later, muscle proteins begin to deteriorate and the rigor mortis disappears.

Myosin continues to pull actin toward the center of the A band in a step-by-step, or ratchetlike, manner as long as there is calcium in the sarcoplasm and sufficient ATP to provide energy. The ATP is needed to energize the myosin and to cause the power stroke and to recombine with myosin to detach the cross-bridges so another cycle can occur.

When there are no more nerve impulses at the neuromuscular junction, muscle impulses stop and calcium is actively transported from the sarcoplasm back into the sarcoplasmic reticulum. Without calcium, the actin and myosin are reconfigured into their noncontracting condition, and the muscle fiber relaxes. The events in the contraction of a skeletal muscle fiber are summarized in Table 7–2.

When stimulation at the neuromuscular junction stops, calcium returns to the sarcoplasmic reticulum and actin and myosin resume their noncontracting positions.

Individual muscle fibers contract according to the **all-or-none principle.** When a muscle fiber receives sufficient stimulus to contract, all the sarcomeres shorten at the same time. A greater stimulus will not elicit a greater contraction. If there is insufficient stimulus, then none of the sarcomeres contract. In other words, it is "all" or "none." The minimum stimulus necessary to cause muscle fiber contraction is a **threshold,** or **liminal, stimulus.** A lesser stimulus, one that is insufficient to cause contraction, is a **subthreshold,** or **subliminal, stimulus.**

Individual muscle fibers contract according to the all-or-none principle.

Contraction of a Whole Muscle

Whereas a single muscle fiber obeys the all-or-none principle, it is obvious that whole muscles do not. Whole muscles have a graded response; they show varying strengths of contraction. A muscle has greater contraction strength when you pick up a 25-pound weight than when you pick up a feather because more muscle fibers are contracting. In-

Relaxed sarcomere

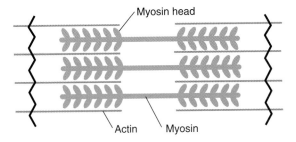

Contracting sarcomere

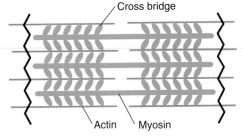

Figure 7–4 Sliding filament theory of muscle contraction.

Table 7–2   Summary of Skeletal Muscle Contraction

1. Nerve impulse travels down the axon to the axon terminals.
2. Acetylcholine is released from the axon terminals.
3. Acetylcholine diffuses across the synaptic cleft and binds with receptor sites on the sarcolemma.
4. Muscle impulse travels along the sarcolemma and into the T tubules.
5. Muscle impulse in the T tubules causes calcium ions to be released from the sarcoplasmic reticulum.
6. Calcium causes a change in the configuration of binding sites on actin and also causes ATP to break down and "energize" the myosin heads.
7. Myosin heads bind with actin to form cross-bridges.
8. Cross-bridges rotate in a "power stroke" that slides actin toward the middle of the myosin to shorten the sarcomere (muscle contraction).
9. A new ATP binds with the myosin, and myosin detaches from actin. Steps 6 through 9 repeat as long as the sarcolemma is stimulated by acetylcholine and there is sufficient ATP.
10. When the nerve impulse stops, calcium ions are actively transported (requires ATP) back into the sarcoplasmic reticulum, and the muscle relaxes with steps 9 and 10.

ATP = adenosine triphosphate.

creased contraction strength is achieved by **motor unit summation** and **wave summation.** Contraction strength is decreased by fatigue, lack of nutrients, and lack of oxygen.

> Single muscle fibers obey the all-or-none principle, but whole muscles show varying strengths of contraction owing to motor unit and wave summation.

Within a muscle, the muscle fibers are organized into motor units. As defined previously, a **motor unit** is a single neuron and all the muscle fibers it stimulates. Because all the muscle fibers in a motor unit receive a threshold stimulus at the same time, a motor unit obeys the all-or-none principle, as does a muscle fiber. A stronger stimulus, however, stimulates more motor units, which increases the contraction strength of the muscle as a whole. This is called **multiple motor unit summation.**

> The contraction strength of a whole muscle can be increased by stimulating more motor units. This is multiple motor unit summation.

A muscle's response to a single threshold stimulus is called a **twitch.** This is not the way a muscle in the body normally functions. This is a laboratory condition, but it gives useful information about muscle action. A myogram, a graphic recording of muscle tension in a twitch, illustrated in Figure 7–5A, shows that there are three distinct phases to the twitch. Initially, just after stimulation, there is no response on the myogram. This is the **lag phase.** Then the **contraction phase** begins and tension in the muscle increases to a peak. If the tension is great enough to overcome a weight load, then movement occurs. This is followed by the **relaxation phase,** when tension decreases until the resting, relaxed state is achieved.

> A muscle twitch, the response to a single stimulus, shows a lag phase, a contraction phase, and a relaxation phase.

If a second stimulus is applied during the relaxation phase, the second twitch is stronger than the first. If the muscle is stimulated at an increasingly faster rate, the relaxation time becomes shorter and shorter. Finally, all evidence of relaxation disappears and the contractions merge into a smooth, sustained contraction called **tetany** (see Fig. 7–5B). Tetany is a form of **multiple wave summation.** This is the usual form of muscle contraction. Neurons normally deliver a rapid succession of impulses that result in tetany, rather than a single impulse that causes a single muscle twitch.

> Rapid repeated stimulation results in a smooth sustained contraction that is stronger than the contraction from a single stimulus of the same intensity. This is multiple wave summation.

The word *tetanus* is often confusing because it means different things to different people. In reference to muscle contraction, the term denotes a wave summation that produces a steady contraction of a muscle fiber, without a relaxation phase. The word also refers to a disease, commonly called "lockjaw," that is caused by the bacterium *Clostridium tetani.* The toxin from the bacteria causes nerves to be highly excitable, which, in turn, causes uncontrollable muscle contractions, or spasms. A third use of the word is to denote a condition caused by a deficiency of calcium ions in the extracellular fluid. The lack of calcium increases nerve excitability with resulting muscle spasms, particularly of the extremities. The word *tetany* is also sometimes used to mean tetanus.

A

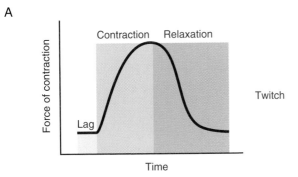

B

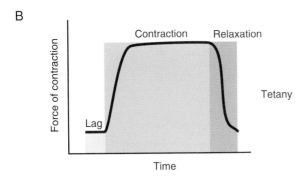

C

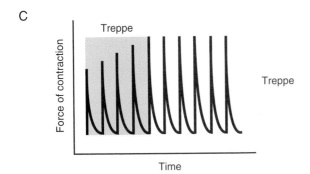

Figure 7–5 Types of contraction in whole muscle. *A,* Twitch. *B,* Tetany. *C,* Treppe.

Treppe (TREP-peh), or staircase effect, is an increase in the force of muscle contraction in response to successive threshold stimuli of the same intensity. This occurs in muscle that has rested for a prolonged period of time. If the muscle is rapidly stimulated with a series of threshold stimuli of the same intensity but not rapidly enough to produce tetanus, the myogram (see Fig. 7–5C) will show that each contraction is slightly stronger than the previous one. The increased force of contraction is due, in part, to the increased availability of calcium ions in the sarcoplasm. Other factors that influence treppe include pH, temperature, and viscosity, which change with cellular activity. Treppe is the basis of the warm-up period for athletes.

Treppe is the staircase effect that is evidenced when repeated stimuli of the same strength produce successively stronger contractions. This is due to changes in the cellular environment.

Muscle tone (tonus) refers to the continued state of partial contraction that is present in muscles. The motor units take turns contracting and relaxing. Some motor units are stimulated to contract whereas others relax. This produces a constant tension in the muscles and keeps them ready for activity. Muscle tone is especially important in maintaining posture. It is responsible for keeping the back and legs straight, the head erect, and the abdomen from protruding and also helps to stabilize joints. Without stimulation to contract, a muscle loses tone, becomes flaccid, and atrophies. Muscle fiber contraction to sustain muscle tone produces heat to maintain body temperature.

Muscle tone refers to the continued state of partial contraction in muscles. It is important in maintaining posture and body temperature.

Not all muscle activity results in shortening the muscle to produce movement. Cross-bridge activity produces tension in the muscle. If this tension exceeds the weight of a load, then the muscle shortens and movement occurs. This is **isotonic contraction.** The tension is constant or the same, but the length of the muscle changes. If, on the other hand, the tension in the muscle increases but never exceeds the weight load, then there is no shortening and no movement. This is **isometric contraction.** If you try to lift a large boulder by yourself, your muscle tension increases but never exceeds the weight of the boulder, so there is no movement. Most body movements are the result of a combination of isotonic and isometric contractions because some muscles stabilize certain joints at the same time other muscles produce movement in different joints.

Isotonic contractions produce movement. Isometric contractions increase muscle tension. Most body movements involve both types of contractions.

Pick this book up off the desk and raise it to shoulder level. That is isotonic muscle contraction because there is movement. Now, hold the book steady in front of you at shoulder height. That is isometric muscle contraction because no movement occurs. The isometric contractions of the shoulder and arm muscles counteract the downward pull of the book. Now lower the book to the desk. Again, this is isotonic contraction because there is movement. Both types of contractions require energy.

Energy Sources and Oxygen Debt

The immediate or initial source of energy for muscle contraction is **ATP** (Fig. 7–6A). Energy from ATP is needed for the cross-bridge power stroke, the detachment of myosin heads from the actin, and the

A

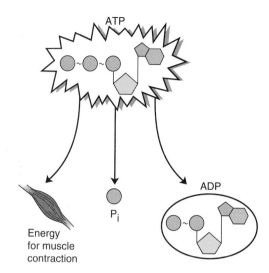

B

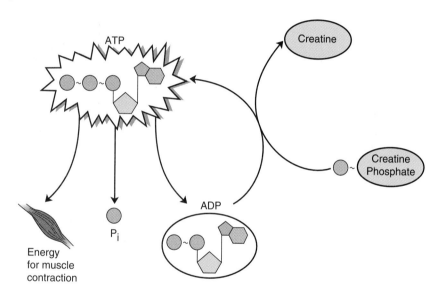

Figure 7–6 Energy sources for muscle contraction. *A,* Initial source is ATP. *B,* ATP is replenished by creatine phosphate.

active transport of calcium from the sarcoplasm into the sarcoplasmic reticulum. Surprisingly, muscles have limited storage facilities for ATP. In working muscles, the stored ATP is depleted in about 6 seconds, and new ATP must be regenerated if muscle contraction is to continue.

> In muscle contraction, energy is needed for the power stroke, the detachment of myosin heads, and the active transport of calcium.

Creatine phosphate (KREE-ah-tin FOS-fate) is a unique high-energy compound that is stored in muscles (see Fig. 7–6B). This compound provides an almost instantaneous transfer of its energy and a phosphate group to ADP molecules to regenerate ATP:

Creatine phosphate + ADP ⟶ creatine + ATP

This reaction is so effective that there is very little change in ATP levels during the initial stages of muscle contraction. When ATP levels are high, this reaction is reversed to form more creatine phosphate. Muscles store enough creatine phosphate to regenerate sufficient ATP to sustain contraction for about 10 seconds.

When muscles are actively contracting for extended periods of time, **fatty acids** and **glucose** become the primary energy sources. Glucose and fatty acids are present in the blood that circulates through the muscles, and glucose is stored in muscles as glycogen. As ATP and creatine phosphate stores are being used, more ATP is produced from the metabolism of glucose and fatty acids.

C

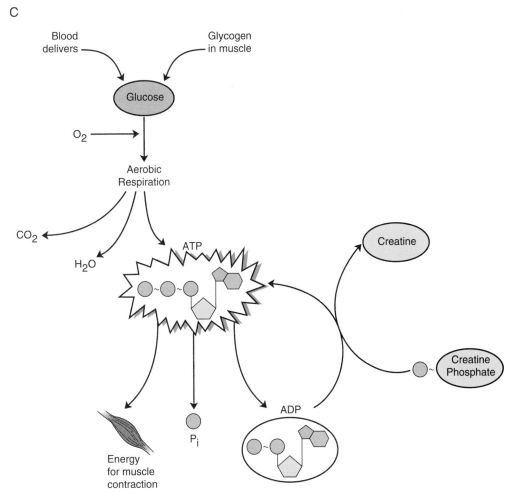

Figure 7-6   *Continued. C*, Aerobic breakdown of glucose and fatty acids provides additional ATP.

> ATP provides the initial energy for muscle contraction. The ATP supply is replenished by creatine phosphate, glucose, and fatty acids.

If adequate oxygen is available, fatty acids and glucose are broken down in the mitochondria by a process called **aerobic respiration** (see Fig. 7–6C). The products are carbon dioxide, water, and large amounts of ATP:

$$\text{Fatty acids or glucose} + \text{oxygen} \longrightarrow \text{carbon dioxide} + \text{water} + \text{ATP}$$

Limited amounts of oxygen can be stored in muscle fibers. Certain fibers, called **red fibers,** contain reddish protein pigment molecules called **myoglobin** (mye-oh-GLOH-bin). This pigment contains iron groups that attract and temporarily bind with oxygen. When the oxygen levels inside the muscle fiber diminish, the oxygen can be resupplied from myoglobin. Muscle fibers that contain very little myoglobin are called **white fibers.**

When muscles are contracting vigorously for long periods of time, myoglobin and the circulatory system are unable to deliver oxygen fast enough to maintain the aerobic pathways. Processes that do not require oxygen are necessary. Under these conditions, glucose is the primary energy source. If adequate oxygen is not available, glucose is broken down by a process called **anaerobic respiration** (see Fig. 7-6D). The products of the anaerobic pathway are lactic acid and a small amount of ATP.

$$\text{Glucose} \longrightarrow \text{lactic acid} + \text{ATP}$$

Some of the lactic acid accumulates in the muscle and causes a burning sensation. Most of it diffuses out of the muscle and into the bloodstream, which takes it to the liver. Later, when sufficient oxygen is available, the liver converts the lactic acid back to glycogen, the storage form of glucose.

> When adequate oxygen is available, glucose is metabolized by aerobic respiration to produce ATP. If adequate oxygen is not available, the mechanism for producing ATP from glucose is anaerobic respiration.

The aerobic pathway produces about 20 times more ATP than the anaerobic pathway. However,

D

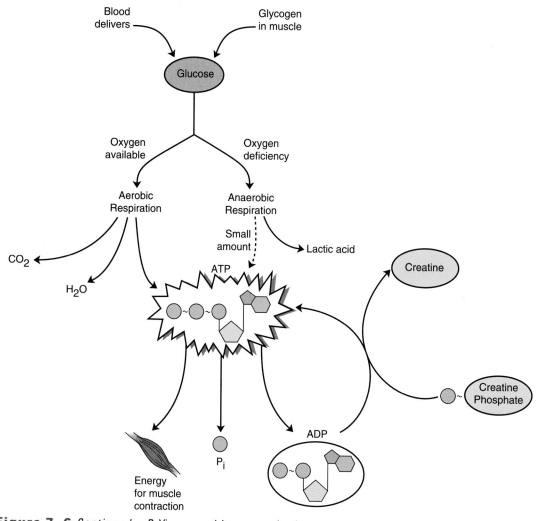

Figure 7–6 *Continued.* D, Vigorous activity may require the anaerobic breakdown of glucose, which produces lactic acid and ATP.

the anaerobic pathway provides ATP about two and one-half times faster than the aerobic pathway. Most of the energy for vigorous activity over a moderate period of time comes from anaerobic respiration. Prolonged activities requiring endurance depend on aerobic mechanisms.

> Aerobic respiration produces nearly 20 times more ATP per glucose than the anaerobic pathway, but anaerobic respiration occurs at a faster rate.

After periods of strenuous exercise that require anaerobic mechanisms to regenerate ATP, there is an accumulation of lactic acid in the muscle. This causes temporary muscular pain and cramping. The ATP and creatine phosphate in the muscle are depleted and need to be replenished. This creates an **oxygen debt** that must be repaid before equilibrium can be restored. Additional oxygen is needed to convert the lactic acid into glycogen, a process that occurs in the liver. Oxygen is also needed to replenish

the ATP and the creatine phosphate in the muscle. Oxygen debt is defined as the additional oxygen that is required after physical activity to restore resting conditions. The debt is paid back by labored breathing that continues after the activity has stopped.

> Oxygen debt occurs when there is an accumulation of lactic acid from anaerobic respiration. Additional oxygen from continued labored breathing is needed to repay the debt and to restore resting conditions.

> Cramps are painful, spastic contractions of muscles. They are usually due to an irritation within the muscles that results in reflex contractions. Local inflammation from the accumulation of lactic acid is one source of irritation.

- What effect would a drug that inactivated acetylcholinesterase have on skeletal muscle contraction?

- What ion is necessary for myosin heads to bind with receptor sites on actin? Why?

- If muscle fibers and motor units obey the all-or-none principle, what accounts for the difference in contraction strength when picking up a feather or a book?

- Which is more effective in terms of ATP produced—anaerobic or aerobic respiration?

Movements

Most intact skeletal muscles are attached to bones by tendons that span joints. When the muscle contracts, one bone (the insertion) moves relative to the other bone (the origin). Frequently muscles work in groups to perform a particular movement. If one muscle has a primary role in providing a movement, it is called a **prime mover.** Muscles that work with, or assist, the prime mover to cause a movement are called **synergists** (SIN-er-jists). Often muscles span more than one joint, and a synergist will stabilize one joint while the prime mover acts on the other joint. For example, the fingers can be flexed to make a fist without bending the wrist because certain muscles fix the wrist in a stabilized position. **Antagonists** are muscles that oppose, or reverse, a particular movement. The biceps brachii muscle on the anterior arm flexes the forearm at the elbow. The triceps brachii muscle on the posterior arm extends the forearm at the elbow. The two muscles are on opposite sides of the humerus and have opposite functions. They are antagonists.

> A prime mover has the major role in producing a specific movement; a synergist assists the prime mover; an antagonist opposes a particular movement.

Bones and muscles work together to perform different types of movement at the various joints. When describing muscular action or movement at joints, you need a frame of reference and descriptive terminology with definite meaning. Some commonly used terms that are used to describe particular movements are defined in Table 7–3.

> Descriptive terminology is used to depict particular movements.

Skeletal Muscle Groups

There are more than 600 skeletal muscles in the body. A discussion of each muscle is certainly beyond the scope of this book. Only the more significant and obvious muscles are identified and described here. These are arranged in groups according to location and/or function. If you iden-

tify and learn the muscles as group associations, it will make them easier to remember. If you can locate a muscle on your own body, you will be able to contract the muscle and describe its action. Learning anatomy in this manner makes it more meaningful.

Naming Muscles

Most skeletal muscles have names that describe some feature of the muscle. Often several criteria are combined into one name. Associating the muscle's characteristics with its name will help you learn and remember them. The following are some terms relating to muscle features that are used in naming muscles:

- **Size:** vastus (huge); maximus (large); longus (long); minimus (small); brevis (short).
- **Shape:** deltoid (triangular); rhomboid (like a rhombus with equal and parallel sides); latissimus (wide); teres (round); trapezius (like a trapezoid, a four-sided figure with two sides parallel).
- **Direction of fibers:** rectus (straight); transverse (across); oblique (diagonal); orbicularis (circular).
- **Location:** pectoralis (chest); gluteus (buttock or rump); brachii (arm); supra- (above); infra- (below); sub- (under or beneath); lateralis (lateral).
- **Number of origins:** biceps (two heads); triceps (three heads); quadriceps (four heads).
- **Origin and insertion:** sternocleidomastoideus (origin on the sternum and clavicle, insertion on the mastoid process); brachioradialis (origin on the brachium or arm, insertion on the radius).
- **Action:** abductor (to abduct a structure); adductor (to adduct a structure); flexor (to flex a structure); extensor (to extend a structure); levator (to lift or elevate a structure); masseter (a chewer).

> Muscle features such as size, shape, direction of fibers, location, number of attachments, origin, insertion, and action are often used in naming muscles.

Muscles of the Head and Neck
(Table 7–4 and Fig. 7–7)

Muscles of Facial Expression

Humans have well-developed muscles in the face that permit a large variety of facial expressions. Because these muscles are used to show surprise, disgust, anger, fear, and other emotions, they are an important means of nonverbal communication. The following are some of the muscles used to produce facial expressions.

The **frontalis** (frun-TAL-is) is over the frontal bone of the forehead. It is attached to the soft tissue of the eyebrow; when it contracts, it raises the eyebrows and wrinkles the forehead. The **orbicularis oris** (oar-BIK-yoo-lair-is OAR-is) is a sphincter that encircles the mouth. This muscle is used to close the

Table 7–3   Types of Body Movements

Flexion (FLEK-shun)

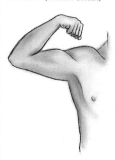

Description: Means to bend. Flexion usually brings two bones closer together and decreases the angle between them. Example: bending the elbow or the knee.

Dorsiflexion (dor-sih-FLEK-shun)

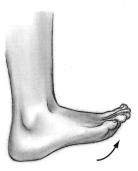

Description: Flexion of the ankle in which the dorsum or top of the foot is lifted upward, decreasing the angle between the foot and leg. Example: standing on your heels.

Extension (ek-STEN-shun)

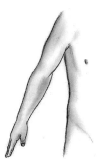

Description: Means to straighten. Extension is the opposite of flexion. It increases the angle between two bones. Example: straightening the elbow or the knee after it has been flexed.

Plantar flexion (PLAN-tar FLEK-shun)

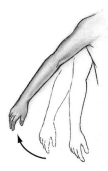

Description: Plantar flexion is movement at the ankle that increases the angle between the foot and leg. Example: standing on your toes.

Hyperextension (hye-per-ek-STEN-shun)

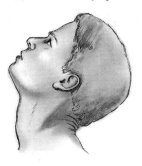

Description: Hyperextension occurs when a part of the body is extended beyond the anatomical position. The joint angle becomes greater than 180°. Example: moving the head backward.

Abduction (ab-DUCK-shun)

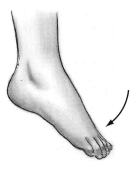

Description: Means to take away. Abduction moves a bone or limb away from the midline or axis of the body. Examples: the outward movement of the legs in "jumping jacks," moving the arms away from the body, or spreading the fingers apart.

mouth, to form words, and to pucker the lips as in kissing. The **orbicularis oculi** (oar-BIK-yoo-lair-is OK-yoo-lye) is another sphincter but is around the eye (oculus). Actions of winking, blinking, and squinting use this muscle. The **buccinator** (BUCK-sin-ay-ter) is the principal muscle in the cheek area and is used to compress the cheek when whistling, sucking, or blowing air out. It is sometimes called the trumpeter's muscle. The **zygomaticus** (zye-goh-MAT-ih-kus) extends from the zygomatic arch to the corners of the mouth. It contracts to raise the corner of the mouth when we smile.

Table 7–3   *Continued*

Adduction (ad-DUCK-shun)

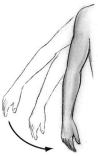

Description: Means to bring together. Adduction is the opposite of abduction. It moves a bone or limb toward the midline of the body. Examples: bringing the arms back to the sides of the body after they have been abducted or moving the legs back to anatomical position after abduction.

Rotation (roh-TAY-shun)

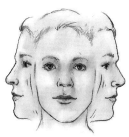

Description: Rotation is the movement of a bone around its own axis in a pivot joint. Example: shaking your head "no."

Supination (soo-pih-NAY-shun)

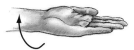

Description: Supination is a specialized rotation of the forearm that turns the palm of the hand forward or anteriorly. If the elbow is flexed, supination turns the palm of the hand upward or superiorly.

Pronation (proh-NAY-shun)

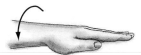

Description: Pronation is the opposite of supination. It is a specialized rotation of the forearm that turns the palm of the hand backward or posteriorly. If the elbow is flexed, pronation turns the palm of the hand downward or inferiorly.

Circumduction (sir-kum-DUCK-shun)

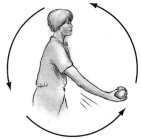

Description: Circumduction is the conelike, circular movement of a body segment. The proximal end of the segment remains relatively stationary while the distal end outlines a large circle. Example: the movement of the arm at the shoulder joint, with the elbow extended, so that the tips of the fingers move in a large circle.

Inversion (in-VER-zhun)

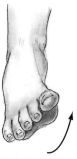

Description: Inversion is the movement of the sole of the foot inward or medially.

Eversion (ee-VER-zhun)

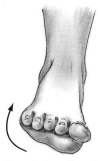

Description: Eversion is the opposite of inversion. It is the movement of the sole of the foot outward or laterally.

◢ **Table 7–4   Muscles of the Head and Neck**

Muscle	Description	Origin	Insertion	Action
Muscles of Facial Expression				
Frontalis (frun-TAL-is)	Flat muscle that covers the forehead	Galea aponeurotica	Skin of eyebrow and nose	Raises eyebrows
Orbicularis oris (oar-BIK-yoo-lair-is OAR-is)	Circular muscle around the mouth	Maxilla and mandible	Skin around the lips	Closes and purses lips
Orbicularis oculi (oar-BIK-yoo-lair-is OK-yoo-lye)	Circular muscle around the eyes	Maxilla and frontal bones	Tissue of the eyelid	Closes eye; winking, blinking, squinting
Buccinator (BUK-sin-ate-ter)	Horizontal cheek muscle; deep to masseter	Maxilla and mandible	Corner of mouth	Compresses cheek; trumpeter's muscle
Zygomaticus (zye-goh-MAT-ih-kus)	Extends diagonally from corner of mouth to cheekbone	Zygomatic bone	Skin and muscle at corner of mouth	Elevates corner of mouth as in smiling
Muscles of Mastication				
Temporalis (tem-por-AL-is)	Flat fan-shaped muscle over temporal bone	Flat portion of the temporal bone	Mandible	Closes jaw
Masseter (MASS-eh-ter)	Covers the lateral aspect of the jaw	Zygomatic arch	Mandible	Closes jaw
Neck Muscles				
Sternocleidomastoid (stir-noh-klye-doh-MAS-toyd)	Straplike muscle that ascends obliquely over the neck	Sternum and clavicle	Mastoid process	Flexes and rotates the head
Trapezius (trah-PEEZ-ee-us)	Large, flat, triangular muscle on the posterior neck and shoulder	Occipital bone and spines of thoracic vertebrae	Scapula	Extends the head; also moves the scapula

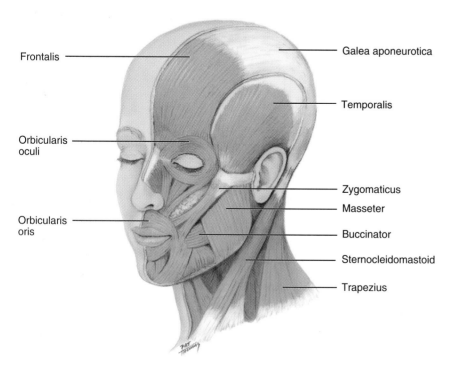

Figure 7–7 Muscles of the head and neck.

The frontalis, orbicularis oris, orbicularis oculi, buccinator, and zygomaticus muscles permit a variety of facial expressions.

Muscles of Mastication

There are four pairs of muscles that are responsible for chewing movements or mastication. All of these muscles insert on the mandible, and they are some of the strongest muscles in the body. Two of the muscles, the **temporalis** (tem-poar-AL-is) and **masseter** (MASS-eh-ter), are superficial and are identified in Table 7–4 and Figure 7–7. The others, the lateral and medial pterygoids, are deep to the mandible and are not shown. The **temporalis** is the largest of the mastication muscles. As the name implies, it has its origin on the temporal bone. The **masseter** is located along the ramus of the mandible and is a synergist of the temporalis.

The masseter and temporalis muscles are responsible for chewing movements.

Neck Muscles

Only two of the more obvious and superficial neck muscles are considered here. There are numerous muscles associated with the throat, the hyoid bone, and the vertebral column, a discussion of which is beyond the scope of this text.

Sternocleidomastoid (stir-no-klye-doh-MAS-toyd) muscles ascend obliquely across the anterior neck from the sternum and clavicle to the mastoid process. When both of these muscles contract together, the neck is flexed and the head is bent toward the chest. When one of the muscles contracts, the head turns toward the direction opposite the side that is contracting. When the left muscle contracts, the head turns to the right. A portion of the **trapezius** (trah-PEEZ-ee-us) muscle is in the neck region and moves the head. Each trapezius muscle extends from the occipital bone at the base of the skull to the end of the thoracic vertebrae and also inserts on the scapula laterally. A portion of this muscle functions to extend the head and is antagonistic to the sternocleidomastoid.

The sternocleidomastoid and trapezius muscles have opposite actions; therefore, they are antagonistic. The sternocleidomastoid flexes the neck whereas the trapezius extends the neck.

Injury to one of the sternocleidomastoid muscles may result in torticollis, or wry neck. This is characterized by a twisting of the neck and an unnatural position of the head.

Muscles of the Trunk

The muscles of the trunk (Table 7–5) include those that move the vertebral column, the muscles that form the thoracic and abdominal walls, and those that cover the pelvic outlet.

Vertebral Column Muscles

The **erector spinae** (ee-REK-ter SPY-nee) group of muscles on each side of the vertebral column is a large muscle mass that extends from the sacrum to the skull. These muscles are primarily responsible for extending the vertebral column to maintain erect posture. Muscle contraction on only one side bends the vertebral column to that side. The **deep back muscles** occupy the space between the spinous and transverse processes of adjacent vertebrae. Each individual muscle is short, but as a group they extend the length of the vertebral column. They are responsible for several movements of the vertebral column.

The erector spinae and deep back muscles are responsible for movements of the vertebral column.

Thoracic Wall Muscles

The muscles of the thoracic wall (Fig. 7–8) are involved primarily in the process of breathing. The intercostal muscles are located in spaces between the ribs. Fibers of the **external intercostal muscles** are directed forward and downward whereas those of the **internal intercostals** are directed backward and downward. The internal intercostal fibers are at right angles to the external intercostal fibers. External intercostal muscles contract to elevate the ribs during the inspiration phase of breathing. The internal intercostals contract during forced expiration.

The **diaphragm** is a dome-shaped muscle that forms a partition between the thorax and the abdomen. It has three openings in it for structures that have to pass from the thorax to the abdomen. One opening is for the inferior vena cava, one is for the esophagus, and one is for the aorta. The diaphragm is responsible for the major movement in the thoracic cavity during quiet relaxed breathing. When the diaphragm contracts, the dome is flattened. This increases the volume of the thoracic cavity and results in inspiration. When the muscle relaxes, it again resumes its dome shape and decreases the volume of the thoracic cavity, which forces air out during expiration.

The diaphragm and intercostal muscles change the size of the thoracic cavity during breathing.

Voluntary forceful contractions of the diaphragm increase intra-abdominal pressure to assist in urination, defecation, and childbirth.

Table 7–5   Muscles of the Trunk

Muscle	Description	Origin	Insertion	Action
Muscles That Move the Vertebral Column				
Erector spinae (ee-REK-ter SPY-nee)	Intrinsic back muscles on each side of the vertebral column	Vertebrae	Superior vertebrae and ribs	Extends vertebral column
Deep back muscles	Short, intrinsic muscles in the space between spinous and transverse processes of vertebrae	Vertebrae	Vertebrae	Move the vertebral column
Muscles of the Thoracic Wall				
External intercostals (inter-KOS-talz)	Short muscles in the intercostal spaces between the ribs	Ribs	Next rib below origin	Inspiration
Internal intercostals (inter-KOS-talz)	Short muscles in the intercostal spaces between the ribs	Ribs	Next rib above origin	Forced expiration
Diaphragm (DYE-ah-fram)	Dome-shaped muscle that forms a partition between the thorax and abdomen	Interior body wall	Central tendon of diaphragm	Inspiration
Abdominal Wall Muscles				
External oblique (ek-STIR-null oh-BLEEK)	Largest and most superficial of the lateral abdominal wall muscles	Rib cage	Iliac crest and fascia	Compresses abdomen
Internal oblique (in-TER-null oh-BLEEK)	Underlies external oblique and fibers are perpendicular to it	Iliac crest and fascia	Lower ribs and fascia	Compresses abdomen
Transversus abdominis (trans-VER-sus ab-DOM-ih-nis)	Deepest muscle of abdominal wall; fibers run horizontally	Fascia and lower ribs	Linea alba and pubis	Compresses abdomen
Rectus abdominis (REK-tus ab-DOM-ih-nis)	Long, straight muscle on each side of linea alba	Pubic bone	Ribs and sternum	Flexes vertebral column and compresses abdomen
Muscles of the Pelvic Outlet				
Pelvic diaphragm; primarily the levator ani muscle	Superior (deep) muscle hammock that forms the floor of the pelvic cavity	Pubis and ischium	Sacrum and coccyx	Supports and maintains position of the pelvic viscera
Urogenital diaphragm	Superficial to the pelvic diaphragm; between the two sides of the pubic arch	Ischium and genitalia	Genitalia and perineum	Supports pelvic viscera and assists in function of the genitalia

Abdominal Wall Muscles

The abdomen, unlike the thorax and pelvis, has no bony reinforcements or protection. The wall consists entirely of four muscle pairs, arranged in layers, and the fascia that envelops them (Fig. 7–9). The aponeuroses of the muscles on opposite sides meet in the anterior midline to form the **linea alba** ("white line"), a band of connective tissue that extends from the sternum to the pubic symphysis. The outer muscle layer is the **external oblique** with fibers that run inferiorly and medially. With fibers oriented perpendicularly to the external oblique, the **internal oblique** lies just underneath it. The deepest layer of muscle is the **transversus abdominis** with its fibers running in a horizontal direction. The arrangement of the muscle layers with the fibers in each layer

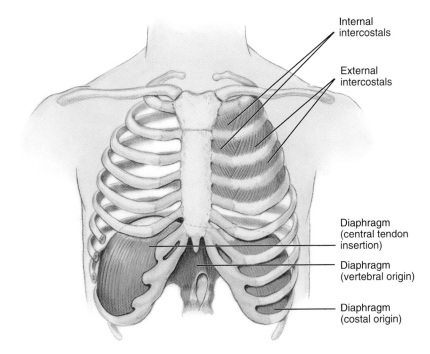

Figure 7–8 Thoracic wall muscles.

going in different directions is similar to the type of construction found in plywood and adds strength to the anterolateral abdominal wall. The fascia of these muscles extends anteriorly to form a broad aponeurosis along much of the anterior aspect of the abdomen. The fascia also envelops the **rectus abdominis** muscle that runs straight up from the pubic bones to the ribs and the sternum on each side of the midline. All of these muscles compress the abdominal wall and increase intra-abdominal pressure. The rectus abdominis also flexes the vertebral column.

> The configuration of the external oblique, internal oblique, transversus abdominis, and rectus abdominis muscles provides strength and support to the abdominal wall.

Pelvic Floor Muscles

The pelvic outlet is formed by two muscular sheets and their associated fascia. The deeper or more superior muscular sheet is the **pelvic diaphragm,** which forms the floor of the pelvic cavity. Most of

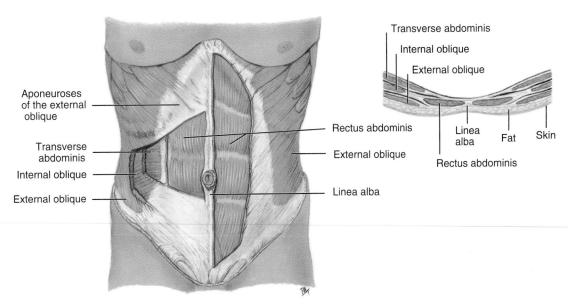

Figure 7–9 Abdominal wall muscles.

the pelvic diaphragm is formed by the two **levator ani** muscles that support the pelvic viscera. They resist increased pressure in the abdominopelvic cavity and thus play a role in the control of the urinary bladder and rectum. The superficial muscle group, the **urogenital diaphragm,** fills the space within the pubic arch and is associated with the genitalia.

> The superficial urogenital diaphragm and the deeper, or more superior, pelvic diaphragm form a covering for the pelvic outlet. The levator ani muscles of the pelvic diaphragm support the pelvic viscera.

Muscles of the Upper Extremity
(Table 7–6 and Fig. 7–10)

The muscles of the upper extremity include those that attach the scapula to the thorax and generally move the scapula, those that attach the humerus to the scapula and generally move the arm, and those that are located in the arm or forearm that move the forearm, wrist, and hand.

Muscles That Move the Shoulder and Arm

The **trapezius** and **serratus anterior** (seh-RAY-tus anterior) are two of the muscles that attach the scap-

Table 7–6   Muscles of the Upper Extremity

Muscle	Description	Origin	Insertion	Action
Muscles That Move the Shoulder and Arm				
Trapezius (trah-PEEZ-ee-us)	Triangular muscle on the posterior neck and shoulder; two together form a trapezoid	Occipital bone and vertebrae	Scapula	Adducts, elevates, and rotates scapula; also extends the head
Serratus anterior (seh-RAY-tus anterior)	Deep and inferior to the pectoral muscles; forms medial wall of axilla; has a serrated appearance	Ribs	Medial border of scapula	Pulls scapula anteriorly and downward
Pectoralis major (pek-tor-AL-iss MAY-jer)	Large, fan-shaped muscle that covers the anterior chest	Sternum, clavicle, ribs	Humerus	Adducts and flexes arm
Latissimus dorsi (lah-TISS-ih-mus DOAR-sye)	Large, broad, flat muscle of the lower back region; swimmer's muscle	Vertebrae	Humerus	Adducts and medially rotates arm
Deltoid (DELL-toyd)	Thick muscle that forms the contour of the shoulder	Clavicle and scapula	Humerus	Abducts the arm
Rotator cuff	A group of four muscles that attaches the humerus to the scapula and forms a cap or cuff over the proximal humerus	Scapula	Humerus	Rotates the arm
Muscles That Move the Forearm and Hand				
Triceps brachii (TRY-seps BRAY-kee-eye)	The only muscle in the posterior compartment of the arm; has three heads of origin	Humerus and scapula	Olecranon of ulna	Extends the forearm
Biceps brachii (BY-seps BRAY-kee-eye)	Major muscle in the anterior compartment of the arm; has two heads of origin	Scapula	Radius	Flexes and supinates forearm
Brachialis (bray-kee-AL-is)	Strong muscle that is deep to the biceps brachii in the anterior compartment of the arm	Humerus	Ulna	Flexes forearm
Brachioradialis (bray-kee-oh-ray-dee-AL-is)	Superficial muscle on lateral forearm	Distal humerus	Distal radius	Flexes forearm

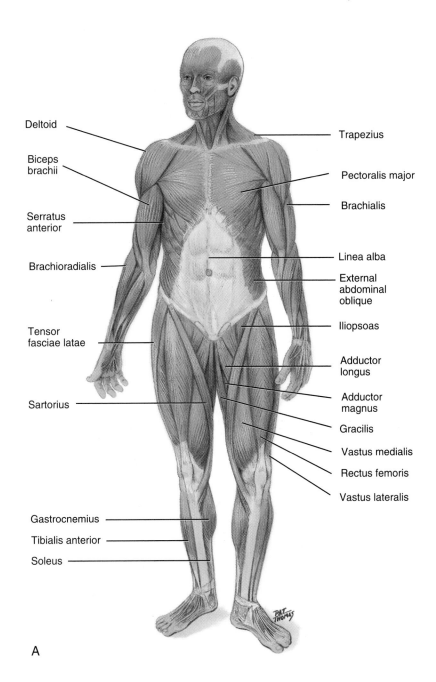

Deltoid

Biceps
brachii

Serratus
anterior

Brachioradialis

Tensor
fasciae latae

Sartorius

Gastrocnemius

Tibialis anterior

Soleus

Trapezius

Pectoralis major

Brachialis

Linea alba

External
abdominal
oblique

Iliopsoas

Adductor
longus

Adductor
magnus

Gracilis

Vastus medialis

Rectus femoris

Vastus lateralis

Figure 7–10   General overview of body
musculature. *A,* Anterior view.

A

ula to the axial skeleton. The trapezius is a large
superficial triangular muscle of the back. It is attached to the thoracic vertebrae and the scapula.
When the trapezius contracts, it adducts and elevates the scapula, as in shrugging the shoulders.
The serratus anterior is located on the side of the
chest where it runs from the ribs to the scapula.
When the serratus anterior contracts, it pulls the
shoulder downward and forward, as in pushing
something.

> The trapezius and serratus anterior muscles move
> the scapula.

Both the **pectoralis major** (pek-tor-AL-iss MAY-
jer) and **latissimus dorsi** (lah-TISS-ih-mus DOR-sye)

muscles attach the humerus to the axial skeleton.
The pectoralis major is a superficial muscle on the
anterior chest. It has a broad origin on the sternum,
costal cartilages, and clavicle, but then the fibers
converge to insert on the humerus by way of a short
tendon. The primary function of the pectoralis major
is to adduct and rotate the arm medially across the
chest. The latissimus dorsi is a large, superficial
muscle located in the lower back region. It has an
extensive origin from the spines of the thoracic vertebrae, ilium, and ribs and then extends upward to
insert on the humerus. The latissimus dorsi adducts
and rotates the arm medially and lowers the shoulder. It is an important muscle in swimming and
rowing motions.

The **deltoid** is a large, fleshy muscle that covers
the shoulder and attaches the humerus to the scap-

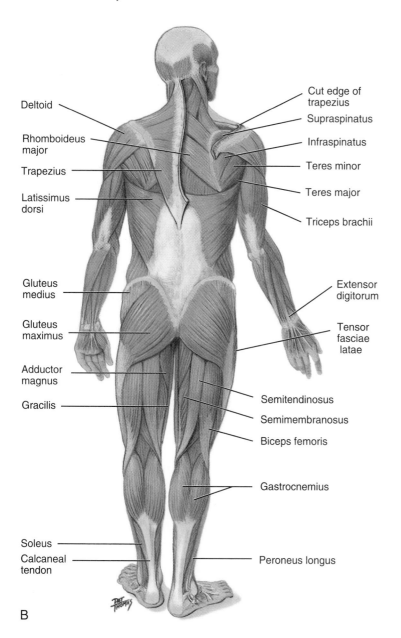

Deltoid

Rhomboideus major

Trapezius

Latissimus dorsi

Gluteus medius

Gluteus maximus

Adductor magnus

Gracilis

Soleus

Calcaneal tendon

Cut edge of trapezius

Supraspinatus

Infraspinatus

Teres minor

Teres major

Triceps brachii

Extensor digitorum

Tensor fasciae latae

Semitendinosus

Semimembranosus

Biceps femoris

Gastrocnemius

Peroneus longus

B

Figure 7–10 *Continued. B, Posterior view.*

ula. This muscle abducts the arm to a horizontal position. It is a common place for administering injections. Another group of four muscles, the **infraspinatus, supraspinatus, subscapularis,** and **teres minor,** attaches the humerus to the scapula and moves the humerus in some way. These muscles, collectively, are called the **rotator cuff muscles** because they form a cuff or cap over the proximal humerus. A rotator cuff injury involves damage to one or more of these muscles or their tendons. The subscapularis is not shown in Figure 7–10 because it is on the costal surface of the scapula and not visible.

> The pectoralis major, latissimus dorsi, deltoid, and rotator cuff muscles insert on the humerus and move the arm.

Muscles That Move the Forearm and Hand

The muscles that move the forearm are located along the humerus. The arm is divided into anterior and posterior muscle compartments. The **triceps brachii,** the primary extensor of the forearm, is the only muscle in the posterior compartment. As the name implies, it has three heads of origin. The anterior muscle compartment contains the **biceps brachii** and **brachialis** (bray-kee-AL-is). These muscles are the primary flexors of the forearm. In addition, the **brachioradialis** (bray-kee-oh-ray-dee-AL-is), a prominent muscle along the lateral side of the forearm, helps to flex the forearm. The brachioradialis extends from the lower part of the humerus to the radius and is generally considered to be a posterior forearm muscle.

The triceps brachii, which extends the forearm, is antagonistic to the biceps brachii and brachialis muscles.

The 20 or more muscles that cause most wrist, hand, and finger movements are located along the forearm. These muscles are divided into anterior and posterior compartments. Most of the anterior compartment muscles flex the wrist and fingers, whereas the posterior muscles cause extension.

Most of the muscles that are located on the forearm act on the wrist, hand, or fingers.

The muscles that flex the fingers and hand are stronger than the extensor muscles. In a normal relaxed position the fingers are slightly flexed because the normal muscle tone is greater in the flexors. Persons who receive a high-voltage electrical shock through the arms flex their hands tightly and "can't let go." All of the flexors and extensors receive the electrical stimulus, but because the flexor muscles are stronger, they contract more forcefully.

Muscles of the Lower Extremity
(Table 7–7 and Fig. 7–10)

The muscles of the lower extremity include those that are located in the hip region and generally move the thigh, those that are located in the thigh and move the leg, and those that are located in the leg and move the ankle and foot.

Muscles That Move the Thigh

The muscles that move the thigh have their origins on some part of the pelvic girdle and their insertions on the femur. The largest muscle mass belongs to the posterior group, the gluteal muscles. The **gluteus maximus** forms the area of the buttocks. The **gluteus medius,** a common site for injections, is superior to the gluteus maximus and then is deep to it. The **gluteus minimus** is the smallest and deepest of the gluteal muscles. It is not illustrated in Figure 7–10. Although the **tensor fasciae latae** (TEN-soar FAH-she-ee LAY-tee) is a superficial muscle on the lateral side of the thigh, its function and innervation associate it with the gluteal muscles. These muscles abduct the thigh; that is, they raise the thigh sideways to a horizontal position. The gluteus maximus also extends or straightens the thigh at the hip for walking or climbing stairs.

The gluteal muscles, as a group, abduct the thigh.

The gluteus medius is a common site for intramuscular injections. Generally, the injection is given in the center of the upper outer quadrant of the buttock, or gluteal, area. The gluteus medius, rather than the gluteus maximus, is used to avoid damaging the sciatic nerve.

The anterior muscle that moves the thigh is the **iliopsoas** (ill-ee-oh-SOH-as). This muscle is formed from the iliacus that originates on the iliac fossa and the psoas that originates on the lumbar vertebrae. The fibers converge into the iliopsoas and insert on the femur. The iliopsoas flexes the thigh, making it antagonistic to the gluteus maximus.

The iliopsoas, an anterior muscle, flexes the thigh.

The medial muscles adduct the thigh and press the thighs together. This group includes the **adductor longus, adductor brevis, adductor magnus,** and **gracilis** (grah-SILL-is) muscles. The adductor brevis is not illustrated in Figure 7–10 because it is deep to the adductor longus.

The muscles in the medial compartment adduct the thigh.

The adductor muscles in the medial compartment are the horse rider's muscles. These muscles adduct, or press the thighs together, to keep a person on a horse.

Muscles That Move the Leg

Muscles that move the leg are located in the thigh region. The **quadriceps femoris** (KWAHD-rih-seps FEM-oar-is) includes four muscles that are on the anterior and lateral sides of the thigh, namely the **vastus lateralis, vastus intermedius, vastus medialis,** and **rectus femoris.** As a group, these muscles are the primary extensors of the leg, straightening the leg at the knee. The vastus intermedius is deep to the rectus femoris and is not illustrated. The other muscle on the anterior surface of the thigh is the long straplike **sartorius** (sar-TOAR-ee-us) that passes obliquely over the quadriceps group. The sartorius, the longest muscle in the body, flexes and medially rotates the leg when you sit cross-legged.

The quadriceps femoris muscle group straightens the leg at the knee.

The quadriceps femoris group is a powerful knee extensor that is used in climbing, running, and rising from a chair.

Table 7–7   Muscles of the Lower Extremity

Muscle	Description	Origin	Insertion	Action
Muscles That Move the Thigh				
Iliopsoas (ill-ee-oh-SOH-as)	Composite of the iliacus and psoas muscles; located in the groin	Iliac fossa and vertebrae	Femur	Flexes and rotates thigh
Tensor fasciae latae (TEN-soar FAH-she-ee LAY-tee)	Most lateral muscle in the hip region	Anterior ilium	Tibia by way of the iliotibial tract	Flexes and abducts thigh; synergist of the iliopsoas
Gluteus maximus (GLOO-tee-us MAK-sih-mus)	Largest and most superficial of the gluteal muscles	Ilium, sacrum, and coccyx	Femur	Extends the thigh; antagonist of the iliopsoas
Gluteus medius (GLOO-tee-us MEE-dee-us)	Thick muscle deep to the gluteus maximus; common site for intramuscular injections	Ilium	Femur	Abducts and rotates thigh
Gluteus minimus (GLOO-tee-us MIN-ih-mus)	Smallest and deepest of the gluteal muscles	Ilium	Femur	Abducts and rotates thigh
Adductor longus (ad-DUCK-toar LONG-us)	Most anterior of the adductor muscles in the medial compartment of the thigh	Pubis	Femur	Adducts thigh
Adductor brevis (ad-DUCK-toar BREH-vis)	Short adductor muscle deep to the adductor longus	Pubis	Femur	Adducts thigh
Adductor magnus (ad-DUCK-toar MAG-nus)	Largest and deepest of the adductor muscles	Pubis	Femur	Adducts thigh
Gracilis (grah-SILL-is)	Long, superficial, straplike muscle on the medial aspect of the thigh	Pubis	Tibia	Adducts thigh; flexes leg
Muscles That Move the Leg				
Sartorius (sar-TOAR-ee-us)	Long, straplike muscle that courses obliquely across the thigh; longest muscle in the body	Ilium	Tibia	Flexes thigh; flexes and rotates leg
Quadriceps femoris (KWAHD-rih-seps FEM-oar-is) Rectus femoris (REK-tus FEM-oar-is) Vastus lateralis (VASS-tus lat-er-AL-is) Vastus medialis (VASS-tus mee-dee-AL-is) Vastus intermedius (VASS-tus in-ter-MEE-dee-us)	A group of four muscles that form the fleshy mass of the anterior thigh; form a common tendon that passes over the patella	Femur; except for rectus femoris, which originates on the ilium	Tibial tuberosity, by way of the patellar tendon	Extends the leg; rectus femoris also flexes the thigh
Hamstrings Biceps femoris (BYE-seps FEM-oar-is) Semimembranosus (sem-ee-MEM-brah-noh-sus) Semitendinosus (sem-ee-TEN-dih-noh-sus)	Large, fleshy muscle mass in the posterior thigh	Ischium; one head of the biceps femoris arises from the femur	Biceps femoris inserts on the fibula; the others on the tibia	Flexes leg and extends thigh; antagonist to the quadriceps femoris

Table 7–7	Muscles of the Lower Extremity *Continued*			
Muscle	**Description**	**Origin**	**Insertion**	**Action**
Muscles That Move the Ankle and Foot				
Tibialis anterior (tib-ee-AL-is an-TEAR-ee-or)	Superficial muscle of the anterior leg	Tibia	Medial cuneiform and first metatarsal	Dorsiflexes foot
Gastrocnemius (gas-trok-NEE-mee-us)	Superficial muscle on posterior surface of leg; forms the curve of the calf	Femur	Calcaneus by way of Achilles tendon	Plantar flexes foot
Soleus (SO-lee-us)	Deep to the gastrocnemius on the posterior leg; has a common tendon for insertion with the gastrocnemius	Tibia and fibula	Calcaneus by way of Achilles tendon	Plantar flexes foot
Peroneus (pear-oh-NEE-us)	Forms the lateral compartment of the leg	Tibia and fibula	Tarsals and metatarsals	Plantar flexes and everts foot

The posterior thigh muscles are called the **hamstrings** and they are used to flex the leg at the knee. All have origins on the ischium and insert on the tibia. Because these muscles extend over the hip joint as well as over the knee joint, they also extend the thigh. The strong tendons of these muscles can be felt behind the knee. These same tendons are present in hogs, and butchers used them to hang the hams for smoking and curing so they were called "ham strings." The hamstring muscles are the **biceps femoris, semimembranosus** (sem-ee-MEM-brah-noh-sus), and **semitendinosus** (sem-ee-TENdih-noh-sus). A "pulled hamstring" is a tear in one or more of these muscles or their tendons.

The hamstrings are antagonists to the quadriceps femoris muscle group.

Muscles That Move the Ankle and Foot

The muscles located in the leg that move the ankle and foot are divided into anterior, posterior, and lateral compartments. The **tibialis anterior** is the primary muscle in the anterior group. Contraction of the muscles in the anterior group, including the tibialis anterior, causes dorsiflexion of the foot. **Peroneus** (pear-oh-NEE-us) muscles occupy the lateral compartment of the leg. Contraction of these muscles everts the foot and also helps in plantar flexion. The **gastrocnemius** (gas-trok-NEE-mee-us) and **soleus** (SOH-lee-us) are the major muscles in the posterior compartment. These two muscles form the fleshy mass in the calf of the leg. They have a common tendon called the **calcaneal tendon** or **Achilles tendon.** These muscles are strong plantar flexors of the foot. They are sometimes called the toe dancer's muscles because they allow you to stand on tiptoe. Numerous other deep muscles in the leg cause flexion and extension of the toes.

The tibialis anterior, which dorsiflexes the foot, is antagonistic to the gastrocnemius and soleus muscles, which plantar flex the foot.

✓ **Quick**Check

● What superficial muscle is a synergist of the temporalis when chewing food?

● What muscle is an antagonist to the biceps brachii?

● The muscle group on the posterior thigh region has what effect on movement at the knee? What is this muscle group? What group acts as an antagonist to this group?

FOCUS ON AGING

One of the most "obvious" age-related changes in skeletal muscles is the loss of muscle mass. This involves a decrease in both the number of muscle fibers and the diameter of the remaining fibers. Because muscle fibers are amitotic, once they are lost they cannot be replaced by new ones. Instead, they are replaced by connective tissue, primarily adipose. The number of muscle cells lost depends on several factors, including the amount of physical activity, the nutritional state of the individual, heredity, and the condition of the motor neurons that supply the muscle tissue. There is an age-related loss of motor neurons to skeletal muscle cells, and this is considered an important cause of muscle atrophy. It is probable that exercise enhances the ability of nerves to stimulate muscle fibers and to reduce atrophy.

As muscle mass decreases, there is a corresponding reduction in muscle strength. The amount of strength loss differs, depending to a large extent on the amount of physical activity. There is evidence that the mitochondria function less effectively in nonexercised muscle cells than in exercised cells. When mitochondria are inefficient, lactic acid accumulates, which contributes to muscle weakness.

There is a tendency for the skeletal muscles of older people to be less responsive, or to respond more slowly, than those of younger people. This is because the latent, contraction, and relaxation phases of muscle action all increase in duration. The increase in response time is less in muscles that are used regularly. Continued physical activity and good nutrition are probably the best deterrents to loss of muscle mass and muscle strength and to increased muscle response time.

DO YOU KNOW THIS ABOUT

Muscles?

Exercise, Bodybuilding, and Steroids

During the past decade, a lot of attention has been given to health, exercise, fitness, and cardiovascular conditioning. Bicycle trails, jogging paths, fitness courses, and health clubs have sprouted up like flowers in spring. Is this just a fad and a lot of "hype" or is there real benefit to exercise? Is all exercise alike? Is one type of exercise better than another? What happens when you don't exercise?

The amount of work, or exercise, that a muscle does is reflected in changes within the muscle itself. During prolonged periods of inactivity, muscles usually shrink in mass and lose their vascularization. This is called atrophy of disuse. Individuals with motor pathway damage, such as paraplegics, may benefit from electrical stimulation therapy. By placing electrodes over the muscle and providing coordinated electrical stimulation impulses, the muscle can be periodically contracted and exercised. This can reduce the atrophy and helps maintain muscle tone and blood vessels.

For individuals with normal motor pathways, exercise may result in an increase in muscle size. This is called hypertrophy. Because the number of muscle fibers within a muscle always remains the same, the change in size is due to a modification in the size of each individual fiber. Other types of exercise may result in greater stamina, or endurance, rather than in hypertrophy.

Aerobic, or **endurance, exercise** increases a muscle's ability to sustain moderate exercise over a long period. Aerobic activities, such as running, bicycling, swimming, and fast walking, increase the number of blood vessels in a muscle without increasing its size. The increased blood flow permits faster delivery of oxygen and glucose to the muscle fibers for more efficient energy production. This type of exercise also increases the number of mitochondria in the fibers, and the fibers synthesize more myoglobin. These changes result in more efficient muscle metabolism, which leads to greater endurance and resistance to fatigue. Aerobic exercise benefits more than just skeletal muscles. It improves neuromuscular coordination, ventilation capabilities of the lungs, gas exchange in the tissues, and cardiac output. It enhances the health and strength of the entire body.

Anaerobic, or **resistance, exercise** is classified as strength training. This is high-intensity exercise that involves contracting muscles against heavy resistance. Weight lifting and similar iso-metric exercise routines result in muscle hyper-trophy. The exercise does not need to be pro-longed to be effective. The key is in forcing the muscles to exert as much force as possible.

Bodybuilding, a sport enjoyed by both men and women, is a prime example of anaerobic exercise. Bodybuilders concentrate on increasing skeletal muscle mass and strength. Their goal is to develop all skeletal muscles to their maximum and to build a well-proportioned body. This re-quires skill and training because it is easy to build some muscles and to ignore others. Early studies showed that this type of training did not provide the equivalent cardiopulmonary benefits that were derived from aerobic regimens. More recent evidence, however, indicates that by com-bining aerobic exercise with their anaerobic rou-tines bodybuilders receive cardiac and respira-tory benefits similar to those derived from aero-bic exercise programs.

Some people try to take a short-cut to increas-ing muscle size and strength by taking synthetic hormones called **anabolic steroids.** These ster-oids are similar to testosterone, a hormone se-creted by the testes. Anabolic steroids cause mus-cle hypertrophy, and people who take them may show an increase in muscle mass and strength and in total body weight. However, using ster-oids is more harmful than beneficial. Harmful side effects of steroid use include irritability, car-diovascular disease, liver dysfunction, sterility, and other disorders. The use of anabolic steroids has been implicated in the death of some known users. Most athletic organizations now prohibit the use of anabolic steroids. They are not worth the price paid in terms of health.

REPRESENTATIVE DISORDERS OF THE MUSCULAR SYSTEM

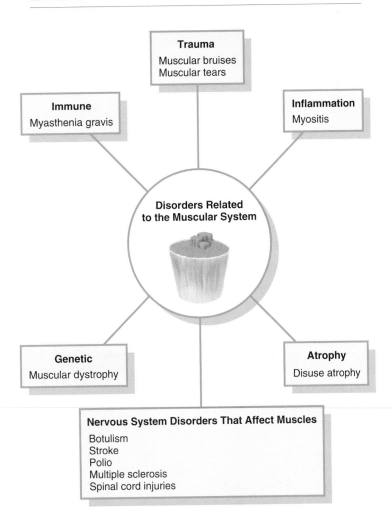

Trauma
Muscular bruises
Muscular tears

Immune
Myasthenia gravis

Inflammation
Myositis

Disorders Related to the Muscular System

Genetic
Muscular dystrophy

Atrophy
Disuse atrophy

Nervous System Disorders That Affect Muscles
Botulism
Stroke
Polio
Multiple sclerosis
Spinal cord injuries

CHAPTER QUIZ

RECALL

Match the definitions on the left with the appropriate term on the right.

1. Connective tissue covering around an individual muscle fiber

2. Broad, flat sheet of tendon

3. Muscle cell membrane

4. More movable attachment of a muscle

5. Functional unit of muscle; from Z line to Z line

6. Neurotransmitter at the neuromuscular junction

7. Minimal stimulus needed to cause contraction

8. High energy compound in muscle

9. Protein pigment molecules in muscle

10. Moving a part away from midline

A. Abduction

B. Acetylcholine

C. Aponeurosis

D. Creatine phosphate

E. Endomysium

F. Insertion

G. Myoglobin

H. Sarcolemma

I. Sarcomere

J. Threshold

THOUGHT

1. Jonathan flexes his elbow by moving his antebrachial region upward toward his brachial region. Which one of the following bones is likely to represent the insertion of the muscle involved?

    a. humerus

    b. ulna

    c. carpal

    d. scapula

2. Arrange the given events in the sequence in which they occur in skeletal muscle contraction: a) calcium released from sarcoplasmic reticulum; b) acetylcholine diffuses across synaptic cleft; c) myosin heads bind with actin; d) impulse travels along sarcolemma and T tubules; e) cross-bridges rotate to shorten sarcomere.

    a. b, d, a, c, e

    b. a, b, d, c, e

    c. d, b, a, c, e

    d. c, a, d, b, e

3. A ballet dancer is standing on her toes. This is an example of

    a. abduction

    b. plantar flexion

    c. circumduction

    d. eversion

4. Which of the following muscles allows you to chew your food?

    a. zygomaticus

    b. sternocleidomastoid

    c. buccinator

    d. masseter

5. When an athlete experiences a "pulled hamstring," which of the following muscles is likely affected?

    a. vastus lateralis

    b. biceps brachii

    c. semimembranosus

    d. soleus

APPLICATION

Clarissa was "daydreaming" in class one day (certainly not an anatomy class!) when the teacher asked her a question. Embarrassed, Clarissa lowered her head, looked at the floor, and shrugged her shoulders to indicate she didn't know the answer. What muscle did she use to lower her head and look down? What muscle did she use to shrug her shoulders?

CHAPTER 8

Nervous System

Outline/Objectives

Functions and Organization of the Nervous System 153

- Outline the organization and functions of the nervous system.

Nerve Tissue 155

- Compare the structure and functions of neurons and neuroglia.

Nerve Impulses 157

- Describe the sequence of events that lead to an action potential when the cell membrane is stimulated and how the impulse is conducted along the length of a neuron.
- Describe the structure of a synapse and how an impulse is conducted from one neuron to another across the synapse.
- List the five basic components of a reflex arc.

Central Nervous System 163

- Describe the three layers of meninges around the central nervous system.
- Locate and identify the major regions of the brain and describe their functions.
- Trace the flow of cerebrospinal fluid from its origin in the ventricles to its return to the blood.
- Describe the structure and functions of the spinal cord.

Peripheral Nervous System 171

- Describe the structure of a nerve.
- List the 12 cranial nerves and state the function of each one.
- Discuss spinal nerves and the plexuses they form.
- Compare the structural and functional differences between the somatic efferent pathways and the autonomic nervous system.
- Distinguish between the sympathetic and parasympathetic divisions of the autonomic nervous system in terms of structure, function, and neurotransmitters.

Key Terms

Action potential

Brain stem

Cerebellum

Cerebrum

Diencephalon

Myelin

Neurilemma

Saltatory conduction

Synapse

Threshold stimulus

Building Vocabulary

WORD PART	MEANING
af-	toward
astro-	star
corpor-	body
dendr-	tree
ef-	away from
encephal-	within the head, brain
esthes-	feeling
-fer-	to carry
gangli-	knot
gli-	glue
gloss-	tongue
lemm-	peel, rind
mening-	membrane
neur-	nerve
peri-	all around
pharyng-	throat
phas-	speech
pleg-	paralysis
plex-	interweave, network
sulc-	furrow, ditch

Functional Relationships of the
Nervous/Sensory System

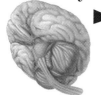

▶ Monitors external and internal environments and mediates adjustments to maintain homeostasis.

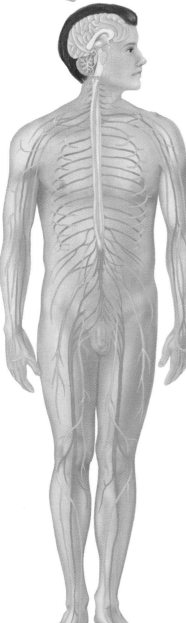

Integument

◀ Provides protection for peripheral nerves; supports peripheral receptors for touch, pressure, pain, and temperature.

▶ Influences secretions of glands in the skin, contraction of arrector pili muscles, and blood flow to skin.

Skeletal

◀ Protects brain and spinal cord; supports ear, eye, and other sensory organs; stores calcium necessary for neural function.

▶ Innervates bones and provides sensory information about joint movement and position.

Muscular

◀ Performs the somatic motor commands that arise in the CNS; muscle spindles provide proprioceptive sense; provides heat to maintain body temperature for neural function.

▶ Coordinates skeletal muscle contraction; adjusts cardiovascular and respiratory systems to maintain cardiac output and oxygen for muscle contraction.

Endocrine

◀ Hormones influence neuronal metabolism and enhance autonomic stimuli.

▶ Regulates secretory activity of anterior pituitary and adrenal medulla; produces ADH and oxytocin.

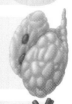

Cardiovascular

◀ Delivers oxygen and nutrients to brain, spinal cord, and other neural and sensory tissue; removes waste products and heat; source of CSF.

▶ Monitors and adjusts heart rate, blood pressure, and blood flow.

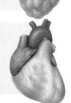

Lymphatic/Immune

◀ Assists in defense against pathogens and repair of neural and sensory tissue following trauma; removes excess fluid from tissues surrounding nerves.

▶ Innervates lymphoid organs and helps regulate the immune response.

Respiratory

◀ Supplies oxygen for brain, spinal cord, and sensory organs; removes carbon dioxide; helps maintain pH.

▶ Stimulates muscle contractions that create pressure changes necessary for ventilation; regulates rate and depth of breathing.

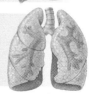

Digestive

◀ Absorbs nutrients for neural growth, maintenance, and repair; provides nutrients for synthesis of neurotransmitters and energy for nerve impulse conduction; liver maintains glucose levels for neural function.

▶ Autonomic nervous system controls motility and glandular activity of the digestive tract.

Urinary

◀ Helps maintain pH and electrolyte balance necessary for neural function; eliminates metabolic wastes harmful to nerve function.

▶ Autonomic nervous system controls renal blood pressure and renal blood flow, which affect rate of urine formation; regulates bladder emptying.

Reproductive

◀ Gonads produce hormones that influence CNS development and sexual behavior; menstrual hormones affect the activity of the hypothalamus.

▶ Regulates sex drive, arousal, and orgasm; stimulates the release of numerous hormones involved in sperm production, menstrual cycle, pregnancy, and parturition.

he nervous system is the major controlling, regulatory, and communicating system in the body. It is the center of all mental activity, including thought, learning, and memory. Together with the endocrine system, the nervous system is responsible for regulating and maintaining homeostasis. Through its receptors, the nervous system keeps us in touch with our environment, both external and internal.

Like other systems in the body, the nervous system is composed of organs, principally the brain, spinal cord, nerves, and ganglia. These, in turn, consist of various tissues, including nerve, blood, and connective tissues. Together these carry out the complex activities of the nervous system.

Functions of the Nervous System

The various activities of the nervous system can be grouped together as three general, overlapping functions:

- Sensory functions
- Integrative functions
- Motor functions

Together these functions keep us in touch with our environments, maintain homeostasis, and account for thought, learning, and memory.

Millions of sensory receptors detect changes, called stimuli, that occur inside and outside the body. They monitor such things as temperature, light, and sound from the external environment. Inside the body, the internal environment, receptors detect variations in pressure, pH, carbon dioxide concentration, and the levels of various electrolytes. All of this gathered information is called **sensory input.**

Sensory input is converted into electrical signals called nerve impulses that are transmitted to the brain. There the signals are brought together to create sensations, to produce thoughts, or to add to memory. Decisions are made each moment based on the sensory input. This is **integration.**

Based on the sensory input and integration, the nervous system responds by sending signals to muscles, causing them to contract, or to glands, causing them to produce secretions. Muscles and glands are called **effectors** because they cause an effect in response to directions from the nervous system. This is the **motor output** or **motor function.**

CLINICAL TERMS

Cerebral concussion (seh-REE-brull kon-KUSH-un) Loss of consciousness as the result of a blow to the head; usually clears within 24 hours; no evidence of permanent structural damage to the brain tissue

Cerebral contusion (seh-REE-brull kon-TOO-shun) Bruising of brain tissue as a result of direct trauma to the head; neurologic problems persist longer than 24 hours

Cerebral palsy (seh-REE-brull PAWL-zee) Partial paralysis and lack of muscular coordination caused by damage to the cerebrum during fetal life, birth, or infancy

Cerebrovascular accident (CVA) (seh-ree-broh-VAS-kyoo-lar AK-sih-dent) Most common brain disorder; may be due to decreased blood supply to the brain or rupture of a blood vessel in the brain; commonly called a stroke

Computed tomography (CT) (kum-PYOO-ted toh-MAHG-rah-fee) Diagnostic procedure in which x-ray images are used to compose a computerized sectional picture of the brain

Electroencephalography (EEG) (e-lek-troh-en-sef-ah-LAHG-rah-fee) Recording the electrical activity of the brain to demonstrate seizures, brain tumors, and other diseases and injury to the brain

Magnetic resonance imaging (MRI) (mag-NET-ick REZ-oh-nans IHM-oh-jing) Use of magnetic waves to create a sectional image of the brain; considered to be more sensitive than computed tomography in diagnosing certain brain lesions

Multiple sclerosis (MS) (MULL-tih-pull skler-OH-sis) A disorder in which there is progressive destruction of the myelin sheaths of central nervous system neurons, interfering with their ability to transmit impulses; characterized by progressive loss of function interspersed with periods of remission; cause is unknown and there is no satisfactory treatment

Positron emission tomography (PET) (PAHZ-ih-tron ee-MIH-shun toh-MAHG-rah-fee) A procedure that uses a radioactive isotope, combined with a form of glucose and injected intravenously, to obtain sectional images that

show how the brain uses glucose and gives information about brain function

Reye's syndrome (RS) (RAYZ SIN-drohm) Brain dysfunction that occurs primarily in children and teenagers and is characterized by edema of the brain that leads to disorientation, lethargy, and personality changes and may progress to a coma; seems to occur after chickenpox and influenza and taking aspirin is a risk factor

Shingles (SHING-gulls) Viral disease affecting peripheral nerves, characterized by blisters and pain spread over the skin in a bandlike pattern that follows the affected nerves; caused by the same herpesvirus that causes chickenpox

Transient ischemic attack (TIA) (TRANS-ee-ent iss-KEE-mik ah-TACK) An episode of temporary cerebral dysfunction due to impaired blood flow to the brain; the onset is sudden and it is of short duration and leaves no long-lasting neurologic impairment; common causes are blood clots and atherosclerosis

The activities of the nervous system include thought, learning, and memory; maintaining homeostasis; and keeping us in touch with our environment. The activities can be grouped into sensory, integrative, and motor functions.

Organization of the Nervous System

There is really only one nervous system in the body, though terminology seems to indicate otherwise. Although each subdivision of the system is also called a "nervous system," all of these smaller systems belong to the single, highly integrated nervous system. Each subdivision has structural and functional characteristics that distinguish it from the others. The nervous system as a whole is divided into two subdivisions: the **central nervous system** (CNS) and the **peripheral nervous system** (PNS) (Fig. 8–1).

The **brain** and **spinal cord** are the organs of the **central nervous system.** Because they are so vitally important, the brain and spinal cord, located in the dorsal body cavity, are encased in bone for protection. The brain is in the cranial vault, and the spinal cord is in the vertebral canal of the vertebral column. Although considered to be two separate organs, the brain and spinal cord are continuous at the foramen magnum.

The organs of the **peripheral nervous system** are the **nerves** and **ganglia.** Nerves are bundles of nerve fibers, much like muscles are bundles of muscle fibers. Cranial nerves (12 pairs) and spinal nerves (31 pairs) extend from the CNS to peripheral organs such as muscles and glands. Ganglia are collections, or small knots, of nerve cell bodies outside the CNS.

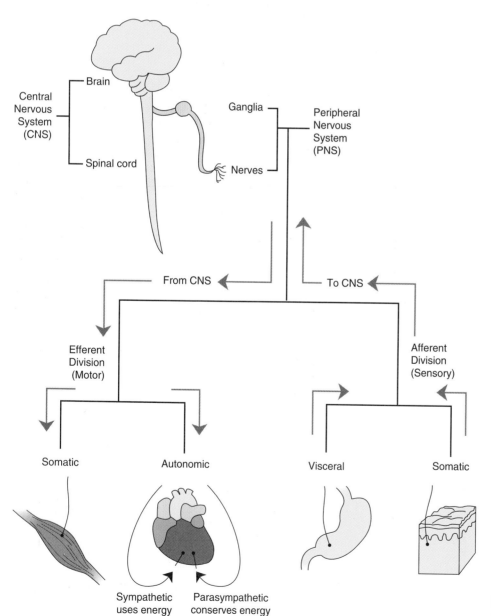

Figure 8–1 Organization of the nervous system.

The CNS consists of the brain and spinal cord. Cranial nerves, spinal nerves, and ganglia make up the PNS.

The PNS is further subdivided into an **afferent (sensory) division** and an **efferent (motor) division.** The afferent or sensory division transmits impulses from peripheral organs to the CNS. The efferent or motor division transmits impulses from the CNS out to the peripheral organs to cause an effect or action.

The afferent division of the PNS carries impulses to the CNS; the efferent division carries impulses away from the CNS.

Finally, the efferent or motor division is again subdivided into the **somatic nervous system** and the **autonomic nervous system.** The somatic nervous system, also called somatomotor or somatic efferent, supplies motor impulses to the skeletal muscles. Because these nerves permit conscious control of the skeletal muscles, the somatic nervous system is sometimes called the **voluntary nervous system.** The autonomic nervous system, also called visceral efferent, supplies motor impulses to cardiac muscle, to smooth muscle, and to glandular epithelium. It is further subdivided into **sympathetic** and **parasympathetic** divisions. Because the autonomic nervous system regulates involuntary or automatic functions, it is sometimes called the **involuntary nervous system.**

The somatic nervous system is an efferent system that carries impulses to skeletal muscles. The autonomic nervous system, also an efferent system, supplies glands and involuntary muscles.

Nerve Tissue

Although the nervous system is very complex, there are only two main types of cells in nerve tissue. The actual nerve cell is the **neuron.** It is the "conducting" cell that transmits impulses. It is the structural unit of the nervous system. The other type of cell is **neuroglia,** or **glial,** cell. The word "neuroglia" means "nerve glue." These cells are nonconductive and provide a support system for the neurons. They are a special type of "connective tissue" for the nervous system.

Neurons are the nerve cells that transmit impulses. Supporting cells are neuroglia.

Neurons

Neurons, or nerve cells, carry out the functions of the nervous system by conducting nerve impulses. They are highly specialized and amitotic. This means that if a neuron is destroyed, it cannot be replaced because neurons do not go through mitosis.

Each neuron has three basic parts:

- **Cell body**
- One or more **dendrites**
- A single **axon**

A neuron is illustrated in Figure 8–2. The main part of the neuron is the **cell body** or **soma.** In many ways, the cell body is similar to other types of cells. It has a nucleus with at least one nucleolus and contains many of the typical cytoplasmic organelles. It lacks centrioles, however. Because centrioles function in cell division, the fact that neurons lack these organelles is consistent with the amitotic nature of the cell. **Dendrites** and **axons** are cytoplasmic extensions, or processes, that project from the cell body. They are sometimes referred to as **fibers.** Dendrites are usually, but not always, short and branching, which increases their surface area to receive signals from other neurons. The number of dendrites on a neuron varies. They are called afferent processes because they transmit impulses to the neuron cell

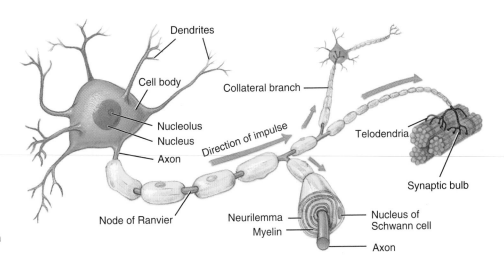

Figure 8–2 Structure of a typical neuron.

body. There is only one axon that projects from each cell body. It is usually elongated; and because it carries impulses away from the cell body, it is called an efferent process.

> The three components of a neuron are a cell body or soma, one or more afferent processes called dendrites, and a single efferent process called an axon.

An axon may have infrequent branches called **axon collaterals.** Axons and axon collaterals terminate in many short branches or **telodendria** (tell-oh-DEN-dree-ah). The distal ends of the telodendria are slightly enlarged to form **synaptic bulbs.** Many axons are surrounded by a segmented, white, fatty substance called **myelin** (MY-eh-lin) or the **myelin sheath.** Myelinated fibers make up the white matter in the CNS, whereas cell bodies and unmyelinated fibers make up the gray matter. The unmyelinated regions between the myelin segments are called the **nodes of Ranvier** (nodes of ron-vee-AY). In the PNS, the myelin is produced by Schwann cells. The cytoplasm, nucleus, and outer cell membrane of the Schwann cell form a tight covering around the myelin and around the axon itself at the nodes of Ranvier. This covering is the **neurilemma** (noo-rih-LEM-mah), which plays an important role in the regeneration of nerve fibers. In the CNS, **oligodendrocytes** (ah-lee-go-DEN-droh-sites) produce myelin, but there is no neurilemma, which is why fibers within the CNS do not regenerate. The structure of an axon and its coverings is illustrated in Figure 8–2.

> Many neurons are surrounded by segmented myelin. The gaps in the myelin are the nodes of Ranvier. An outer covering, the neurilemma, plays a role in nerve regeneration.

Functionally, neurons are classified as afferent, efferent, or interneurons (association neurons) according to the direction in which they transmit impulses relative to the CNS (Table 8–1). **Afferent,** or **sensory, neurons** carry impulses from peripheral sense receptors to the CNS. They usually have long dendrites and relatively short axons. **Efferent,** or **motor, neurons** transmit impulses from the CNS to effector organs such as muscles and glands. Efferent neurons usually have short dendrites and long axons. **Interneurons,** or **association neurons,** are located entirely within the CNS in which they form the connecting link between the afferent and efferent neurons. They have short dendrites and may have either a short or long axon.

> Afferent neurons are sensory, efferent neurons are motor, and association neurons form the connection between the other two.

Neuroglia

Neuroglia cells do not conduct nerve impulses, but, instead, they support, nourish, and protect the neurons. They are far more numerous than neurons and, unlike neurons, are capable of mitosis. Table 8–2 describes the six types of neuroglia cells. Some authorities classify only the four supporting cell types found in the CNS as true neuroglia.

> Neuroglia cells support, protect, and nourish the neurons. Neuroglia cells are capable of mitosis.

Because neurons are not capable of mitosis, primary malignant tumors of the brain are tumors of the glial cells, rather than of the neurons themselves. These tumors, called gliomas, have extensive roots, making them extremely difficult to remove.

Table 8–1 Types of Neurons Classified According to Function		
Type of Neuron	**Structure**	**Function**
Afferent (Sensory)	Long dendrites and a short axon; cell body located in ganglia in the PNS; dendrites in the PNS; axon extends into the CNS	Transmits impulses from peripheral sense receptors to the CNS
Efferent (Motor)	Short dendrites and a long axon; dendrites and cell body located within the CNS; axons extend to PNS	Transmits impulses from the CNS to effectors such as muscles and glands in the periphery
Association (Interneurons)	Short dendrites; axon may be short or long; located entirely within the CNS	Transmits impulses from afferent neurons to efferent neurons

PNS = peripheral nervous system; CNS = central nervous system.

Table 8–2 Neuroglial Cell Types

Cell Type	Location	Description	Special Function
Astrocytes	CNS	Star shaped; numerous radiating processes with bulbous ends for attachment	Bind blood vessels to nerves; regulate the composition of fluid around neurons
Ependymal cells	CNS (line the ventricles of the brain and central canal of spinal cord)	Columnar cells with cilia	Active role in formation and circulation of cerebrospinal fluid
Microglia	CNS	Small cells with long processes; modified macrophages	Protection; become mobile and phagocytic in response to inflammation
Oligodendrocytes	CNS	Small cells with few, but long, processes that wrap around axons	Form myelin sheaths around axons in the CNS
Schwann cells*	PNS	Flat cells with a long, flat process that wraps around an axon in the PNS	Form myelin sheaths around axons in PNS; active role in nerve fiber regeneration
Satellite cells*	PNS	Flat cells, similar to Schwann cells	Support nerve cell bodies within ganglia

CNS = central nervous system; PNS = peripheral nervous system.
*Some authorities do not consider these to be neuroglia because they are in the PNS.

Neuroglia, particularly astrocytes, form a wall around the outside of the blood vessels in the nervous system. This astrocyte wall plus the blood vessel wall forms the blood–brain barrier. Water, oxygen, carbon dioxide, alcohol, and a few other substances are able to pass through this barrier and move between the blood and brain tissue. Other substances such as toxins, pathogens, and certain drugs cannot pass through this barrier. This is a protective mechanism to keep harmful substances out of the brain. It has clinical significance because drugs, such as penicillin, that may be used to treat disorders in other parts of the body have no effect in the brain because they do not cross the blood–brain barrier.

 QuickCheck

- What type of neurons are located entirely within the CNS?
- Defective oligodendrocytes interfere with the production of what substance?
- What function is impaired if there is damage to afferent neurons?

Nerve Impulses

The functional characteristics of neurons are **excitability** and **conductivity**. Excitability is the ability to respond to a stimulus; conductivity is the ability to transmit an impulse from one point to another. All the functions associated with the nervous system, including thought, learning, and memory, are based on these two characteristics. These functional characteristics are the result of structural features of the cell membrane.

> The ability to respond to a stimulus (excitability) and to transmit an impulse (conductivity) are two functional characteristics of neurons.

Resting Membrane

A **resting membrane** is the cell membrane of a nonconducting, or resting, neuron. The membrane is impermeable to the passive diffusion of sodium (Na^+) and potassium (K^+) ions. An active transport mechanism, the sodium-potassium pump, maintains a difference in concentration of these ions on the two sides of the membrane. Sodium ions are concentrated in the extracellular fluid whereas the potassium ions are inside the cell, as illustrated in Figure 8–3A. The intracellular fluid also contains proteins and other negatively charged ions. The result is a polarized membrane with more positive charges outside the cell and more negative charges inside the cell. This difference in charges on the two sides of the resting membrane is the **resting membrane potential**. Electrical measurements show the resting membrane potential to be about −70 millivolts (mV), which means that the inside of the membrane is 70 mV less positive (more negative) than the outside.

> The cell membrane of a nonconducting neuron is polarized with an abundance of sodium ions outside the cell and an abundance of potassium ions and negatively charged proteins inside the cell. The inside of the membrane is approximately 70 mV negative to the outside.

A Resting Membrane

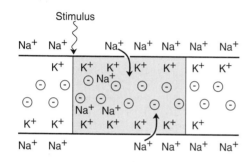

The resting membrane is polarized with the inside negative to the outside. Sodium ions are concentrated on the outside and potassium ions on the inside.

B Depolarizing membrane

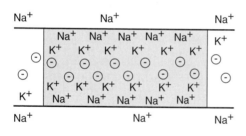

When stimulus is applied, membrane becomes permeable to sodium, which diffuses inward and makes the inside more positive.

C Reverse polarization

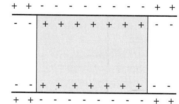

The rapid inward movement of sodium makes the inside of the membrane positive to the outside.

D Repolarization

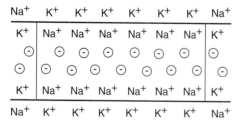

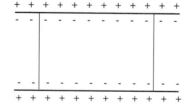

Sodium channels close and potassium channels open, which allows potassium to diffuse out of the cell. This restores the polarity of the membrane. Active transport mechanisms restore sodium and potassium to resting conditions.

Figure 8–3 Generation of an action potential.

Stimulation of a Neuron

A stimulus is a physical, chemical, or electrical event that alters the neuron cell membrane and reduces its polarization for a brief time. The stimulus changes the membrane so that it becomes permeable to so-

dium ions, which diffuse into the cell. If the stimulus is weak, the membrane is only slightly permeable and the inward movement of sodium is offset by an outward movement of potassium. In this case, the resting membrane potential is maintained and no response is initiated.

> A stimulus alters the permeability of the cell membrane.

If the stimulus is strong enough, the membrane becomes highly permeable to sodium at the point of the stimulation. Positively charged sodium ions rapidly diffuse through the membrane to the inside of the cell. This movement is driven by the concentration gradient and the electrical gradient. (Remember, the inside is negatively charged, which attracts the positive sodium ions.) As the positive ions enter the cell, the inside of the membrane becomes more positively charged, reducing the polarization found in the resting membrane (Fig. 8–3B). This is **depolarization.**

> Some anesthetics produce their effects by inhibiting the diffusion of sodium through the cell membrane and thus blocking the initiation and conduction of nerve impulses.

For just an instant the influx of sodium ions reverses the membrane polarity with more positive charges inside the cell than outside. This is **reverse polarization** (Fig. 8–3C).

> In response to a stimulus, the cell membrane becomes permeable to sodium ions, so they rapidly enter the cell and depolarize the membrane. This is followed by reverse polarization.

Very quickly, the membrane again becomes impermeable to sodium, with the sodium ions trapped inside the cell. Next the membrane becomes permeable to the intracellular potassium ions for a fraction of a millisecond, and they rapidly diffuse down the concentration gradient to the outside of the cell. Because these are positive ions, this action removes the intracellular positive charge and restores the resting membrane potential of -70 mV. This process is called **repolarization** (Fig. 8–3D).

> Reverse polarization is followed by repolarization as potassium ions diffuse out of the cell.

The rapid sequence of events in response to a stimulus, namely depolarization, reverse polarization, and repolarization, is called the **action potential.** Electrical measurements show the action potential to peak at approximately $+30$ mV (Fig. 8–4). At the conclusion of the action potential, the sodium-potassium pump actively transports sodium ions out of the cell and potassium ions into the cell to completely restore resting conditions.

> After the action potential, active transport mechanisms move sodium and potassium to restore resting conditions.

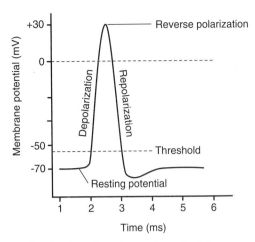

Figure 8–4   Recording of an action potential.

The minimum stimulus necessary to initiate an action potential is called a **threshold (liminal) stimulus.** A weaker stimulus, called a **subthreshold (subliminal) stimulus,** does not cause sufficient depolarization to elicit an action potential.

Conduction Along a Neuron

Once a threshold stimulus has been applied and an action potential generated, it must be conducted along the total length of the neuron either to an effector or to another neuron.

Propagated Action Potentials

The threshold stimulus causes a localized area of reverse polarization on the membrane. In that one area, the membrane is negative on the outside and positive on the inside. The rest of the membrane is in the resting condition. When a given area reverses its polarity, the difference in potential between that area and the adjacent area creates a current flow that depolarizes the second point (Fig. 8–5A). When the second point reverses its polarity, current flow between the second point and the third point depolarizes the third point. This continues point by point, in domino fashion, along the entire length of the neuron, creating a **propagated action potential,** or **nerve impulse.** The following list summarizes the events that occur during nerve impulse conduction:

- Resting membrane has sodium ions on the outside and potassium ions on the inside. Intracellular negative ions produce a resting membrane potential of -70 mV.
- Receptors are stimulated by a physical, chemical, or electrical event.
- Stimulus alters permeability of neuron cell membrane; sodium channels open and sodium ions diffuse to the inside of the cell.
- Influx of sodium ions depolarizes the cell membrane.

A

Unmyelinated fiber (continuous)

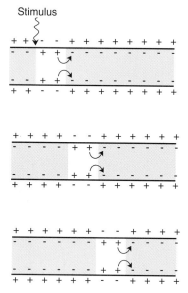

B

Myelinated fiber (saltatory)

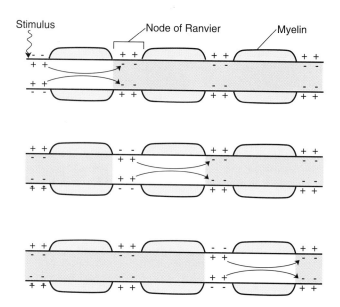

Figure 8-5 Propagation of an action potential.

- Sodium ions continue inward diffusion to reverse the membrane's polarity to +30 mV.
- Sodium channels close and potassium channels open.
- Potassium ions diffuse out of the cell.
- Outward diffusion of potassium ions restores resting membrane potential of −70 mV.
- Sodium-potassium pump transports sodium ions out of the cell and potassium ions back into the cell to restore resting conditions.
- Reverse polarity at one point is the stimulus that depolarizes an adjacent point to propagate the action potential.

> An action potential at a given point stimulates depolarization at an adjacent point to create a propagated action potential, or nerve impulse, that continues along the entire length of the neuron.

Saltatory Conduction

The conduction described in the previous paragraphs is representative of an unmyelinated axon. Because myelin is an insulating substance, it inhibits the flow of current from one point to another. In myelinated fibers, depolarization occurs only at the places where there is no myelin, at the nodes of Ranvier (Fig. 8–5B). The action potential "jumps" from node to node. This "jumping" is **saltatory** (SAL-tah-toar-ee) **conduction,** which is faster than conduction in unmyelinated fibers.

> Saltatory conduction occurs in myelinated fibers where the action potential "jumps" from node to node.

Refractory Period

The period of time during which a point on the cell membrane is "recovering" from depolarization is called the **refractory period.** While the membrane is permeable to sodium ions, it cannot respond to a second stimulus, no matter how strong the stimulus. This is the **absolute refractory period.** For a brief period after the absolute refractory period, roughly comparable to the time of altered membrane permeability to potassium, it takes a stronger than normal stimulus to reach threshold. This is the **relative refractory period.**

> The absolute refractory period is the time during which a neuron cannot respond to a second stimulus. During the relative refractory period, it takes a stronger than normal stimulus to initiate an action potential.

All-or-None Principle

Nerve fibers, like muscle fibers, obey the **all-or-none principle.** If a threshold stimulus is applied, an action potential is generated and propagated along the entire length of the neuron at maximum strength and speed for the existing conditions. A stronger

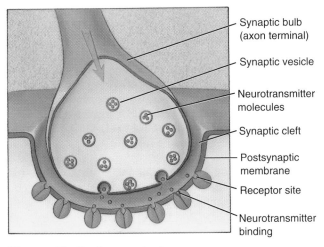

Synaptic bulb (axon terminal)

Synaptic vesicle

Neurotransmitter molecules

Synaptic cleft

Postsynaptic membrane

Receptor site

Neurotransmitter binding

Figure 8-6 Components of a synapse.

stimulus does not increase the strength of the action potential or change the rate of conduction. A weaker stimulus is subthreshold and does not evoke an action potential. If a stimulus is threshold or greater, an impulse is conducted. If the stimulus is subthreshold, there is no conduction.

▌ Nerve fibers operate on the all-or-none principle.

Conduction Across a Synapse

A nerve impulse, or propagated action potential, travels along a nerve fiber until it reaches the end of the axon, then it must be transmitted to the next neuron. The region of communication between two neurons is called a **synapse** (SIN-aps). A synapse has three parts (Fig. 8-6):

• Synaptic knob
• Synaptic cleft
• Postsynaptic membrane

The first neuron, the one preceding the synapse, is called the **presynaptic neuron;** the second neuron, the one following the synapse, is called the **postsynaptic neuron.** Synaptic knobs are tiny bulges at the end of the telodendria on the presynaptic neuron. Small sacs within the synaptic knobs, called **synaptic vesicles,** contain chemicals known as **neurotransmitters** (noo-roh-TRANS-mitters).

When a nerve impulse reaches the synaptic knob, a series of reactions releases neurotransmitters into the synaptic cleft. The neurotransmitters diffuse across the synaptic cleft and react with receptors on the postsynaptic cell membrane. This is synaptic transmission. To prevent prolonged reactions with the postsynaptic receptors, the transmitters are very quickly inactivated by enzymes. One of the best known neurotransmitters is **acetylcholine** (ah-see-till-KOH-leen), which is inactivated by the enzyme **cholinesterase** (koh-lin-ES-ter-ase). Table 8-3 lists some of the common neurotransmitters.

▌ At the synapse, a neurotransmitter, such as acetylcholine, diffuses across the synaptic cleft to the postsynaptic membrane.

Table 8-3 Some Common Neurotransmitters

Neurotransmitter	Location	Function	Comments
Acetylcholine	CNS and PNS	Generally excitatory but is inhibitory to some visceral effectors	Found in skeletal neuromuscular junctions and in many ANS synapses
Norepinephrine	CNS and PNS	May be excitatory or inhibitory depending on the receptors	Found in visceral and cardiac muscle neuromuscular junctions; cocaine and amphetamines exaggerate the effects
Epinephrine	CNS and PNS	May be excitatory or inhibitory depending on the receptors	Found in pathways concerned with behavior and mood
Dopamine	CNS and PNS	Generally excitatory	Found in pathways that regulate emotional responses; decreased levels in Parkinson's disease
Serotonin	CNS	Generally inhibitory	Found in pathways that regulate temperature, sensory perception, mood, onset of sleep
Gamma-aminobutyric acid (GABA)	CNS	Generally inhibitory	Inhibits excessive discharge of neurons
Endorphins and enkephalins	CNS	Generally inhibitory	Inhibit release of sensory pain neurotransmitters; opiates mimic the effects of these peptides

CNS = central nervous system; PNS = peripheral nervous system; ANS = autonomic nervous system.

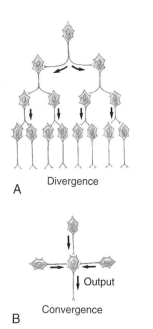

A Divergence

B Convergence

↓ Output

Figure 8–7   Divergence and convergence in neuronal pools.

In **excitatory transmission,** the neurotransmitter–receptor reaction on the postsynaptic membrane depolarizes the membrane and initiates an action potential. This is excitation or stimulation. Acetylcholine is typically an excitatory neurotransmitter. Some neurotransmitters result in **inhibitory transmission.** In this case, the reaction between the neurotransmitter and the receptor opens potassium channels in the membrane so that potassium diffuses out of the cell but has no effect on the sodium channels. This action makes the inside of the membrane even more negative than it is in the resting condition; it **hyperpolarizes** the membrane, which makes it more difficult to generate an action potential. This is inhibition. Gamma-aminobutyric acid (GABA) is an inhibitory neurotransmitter in the CNS.

Synaptic transmission may be either excitatory or inhibitory.

The billions of neurons in the CNS are organized into functional groups called **neuronal pools.** The neuronal pools receive information, process and integrate that information, then transmit it to some other destination. Neuronal pools are arranged in pathways, or circuits, over which the nerve impulses are transmitted. The simplest pathway is the **simple series circuit** in which a single neuron synapses with another neuron, which in turn synapses with another, and so on. Most pathways are more complex. In a **divergence circuit** (Fig. 8–7A), a single neuron synapses with multiple neurons within the pool. This permits the same information to diverge or to go along different pathways at the same time.

This type of pathway is important in muscle contraction when many muscle fibers, or even several muscles, must contract at the same time. Another type of pathway is the **convergence circuit** (Fig. 8–7B). In this case, several presynaptic neurons synapse with a single postsynaptic neuron. This accounts for the fact that many different stimuli may have the same ultimate effect. For example, thinking about food, smelling food, and seeing food all have the same effect, the flow of saliva.

Neuronal pools are functional groups within the CNS. These may contain simple series circuits, divergence circuits, or convergence circuits.

Reflex Arcs

The neuron is the structural unit of the nervous system; the **reflex arc** is the functional unit. The reflex arc is a type of conduction pathway. It is like a one-way street because it allows impulses to travel in only one direction. The simplest reflex arc consists of two neurons, but most have three or more neurons in the conduction pathway. Figure 8–8 illustrates a three-neuron reflex arc. There are five basic components in a reflex arc (Table 8–4):

- Receptor
- Sensory neuron
- Center
- Motor neuron
- Effector

A reflex is an automatic, involuntary response to some change, either inside or outside the body. Reflexes are important in maintaining homeostasis by making adjustments to heart rate, breathing rate,

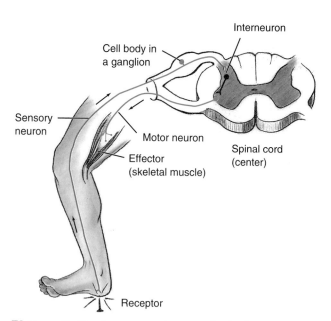

Figure 8–8   Components of a generalized reflex arc.

Table 8–4 Components of a Reflex Arc

Component	Description	Function
Receptor	Site of stimulus action; receptor end of a dendrite or special cell in receptor organ	Responds to some change in the internal or external environment
Sensory neuron	Afferent neuron; cell body is in ganglion outside the CNS; axon extends into the CNS	Transmits nerve impulses from receptor to the CNS
Integration center	Always within the CNS; in simplest reflexes, it consists of a synapse between sensory and motor neuron; more commonly one or more interneurons are involved	Processing center; region in CNS where incoming sensory impulses generate appropriate outgoing motor impulses
Motor neuron	Efferent neuron; dendrites and cell body are in the CNS; axon extends to the periphery	Transmits nerve impulses from the integration center in the CNS to the effector organ
Effector	Muscle or gland outside the CNS	Responds to the impulses from the motor neuron to produce an action such as contraction or secretion

CNS = central nervous system.

and blood pressure. Reflexes are also involved in coughing, sneezing, and reactions to painful stimuli. Everyone is familiar with the withdrawal reflex. When you step on a tack or touch a hot iron, you immediately, without conscious thought, withdraw the injured foot or hand from the source of the irritation. Clinicians frequently test an individual's reflexes to determine if the nervous system is functioning properly.

 The reflex arc is a simple conduction pathway that utilizes a receptor, sensory neuron, center, motor neuron, and effector.

✓ QuickCheck

- What is the response to a threshold stimulus on a neuron?

- What is a distinguishing feature of a neuron on which saltatory conduction occurs?

- Many muscle fibers must contract at the same time. What type of neuronal circuit permits this?

Central Nervous System

The CNS consists of the brain and spinal cord, which are located in the dorsal body cavity. These are vital to our well-being and are enclosed in bone for protection. The brain is surrounded by the cranium, and the spinal cord is protected by the vertebrae. The brain is continuous with the spinal cord at the foramen magnum. In addition to bone, the CNS is surrounded by connective tissue membranes, called **meninges,** and by **cerebrospinal fluid** (CSF).

Meninges

Three layers of meninges (men-IN-jeez) surround the brain and spinal cord (Fig. 8–9). The outer layer, the **dura mater** (DOO-rah MAY-ter), is tough white

fibrous connective tissue. It is just inside the cranial bones and lines the vertebral canal. The dura mater contains channels, called **dural sinuses,** that collect venous blood to return it to the cardiovascular system. The **superior sagittal sinus,** located in the midsagittal line over the top of the brain, is the largest of the dural sinuses.

The middle layer of meninges is the **arachnoid** (ah-RAK-noyd). The arachnoid, which resembles a cobweb in appearance, is a thin layer with numerous threadlike strands that attach it to the innermost layer. The space under the arachnoid, the **subarachnoid space,** is filled with CSF and contains blood vessels.

The **pia mater** (PEE-ah MAY-ter) is the innermost layer of meninges. This thin, delicate membrane is tightly bound to the surface of the brain and spinal cord and cannot be dissected away without damaging the surface. It closely follows all surface contours.

 There are three layers of meninges around the brain and spinal cord. The outer layer is dura mater, the middle layer is arachnoid, and the innermost layer is pia mater.

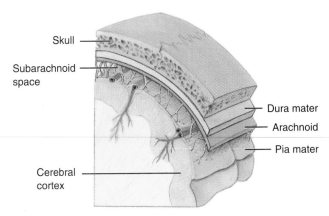

Figure 8–9 Meninges of the central nervous system.

Meningitis is an acute inflammation of the pia mater and the arachnoid. It is most commonly caused by bacteria. However, viral infections, fungal infections, and tumors may also cause inflammation of the meninges. Depending on the primary cause, meningitis may be mild or it may progress to a severe and life-theatening condition.

Brain

The brain is divided into the cerebrum, diencephalon, brain stem, and cerebellum.

Cerebrum

The largest and most obvious portion of the brain is the **cerebrum** (seh-REE-brum), which is divided by a deep **longitudinal fissure** (FISH-ur) into two **cerebral hemispheres.** The two hemispheres are two separate entities but are connected by an arching band of white fibers, called the **corpus callosum** (KOR-pus kah-LOH-sum), that provides a communication pathway between the two halves. An extension of dura mater, the **falx cerebri** (FALKS SAYR-eh-brye), projects into the longitudinal fissure down to the corpus callosum. The superior sagittal sinus, a dural sinus mentioned earlier, is in the superior margin of the falx cerebri. The surface of the cerebrum is marked by convolutions, or **gyri** (JYE-rye), separated by grooves, or **sulci** (SULL-see). The pia mater closely follows the convolutions and goes deep into the sulci, then up and over the gyri.

Each cerebral hemisphere is divided into five lobes, as illustrated in Figure 8–10. Four of the lobes have the same name as the bone over them. The **frontal lobe,** under the frontal bone, is the most anterior portion of each hemisphere. The posterior boundary of the frontal lobe is the **central sulcus.** The **parietal lobe** is immediately posterior to the central sulcus, under the parietal bone. The **occipital lobe,** under the occipital bone, is the most posterior portion of the cerebral hemisphere. Laterally, the **temporal lobe** is inferior to the frontal and parietal lobes. The **lateral sulcus** (fissure) separates the temporal lobe from the two lobes that are superior to it. A fifth lobe, the **insula** (IN-sull-ah) or **Island of Reil,** lies deep within the lateral sulcus. It is covered by parts of the frontal, parietal, and temporal lobes.

Each cerebral hemisphere is divided into frontal, parietal, occipital, and temporal lobes and an insula.

The cerebral hemispheres consist of gray matter and white matter. A thin layer of **gray matter,** the **cerebral cortex,** forms the outermost portion of the cerebrum. Gray matter consists of neuron cell bodies and unmyelinated fibers. Nearly three fourths of the neuron cell bodies in the entire nervous system are found in the cerebral cortex. Additional regions of gray matter, the **basal ganglia,** are scattered throughout the white matter. The **white matter,** which makes up the bulk of the cerebrum, is just beneath the cerebral cortex. White matter is myeli-

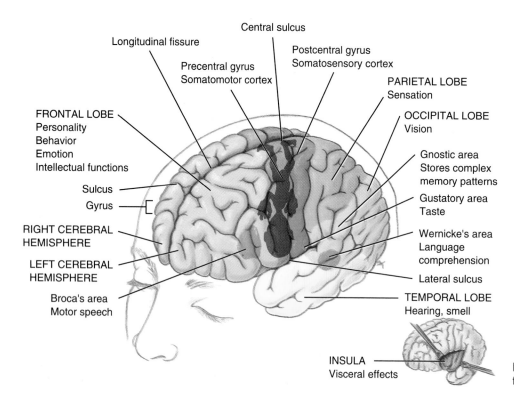

Central sulcus
Longitudinal fissure
Precentral gyrus
Somatomotor cortex
Postcentral gyrus
Somatosensory cortex

PARIETAL LOBE
Sensation

OCCIPITAL LOBE
Vision

FRONTAL LOBE
Personality
Behavior
Emotion
Intellectual functions

Gnostic area
Stores complex
memory patterns

Gustatory area
Taste

Sulcus
Gyrus

RIGHT CEREBRAL
HEMISPHERE

LEFT CEREBRAL
HEMISPHERE

Wernicke's area
Language
comprehension

Lateral sulcus

Broca's area
Motor speech

TEMPORAL LOBE
Hearing, smell

INSULA
Visceral effects

Figure 8–10 Lobes and functional areas of the cerebrum.

nated nerve fibers that form three types of communication pathways in the cerebrum (Table 8–5).

> Gray matter consists of neuron cell bodies; white matter is myelinated nerve fibers.

The cerebral cortex is the neural basis of what makes us "human." It is the center for sensory and motor functions. It is concerned with memory, language, reasoning, intelligence, personality, and all the other factors that we associate with human life. Even though the two cerebral hemispheres are nearly symmetrical in structure, they are not always equal in function; instead, there are areas of specialization. However, there is considerable overlap in these regions and no area really works alone but all are dependent on each other for mental "consciousness," those abilities that involve higher mental processing such as memory, reasoning, logic, and judgment.

> In most people (about 90 percent), the left cerebral hemisphere dominates for language and mathematical abilities. It is the reasoning and analytical side of the brain. The right cerebral hemisphere is involved with motor skills, intuition, emotion, art, and music appreciation. It is the poetic and creative side of the brain. These people are generally right-handed. In about 10 percent of the people these sides are reversed. In some cases, neither hemisphere dominates. This may result in "confusion" and learning disabilities.

It is possible to identify regions of the cerebral cortex that have specific functions. Some of these regions are illustrated in Figure 8–10. **Sensory areas** in the parietal, occipital, and temporal lobes receive information from the various sense organs and receptors throughout the body. The primary sensory area, the **somatosensory** (soh-mat-oh-SEN-soar-ee) **cortex,** is located in the **postcentral gyrus** of the parietal lobe, immediately posterior to the central sulcus. This region receives sensory input from sensory receptors in the skin and skeletal muscles. The right side of the somatosensory cortex receives input

from the left side of the body and vice versa. The somatosensory cortex is highly organized with specific regions responsible for receiving sensory input from specific parts of the body. This organizational mapping is illustrated by the distorted figure of the body (homunculus) superimposed on Figure 8–10. Note that larger areas of the cortex are devoted to the face and hands than to other parts of the body. Other areas of the cerebrum are responsible for vision, hearing, taste, and smell.

Motor areas responsible for muscle contraction are located in the frontal lobe. The primary motor area, the **somatomotor** (soh-mat-oh-MOH-ter) **cortex,** is in the **precentral gyrus,** immediately anterior to the central sulcus. Neurons in this area allow us to consciously control our skeletal muscles. The right primary motor gyrus controls muscles on the left side of the body and vice versa. The primary motor cortex is also highly organized in a manner similar to the primary sensory cortex, with neurons in a specific region responsible for controlling movement in a specific part of the body (see Fig. 8–10).

Association areas of the cerebral cortex are involved in the process of recognition. They analyze and interpret sensory information, based on previous experiences, then integrate appropriate responses through the motor areas. Table 8–6 describes some of the specific functional areas of the cerebral cortex.

> The primary sensory area of the brain is the postcentral gyrus in the parietal lobe. The primary motor area is the precentral gyrus in the frontal lobe. Association areas that analyze, interpret, and integrate information are scattered throughout the cortex

The **basal ganglia** are functionally related regions of gray matter that are scattered throughout the white matter of the cerebral hemispheres. These regions function as relay stations, or areas of synapse, in pathways going to and from the cortex. The major effects of the basal ganglia are to decrease muscle tone and to inhibit muscular activity. Because of these effects, they play an important role in posture and coordinating motor movements. Also, nearly all the inhibitory neurotransmitter, dopamine, is produced in the basal ganglia.

> Parkinson's disease is a condition in which the basal ganglia do not produce enough of the inhibitory transmitter dopamine. Without dopamine, there is an excess of excitatory signals that affect certain voluntary muscles, producing rigidity and tremors.

Diencephalon

The **diencephalon** (dye-en-SEF-ah-lon) is centrally located and is nearly surrounded by the cerebral hemispheres. It includes the **thalamus, hypothala-**

Table 8–5	Pathways of White Matter in the Cerebrum
Type of Fibers	**Function**
Association	Transmit impulses from one gyrus to another within the same hemisphere
Commissural	Transmit impulses from one cerebral hemisphere to the other; allow one side to know what the other side is doing; corpus callosum is a large band of commissural fibers
Projection	Transmit impulses from the cerebrum to other parts of the central nervous system

Table 8–6   Functional Regions of the Cerebral Cortex

Functional Region	Location	Description	Comments
Primary sensory cortex (somatosensory cortex)	Postcentral gyrus in the parietal lobe	Receives sensory input from receptors in the skin and skeletal muscles	Functions in sensations of temperature, touch, pressure, and pain
Somatosensory association area	Parietal lobe, immediately posterior to the primary sensory cortex	Integrates and analyzes input received by the primary sensory cortex	Analyzes and interprets current sensory information and compares it with previous experience to form a basis for recognition
Primary visual cortex	Posterior region of the occipital lobe	Receives sensory input from the retina of the eye	Perceives current visual image
Visual association area	Anterior to the primary visual cortex in the occipital lobe	Integrates and analyzes input received by the primary visual cortex	Compares present visual information with previous experience as a basis for recognition; attaches significance to what you see
Auditory cortex	Superior margin of the temporal lobe, along the lateral sulcus	Receives auditory impulses related to pitch, rhythm, and loudness from the inner ear	Allows you to hear "sounds"
Auditory association area	Adjacent to the primary auditory area in the temporal lobe	Integrates and analyzes input received by the primary auditory area	Permits recognition of sounds (e.g., speech, music, noise); involved in memory of music
Olfactory cortex	Medial aspect of the temporal lobe	Receives input from the olfactory (smell) receptors in the nasal cavity	Permits perception of different odors
Gustatory cortex	Parietal lobe where it is overlapped by the temporal lobe	Receives input from the taste buds on the tongue	Permits perception of different tastes
Wernicke's area	Posterior aspect of the temporal lobe of one hemisphere, usually the left	Receives input from auditory and visual association areas	Permits comprehension of spoken and written language
Primary motor cortex (somatomotor cortex)	Precentral gyrus in the frontal lobe	Initiates efferent action potentials that control voluntary movements	Permits skeletal muscle contraction
Premotor cortex	Anterior to the primary motor cortex in the frontal lobe	Controls learned motor skills that involve skeletal muscles, either simultaneously or sequentially	Examples of learned motor skills are playing the piano, typing, writing
Broca's area (motor speech area)	Inferior portion of the frontal lobe in one hemisphere, usually the left	Programs and coordinates the muscular movements necessary to articulate words	A person with injury in this area is able to understand words but is unable to speak because of the inability to coordinate the muscles necessary to form words
Prefrontal cortex	Anterior portion of the frontal lobes	Involved with thought, reasoning, intelligence, judgment, planning, conscience	This area is well developed only in humans
Gnostic area (general interpretation area)	Region where parietal, temporal, and occipital lobes meet; found in one hemisphere (usually left)	Integrates sensory interpretations from the adjacent association areas to form thoughts, then transmits signals for appropriate responses	Stores complex memory patterns; allows a person to recognize words and arrange them appropriately to express thoughts or to read and understand written ideas

mus, and **epithalamus.** Regions of the diencephalon are illustrated in Figure 8–11.

The **thalamus** (THAL-ah-mus), about 80 percent of the diencephalon, consists of two oval masses of gray matter that serve as relay stations for sensory impulses, except for the sense of smell, going to the cerebral cortex. When the impulses reach the thalamus, there is a general awareness and crude recog-

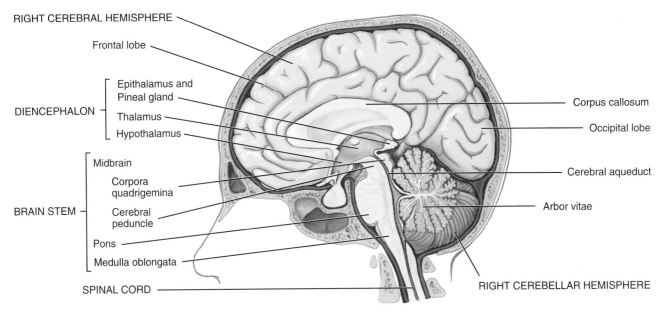

RIGHT CEREBRAL HEMISPHERE

Frontal lobe

DIENCEPHALON
- Epithalamus and Pineal gland
- Thalamus
- Hypothalamus

BRAIN STEM
- Midbrain
  - Corpora quadrigemina
  - Cerebral peduncle
- Pons
- Medulla oblongata

SPINAL CORD

Corpus callosum

Occipital lobe

Cerebral aqueduct

Arbor vitae

RIGHT CEREBELLAR HEMISPHERE

Figure 8–11   Midsagittal section of the brain showing the major portions of the diencephalon, brain stem, and cerebellum.

nition of sensation. The thalamus channels the impulses to the appropriate region of the cortex for discrimination, localization, and interpretation.

The **hypothalamus** (HYE-poh-thal-ah-mus) is a small region below the thalamus. It plays a key role in maintaining homeostasis because it regulates many visceral activities. The hypothalamus also serves as a link between the nervous and endocrine systems because it regulates secretion of hormones from the pituitary gland. A slender stalk, the **infundibulum,** extends from the floor of the hypothalamus to the pituitary gland and acts as a connector between the two structures. Two visible "bumps" on the posterior portion of the hypothalamus, the **mamillary bodies,** are involved in memory and emotional responses to different odors (see Functions of the Hypothalamus).

Functions of the Hypothalamus

▶ **Regulates and integrates the autonomic nervous system.**
  The hypothalamus influences the autonomic centers in the brain stem and spinal cord. In this way it regulates many visceral activities such as heart rate, blood pressure, respiratory rate, and motility of the digestive tract.

▶ **Regulates emotional responses and behavior.**
  The hypothalamus acts through the autonomic nervous system to mediate the physical responses to emotion and mind-over-body phenomena. Nuclei involved in feelings of rage, aggression, fear, pleasure, and the sex drive are localized in the hypothalamus.

▶ **Regulates body temperature.**
  Certain cells of the hypothalamus act as a body thermostat and activate appropriate responses.

▶ **Regulates food intake.**
  The feeding or hunger center in the hypothalamus is responsible for hunger sensations. After food ingestion, the satiety center inhibits the hunger center.

▶ **Regulates water balance and thirst.**
  Osmoreceptors in the hypothalamus monitor the volume and concentration of body fluids, then initiate appropriate responses from the thirst center and antidiuretic hormone.

▶ **Regulates sleep–wake cycles.**
  Centers in the hypothalamus act with other brain centers to maintain alternating periods of sleep and wakefulness.

▶ **Regulates endocrine system activity.**
  The hypothalamus produces releasing factors that control the release of hormone from the anterior pituitary gland. It also produces two hormones, antidiuretic hormone and oxytocin, which are stored in the posterior pituitary gland.

The **epithalamus** (ep-ih-THAL-ah-mus) is the most dorsal, or superior, portion of the diencephalon. The **pineal** (PIE-nee-al) **gland,** or **body,** extends from its posterior margin. This small gland is involved with the onset of puberty and rhythmic cycles in the body. It is like a biological clock.

> The diencephalon includes the thalamus, hypothalamus, and epithalamus. These areas integrate and regulate a variety of body functions.

The **limbic system** consists of scattered but interconnected regions of gray matter in the cerebral hemispheres and diencephalon. The limbic system is involved in memory and in emotions such as sadness, happiness, anger, and fear. It is our emotional brain.

Brain Stem

The **brain stem** is the region between the diencephalon and the spinal cord. It consists of three regions:

- Midbrain
- Pons
- Medulla oblongata

Regions of the brain stem are illustrated in Figure 8-11.

The **midbrain** is the most superior portion of the brain stem, the region next to the diencephalon. Two **cerebral peduncles** (seh-REE-brull pee-DUNK-als) form the ventral aspect of the midbrain. These bundles of myelinated fibers contain the voluntary motor tracts that descend from the cerebral cortex. On the dorsal aspect of the midbrain, four rounded protuberances form the **corpora quadrigemina** (KOR-poar-ah kwad-rih-JEM-ih-nah). The two superior bodies, the **superior colliculi** (soo-PEER-ee-or koh-LIK-yoo-lye), function as visual reflex centers. The other two, the **inferior colliculi,** contain auditory reflex centers. A narrow channel, the **cerebral aqueduct** (seh-REE-brull AH-kweh-dukt), descends through the center of the midbrain.

The **pons** is the bulging middle portion of the brain stem. This region primarily consists of nerve fibers that form conduction tracts between the higher brain centers and the spinal cord. Four cranial nerves originate in the pons. It also contains the **pneumotaxic** (noo-moh-TACK-sik) and **apneustic** (ap-NOO-stick) **areas** that help regulate breathing movements.

The **medulla oblongata** (meh-DULL-ah ahb-long-GAH-tah), or simply **medulla,** extends inferiorly from the pons. It is continuous with the spinal cord at the foramen magnum. All the ascending (sensory) and descending (motor) nerve fibers connecting the brain and spinal cord pass through the medulla. Most of the descending fibers cross over from one side to the other. In other words, fibers descending on the left side cross over to the right and vice versa. This is called **decussation** (dee-kuh-SAY-shun). Because the fibers decussate, or cross over, the brain controls motor functions on the opposite side of the body. Five pairs of cranial nerves originate in the medulla. In addition, it contains three vital centers that control visceral activities. The **cardiac center** adjusts the heart rate and contraction strength to meet body needs. The **vasomotor center** regulates blood pressure by effecting changes in blood vessel diameter. The **respiratory center** acts with the centers in the pons to regulate the rate, rhythm, and depth of breathing. Other centers are involved in coughing, sneezing, swallowing, and vomiting.

> The midbrain, pons, and medulla oblongata form the brain stem. This region contains numerous centers, some essential to life, that control visceral activities.

The **reticular formation** consists of scattered, but interconnected neurons and fiber pathways in the midbrain and brain stem. It is a functional system that maintains alertness and filters out repetitive stimuli. Motor portions of the reticular formation help coordinate skeletal muscle activity and maintain muscle tone.

Cerebellum

The **cerebellum** (sair-eh-BELL-um), second largest portion of the brain, is located below the occipital lobes of the cerebrum and is separated from them by the **transverse fissure.** It consists of two **cerebellar hemispheres** connected in the middle by a structure called the **vermis.** An extension of dura mater, the **falx cerebelli** (FALKS sair-eh-BELL-eye), forms a partial partition between the hemispheres. Another extension of dura mater, the **tentorium cerebelli** (ten-TOAR-ee-um sair-eh-BELL-eye), is found in the transverse fissure between the cerebellum and the occipital lobes of the cerebrum.

Like the cerebrum, the cerebellum consists of white matter surrounded by a thin layer of gray matter, the **cerebellar cortex.** Because the surface convolutions are less prominent in the cerebellum than in the cerebrum, the cerebellum has proportionately less gray matter. The branching arrangement of white matter is called **arbor vitae** (AR-bor vye-tay).

Three paired bundles of myelinated nerve fibers, called **cerebellar peduncles,** form communication pathways between the cerebellum and other parts of the CNS. The **superior cerebellar peduncles** connect the cerebellum to the midbrain; the **middle cerebellar peduncles** communicate with the pons; and the **inferior cerebellar peduncles** consist of pathways between the cerebellum and the medulla oblongata and spinal cord.

> Cerebellar peduncles connect the cerebellum to other parts of the CNS.

The cerebellum functions as a motor area of the brain that mediates subconscious contractions of skeletal muscles necessary for **coordination, posture, and balance.** The cerebellum coordinates skeletal muscles to produce smooth muscle movement rather than jerky, trembling motion. When the cerebellum is damaged, movements such as running, walking, and writing become uncoordinated. Posture is dependent on muscle tone, which is mediated by the cerebellum. Impulses from the inner ear concerning position and equilibrium are directed to the cerebellum, which uses that information to maintain balance.

> The cerebellum is a motor area that coordinates skeletal muscle activity and is important in maintaining muscle tone, posture, and balance.

Ventricles and Cerebrospinal Fluid

A series of interconnected, fluid-filled cavities are found within the brain (Fig. 8–12A). These cavities are the **ventricles** of the brain, and the fluid is **cerebrospinal** (seh-ree-broh-SPY-null) **fluid (CSF).** The **lateral ventricles** in the cerebrum are the largest of these cavities. There is one lateral ventricle in each cerebral hemisphere. A single, narrow, slitlike, midline **third ventricle** is enclosed by the diencephalon. The two lateral ventricles open into the third ventricle through the **interventricular foramina.** The **fourth ventricle** is at the level of the cerebellum and pons. A long, narrow channel, the **cerebral aqueduct,** passes through the midbrain to connect the third and fourth ventricles. The fourth ventricle is continuous with the central canal of the spinal cord. Openings in the wall of the fourth ventricle permit CSF to enter the subarachnoid space.

> Four interconnected cavities, called ventricles, contain CSF within the brain.

In hydrocephalus, an obstruction in the normal flow of CSF causes the fluid to accumulate in the ventricles. The obstruction may be a congenital defect or an acquired lesion such as a tumor. As the fluid accumulates, it causes the ventricles to enlarge and CSF pressure to increase. When this happens in an infant, before the cranial bones ossify, the cranium enlarges. In an older child or adult, the pressure damages the soft brain tissue.

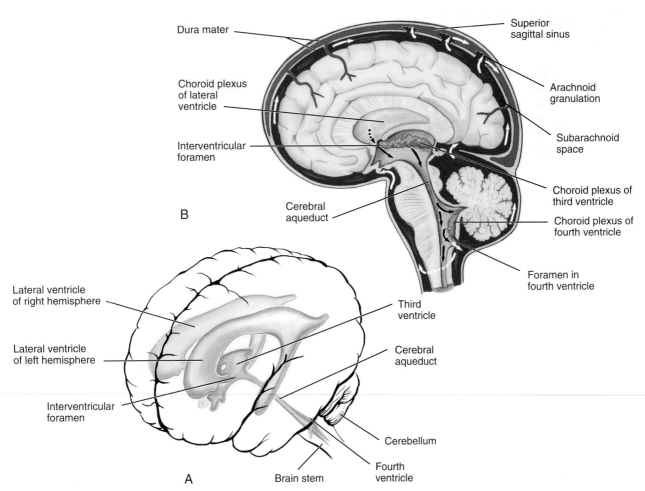

Figure 8–12 *A,* Ventricles of the brain. *B,* Circulation of cerebrospinal fluid.

The CSF is a clear fluid that forms as a filtrate from the blood in specialized capillary networks, the **choroid plexus** (KOR-oyd PLEKS-us), within the ventricles. The circulation of the CSF is illustrated in Figure 8–12B. Ependymal cells, a type of neuroglia cell, aid in the circulation of CSF through the ventricles and central canal. CSF then enters the subarachnoid space through foramina in the fourth ventricle. From the subarachnoid space, CSF carrying waste products filters through **arachnoid granulations** (villi) into the dural sinuses and is returned to the blood. In addition to providing support and protection for the CNS, the CSF helps to nourish the brain and maintain constant ionic conditions for the brain and spinal cord, and provides a pathway for removal of waste products.

> CSF is formed from the blood in the choroid plexus of the ventricles, circulates through the ventricles and subarachnoid space, then returns to the blood in the dural sinuses.

Spinal Cord

The **spinal cord,** illustrated in Figure 8–13, extends from the foramen magnum at the base of the skull to the level of the first lumbar vertebra, a distance of about 43 to 46 centimeters (17 or 18 inches). The cord is continuous with the medulla oblongata at the foramen magnum. Distally, it terminates in the **conus medullaris** (KOH-nus med-yoo-LAIR-is). Like the brain, the spinal cord is surrounded by bone, meninges, and CSF. Unlike the dura mater around the brain, the spinal dura is separated from the vertebral bones by an **epidural space** (Fig. 8–14). This space is filled with loose connective tissue and adipose. The meninges extend beyond the end of the spinal cord, down to the upper part of the sacrum. From there, a fibrous cord of pia mater, the **filum terminale** (FYE-lum term-ih-NAL-ee), extends down to the coccyx where it is anchored.

> The spinal cord begins at the foramen magnum as a continuation of the medulla oblongata and extends to the first lumbar vertebra.

The spinal cord is divided into 31 segments with each segment giving rise to a pair of spinal nerves. At the distal end of the cord, many spinal nerves extend beyond the conus medullaris to form a collection that resembles a horse's tail. This is the **cauda equina** (KAW-dah ee-KWYNE-ah). There are two enlargements in the cord, one in the cervical region and one in the lumbar region. The **cervical enlargement** gives rise to the nerves that supply the upper extremity. Nerves from the **lumbar enlargement** supply the lower extremity.

> A lumbar puncture is the withdrawal of some CSF from the subarachnoid space in the lumbar region of the spinal cord. The extension of the meninges beyond the end of the cord makes it possible to do this without injury to the spinal cord. The needle is usually inserted just above or just below the fourth lumbar vertebra and the spinal cord ends at the first lumbar vertebra. The CSF that is removed can be tested for abnormal characteristics that may indicate an injury or infection.

In cross section, the spinal cord appears oval (see Fig. 8–14). A narrow, deep, **dorsal (posterior) median sulcus** and a shallower, but wider, **ventral (anterior) median fissure** partially divide the cord into right and left halves. Peripheral white matter surrounds a core of gray matter that resembles a butterfly or the letter H. Each side of the gray matter is divided into **dorsal, lateral,** and **ventral horns.** These contain the terminal portions of sensory neuron axons, entire interneurons, and the dendrites and cell bodies of motor neurons. The central connecting bar between the two large areas of gray matter is the **gray commissure** (KOM-ih-shur). This surrounds the **central canal,** which contains CSF. The gray matter divides the surrounding white matter into three regions on each side. These regions are the **dorsal, lateral,** and **ventral funiculi** (fuh-NIK-

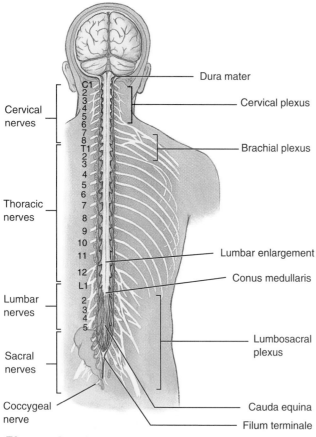

Cervical nerves

Thoracic nerves

Lumbar nerves

Sacral nerves

Coccygeal nerve

C1
2
3
4
5
6
7
8
T1
2
3
4
5
6
7
8
9
10
11
12
L1
2
3
4
5

Dura mater

Cervical plexus

Brachial plexus

Lumbar enlargement

Conus medullaris

Lumbosacral plexus

Cauda equina

Filum terminale

Figure 8–13 Gross anatomy of the spinal cord.

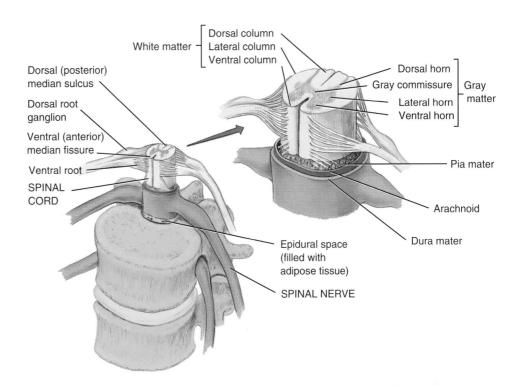

Figure 8–14 Cross section of the spinal cord.

yoo-lee) or **columns.** The white matter contains longitudinal bundles of myelinated nerve fibers, called **nerve tracts.**

> The central core of the spinal cord is gray matter, which is divided into regions called horns. This is surrounded by white matter, which is divided into columns or funiculi.

The spinal cord has two main functions. It is a conduction pathway for impulses going to and from the brain, and it serves as a reflex center.

The conduction pathways that carry sensory impulses from body parts to the brain are called **ascending tracts.** Pathways that carry motor impulses from the brain to muscles and glands are **descending tracts.** Tracts are often named according to their points of origin and termination. For example, **spinothalamic** (spy-noh-tha-LAM-ik) **tracts** are ascending (sensory) tracts that begin in the spinal cord and conduct impulses to the thalamus. They function in the sensations of touch, pressure, pain, and temperature. **Corticospinal** (kor-tih-koh-SPY-null) **tracts,** also called **pyramidal** (pih-RAM-ih-dal) **tracts,** are descending (motor) tracts that begin in the cerebral cortex and end in the spinal cord. These tracts function in the control of skeletal muscle movement. All other descending tracts are grouped together as **extrapyramidal** (eks-trah-pih-RAM-ih-dal) **tracts,** and they function in muscle movements associated with posture and balance.

In addition to serving as a conduction pathway, the spinal cord functions as a center for spinal reflexes. The reflex arc, described earlier in this chapter and illustrated in Figure 8–9, is the functional unit of the nervous system. Reflexes are responses to stimuli that do not require conscious thought and, consequently, they occur more quickly than reactions that require thought processes. For example, with the withdrawal reflex, the reflex action withdraws the affected part before you are aware of the pain. Many reflexes are mediated in the spinal cord without going to the higher brain centers. Table 8–7 describes some clinically significant reflexes.

> The spinal cord functions as a conduction pathway and as a reflex center. Sensory impulses travel to the brain on ascending tracts in the cord. Motor impulses travel on descending tracts.

✓ Quick**Check**

- In which cerebral lobe is the primary somatosensory area located?
- What comprises the white matter of the brain and spinal cord?
- In which ventricle will CSF accumulate if there is a constriction or blockage in the cerebral aqueduct?
- What type of impulses are transmitted by the spinothalamic tracts of the spinal cord?

Peripheral Nervous System

The PNS consists of the nerves that branch out from the brain and spinal cord. These nerves form the communication network between the CNS and the

Table 8–7	Some Clinically Significant Reflexes	
Reflex	**Description**	**Indications**
Patellar (Knee-jerk reflex)	Stretch reflex; two-neuron path; reflex hammer strikes patellar tendon just below the knee; receptors in quadriceps femoris muscle are stretched; reflex results in an immediate "kick"	Reflex is blocked by damage to the nerves involved and by damage to lumbar segments of the spinal cord; also absent in people with chronic diabetes mellitus and neurosyphilis
Achilles tendon (Ankle-jerk reflex)	Stretch reflex; two-neuron path; reflex hammer strikes Achilles tendon just above the heel; gastrocnemius and soleus muscles contract to plantar flex the foot	Weak or no reflex action indicates damage to the nerves involved or to the L5–S2 segments of the spinal cord; also absent in chronic diabetes, neurosyphilis, and alcoholism
Abdominal	Stroking the lateral abdominal wall produces a reflex action that compresses the abdominal wall and moves the umbilicus toward the stimulus	Absent in lesions of peripheral nerves, lesions in the thoracic segments of the spinal cord, and in multiple sclerosis
Babinski's	Lateral sole of the foot is stroked from heel to toe; positive sign results in dorsiflexion of the big toe and spreading of other toes; negative sign results in toes curling under with slight inversion of the foot	Positive Babinski's sign is normal in children younger than 18 months of age; negative sign is normal after 18 months of age; if motor tracts in the spinal cord are damaged, positive Babinski's sign reappears

body parts. The PNS is further subdivided into the **somatic nervous system** and the **autonomic nervous system**. The somatic nervous system consists of nerves that go to the skin and muscles and is involved in conscious activities. The autonomic nervous system consists of nerves that connect the CNS to the visceral organs such as the heart, stomach, and intestines. It mediates unconscious activities.

> The cranial and spinal nerves form the peripheral nervous system.

Structure of a Nerve

A nerve contains bundles of nerve fibers, either axons or dendrites, surrounded by connective tissue. **Sensory nerves** contain only afferent fibers, long dendrites of sensory neurons. **Motor nerves** have only efferent fibers, long axons of motor neurons. **Mixed nerves** contain both types of fibers.

Each nerve is surrounded by a connective tissue sheath called the **epineurium** (ep-ih-NOO-ree-um). Portions of the epineurium project inward to divide the nerve into compartments, each containing a bundle of nerve fibers. Each bundle of nerve fibers is called a **fasciculus** and is surrounded by a layer of connective tissue called the **perineurium** (pair-ih-NOO-ree-um). Within the fasciculus, each individual nerve fiber, with its myelin and neurilemma, is surrounded by connective tissue called the **endoneurium** (end-oh-NOO-ree-um). A nerve may also have blood vessels enclosed in its connective tissue wrappings (Fig. 8–15).

> Nerves are bundles of nerve fibers with connective tissue wrappings. Most nerves are mixed nerves because they have both sensory and motor components.

Cranial Nerves

Twelve pairs of cranial nerves, illustrated in Figure 8–16, emerge from the inferior surface of the brain. All of these nerves, except the vagus nerve, pass through foramina of the skull to innervate structures in the head, neck, and facial region. The vagus nerve, cranial nerve X, has numerous branches that

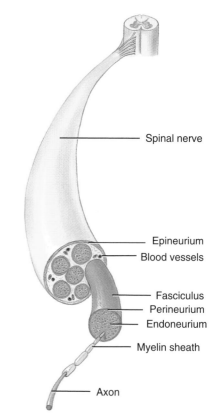

Figure 8–15 Structure of a nerve.

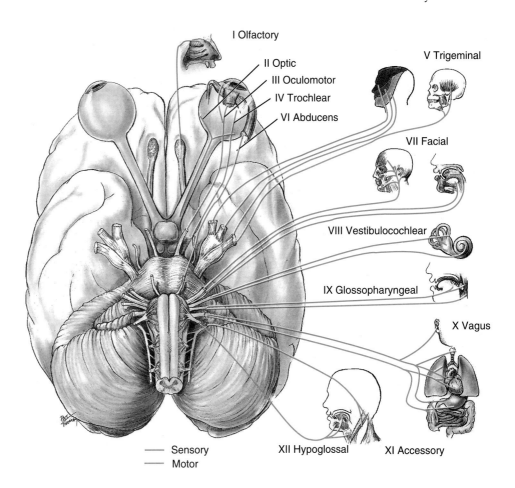

I Olfactory

II Optic
III Oculomotor
IV Trochlear
VI Abducens

V Trigeminal

VII Facial

VIII Vestibulocochlear

IX Glossopharyngeal

X Vagus

XII Hypoglossal

XI Accessory

—— Sensory
—— Motor

Figure 8–16 Cranial nerves.

supply the viscera in the body. When sensory fibers are present in a cranial nerve, the cell bodies of these neurons are located in groups, called **ganglia**, outside the brain. Motor neuron cell bodies are typically located in the gray matter of the brain.

The cranial nerves are designated both by name and by Roman numerals, according to the order in which they appear on the inferior surface of the brain. Most of the nerves have both sensory and motor components. Three of the nerves (I, II, VIII) are associated with the special senses of smell, vision, hearing, and equilibrium and have only sensory fibers. Five other nerves (III, IV, VI, XI, XII) are primarily motor in function but do have some sensory fibers for proprioception. The remaining four nerves (V, VII, IX, X) consist of significant amounts of both sensory and motor fibers. Table 8–8 itemizes the cranial nerves.

Twelve pairs of cranial nerves emerge from the brain. Three of these have only sensory fibers.

Spinal Nerves

Thirty-one pairs of spinal nerves emerge laterally from the spinal cord. Each pair of nerves corre-

sponds to a segment of the cord and they are named accordingly. This means there are **8 cervical nerves** (C1–C8), **12 thoracic nerves** (T1–T12), **5 lumbar nerves** (L1–L5), **5 sacral nerves** (S1–S5), and **1 coccygeal nerve** (Co).

There is a close relationship between a spinal nerve, its source from the spinal cord, and the region it innervates. The skin surface area supplied by a single spinal nerve is called a dermatome.

Each spinal nerve is connected to the spinal cord by a **dorsal root** and a **ventral root** (see Fig. 8–14). The dorsal root can be recognized by an enlargement, the **dorsal root ganglion.** The dorsal root has only sensory fibers, and the ventral root has only motor fibers. The cell bodies of the sensory neurons are in the dorsal root ganglion, but the motor neuron cell bodies are in the gray matter. The two roots join to form the spinal nerve just before the nerve leaves the vertebral column. Because all spinal nerves have both sensory and motor components, they are all mixed nerves.

Immediately after they leave the vertebral col-

Table 8–8 Summary of Cranial Nerves

Number	Name	Type	Function
I	Olfactory	Sensory	Sense of smell
II	Optic	Sensory	Vision
III	Oculomotor	Primarily motor	Movement of eyes and eyelids
IV	Trochlear	Primarily motor	Movement of the eyes
V	Trigeminal	Mixed	
	Ophthalmic branch		**Sensory fibers** from the cornea, skin of nose, forehead, scalp
	Maxillary branch		**Sensory fibers** from the cheek, nose, upper lip, and teeth
	Mandibular branch		**Sensory fibers** from the skin over the mandible, lower lip, and teeth
			Motor fibers to the muscles of mastication
VI	Abducens	Primarily motor	Eye movement
VII	Facial	Mixed	**Sensory fibers** from taste receptors on the anterior two thirds of the tongue
			Motor fibers to the muscles of facial expression, lacrimal glands, and salivary glands
VIII	Vestibulocochlear	Sensory	Hearing and equilibrium
IX	Glossopharyngeal	Mixed	**Sensory fibers** from taste receptors on the posterior one third of the tongue
			Motor fibers to the muscles used in swallowing and to the salivary glands
X	Vagus	Mixed	**Sensory fibers** from the pharynx, larynx, esophagus, and visceral organs
			Somatic motor fibers to the muscles of the pharynx and larynx
			Autonomic motor fibers to the heart, smooth muscles, and glands to alter gastric motility, heart rate, respiration, and blood pressure
XI	Accessory	Primarily motor	Contraction of trapezius and sternocleidomastoid muscles
XII	Hypoglossal	Primarily motor	Contraction of muscles of tongue

umn, the spinal nerves divide into several branches that provide the nerve supply to the muscles and the skin of the body wall. In the thoracic region, the main portions of the nerves go directly to the thoracic wall where they are called **intercostal nerves.** In other regions, the main portions of the nerves form complex networks called **plexuses** (see Fig. 8–13). In the plexus, the fibers are sorted and recombined so that the fibers associated with a particular body part are together even though they may originate from different regions of the cord (Table 8–9).

Thirty-one pairs of spinal nerves emerge from the spinal cord. All spinal nerves are mixed nerves. In all except the thoracic region, spinal nerves form complex networks called plexuses.

Carpal tunnel syndrome is a common occupational injury to the hand and wrist that is associated with repetitive hand motions. It is also associated with several diseases, including arthritis, diabetes, and gout. Symptoms, which include tingling of the thumb and fingers, result from the compression of the median nerve due to the inflammation and swelling of the tendons within the carpal tunnel.

Autonomic Nervous System

General Features

The **autonomic nervous system** (ANS) is a visceral efferent system, which means it sends motor im-

Table 8–9   Spinal Nerve Plexuses

Plexus	Location	Spinal Nerves Involved	Region Supplied	Major Nerves Leaving Plexus
Cervical	Deep in the neck, under the sternocleidomastoid muscle	C1–C4	Skin and muscles of neck and shoulder; diaphragm	Phrenic
Brachial	Deep to the clavicle, between the neck and axilla	C5–C8, T1	Skin and muscles of upper extremity	Musculocutaneous Ulnar Median Radial Axillary
Lumbosacral	Lumbar region of the back	T12, L1–L5, S1–S4	Skin and muscles of lower abdominal wall, lower extremity, buttocks, external genitalia	Obturator Femoral Sciatic Pudendal

pulses to the visceral organs. It functions automatically and continuously, without conscious effort, to innervate smooth muscle, cardiac muscle, and glands. It is concerned with heart rate, breathing rate, blood pressure, body temperature, and other visceral activities that work together to maintain homeostasis.

In the somatic motor pathways, typically there is one neuron that extends from the brain or spinal cord to the effector that is innervated. Autonomic pathways have two neurons between the CNS and the visceral effector (Fig. 8–17). The first neuron's cell body is in the brain or spinal cord. Its axon, the **preganglionic fiber,** leaves the CNS and synapses with a second neuron in an **autonomic ganglion.** The cell body of the second neuron is located in the autonomic ganglion. The axon of the second neuron, the **postganglionic fiber,** leaves the ganglion and goes to the effector organ.

The ANS has two parts, the **sympathetic division** and the **parasympathetic division** (Table 8–10). Many visceral organs are supplied with fibers from both divisions (**dual innervation**). In this case, one

stimulates and the other inhibits. This antagonistic functional relationship serves as a balance to help maintain homeostasis.

> The ANS, which contains visceral efferent nerves, is divided into sympathetic and parasympathetic divisions. Autonomic pathways have two neurons between the CNS and the effector organ.

Sympathetic Division

The sympathetic division, illustrated in Figure 8–18, is concerned primarily with preparing the body for stressful or emergency situations. Sometimes called the fight-or-flight system, it is an energy-expending system. It stimulates the responses that are needed to meet the emergency and inhibits the visceral activities that can be delayed momentarily. For example, during an emergency, the sympathetic system increases breathing rate, heart rate, and blood flow to skeletal muscles. At the same time, it decreases activity in the digestive tract because that is not needed to meet the emergency.

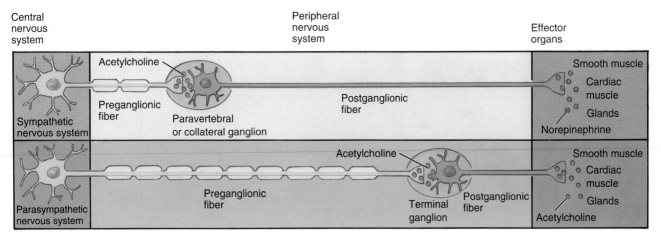

Figure 8–17   Preganglionic and postganglionic fibers in the autonomic nervous system.

Table 8–10 Comparison of Sympathetic and Parasympathetic Actions on Selected Visceral Effectors

Visceral Effectors	Sympathetic Action	Parasympathetic Action
Pupil of the eye	Dilates	Constricts
Lens of the eye	Lens flattens for distance vision	Lens bulges for near vision
Sweat glands	Stimulates	No innervation
Arrector pili muscles of hair	Stimulates contraction; goosebumps	No innervation
Heart	Increases heart rate	Decreases heart rate
Bronchi	Dilates	Constricts
Digestive glands	Decreases secretion of digestive enzymes	Increases secretion of digestive enzymes
Digestive tract	Decreases peristalsis	Increases peristalsis
Digestive tract sphincters	Stimulates—closes sphincters	Inhibits—opens sphincters
Blood vessels to digestive organs	Constricts	No innervation
Blood vessels to skeletal muscles	Dilates	No innervation
Blood vessels to skin	Constricts	No innervation
Adrenal medulla	Stimulates secretion of epinephrine	No innervation
Liver	Increases release of glucose	No innervation
Urinary bladder	Relaxes bladder and closes sphincter	Contracts bladder and opens sphincter

The sympathetic division is an energy-expending, fight-or-flight system that helps meet emergencies.

The sympathetic preganglionic fibers arise from the thoracic and lumbar regions of the spinal cord; thus, the sympathetic division is sometimes called the **thoracolumbar** (thoar-ah-koh-LUM-bar) **division.** These fibers almost immediately terminate in one of the **paravertebral** (pair-ah-ver-TEE-brull) **ganglia.** A chain of these ganglia, the sympathetic chain, extends longitudinally along each side of the vertebral column. Some fibers synapse in **collateral ganglia** outside the sympathetic chain but still close to the

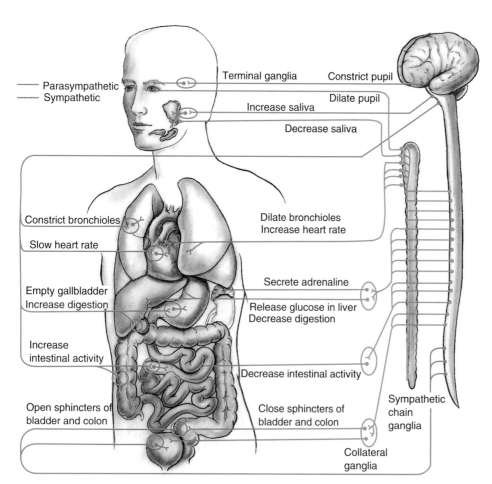

Figure 8–18 Structure and function of autonomic nervous system.

Table 8-11 Some Comparisons Between the Sympathetic and Parasympathetic Divisions of the Autonomic Nervous System

Feature	Sympathetic Division	Parasympathetic Division
General effect	Fight or flight; stress and emergency	Rest and repose; normal activity
Extent of effect	Widespread	Localized
Duration of effect	Long lasting	Short duration
Energy	Expends energy	Conserves energy
Origin of ouflow	Thoracolumbar	Craniosacral
Ganglia	Paravertebral and collateral	Terminal
Preganglionic fibers	Short	Long
Postganglionic fibers	Long	Short
Neurotransmitters	Preganglionic fibers are cholinergic; most postganglionic fibers are adrenergic	Fibers are all cholinergic
Divergence	Great divergence; a preganglionic fiber synapses with several postganglionic fibers	Little divergence; a preganglionic fiber synapses with few postganglionic fibers

vertebral column. Thus, in the sympathetic division, the preganglionic fiber is short, but the postganglionic fiber that makes contact with the effector organ is long.

> The sympathetic fibers arise in the spinal cord, and the ganglia between the neurons are located near the vertebral column.

A sympathetic preganglionic fiber typically synapses with many postganglionic fibers in the ganglion. The postganglionic fibers then go to numerous organs to give a widespread, diffuse effect. At the synapses in the ganglia, the preganglionic fibers release the neurotransmitter **acetylcholine.** For this reason they are called **cholinergic** (koh-lih-NER-jik) **fibers.** Most of the postganglionic fibers release **norepinephrine** (noradrenaline) and are called **adrenergic** (add-rih-NER-jik) **fibers.** Because norepinephrine is inactivated rather slowly these fibers provide a long-lasting effect. Table 8-11 summarizes the features of the sympathetic nervous system.

> Sympathetic preganglionic fibers are cholinergic, and most of the postganglionic fibers are adrenergic.

Parasympathetic Division

The parasympathetic division is most active under ordinary, relaxed conditions (see Fig. 8-18). It also brings the body's systems back to a normal state after an emergency by slowing the heart rate and the breathing rate, decreasing blood pressure, decreasing blood flow to skeletal muscles, and increasing digestive tract activity. Sometimes called the rest-and-repose system, it is an energy-conserving system.

> The parasympathetic division conserves energy and is most active under ordinary, relaxed conditions.

The parasympathetic preganglionic fibers arise from the brain stem and sacral region of the spinal cord; thus it is sometimes called the **craniosacral** (kray-nee-oh-SAY-kral) **division.** The ganglia, called **terminal ganglia,** are located near or within the visceral organs. This makes the preganglionic fiber long and the postganglionic fiber short. Typically, a parasympathetic preganglionic fiber synapses with only a few postganglionic fibers so the effect is localized. Both the preganglionic and postganglionic fibers are **cholinergic,** which means they secrete acetylcholine at the synapses. Because acetylcholine is readily inactivated, the parasympathetic effect is short term. Table 8-11 summarizes the features of the parasympathetic nervous system and compares them with the features of the sympathetic nervous system.

> Nerve fibers in the parasympathetic division arise in the brain stem and sacral region of the spinal cord. The ganglia between the neurons are near the visceral effectors, and the fibers are cholinergic.

☑ QuickCheck

- The ability to smile, frown, and produce tears is due to which cranial nerve?

- Which division of the autonomic nervous system has adrenergic fibers and increases heart rate?

- What accounts for the localized, short-term effect of the parasympathetic nervous system?

FOCUS ON AGING

Aging of the nervous system is of major importance because changes in this system affect organs in other systems and can cause disturbances of many body functions. For example, changes in nerves decrease stimulation of skeletal muscle, which contributes to muscle atrophy with age. Because of its widespread consequences, aging of the nervous system is one of the most distressing aspects of growing old.

Like other cells, nerve cells are lost as a person ages, even in the absence of disease processes. Because neurons are amitotic, those that are lost are not replaced. Loss of neurons is largely responsible for the decrease in brain mass that occurs with aging. Fortunately, the brain has a large reserve supply of neurons, many more than are needed to carry out its functions, so the decrease in neuron number alone is not devastating. The loss of neurons is not constant in all areas of the brain. For example, about 25 percent of the specialized cells in the cerebellum, which are responsible for coordinated movements, are lost during aging. This may affect balance and cause difficulty in coordinating fine movements. There are other areas of the brain in which the number of neurons remains essentially constant throughout life.

It is generally accepted that there is a decline in intelligence with aging, and this is thought to be associated with the loss of neurons. However, it is important to remember that there are wide variations in individuals regarding changes in intellect with age. Because a person is old does not mean that person is "dumb." Many elderly people retain a keen intellect until death. Along with the decline in intelligence, there is a general decline in memory. Again, this varies from person to person. In general, short-term memory seems to be affected more than long-term memory. Intellect and memory appear to be retained better in people who remain mentally and physically active.

Another change observed in older people is a decrease in the rate of impulse conduction along an axon and across a synapse. A reduction in the amount of myelin around the axon probably accounts for the diminished conduction rate along the axon. Decreases in the quantity of neurotransmitter and in the number of receptor sites cause slower conduction across the synapses. These factors contribute to the slower reflexes and the longer time required to process information that are observed in many elderly people.

DO YOU KNOW THIS ABOUT THE

Nervous System?

Alzheimer's Disease

Alzheimer's disease is a debilitating and cruel neurologic disorder that afflicts nearly 4 million Americans. It strikes almost 10 percent of the people older than age 65 and over 30 percent of those older than age 80. Although it generally affects older people, Alzheimer's disease is not a normal phenomenon of aging. It is a dementia that goes far beyond the dulling of the senses and fading memory that usually are associated with the normal aging process. As the number of aging Americans increases, Alzheimer's disease will become more of a problem as families and health care facilities try to cope with patients who no longer can care for themselves, cannot be left alone, have no sense of reality or reason, and may be violent.

Alzheimer's disease has apparently plagued humanity for a long time. Sophocles wrote about an unnamed condition like Alzheimer's in the fifth century BC. In 1906, the German neurologist

Alois Alzheimer linked the dementia of one of his female patients to the destruction he found in her brain after she died. Now, as more people live longer and there are more cases to study, it is recognized as a complex and perplexing disease entity.

Over a period lasting from 5 to 20 years, the disorder destroys the brain and results in increasingly abnormal behavior. The destruction of neurons in the brain appears to correspond with the victim's behavior. The first area to be destroyed is the hippocampus, located deep within the brain and part of the limbic system, which controls emotions and memory. At first, memories fade. Patients in the early stages forget things that happened yesterday or last week. Next, as longer-term memory diminishes, they become more confused and forgetful, fail to recognize familiar places and people, and become depressed. As the disease progresses, destruction reaches the cerebral cortex, the thinking part of the brain. This is when delusions, hallucinations, violent mood swings, and paranoia appear. If the patient lives long enough, the nerve cells in the motor cortex die and the patient loses the ability to walk, talk, or swallow. Death is often from pneumonia that sets in when the patient breathes bits of food.

Two types of abnormalities, called plaques and tangles, are present in the brains of Alzheimer's victims. **Plaques,** which appear on the outside of neurons, are clumps of an abnormal protein, called beta amyloid, mixed with dead branches of surrounding nerves. **Tangles** appear as insoluble clots of protein fibrils inside the nerve cells. It is not known whether these abnormalities cause the neuron destruction or if they are the result, or byproducts, of the devastation.

No one really knows what causes this assault on brain tissue. There is sketchy evidence that aluminum may have some role. Neurons with tangles appear to have from 10 to 50 times more aluminum than normal neurons. However, many researchers remain skeptical about aluminum because, even though it is toxic to cells, it does not cross the blood–brain barrier and the kidneys readily excrete it. There is considerable evidence, and researchers are quite certain, that defective genes have a dominant role in the development of the disease. A defective gene has been identified that codes for the beta amyloid protein. In normal brains, the protein does not exist, but it is present in many Alzheimer's disease patients. Another clue may be in the tangles present inside the nerve cells, but these are insoluble, which makes them difficult to analyze.

There is no proven effective treatment for Alzheimer's disease at present. The hope for the future, for the 21st century, is that teams of scientists, working together, will be able to unravel the biochemical mysteries of Alzheimer's disease. After that, research holds promise for a treatment and maybe a cure.

Representative Disorders of the Nervous System

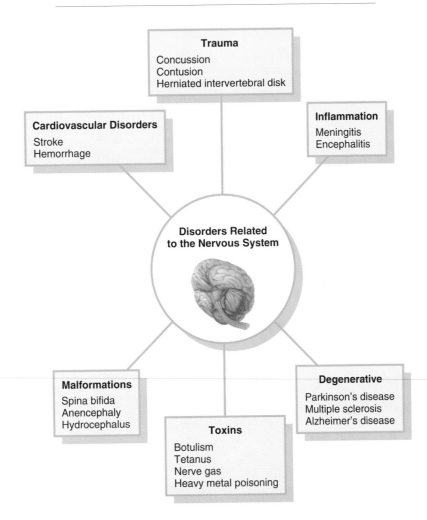

CHAPTER QUIZ

RECALL

Match the definitions on the left with the appropriate term on the right.

1. Outermost covering of the CNS

2. Produces cerebrospinal fluid

3. Occurs along myelinated axons

4. Supporting cells of the nervous system

5. White, fatty covering of axons

6. Controls contraction of skeletal muscles

7. Lowest part of the brain stem

8. Contains visual cortex

9. Efferent process of a neuron

10. Contains somatosensory cortex

A. Axon

B. Choroid plexus

C. Dura mater

D. Medulla oblongata

E. Myelin

F. Neuroglia

G. Occipital lobe

H. Parietal lobe

I. Saltatory conduction

J. Somatic nervous system

THOUGHT

1. Neurons located entirely within the CNS are

   a. motor neurons

   b. association neurons

   c. efferent neurons

   d. sensory neurons

2. Selected events in impulse conduction are given. Arrange these events in the order in which they occur: 1) sodium gates open; 2) potassium gates open; 3) stimulus alters membrane permeability; 4) active transport of sodium and potassium; 5) reverse polarization.

   a. 3, 1, 2, 4, 5

   b. 3, 1, 5, 4, 2

   c. 3, 4, 1, 5, 2

   d. 3, 1, 5, 2, 4

3. White matter

   a. forms the cerebral cortex

   b. consists of neuron cell bodies

   c. forms the outer covering of the brain

   d. consists of myelinated fibers

4. The three regions of the brain stem are the

   a. thalamus, hypothalamus, pineal body

   b. thalamus, pons, cerebellum

   c. midbrain, pons, medulla oblongata

   d. thalamus, midbrain, cerebral peduncles

5. Three cranial nerves that have only sensory functions are

   a. optic, olfactory, and trigeminal

   b. optic, olfactory, and vestibulocochlear

   c. optic, oculomotor, and glossopharyngeal

   d. vagus, trigeminal, and facial

APPLICATION

A medical student is practicing technique on an anesthetized animal and accidentally severs the left phrenic nerve. What effect will this have on the animal?

Which cranial nerve conveys pain impulses to the brain:

a) when you bite the tip of your tongue?

b) when a piece of dirt blows into your eye?

c) when you have a toothache from an upper molar?

CHAPTER 9

Sensory System

Outline/Objectives

Receptors and Sensations 184
- Distinguish between general senses and special senses.
- Classify sense receptors into five groups.

General Senses 185
- Describe the sense receptors for touch, pressure, proprioception, temperature, and pain.

Gustatory Sense 186
- Locate the four different taste sensations and follow the impulse pathway from stimulus to the cerebral cortex.

Olfactory Sense 187
- Locate the sense receptors for smell and trace the impulse pathway to the cerebral cortex.

Visual Sense 188
- Describe the structure of the eye and the significance of each component.
- Explain how light focuses on the retina.
- Identify the photoreceptor cells in the retina, describe the mechanism by which nerve impulses are triggered in response to light, and trace the impulse to the visual cortex.

Auditory Sense 194
- Describe the structure of the ear and the contribution each region makes to the sense of hearing.

- Summarize the sequence of events in the initiation of auditory impulses and trace these impulses to the auditory cortex.

Sense of Equilibrium 197
- Identify and describe the structure of the components of the ear involved in static equilibrium and those involved in dynamic equilibrium.
- Summarize the events in the initiation of impulses for static equilibrium and for dynamic equilibrium and identify the cranial nerve that transmits these impulses to the cerebral cortex.

Key Terms

Accommodation

Chemoreceptor

Mechanoreceptor

Nociceptor

Photoreceptor

Proprioception

Sensory adaptation

Thermoreceptor

Building Vocabulary

WORD PART	MEANING
audi-	to hear
coch-	snail
fove-	pit
gust-	taste
irid-	iris
kerat-	cornea
lacr-	tears
lith-	stone
lute-	yellow
macul-	spot
meat-	passage
ocul-	eye
olfact-	smell
op-	eye
ophthalm-	eye
ot-	ear
presby-	old
scler-	hard
tympan-	drum
vitre-	glass

Sense perception depends on sensory receptors that respond to various stimuli. When a stimulus triggers an impulse in a receptor, the action potentials travel to the cerebral cortex, where they are processed and interpreted. Only after this occurs is a particular sensation perceived. Some senses, such as pain, touch, pressure, and proprioception, are widely distributed in the body. These are called **general senses.** Other senses, such as taste, smell, hearing, and sight, are called **special senses** because their receptors are localized in a particular area.

> Receptors for the general senses are widely distributed in the body. Receptors for the special senses are localized.

Receptors and Sensations

Although there are many different kinds of sense receptors, they can be grouped into five types. The basis for these receptor types is the kind of stimulus to which they are sensitive or have a low threshold. The five types of receptors are **chemoreceptors, mechanoreceptors, nociceptors, thermoreceptors,** and **photoreceptors** (Table 9–1).

Perceived sensation occurs only after impulses are interpreted by the brain. Steps involved in sensory perception include the following:

1. There must be a **stimulus.**

2. A **receptor** must detect the stimulus and create an action potential.

3. The action potential (impulse) must be **conducted** to the central nervous system (CNS).

4. Within the CNS, the impulse must be **translated** into information.

5. Information must be **interpreted** in the CNS into an awareness or perception of the stimulus.

The impulses from all the receptors are alike. The difference in perception is where they are interpreted in the brain. For example, all impulses going to one particular region are interpreted as sound, whereas those going to another region are interpreted as taste. As the brain interprets a sensation, it projects that sense back to its original source so that the "feeling" seems to come from the receptors that are stimulated. This projection allows us to locate the source of the stimulus.

> The way in which a particular sensation is perceived depends on where it is interpreted in the brain.

Some sense receptors, when they are continually stimulated, undergo **sensory adaptation.** They have a decreased sensitivity to a continued stimulus and trigger impulses only if the strength of the stimulus is increased.

> Some sense receptors undergo sensory adaptation when they are continually stimulated.

CLINICAL TERMS

Astigmatism (ah-STIG-mah-tizm) Defective curvature of the cornea or lens of the eye resulting in a distorted image on the retina

Audiometry (aw-dee-AHM-eh-tree) Hearing test

Blepharitis (bleff-ahr-EYE-tis) Inflammation of the edges of the eyelid

Diplopia (dip-LOH-pee-ah) Double vision

Emmetropia (emm-eh-TROH-pee-ah) Normal or perfect vision

Hyperopia (hye-per-OH-pee-ah) A defect in vision in which light rays focus beyond the retina; farsightedness

Myopia (my-OH-pee-ah) A defect in vision in which light rays focus in front of the retina; nearsightedness

Nyctalopia (nick-tah-LOH-pee-ah) A condition in which the individual has difficulty seeing at night; night blindness

Otalgia (oh-TAL-jee-ah) Earache

Otosclerosis (oh-toe-sklee-ROH-sis) Progressive formation of bony tissue around the oval window, immobilizing the stapes; results in conduction deafness

Otoscopy (oh-TAHS-koh-pee) Visual examination of the external auditory canal and the tympanic membrane using an otoscope

Presbycusis (prez-bih-KUS-is) Impairment of hearing due to aging

Presbyopia (prez-bih-OH-pee-ah) Impairment of vision due to aging

Snellen chart (SNELL-en chart) A chart, printed with lines of black letters that are graduated in size from smallest on the bottom to largest on the top, used for testing visual acuity

Tinnitus (tin-EYE-tus) A ringing or buzzing sound in the ears

Tonometry (toh-NAHM-eh-tree) Measurement of the tension or pressure within the eye, which is useful in detecting glaucoma

Tympanitis (tim-pan-EYE-tis) Inflammation of the tympanic membrane

Vertigo (VER-tih-goh) A feeling of dizziness and lightheadedness caused by a disturbance of the semicircular canals, utricle, saccule, or vestibular nerve

Table 9–1	Types of Sense Receptors	
Receptor	**Stimulus**	**Example**
Chemoreceptors	Changes in chemical concentration of substances	Taste and smell
Mechanoreceptors	Changes in pressure or movement in fluids	Proprioceptors in joints, receptors for hearing and equilibrium
Nociceptors	Tissue damage	Pain receptors
Thermoreceptors	Changes in temperature	Heat and cold
Photoreceptors	Light energy	Vision

Nearly everyone is familiar with sensory adaptation in the sense of smell. A particular odor becomes unnoticed after a short time even though the odor molecules are still present in the air because the system quickly adapts to the continued stimulation.

General Senses

General senses, or **somatic senses,** are those that are found throughout the body. They are associated with the visceral organs as well as the skin, muscles, and joints and include the following:

- Touch
- Pressure
- Proprioception
- Temperature
- Pain

Touch and Pressure

As a group, the receptors for touch and pressure are mechanoreceptors that are sensitive to forces that deform or displace tissues. They are widely distrib- uted in the skin. Three of the receptors involved in touch and pressure are **free nerve endings, Meissner's corpuscles** (MYZE-ners KOAR-pus-als), and **pacinian (lamellated) corpuscles** (pah-SIN-ee-an KOAR-pus-als) (Fig. 9–1).

Free nerve endings are the dendritic ends of sensory neurons that are interspersed between the cells in epithelial tissue. They do not have a connective tissue covering. They are important in sensing objects, such as clothing, that are in continuous contact with the skin. Meissner's corpuscles consist of the ends of sensory nerve fibers surrounded by connective tissue and are very specific in localizing tactile sensations. They are located in the dermal papillae, just beneath the epidermis, where they are important in sensing light discriminative touch stimuli. Pacinian corpuscles are called lamellated corpuscles because several layers of connective tissue surround the nerve endings. These are common in deeper dermis and subcutaneous tissues, tendons, and ligaments. They are stimulated by heavy pressure.

> Mechanoreceptors that are sensitive to touch and pressure include free nerve endings, Meissner's corpuscles, and pacinian corpuscles.

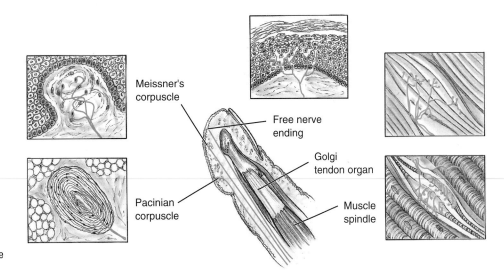

Meissner's corpuscle

Free nerve ending

Golgi tendon organ

Pacinian corpuscle

Muscle spindle

Figure 9–1 General sense receptors.

Proprioception

Proprioception (proh-pree-oh-SEP-shun) is the sense of position or orientation. It allows us to sense the location and rate of movement of one body part relative to another. **Golgi tendon organs,** found at the junction of a tendon with a muscle, and **muscle spindles**, located in skeletal muscles, are important mechanoreceptors for proprioception. They are illustrated in Figure 9–1.

| Golgi tendon organs and muscle spindles function in sensing the orientation of one body part to another.

Temperature

Thermoreceptors are located immediately under the skin and are widely distributed throughout the body. They are most numerous on the lips and are least numerous on some of the broad surfaces of the trunk. Thermoreceptors include at least two types of free nerve endings that are sensitive to temperature changes. In general, there are up to 10 times more **cold receptors** in a given area than **heat receptors.** Extremes in temperature stimulate pain receptors. Below 10°C, pain receptors produce a freezing sensation. As the temperature increases above 10°C, pain impulses cease but **cold receptors** begin to be stimulated. At temperatures about 25°C, **heat receptors** begin to be stimulated and cold receptors fade out. Finally, as temperatures approach 45°C, heat receptors fade out and pain receptors are stimulated to produce a burning sensation. A person determines gradations in temperatures by the degree of stimulation of each type of receptor. Extreme cold and extreme heat feel almost the same—both are painful—because the pain receptors are being stimulated. Thermoreceptors are strongly stimulated by abrupt changes in temperature and then fade after a few seconds or minutes. In other words, thermoreceptors show rapid **sensory adaptation.**

| Temperature changes are detected by thermoreceptors that are free nerve endings. They show sensory adaptation.

When a person first enters a cool swimming pool on a hot day, there is an abrupt change in temperature; therefore, the cold receptors are strongly stimulated and there is a feeling of discomfort. After a brief time, the receptors adapt, the stimulation fades, and the cool water feels comfortable.

Pain

The sense of pain is initiated by **nociceptors** (noh-see-SEP-tors), which are free nerve endings that are stimulated by tissue damage. They are widely distributed throughout the skin and in the tissues of the internal organs. There are no pain receptors in the nervous tissue of the brain; however, other tissues in the head, including the meninges and blood vessels, have an abundant supply. Pain receptors have a protective function because pain is usually perceived as unpleasant and is a signal to locate and to remove the source of the tissue damage. Nociceptors usually do not adapt and may continue to send signals after the stimulus is removed.

| Tissue damage stimulates free nerve endings called nociceptors to initiate the sensation of pain.

✓ QuickCheck

● Why is taste considered a special sense and temperature a general sense?

● What are the most sensitive receptors for touch and where are they located?

If there are no pain receptors in the nervous tissue of the brain, what are headaches? Headaches are a type of referred pain, pain that is referred to the surface of the head from deeper structures. The pain stimuli may originate in the meninges or blood vessels within the cranium. Other pain stimuli may originate outside the cranium from muscular spasms, the nasal sinuses, or the eyes.

Gustatory Sense

The **gustatory sense**, or **taste**, is one of the special senses. The organs of taste, the **taste buds**, are localized in the mouth region, primarily on the surface of the tongue, where they lie along the walls of projections called **papillae** (Fig. 9–2). The receptors belong to the **chemoreceptor** (kee-moh-ree-Sep-tor) category because they are sensitive to chemicals in the food we eat. In order for these chemicals to be detected by a chemoreceptor, they must be dissolved in water.

Within the taste bud, specialized epithelial cells called **taste cells** or **gustatory cells** are interspersed with supporting cells and nerve fibers (Fig. 9–2). The entire taste bud opens to the surface through a **taste pore.** Tiny **taste hairs** (microvilli) project from the taste cells through the taste pore, and it is these hairs on the taste cells that function as the receptors.

| The receptors for taste are taste hairs that project from the taste buds on the surface of the tongue.

Although all the taste receptors appear to be alike, there are at least four different types, each one sensitive to a particular kind of stimulus. Consequently, there are four different taste sensations:

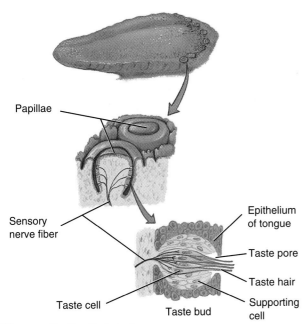

Papillae

Sensory
nerve fiber

Epithelium
of tongue

Taste pore

Taste hair

Supporting
cell

Taste cell

Taste bud

Figure 9-2 Taste buds.

Olfactory Sense

The receptors for **olfaction** (sense of smell) are bipolar neurons surrounded by supporting columnar epithelial cells in the **olfactory epithelium** of the nasal cavity (Fig. 9–4). The **olfactory neurons** are concentrated in the superior region of the cavity. The olfactory neurons have long cilia that extend to the surface and project into the nasal cavity. The cilia are believed to be the sensitive receptors of the neuron.

Like those for taste, the olfactory receptors are **chemoreceptors.** They are stimulated by chemicals dissolved in liquids. In this case, airborne molecules responsible for odors dissolve in the fluid on the surface of the olfactory epithelium and then bind to the receptors and trigger impulses.

> The sense of smell is called olfaction. The receptors for the sense of smell are chemoreceptors and are located in the olfactory epithelium of the nasal cavity.

Axons from the olfactory neurons pass through foramina in the cribriform plate of the ethmoid bone and enter the **olfactory bulb.** Here they synapse with association neurons that conduct the impulses through the **olfactory tract** to the brain. The olfactory tracts terminate in the **olfactory cortex** in the temporal lobe.

The senses of taste and smell are closely related and complement each other. They often have a combined effect when they are interpreted in the cere-

• Salty
• Sweet
• Sour
• Bitter

Instead of being evenly distributed over the surface of the tongue, each one of the four tastes is concentrated in a specific region, as illustrated in Figure 9–3.

When the microvilli, or taste hairs, are stimulated, an impulse is triggered on a nearby nerve fiber. Impulses from the anterior two thirds of the tongue travel along the **facial nerve,** and those from the posterior one third travel along the **glossopharyngeal** (glos-so-fah-RIN-jee-al) **nerve** to the medulla oblongata (see Table 8–8). From the medulla oblongata they travel to the thalamus, then to the sensory cortex on the parietal lobe, near the lateral sulcus.

> Salty, sweet, sour, and bitter are the four different taste sensations. Impulses for taste are conducted along the facial nerve or the glossopharyngeal nerve and are interpreted in the sensory cortex of the parietal lobe.

The taste receptors with the highest degree of sensitivity are those that are stimulated by bitter substances, and a highly intense bitter taste usually causes a person to reject that substance. This is probably an important protective mechanism because many of the deadly toxins found in poisonous plants have an intensely bitter taste.

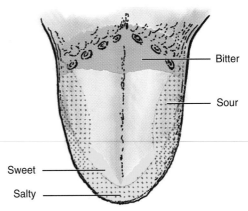

Bitter

Sour

Sweet

Salty

Figure 9-3 Regions of the tongue sensitive to various tastes.

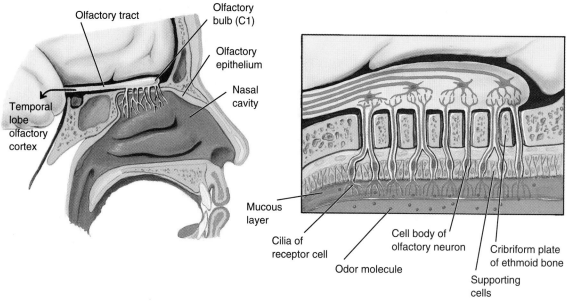

Figure 9-4 Structure of the olfactory receptors.

bral cortex. This implies that part of what we "taste" is really smell. Also, part of what we "smell" is taste because some airborne molecules move from the nose down to the mouth and stimulate taste buds.

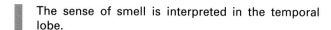

| The sense of smell is interpreted in the temporal lobe.

✓ QuickCheck

● Damage to the facial and/or glossopharyngeal nerves will interfere with which special sense?

● What two special senses are detected by chemoreceptors?

> Odors have the quality of being interpreted as pleasant or unpleasant. Because of this the sense of smell is as important as taste in the selection of food. For example, a person who has became sick after eating a certain type of food is often nauseated by the smell of that same food at a later occasion.

Visual Sense

Most of us consider vision to be one of the most important senses we have. The eyes, which contain the photoreceptors, are the organs of vision. They are protected by a bony socket and are assisted in their function of vision by accessory structures that protect and move them.

Protective Features and Accessory Structures of the Eye

Only a small portion of the eye is visible from the exterior. Most of it is surrounded by a protective bony **orbit,** or socket, formed by portions of seven cranial bones: frontal, lacrimal, ethmoid, maxilla, zygomatic, sphenoid, and palatine. It also contains fat, various connective tissues, blood vessels, and nerves.

| The socket for the eye is formed by the frontal, lacrimal, ethmoid, maxilla, zygomatic, sphenoid, and palatine bones.

Eyebrows help to keep perspiration, which can be an irritant, out of the eyes. **Eyelids** function to open and close the eye and to keep foreign objects from entering the eye. The eyelids are composed of skin, connective tissue, muscle, and **conjunctiva** (kon-junk-TYE-vah). The muscles associated with the eyelids are the **orbicularis oculi,** which is a sphincter that closes the eye, and the **levator palpebrae superioris,** which elevates the eyelid to open the eye. The conjunctiva, a thin mucous membrane, lines the eyelid and then folds back to cover the anterior portion of the eyeball, except for the central portion, which is the cornea. Mucus from the conjunctiva helps keep the eye from drying out. **Eyelashes** line the margin of the eyelid and help trap foreign particles. **Sebaceous glands** associated with the eyelashes secrete an oily fluid that helps lubricate the region. Inflammation of the sebaceous glands is called a **stye.**

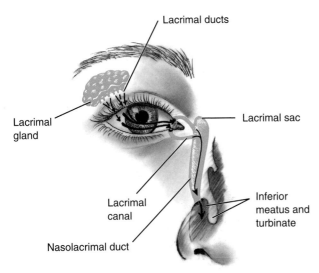

Lacrimal ducts

Lacrimal gland

Lacrimal sac

Lacrimal canal

Inferior meatus and turbine

Nasolacrimal duct

Figure 9-5 Lacrimal apparatus of the eye. (From Jarvis C: Physical Examination and Health Assessment. Philadelphia, WB Saunders, 1992.)

Conjunctivitis is an inflammation of the conjunctiva. This may be due to irritation, allergies, or bacterial infections. One example, caused by bacteria is acute contagious conjunctivitis, or pinkeye.

The **lacrimal** (LACK-rih-mal) **apparatus,** shown in Figure 9–5, consists of the lacrimal gland and vari-

ous ducts. The **lacrimal gland** is located in the superior and lateral region of the orbit. Tears produced by the lacrimal gland flow through **lacrimal ducts** and across the surface of the eye to the medial side, where they drain into two small **lacrimal canals** (canaliculi). From the lacrimal canals, the tears flow into the **lacrimal sac,** then into the **nasolacrimal duct,** which opens into the nasal cavity. Tears moisten, lubricate, and cleanse the anterior surface of the eye. They also contain an enzyme (lysozyme) that helps destroy bacteria and prevent infections.

Tears are produced by the lacrimal apparatus. Tears moisten and cleanse the eye and help destroy bacteria that may cause eye infections.

The eye blinks 6 to 30 times a minute. Blinking stimulates the lacrimal glands to secrete a sterile fluid, or "tears," and helps move the fluid across the eyes.

There are six muscles associated with movements of the eyeball. These muscles all originate from the bones of the orbit and insert on the tough outer layer of the eyeball. The six extrinsic eye muscles are listed in Table 9–2 along with their nerve supply and actions.

Table 9-2 Muscles of the Eye

Muscle	Controlling Nerve	Function
Extrinsic (Skeletal) Muscles		
Superior rectus	Oculomotor (III)	Elevates eye or rolls it superiorly and toward the midline
Inferior rectus	Oculomotor (III)	Depresses eye or rolls it inferiorly and toward the midline
Medial rectus	Oculomotor (III)	Moves eye medially, toward the midline
Lateral rectus	Abducens (VI)	Moves eye laterally, away from the midline
Superior oblique	Trochlear (IV)	Depresses eye and turns it laterally, away from the midline
Inferior oblique	Oculomotor (III)	Elevates eye and turns it laterally, away from the midline
Intrinsic (Smooth) Muscles		
Ciliary	Oculomotor (III) Parasympathetic fibers	Causes suspensory ligament to relax, lens becomes more convex for close vision
Iris, circular muscles	Oculomotor (III) Parasympathetic fibers	Decreases the size of the pupil to allow less light to enter the eye
Iris, radial muscles	Sympathetic fibers from spinal nerves	Increases the size of the pupil to allow more light to enter the eye

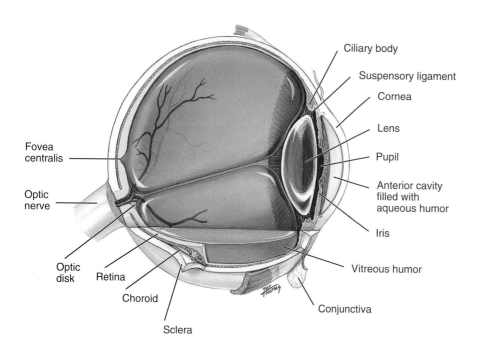

Fovea
centralis

Optic
nerve

Optic
disk

Retina

Choroid

Sclera

Ciliary body

Suspensory ligament

Cornea

Lens

Pupil

Anterior cavity
filled with
aqueous humor

Iris

Vitreous humor

Conjunctiva

Figure 9-6 Anatomy of the eye.

Structure of the Eyeball

The eyeball, or **bulbus oculi** (BUL-bus AHK-yoo-lye), is somewhat spherical, is 2 to 3 centimeters in diameter, and has an anterior bulge. It is surrounded by orbital fat within the orbital cavity. Figure 9–6 illustrates the structure of the bulbus oculi.

The wall of the eyeball is made up of three concentric coats or tunics. The outermost layer is the **fibrous tunic.** It consists of the white opaque **sclera** (SKLEE-rah) and the transparent **cornea.** The sclera, the white part of the eye, covers the posterior five sixths of the eyeball, and the muscles that move the eye are attached to it. The transparent cornea, which covers the anterior one sixth of the eyeball, is the "window" of the eye. It helps focus light rays entering the eye.

> The sclera and cornea are parts of the fibrous tunic of the eye.

The cornea was one of the first organs transplanted. Surgical removal of deteriorating corneas and replacement with donor corneas is a common medical procedure for several reasons. The cornea is readily accessible and relatively easy to remove. The tissue is avascular, so there is no bleeding problem or difficulty in establishing circulatory pathways. Corneas are less active than other tissues immunologically and are less likely to be rejected. Long-term success after corneal implant surgery is excellent.

The middle layer of the eyeball is the **vascular tunic.** It consists of the **choroid** (KOAR-oyd), **ciliary body,** and **iris.** The **choroid** is a highly vascular, brown pigmented layer located between the sclera and the retina in the posterior portion of the eye. It is the largest part of the middle tunic and lines most of the sclera, although it is only loosely connected to the fibrous coat and can be stripped away easily. The choroid is, however, firmly attached to the retina. The brown pigment in the choroid absorbs excess light rays that might interfere with vision. The blood vessels nourish the interior of the eye. Anteriorly, the choroid is continuous with the **ciliary body.** Numerous fingerlike **ciliary processes** within the ciliary body secrete aqueous humor, a fluid in the anterior portion of the eye. The ciliary body also contains **ciliary muscle. Suspensory ligaments** connect the ciliary body to the transparent, biconvex **lens** of the eye. When the ciliary muscle contracts, the suspensory ligaments relax, and the lens bulges to allow focusing for close vision. The **iris** is the conspicuous, colored portion of the eye. It is a doughnut-shaped diaphragm with a central aperture, called the **pupil.** The iris contains two groups of smooth muscles, a radial group and a circular group. When the radial muscles contract, the pupil dilates; when the circular group contracts, the pupil gets smaller. These muscles of the iris continually contract and relax to change the size of the pupil, which regulates the amount of light entering the eye.

> The vascular tunic includes the choroid, ciliary body, and iris. The choroid absorbs excess light rays; the ciliary body changes the shape of the lens; and the iris regulates the size of the pupil.

In addition to regulating the amount of light that enters the eye, pupillary reflexes may also reflect interest or emotional state. For example, frequently the pupils dilate during problem solving or when the subject is appealing. If the subject is boring or repulsive the pupils constrict.

The innermost coat of the eyeball is the **nervous tunic,** or **retina** (RET-ih-nah), which is found only in the posterior portion of the eye. It ends at the posterior margin of the ciliary body. The retina contains several layers. The outer layer is deeply pigmented and firmly attached to the choroid. The layer next to the pigmented layer contains the **rods and cones,** which are the receptor (photoreceptor) cells. Other layers consist of bipolar neurons and ganglion cells. The axons of the ganglion cells converge to form the **optic nerve,** which penetrates the tunics at the **optic disk** and passes through the apex of the orbital cavity to reach the brain. Because there are no receptor cells in the optic disk, it is commonly referred to as the "blind spot" of the eye. Just lateral to the optic disk, near the center of the retina, there is a yellow spot called the **macula lutea** (MACK-yoo-lah LOO-tee-ah). The region of the retina that produces the sharpest image is a depression, the **fovea centralis** (FOE-vee-ah sen-TRAL-is), in the center of the macula lutea.

> The retina is the innermost layer, the nervous tunic, of the eye. It contains the rods and cones, which are the receptor cells for vision.

The lens, suspensory ligaments, and ciliary body form a partition that divides the interior of the eyeball into two cavities. The space anterior to the lens, between the cornea and the lens, is the anterior cavity and is filled with **aqueous humor** secreted by the ciliary body. Aqueous humor helps maintain the shape of the anterior part of the eye and nourishes the structures in that region. It is largely responsible for the internal pressure of the eye. The aqueous humor circulates through the anterior cavity and then is reabsorbed into blood vessels at the junction of the sclera and cornea. The posterior cavity, between the lens and the retina, is filled with a colorless, transparent, gel-like **vitreous humor.** The vitreous humor presses the retina firmly against the wall of the eye, supports the internal parts of the eye, and helps maintain its shape.

Sometimes the sensory portion of the retina breaks away from the pigmented layer, resulting in a **detached retina.** This may be due to trauma, such as a blow to the head, or to certain eye disorders. If allowed to progress, the result is distorted vision and, eventually, blindness. In many cases, the retina can be reattached by laser surgery.

The space between the cornea and the lens, the anterior cavity of the eye, is filled with aqueous humor. The space posterior to the lens is the posterior cavity and is filled with vitreous humor.

Pathway of Light and Refraction

Vision depends on light rays. When a person sees an object, light rays from the object enter the eye. Light rays have two important properties—they travel in a straight line and they can be bent. When light rays travel from one substance to another that has a different optical density, the rays bend. The bending of light rays is called **refraction.** When light rays hit a concave surface, they scatter or diverge. When the rays meet a convex surface, they get closer together or converge. There are four refractive surfaces and media in the eyes. In a normal eye, the cornea, aqueous humor, lens, and vitreous humor bend the light rays so that they focus on the retina. The image that forms on the retina is upside down and backward (Fig. 9–7), but somehow the brain turns it around and interprets the image in the correct position.

> The cornea, aqueous humor, lens, and vitreous humor are refractive surfaces and media that bend light rays to focus on the retina.

Glaucoma is a disorder that involves an increase in intraocular pressure due to an accumulation of aqueous humor. This may be because there is a blockage in the canal of Schlemm so the aqueous humor doesn't drain out of the eye or it may be due to an overproduction of aqueous humor. If untreated, the increased pressure causes damage to the retina and optic nerve.

When an object is at least 20 feet away, the normal relaxed eye is able to focus the image on the retina. When the object is closer than 20 feet, the eye must make adjustments to focus the image. These adjustments are called accommodation. The primary action in accommodation, illustrated in Figure 9–8, is changing the shape of the lens. For distance vision, the ciliary muscle is relaxed, the suspensory ligaments are taut, and the lens is flat. When the eyes accommodate for close vision, the ciliary mus-

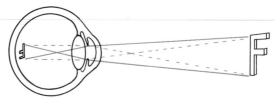

Figure 9-7 Formation of images on the retina.

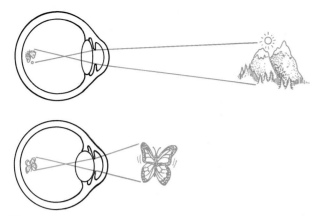

Figure 9–8 Accommodation.

cle contracts, the suspensory ligaments become loose or relaxed, and the lens bulges or becomes more convex. The closer the object, the more the light rays have to bend to focus and the greater the curvature of the lens.

> When the eyes accommodate for close vision, the lens becomes more convex so that light rays have sufficient refraction to focus on the retina.

Photoreceptors

The retina, illustrated in Figure 9–9, contains two kinds of photoreceptor cells: rods and cones. These cells are next to the outermost retina layer of pigmented epithelium. **Rods,** thin cells with slender rodlike projections, are sensitive to dim light. Even though rods are much more numerous than cones, they are absent in the fovea centralis and their number increases proportionately to the distance away from the fovea centralis. Many rods synapse with a single sensory fiber (convergence); thus, vision with rods lacks fine detail. **Cones,** the receptors for color vision and visual acuity, are located primarily in the fovea centralis. They are thicker cells with short, blunt projections. Cones exhibit less convergence than rods, so in addition to color, cones provide sharp images and fine detail. Table 9–3 compares the rods and cones.

> Rods are the photoreceptors for black and white vision and for vision in dim light. Cones are the photoreceptors for color vision and visual acuity.

Rods contain a substance, **rhodopsin** (roe-DOP-sin) (visual purple), that is very light sensitive. When even small amounts of light focus on the rods, rhodopsin breaks down into its component parts, opsin (a protein) and a derivative of vitamin A, retinal (retinene). This reaction triggers a nerve impulse. Rhodopsin is resynthesized from opsin and retinal to prepare the rods for receiving subsequent stimuli. The more rhodopsin there is in the rods, the greater the sensitivity to light. In bright light, nearly all the rhodopsin in the rods is decomposed. After entering a dimly lit area, it takes some time for the eyes to adapt to the dim light. During this period, rhodopsin is regenerated in the rods so that they become more sensitive.

> Rods contain rhodopsin, which breaks down into opsin and retinal when it is exposed to light. This reaction triggers a nerve impulse.

Cones function in a manner that is similar to rods. Light-sensitive pigments break down into component parts, and the reaction triggers nerve impulses. There are three different types of cones, each

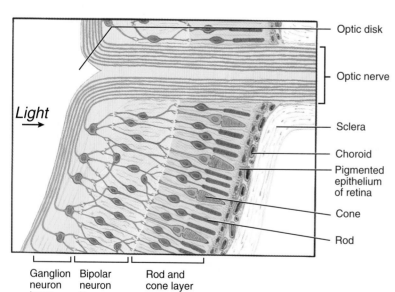

Light →

Optic disk

Optic nerve

Sclera

Choroid

Pigmented epithelium of retina

Cone

Rod

Ganglion neuron layer Bipolar neuron layer Rod and cone layer

Figure 9–9 Structure of the retina showing the rods and cones.

Table 9–3   Comparison of Rods and Cones

Feature	Rods	Cones
Shape	Long, slender projections	Short, thick projections
Location	None in fovea centralis; increase in density away from fovea centralis	Concentrated in fovea centralis; decrease in density away from fovea centralis
Quantity	More numerous than cones	Less numerous than rods
Convergence	High degree of convergence	Less convergence
Pigments	Single pigment—rhodopsin	Three pigments—one each for red, green, blue
Functions	Black and white vision; dim light; night vision; lacks detail	Color vision; bright light; precise vision with fine detail

with a different visual pigment. All the pigments contain retinal, but the protein portion is different. One type responds best to green light, another responds best to blue light, and a third type responds best to red light. The perceived color of an object depends on the quantity and combination of cones that are stimulated. If all the pigments are stimulated, the person senses white. If none are stimulated, the person senses black.

> There are three types of cones. One is sensitive to green light, one is sensitive to blue light, and one responds to red light. The way they function is similar to rods.

Color blindness occurs because there is an absence or deficiency of one or more of the visual pigments in the cones, and the person cannot distinguish certain colors. In the most common form, red-green color blindness, the cones lack the red pigment and the person is unable to distinguish red from green. Most color blindness is inherited and occurs more frequently in males.

Visual Pathway

Visual impulses generated in the rods and cones of the retina leave the eyes in the axons that form the **optic nerves.** Just anterior to the pituitary gland, these nerves form an X-shaped structure, the **optic chiasma** (OP-tik kye-AZ-mah). Within the optic chiasma, the axons from the medial portion of each retina cross over to enter the **optic tract** on the opposite side (Fig. 9–10). The right optic tract contains the fibers from the lateral portion of the right eye and the medial portion of the left eye. The left optic tract contains the fibers from the lateral portion of the left eye and the medial portion of the right eye. The optic tracts lead to the **thalamus.** Just before they reach the thalamus, a few fibers leave the tracts and enter the nuclei that function in visual reflexes

(superior colliculi). Most of the fibers enter the thalamus, where they synapse with neurons that carry the impulses in the **optic radiations** to the visual cortex of the occipital lobes. Because some of the fibers cross over to the other side in the optic chiasma, each occipital lobe receives an image of the entire object from each eye but from slightly different perspectives. This enables vision in three dimensions.

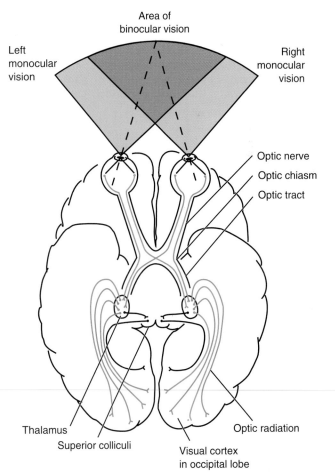

Figure 9–10   Visual pathway.

The visual pathway begins with impulses that are triggered by the rods and cones and ends with interpretation in the visual cortex of the occipital lobe.

☑ **Quick**Check

- Why is it important that images of objects being examined for fine detail fall on the fovea centralis?

- Why is the optic disk called the blind spot?

- What structure in the eye accommodates for close vision by adjusting the amount of refraction?

Auditory Sense

The **ear** is the organ of hearing (auditory or acoustic organ). It is also the organ for the sense of equilibrium, which is covered later in this chapter. The receptors for hearing, located within the ear, are **mechanoreceptors** (mek-ah-noh-ree-SEP-tors). Physical forces, in the form of sound vibrations, are responsible for initiating impulses that are interpreted as sound.

The receptors for hearing are mechanoreceptors.

Structure of the Ear

The "ears" on the sides of the head are only a portion of the actual organ of hearing. A large part of the organ, actually the most important part, lies hidden from view in the temporal bone. Anatomically,

the organ of hearing is divided into the external ear, middle ear, and inner ear. The anatomy of the ear is illustrated in Figure 9–11.

External Ear

The **external ear** consists of an auricle, or pinna, and the external auditory meatus (canal). The **auricle,** or pinna, is the fleshy part of the external ear that is visible on the side of the head and surrounds the opening into the external auditory meatus. The auricle collects sound waves and directs them toward the auditory meatus.

The **external auditory meatus** is an S-shaped tube, about 2.5 cm long, that extends from the auricle to the **tympanic membrane.** The skin that lines the meatus has numerous hairs and **ceruminous glands,** which secrete a waxy substance called **cerumen.** The hairs and cerumen help prevent foreign objects from reaching the eardrum. The external ear ends at the tympanic membrane.

The external ear, which includes the auricle and external auditory meatus, ends at the tympanic membrane.

Surprisingly, a branch of the facial nerve passes along the inner surface of the tympanic membrane. This nerve has nothing to do with hearing but rather carries taste impulses from the tongue. The nerve may be damaged by middle ear infection or during ear surgery.

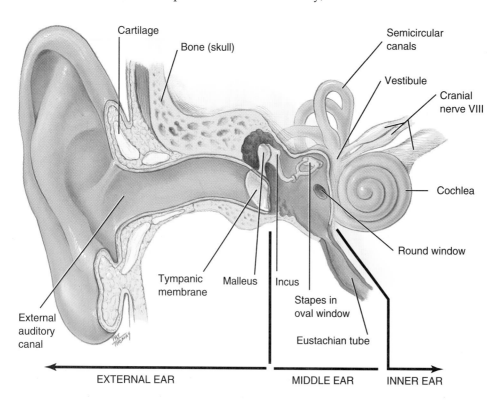

Cartilage

Bone (skull)

Semicircular canals

Vestibule

Cranial nerve VIII

Cochlea

Round window

Tympanic membrane

Malleus

Incus

Stapes in oval window

Eustachian tube

External auditory canal

EXTERNAL EAR

MIDDLE EAR

INNER EAR

Figure 9–11 Anatomy of the ear. (From Jarvis C: Physical Examination and Health Assessment. Philadelphia, WB Saunders, 1992.)

Middle Ear

The **middle ear** is an air-filled cavity, called the **tympanic cavity,** in the temporal bone. It begins at the tympanic membrane, contains the auditory ossicles, and has an opening into the eustachian tube. The **oval window** and the **round window** in the medial wall of the middle ear connect the middle ear with the inner ear. The oval window is closed by the stapes, one of the bones in the middle ear. The round window is closed by a membrane.

The **tympanic membrane,** or eardrum, is a thin membrane that separates the external ear from the middle ear. Sound waves cause the tympanic membrane to vibrate.

> The eardrum is sometimes ruptured, or perforated, by shock waves from an explosion, scuba diving, trauma, or acute middle ear infections. A perforated eardrum is characterized first by acute pain, then by noise in the affected ear, and then by hearing impairment.

An **auditory tube** (eustachian tube) connects each middle ear with the throat. Its purpose is to equalize the pressure between the outside air and the middle ear cavity, a condition necessary for normal hearing. Throat infections may spread to the middle ear through the auditory tube.

> **Otitis media,** infection of the middle ear, occurs frequently in children. The infection usually starts in the throat, then spreads through the auditory tube into the middle ear.

The **auditory ossicles** are three tiny bones: the **malleus** (hammer), **incus** (anvil), and **stapes** (stirrup). These bones are linked together by tiny ligaments and form a bridge across the space of the tympanic cavity. The malleus is attached to the tympanic membrane, and the stapes is attached to the oval window between the middle ear and the inner ear. The incus is between the malleus and stapes. When the tympanic membrane vibrates, the ossicles transmit the vibrations across the cavity to the oval window, which transfers the motion to the fluids in the inner ear. This fluid motion excites the receptors for hearing.

> The middle ear contains the malleus, incus, and stapes, which transmit sound vibrations from the tympanic membrane to the oval window.

Inner Ear

The **inner ear** consists of a bony labyrinth and a membranous labyrinth (Fig. 9–12). The **bony** (osseous) **labyrinth** is a series of interconnecting chambers in the temporal bone. The **membranous laby-**

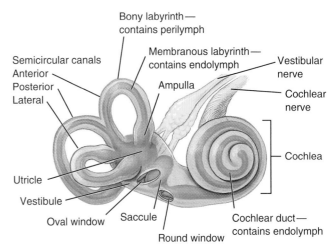

Figure 9–12 Labyrinths of the inner ear.

rinth, located inside the bony labyrinth, is a system of membranous tubes that are similar to the bony labyrinth in shape but smaller. A clear fluid called **endolymph** fills the membranous labyrinth. The space between the bony and the membranous labyrinths contains a fluid called **perilymph.** The inner ear is divided into the vestibule, semicircular canals, and cochlea. The vestibule and semicircular canals function in the sense of equilibrium. The cochlea functions in the sense of hearing.

> The inner ear consists of a bony labyrinth that surrounds a membranous labyrinth. It includes the vestibule, semicircular canals, and cochlea.

The **cochlea** (KOK-lee-ah) is the coiled portion of the bony labyrinth. The **cochlear duct** is the membranous labyrinth inside the bony labyrinth. Figure 9–13 shows that the inside of the cochlea is divided into three regions by the **vestibular membrane** and the **basilar membrane.** The region above the vestibular membrane is the **scala vestibuli** (SKAY-lah ves-TIB-yoo-lee), which contains perilymph. It extends from the oval window to the apex of the cochlea. The region below the basilar membrane is the **scala tympani** (SKAY-lah TIM-pah-nee), which extends from the apex of the cochlea to the round window. It is continuous with the scala vestibuli at the apex and also contains perilymph. The basilar membrane contains thousands of stiff fibers that gradually increase in length from the base to the apex. The arrangement is similar to the reeds in a harmonica or the bars on a marimba. The fibers vibrate when activated by sound. The middle region of the cochlea, between the scala vestibuli and the scala tympani, is the cochlear duct, which ends as a closed sac at the apex of the cochlea. The cochlear duct contains endolymph.

> The membranous labyrinth of the cochlea is the cochlear duct, which contains endolymph.

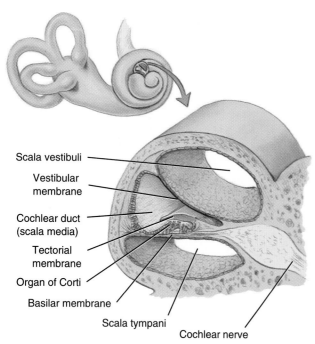

Scala vestibuli

Vestibular
membrane

Cochlear duct
(scala media)

Tectorial
membrane

Organ of Corti

Basilar membrane

Scala tympani

Cochlear nerve

Figure 9–13 Section through the cochlea.

The **organ of Corti** (KOAR-tee), which contains the receptors for sound, is located on the upper surface of the basilar membrane, within the cochlear duct (Fig. 9–14). It consists of supporting cells and **hair cells.** The hair cells are specialized sensory cells that have hairlike projections (microvilli) extending from their free surface. The tips of the projections contact a gelatinous **tectorial** (tek-TOE-ree-al) **membrane** that extends over them. Hair cells have no axons, but they are surrounded by sensory nerve fibers that form the **cochlear branch** of the **vestibulocochlear nerve** (cranial nerve VIII).

> The organ of Corti, located on the basilar membrane in the cochlear duct, contains the receptors for sound.

Physiology of Hearing

Sound travels through the atmosphere in waves of alternating compressions and decompressions of molecules. Low-pitched tones create low-frequency sound waves; high-pitched tones create high-frequency sound waves. Although the human ear can detect sound waves with frequencies ranging from 20 to 20,000 vibrations per second, hearing is most acute with frequencies between 2,000 and 3,000 vibrations per second.

Initiation of Impulses

The process of hearing begins when sound waves enter the external auditory meatus. As the waves travel through the external ear, they hit the tympanic membrane and cause it to vibrate. Because the malleus is attached to the membrane, the vibrations

are transferred from the tympanic membrane to the malleus, then to the incus, then to the stapes, which creates vibrations in the membrane of the oval window. Movement of the oval window passes the vibrations to the perilymph in the inner ear.

> **Otosclerosis** is an ear disorder in which spongy bone grows around the oval window and fuses with the stapes. This immobilizes the stapes and results in a form of conduction deafness.

Figure 9–15 illustrates an uncoiled cochlea to show the relationships of its components. The vibrations in the perilymph, caused by movement of the oval window, travel through the scala vestibuli, around the apex, and through the scala tympani to the round window. Thus, every time the stapes pushes the oval window inward toward the inner ear, movement in the perilymph pushes the round window outward toward the middle ear to relieve the pressure in the fluid. As vibrations travel through the perilymph, they create corresponding oscillations in the vestibular membrane, which causes movement of the endolymph within the scala media (cochlear duct), and finally the vibrations are transferred to the basilar membrane.

When the basilar membrane moves up and down, the organ of Corti moves with it and the hairs on the hair cells rub against the tectorial membrane. As the hairs contact the membrane, they bend, and this mechanical deformation initiates the nerve impulses that result in hearing. The list below summarizes the sequence of events in the initiation of auditory impulses.

1. The tympanic membrane vibrates in response to sound waves.

2. The malleus, incus, and stapes transfer vibrations to the oval window membrane.

3. Movement of the oval window membrane starts oscillations in the perilymph in the cochlea.

4. Oscillations in the perilymph cause vibrations in the vestibular and basilar membranes.

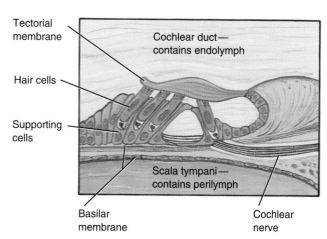

Tectorial membrane

Hair cells

Supporting cells

Cochlear duct— contains endolymph

Scala tympani— contains perilymph

Basilar membrane

Cochlear nerve

Figure 9–14 Organ of Corti.

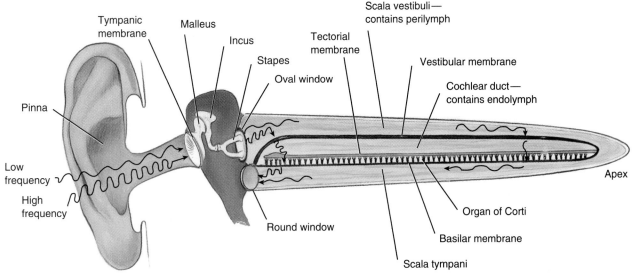

Figure 9-15 Uncoiled cochlea showing the pathway of pressure waves.

5. When the basilar membrane moves, the hairs on the hair cells in the organ of Corti rub against the tectorial membrane and bend.

6. Bending of the hairs on the hair cells stimulates the formation of impulses.

7. Impulses are transmitted to the auditory cortex of the temporal lobe on the cochlear branch of cranial nerve VIII, the vestibulocochlear nerve.

Pitch and Loudness

Hair cells along the length of the organ of Corti have varying sensitivities to different frequencies. Also, different regions of the basilar membrane vibrate in response to different frequencies. The portion of the membrane near the base of the cochlea vibrates in response to high frequencies. Near the apex of the cochlea, the basilar membrane responds to low frequencies. Pitch is detected by the portion of the basilar membrane that vibrates in response to the sound and the sensitivity of the hair cells.

Loudness is determined by the intensity of the sound waves. The basilar membrane vibrates more, i.e., has a greater magnitude of oscillation, in response to loud sounds. This means that more hair cells are stimulated and more impulses travel to the auditory cortex.

> The interpretation of pitch is mediated by the portion of the basilar membrane that vibrates in response to the sound. Loudness is interpreted by the number of hair cells that are stimulated.

Auditory Pathway

Auditory impulses leave the cochlea on the **cochlear nerve,** a branch of cranial nerve VIII, the **vestibulocochlear nerve.** The fibers synapse in the **medulla,** where some cross over to the opposite side, then continue to the inferior colliculi of the **midbrain** for auditory reflexes. Next the impulses are transmitted to the **thalamus,** where they synapse with neurons that transmit the impulses to the auditory cortex of the **temporal lobe.**

> Cranial nerve VIII transmits auditory impulses to the medulla oblongata. From there, the impulses travel to the thalamus and then to the auditory cortex of the temporal lobe.

Sense of Equilibrium

The sense of equilibrium is a combination of two different senses: the sense of **static equilibrium** and the sense of **dynamic equilibrium.** Static equilibrium is involved in evaluating the position of the head relative to gravity. It occurs when the head is motionless or moving in a straight line. Dynamic equilibrium occurs when the head is moving in a rotational or angular direction.

> Static equilibrium occurs when the head is motionless or moving in a straight line. Dynamic equilibrium is in response to rotational or angular movement.

Static Equilibrium

The organs of static equilibrium are located in the **vestibule** portion of the bony labyrinth of the inner ear. The membranous labyrinth inside the vestibule is divided into two saclike structures, the **utricle** (YOO-trih-kull) and the **saccule** (SACK-yool) (see Fig. 9-12). Each of these contains a small structure called a **macula** (MACK-yoo-lah), which is the organ of static equilibrium. The macula consists of sensory

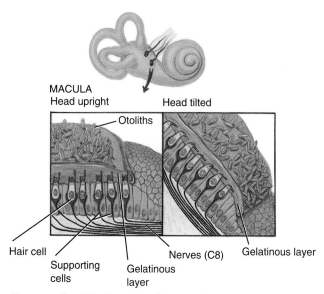

MACULA
Head upright   Head tilted

Otoliths

Hair cell
Supporting cells
Gelatinous layer
Nerves (C8)
Gelatinous layer

Figure 9–16   Structure of the macula.

hair cells, similar to those in the organ of Corti, and supporting cells (Fig. 9–16). The projections, or hairs, of the hair cells are embedded in a gelatinous mass that covers the macula. Grains of calcium carbonate, called **otoliths** (OH-toe-liths), are embedded on the surface of the gelatinous mass.

When the head is in an upright position, the hairs are straight. When the head tilts or bends forward, the otoliths and the gelatinous mass move in response to gravity. As the gelatinous mass moves, it bends some of the hairs on the receptor cells. This action initiates an impulse that travels to the CNS by way of the vestibular branch of the vestibulocochlear nerve. The CNS interprets the information and sends motor impulses out to appropriate muscles to maintain balance.

> The receptors for static equilibrium are in the membranous utricle and saccule, which are located in the bony vestibule of the inner ear. The vestibulocochlear nerve transmits the impulses to the cerebral cortex.

Dynamic Equilibrium

The sense organs for dynamic equilibrium, the equilibrium of rotational or angular movements, are located in the membranous labyrinth of the **semicircular canals.** There are three semicircular canals, positioned at right angle to each other, in three different planes (see Fig. 9–12). Each membranous canal is surrounded by perilymph and contains endolymph. At the base of each canal, near where it attaches to the utricle, there is a swelling called the **ampulla.** The sensory organs of the semicircular canals are located within the ampullae. Each of these

organs, called a **crista ampullaris** (KRIS-tah amp-yoo-LAIR-is), contains sensory hair cells and supporting cells (Fig. 9–17). The crista ampullaris is covered by a dome-shaped gelatinous mass called the **cupula** (KEW-pew-lah). The hairs of the hair cells are embedded in the cupula.

> The receptors for dynamic equilibrium are located in the crista ampullaris within the ampullae at the base of the semicircular canals.

When the head turns rapidly, the semicircular canals move with the head but the endolymph tends to remain stationary. The fluid pushes against the cupula, and it tilts to one side. As the cupula tilts, it bends some of the hairs on the hair cells, which triggers a sensory impulse. Because the three canals are in different planes, their cristae are stimulated differently by the same motion. This creates a mosaic of impulses that are transmitted to the CNS on the **vestibular branch** of the **vestibulocochlear nerve.** The CNS interprets the information and initiates appropriate responses to maintain balance. The cerebellum is particularly important in mediating the sense of balance and equilibrium.

> The vestibulocochlear nerve transmits the impulses for dynamic equilibrium from the receptors to the cerebral cortex.

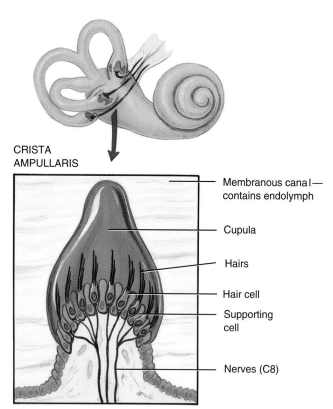

CRISTA AMPULLARIS

Membranous canal—contains endolymph

Cupula

Hairs

Hair cell

Supporting cell

Nerves (C8)

Figure 9–17   Structure of the crista ampullaris.

QuickCheck

- Anything that interferes with movement of the malleus, incus, and stapes impairs hearing. Why?

- Which portion of the cochlea is sensitive to high-frequency sounds?

- Identify two locations for the equilibrium receptors.

Motion sickness is nausea and vomiting due to repetitive and excessive stimulation of the equilibrium receptors. Some people are more susceptible than others.

 FOCUS ON AGING

There is a general decline in all of the special senses with age. The most significant changes in the eye occur in the lens. It tends to become thicker and less elastic, which makes it less able to change shape to accommodate for near vision. This condition, called **presbyopia** or farsightedness of aging, probably is the most common age-related dysfunction of the eye. The lens also tends to become cloudy or opaque, forming cataracts. About 90 percent of people older than age 70 have some degree of cataract formation; however, it is not always significant enough to affect vision. The cornea tends to become more translucent and less spherical, which contributes to an increase in astigmatism in older people. Older people require more light to see well because atrophy of the muscles in the iris reduces the ability of the pupil to dilate and decreases the amount of light that reaches the retina. The chemical processes that rebuild the visual pigment, rhodopsin, are slower in older people, so dark adaptation takes longer and is not as complete as in young people.

Most age-related changes in the external ear and middle ear have little effect on hearing. A buildup of cerumen, or earwax, in the external ear may contribute to hearing loss in the low-frequency range. The joints between the auditory ossicles in the middle ear may become less movable, which interferes with the transmission of sound waves to the inner ear, but generally it is not clinically significant. Most of the gradual loss of hearing that usually begins by the age of 40 is due to degeneration of the receptor cells in the spiral organ of Corti in the inner ear. Another factor is the decrease in the number of nerve fibers in the vestibulocochlear nerve. The reduction in fibers in the cochlear branch contributes to hearing loss. A decrease in vestibular fibers affects balance and equilibrium.

Taste and smell, both chemical senses, show a decline with age; however, the mechanism is unclear. Diminished perception may be due to degeneration of the receptor cells, to changes in the way the impulses are processed in the brain, or to other factors. It is likely that decreases in sensory perception are due to a combination of several factors.

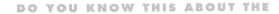

DO YOU KNOW THIS ABOUT THE

Special Senses?

To Hear or Not To Hear (Deafness)

The ability to hear sounds clearly and distinctly is taken for granted by many people with normal hearing. Little thought is given to things that might damage the ear. Many people try to protect their eyes with sunglasses, goggles, and the like, yet bombard their ears with noise levels that damage the hearing receptors. Hearing ability slowly, but steadily, declines beginning in early childhood. Several factors account for this normal process. The basilar membrane in the cochlea appears to lose some of its elasticity. Harmful calcium deposits form around the auditory ossi-

cles and oval window in the middle ear. Receptor hair cells and supporting cells in the spiral organ of Corti begin to degenerate. This hearing loss that occurs with aging, even in people living in a quiet environment, is called **presbycusis.**

Hearing loss varies from the inability to detect a specific pitch or intensity to a complete inability to detect any type of sound. Sensitivity to high-frequency tones usually disappears first. Words sound garbled because it is harder to hear consonants, which are higher pitched, than to hear vowels. The normal loss that occurs with

Continued on following page

aging is accelerated by exposure to high-intensity sounds because the hair cells in the spiral organ of Corti are easily damaged by them. Noise, or high-intensity sound, is stressful to the body. It causes constriction of blood vessels, high blood pressure, and increased heart rate. Vascular constriction reduces oxygen and nutrients to cells in the ear. As a result, the hair cells become disorganized and supporting cells degenerate.

Sound intensity is measured in units called decibels (dB). Each difference of 10 decibel units represents a doubling of the intensity. For example, a sound of 50 dB is twice as loud as a 40-dB sound. A library or water dripping from a faucet measures about 40 dB; normal conversation and the singing of birds measure about 60 dB. Because there is a difference of 2 increments of 10 dB (40 to 50 and 50 to 60), the singing birds are 4 times as loud as the dripping faucet. A jackhammer measures 100 dB, and a live rock band concert averages about 110 dB. Therefore, the live rock band concert has double the sound intensity of a jackhammer or 32 times the noise level of normal conversation.

The extent of ear damage from high-intensity sound depends on the length of exposure as well as on the intensity. For example, it is estimated that 16 hours of hearing a food blender in operation (90 dB) potentially produces some hearing loss. On the other hand, it takes only 2 hours of jackhammer noise or 26 minutes of a live rock band concert to produce an equivalent loss. Unfortunately, the deficiency often is not detected until the destruction is extensive, which is why U.S. employers must require their employees to wear ear protectors when occupational noise levels exceed 90 dB.

Deafness is classified as either conduction or sensorineural, according to its cause. **Conduction deafness** occurs when something interferes with the transmission of sound waves from the external ear to the fluids in the cochlea. For example, impacted earwax and foreign objects prevent the sound waves from reaching the tympanic membrane. A ruptured tympanic membrane keeps the vibrations from being transferred to the ossicles. Tumors may interfere with conduction in either the external ear or the middle ear. Temporary impairment often results from middle ear infections. When the ossicles fuse together or the stapes fuses in the oval window as a result of otosclerosis, the sound waves are not transmitted to the inner ear. Conduction deafness sometimes may be treated by removing the blockage. Surgery to mobilize the ossicles has some success. A hearing aid that transmits sound waves to the inner ear through the bones of the skull can make hearing almost normal in this type of deafness.

Sensorineural deafness results from damage along any part of the auditory pathway from the receptor cells in the cochlea to the auditory cortex of the cerebrum. This type of deafness, which may be partial or complete, typically results from a gradual loss of hearing throughout life. Tumors, cerebral damage along the pathway, and degenerative lesions of the nerves are other causes. Noise damage to the receptor cells in the cochlea is also in this category. Sensorineural deafness caused by age and noise-related damage to the cochlea may be helped by **cochlear implants,** or artificial ears. These are tiny electronic devices that convert sound waves into nerve impulses in the cochlear nerve. The sounds perceived in this way are crude compared with normal hearing, but many consider this sound better than nothing.

Representative Disorders of the Special Senses

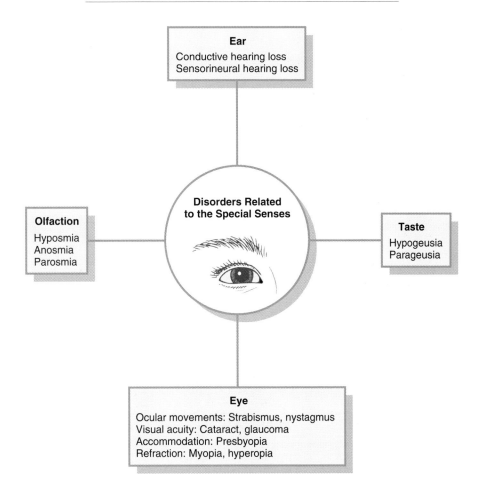

Ear
Conductive hearing loss
Sensorineural hearing loss

**Disorders Related
to the Special Senses**

Olfaction
Hyposmia
Anosmia
Parosmia

Taste
Hypogeusia
Parageusia

Eye
Ocular movements: Strabismus, nystagmus
Visual acuity: Cataract, glaucoma
Accommodation: Presbyopia
Refraction: Myopia, hyperopia

CHAPTER QUIZ

RECALL

Match the definitions on the left with the appropriate term on the right.

1. Sense of position or orientation

2. Free nerve endings for sense of pain

3. Gland that produces tears

4. Contains intrinsic eye muscles

5. Bending of light rays

6. Light-sensitive pigment

7. Ossicle adjacent to oval window

8. Contains auditory receptors

9. Sense organ for dynamic equilibrium

10. Fluid within membranous labyrinth

A. Cochlear duct

B. Crista ampullaris

C. Endolymph

D. Iris

E. Lacrimal

F. Nociceptor

G. Proprioception

H. Refraction

I. Rhodopsin

J. Stapes

THOUGHT

1. Which of the following is NOT a general sense?

   a. taste

   b. touch

   c. pressure

   d. pain

2. Damage to which cranial nerve will interfere with the sense of taste from the tip of the tongue?

   a. gustatory

   b. facial

   c. glossopharyngeal

   d. hypoglossal

3. In what lobe of the brain is the sense of smell interpreted?

   a. frontal

   b. parietal

   c. occipital

   d. temporal

4. Dr. Ike Ular, an ophthalmologist, suspects that his patient might have glaucoma. One of the tests he performed was to measure the pressure in the anterior cavity of the eye. The fluid in this cavity is

   a. endolymph

   b. vitreous humor

   c. aqueous humor

   d. perilymph

5. Which of the following is the first to vibrate in response to sound waves?

   a. tectorial membrane

   b. tympanic membrane

   c. vestibular membrane

   d. basilar membrane

APPLICATION

Ima Student went to see an otolaryngologist because she had difficulty hearing. A week previously she had a sinus infection and sore throat but apparently that condition had resolved. After performing numerous tests, the doctor explained that she had a middle ear infection with an accumulation of fluid and that it was the result of the sinus infection and sore throat.

a) How would fluid in the middle ear reduce the ability to perceive sound?

b) Explain how a sore throat and sinus infection can result in a middle ear infection.

CHAPTER 10

Endocrine System

Outline/Objectives

Introduction to the Endocrine System 205
- Compare the actions of the nervous system and the endocrine system.

Characteristics of Hormones 205
- Compare the major chemical classes of hormones.
- Discuss the general mechanisms of hormone action.

Endocrine Glands and Their Hormones 207
- Identify the major endocrine glands and discuss their hormones and functions: pituitary, thyroid, parathyroid, adrenal, pancreas, gonads, thymus, pineal.
- Name and describe the function of at least one hormone from the (a) gastric mucosa; (b) small intestine; (c) heart; and (d) placenta.

Prostaglandins 220
- Differentiate between hormones and prostaglandins.

Key Terms

Adenohypophysis
Endocrine gland
Exocrine gland
Hormone
Negative feedback
Neurohypophysis
Target tissue

Building Vocabulary

WORD PART	MEANING
ad-	toward
aden-	gland
-agon	assemble, gather together
andr-	male, maleness
cortic-	outer region, cortex
crin-	to secrete
di-	passing through
dips-	thirst
-gen-	to produce
-gest-	to carry, pregnancy
lact-	milk
oxy-	swift, rapid
para-	beside
pin-	pine cone
-ren-	kidney
ster-	steroid
test-	eggshells, eggs
-toc-	birth
trop-	to change, influence
-uria	urine condition

Functional Relationships of the
Endocrine System

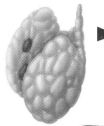

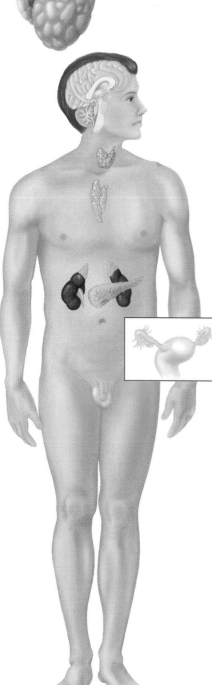

► Influences development and growth; adjusts rates of metabolism.

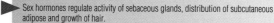

Integument
► Provides barrier against entry of pathogens; mechanical protection of superficial glands.
► Sex hormones regulate activity of sebaceous glands, distribution of subcutaneous adipose and growth of hair.

Skeletal
► Protects glands in head, thorax, and pelvis.
► Hormones from the pituitary, thyroid, and gonads stimulate bone growth; calcitonin and parathyroid hormone regulate calcium uptake and release from bone.

Muscular
► Provides protection for some endocrine glands.
► Hormones influence muscle metabolism, mass, and strength; epinephrine and norepinephrine adjust cardiac and smooth muscle activity.

Nervous
► Regulates secretory activity of anterior pituitary and adrenal medulla; produces ADH and oxytocin.
► Hormones influence neuronal metabolism and enhance autonomic stimuli.

Cardiovascular
► Delivers oxygen and nutrients to endocrine glands; removes carbon dioxide and heat; transports hormones from glands to target tissue; heart secretes atrial natriuretic hormone.
► Hormones adjust heart rate, contraction strength, blood volume, blood pressure, and red blood cell production.

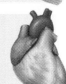

Lymphatic/Immune
► Assists in defense against infections in endocrine glands.
► Hormones from thymus influence development of lymphocytes; glucocorticoids suppress immune respone.

Respiratory
► Supplies oxygen, removes carbon dioxide, and helps maintain pH for metabolism in endocrine glands; converts angiotensin I into active angiotensin II.
► Epinephrine promotes bronchodilation; thyroxine and epinephrine stimulate cell respiration.

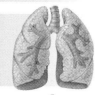

Digestive
► Absorbs nutrients for endocrine metabolism and hormone synthesis.
► Hormones influence motility and glandular activity of the digestive tract, gallbladder secretion, and secretion of enzymes from the pancreas; insulin and glucagon adjust glucose metabolism in the liver.

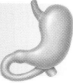

Urinary
► Helps maintain pH and electrolyte balance necessary for endocrine function; eliminates inactivated hormones and other metabolic wastes; releases renin and erythropoietin.
► Aldosterone, ADH, and atrial natriuretic hormone regulate urine formation in the kidneys.

Reproductive
► Gonads produce hormones that feedback to influence pituitary function.
► Hormones have a major role in differentiation and development of reproductive organs, sexual development, sex drive, gamete production, menstrual cycle, pregnancy, parturition, and lactation.

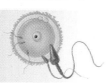

The organs that make up the endocrine system are the glands that secrete hormones into the blood. Unlike the organs in other systems, endocrine glands are scattered throughout the body. In addition, they are small and unimpressive; but as you study this chapter, you will discover that they are extremely important. The study of endocrine glands and hormones is called endocrinology.

Introduction to the Endocrine System

Comparison of the Endocrine and Nervous Systems

The endocrine system, along with the nervous system, functions in the regulation of body activities. The nervous system acts through electrical impulses and neurotransmitters to cause muscle contraction and glandular secretion. The effect is of short duration, measured in seconds, and localized. The endocrine system acts through chemical messengers called hormones that influence growth, development, and metabolic activities. The action of the endocrine system is measured in minutes, hours, or weeks and is more generalized than the action of the nervous system.

> Chemical messengers from the endocrine system help regulate body activities. Their effect is of longer duration and is more generalized than that of the nervous system.

Comparison of Exocrine and Endocrine Glands

There are two major categories of glands in the body—**exocrine** and **endocrine.** Exocrine glands have ducts that carry their secretory product to a surface. These have a variety of functions and include the sweat, sebaceous, and mammary glands and the glands that secrete digestive enzymes. The endocrine glands do not have ducts to carry their product to a surface. They are called ductless glands. The word "endocrine" is derived from the Greek terms *endo,* meaning "within," and *krine,* meaning "to separate or secrete." The secretory products of endocrine glands are called **hormones** and are secreted directly into the blood and then carried throughout the body where they influence only those cells that have receptor sites for that hormone. Other cells are not affected. Endocrine glands have an extensive network of blood vessels, and organs with the richest blood supply include some of the endocrine glands such as the thyroid and adrenal gland.

> Endocrine glands secrete hormones directly into the blood, which transports the hormones throughout the body.

Characteristics of Hormones

Each hormone produced in the body is unique. Each one is different in its chemical composition, structure, and action. In spite of the differences, there are similarities in these molecules.

Chemical Nature of Hormones

Chemically, hormones may be classified as either **proteins** or **steroids.** All of the hormones in the human body, except the sex hormones and those from the adrenal cortex, are proteins or protein derivatives. This means that their fundamental building blocks are **amino acids.** Protein hormones are difficult to administer orally because they are quickly inactivated by the acid and pepsin in the stomach. These hormones must be administered by injection. Sex hormones and those from the adrenal cortex are steroids, which are lipid derivatives. These lipid-soluble hormones may be taken orally.

> Hormones are either proteins or steroids.

> Insulin is a small protein molecule. It cannot be taken by mouth because it is rapidly inactivated by digestive enzymes.

CLINICAL TERMS

Acromegaly (ack-roh-MEG-ah-lee) Enlargement of the extremities caused by excessive growth hormone in the adult

Adenoma (add-eh-NOH-mah) A tumor of a gland

Cretinism (KREE-tin-izm) Dwarfism caused by a deficiency of thyroid hormone in childhood and usually accompanied by mental retardation

Endocrinology (en-doh-krin-AHL-oh-jee) Study of the endocrine glands

Exophthalmic (eks-off-THAL-mick) Pertaining to an abnormal protrusion or bulging of the eye

Glucose tolerance test (GTT) (GLOO-kohs TAHL-er-ans test) A blood sugar test performed at specified intervals after the patient has been given a certain amount of glucose. Blood samples are drawn, and the blood glucose level of each sample is determined.

Myxedema (miks-eh-DEE-mah) A condition of swelling due to an accumulation of mucus in the skin; results from deficiency of thyroid hormone in the adult

Progeria (pro-JEER-ih-ah) A condition of premature old age occurring in childhood, which may be due to hormone dysfunction

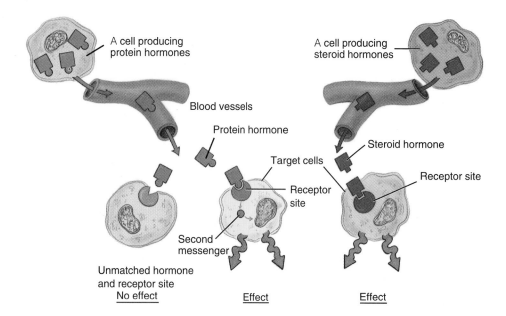

Figure 10–1 Hormone-receptor action.

Mechanism of Hormone Action

Hormones are carried by the blood throughout the entire body, yet they affect only certain cells. The specific cells that respond to a given hormone have **receptor sites** for that hormone. This is sort of a lock and key mechanism. If the key fits the lock, then the door will open. If a hormone fits the receptor site, then there will be an effect (Fig. 10–1). If a hormone and a receptor site do not match, then there is no reaction. All the cells that have receptor sites for a given hormone make up the **target tissue** for that hormone. In some cases, the target tissue is localized in a single gland or organ. In other cases, the target tissue is diffuse and scattered throughout the body so that many areas are affected. Hormones bring about their characteristic effects on target cells by modifying cellular activity.

> Cells in a target tissue have receptor sites for specific hormones.

Receptor sites may be located on the **surface of the cell membrane** or in the **interior of the cell.** Protein hormones, in general, are unable to diffuse through the cell membrane and react with receptor sites on the surface of the cell. The hormone-receptor reaction on the cell membrane activates an enzyme within the membrane, called adenyl cyclase, which diffuses into the cytoplasm. Within the cell, adenyl cyclase catalyzes the removal of phosphates from adenosine triphosphate to produce cyclic adenosine monophosphate (AMP). Cyclic AMP activates enzymes within the cytoplasm that alter the cellular activity. The protein hormone, which reacts at the cell membrane, is called the **first messenger.** Cyclic AMP, which brings about the action attributed to the hormone, is called the **second messenger.** This type of action is relatively rapid because the precursors are already present and they just need to be activated in some way.

Steroids, which are lipid soluble, diffuse through the cell membrane and react with receptors inside the cell. The hormone-receptor complex that is formed enters the nucleus, where it has a direct effect on specific genes within the DNA. These genes act as templates for the synthesis of messenger RNA (mRNA), which diffuses into the cytoplasm. The mRNA in the cytoplasm directs the synthesis of proteins at the ribosomes. The proteins that are formed represent the cell's response to the hormone. This method of hormone action is relatively slow because mRNA and proteins actually have to be synthesized rather than just activated.

> Protein hormones react with receptors on the surface of the cell, and the sequence of events that results in hormone action is relatively rapid. Steroid hormones typically react with receptor sites inside a cell. Because this method of action actually involves synthesis of proteins, it is relatively slow.

Control of Hormone Action

Hormones are very potent substances, which means that very small amounts of a hormone may have profound effects on metabolic processes. Because of their potency, hormone secretion must be regulated within very narrow limits to maintain homeostasis in the body.

Many hormones are controlled by some form of a negative feedback mechanism. In this type of system, a gland is sensitive to the concentration of a substance that it regulates. The interaction between insulin from the pancreatic islets of Langerhans and the concentration of glucose in the blood is an example of a physiologic negative feedback system (Fig. 10–2). The islets of Langerhans in the pancreas secrete insulin, which causes a decrease in the amount of glucose in the blood. The decrease in glucose concentration inhibits the production of in-

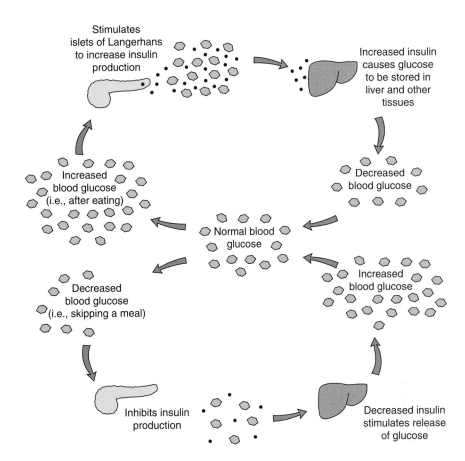

Figure 10–2   Interaction of blood glucose and insulin.

sulin, which causes an increase in the amount of glucose in the blood. A negative feedback system causes a reversal of increases and decreases in body conditions to maintain a state of stability or homeostasis.

Some endocrine glands secrete hormones in response to **other hormones.** The hormones that cause secretion of other hormones are called **tropic** hormones. A hormone from gland A causes gland B to secrete its hormone. For example, thyroid-stimulating hormone from the anterior pituitary gland (gland A) causes the thyroid gland (gland B) to secrete the hormone thyroxin.

A third method of regulating hormone secretion is by direct **nervous stimulation.** A nerve stimulus causes gland A to secrete its hormone. A physiologic example of this mechanism is the adrenal medulla, which secretes epinephrine (adrenaline) in response to stimulation by sympathetic nerves.

> Many hormones are regulated by a negative feedback mechanism; some are controlled by other hormones; and others are affected by direct nerve stimulation.

✓ QuickCheck

- What is the difference in location of receptor sites for protein hormones and the receptor sites for steroid hormones?
- What is a tropic hormone?

Endocrine Glands and Their Hormones

The endocrine system is made up of the endocrine glands that secrete hormones. Figure 10–3 illustrates that the eight major endocrine glands are scattered throughout the body; however, they are still considered to be one system because they have similar functions, similar mechanisms of influence, and many important interrelationships. Some glands also have nonendocrine regions that have functions other than hormone secretion. The pancreas is one of these. It has a major exocrine portion that secretes digestive enzymes and an endocrine portion that secretes hormones. The ovaries and testes secrete hormones and also produce the ova and sperm. Some organs, such as the stomach, intestines, and heart, produce hormones, but their primary function is not hormone secretion. These organs are discussed in more detail in the chapters dealing with their predominant function. Table 10–1 summarizes the major endocrine glands and their hormones.

> Even though the endocrine glands are scattered throughout the body, they have numerous interrelationships and similar mechanisms of action.

Pituitary Gland

The **pituitary gland** or **hypophysis** is a small gland about 1 centimeter in diameter or the size of a pea.

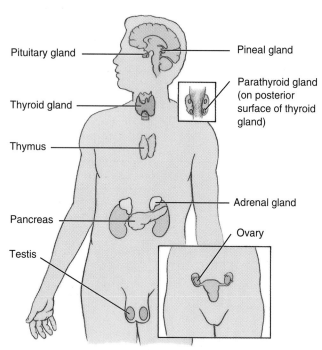

Figure 10-3 Major endocrine glands.

made up of neurons and neuroglia. It is called the **neurohypophysis** (noo-roh-hye-PAH-fih-sis).

> The pituitary gland is divided into an adenohypophysis and a neurohypophysis.

Just as there are two distinct regions or lobes with different embryonic derivations, there are separate regulating mechanisms that influence the secretory activity of the two parts. The activity of the anterior lobe is controlled by releasing and inhibitory hormones secreted by the hypothalamus of the brain. The releasing and inhibitory hormones, secreted in response to neural stimulation, enter capillaries in the hypothalamus and are transported by veins along the infundibulum to another capillary network in the anterior lobe. The two sets of capillaries and the veins between them are called the hypothalamic-pituitary portal system. Within the adenohypophysis, the releasing hormones affect the glandular epithelium to cause secretion of anterior pituitary hormones. Inhibitory hormones have the opposite effect.

Some of the neurosecretory cells in the hypothalamus have long axons that descend through the infundibulum and terminate in the posterior lobe. A stimulus to the nerve cell in the hypothalamus triggers the axon end in the posterior lobe to secrete a hormone that enters blood vessels and is transported to the target tissue. These hormones actually are made in the neuron cell bodies within the hypothalamus, then they travel down the axon to the neurohypophysis, where they are stored and subsequently released. Figure 10–4 illustrates the relationship of the hypothalamus to the anterior and posterior lobes of the pituitary gland.

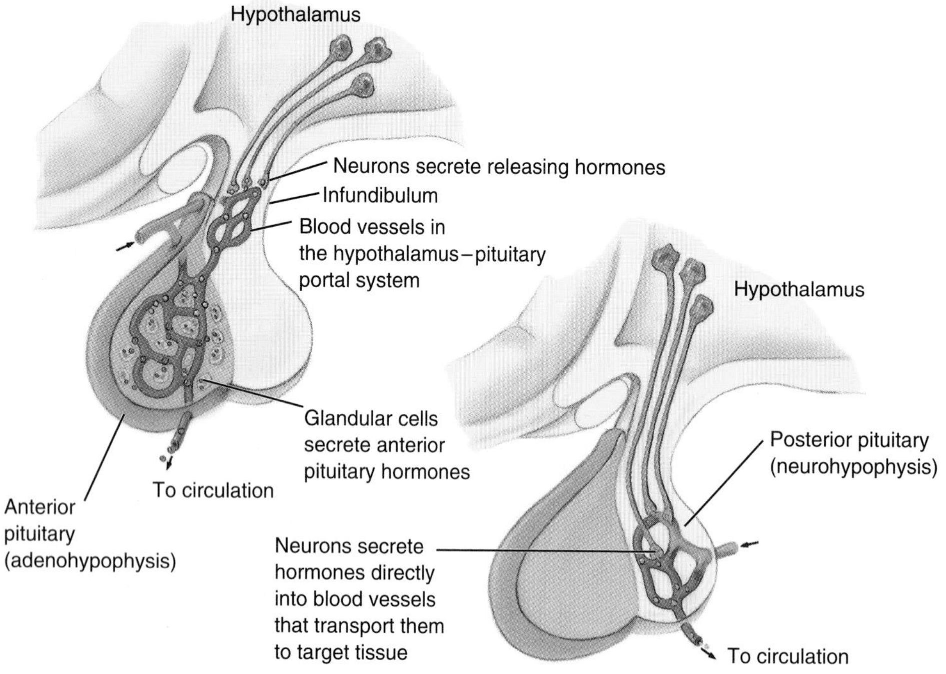

It is nearly surrounded by bone as it rests in the sella turcica, a depression in the sphenoid bone. The gland is connected to the hypothalamus of the brain by a slender stalk called the infundibulum (Fig. 10–4). There are two distinct regions in the gland. The anterior portion consists of epithelial cells derived from the embryonic oral cavity and is called the **adenohypophysis** (add-eh-noe-hye-PAH-fih-sis). The posterior region is an extension of the brain and is

Figure 10-4 Relationship of hypothalamus to pituitary gland.

Table 10–1	The Principal Endocrine Glands and Their Hormones		
Gland	**Hormone**	**Target Tissue**	**Principal Actions**
Hypothalamus	Releasing and inhibiting hormones	Anterior lobe of pituitary gland	Stimulates or inhibits secretion of specific hormones
Anterior lobe of pituitary	Growth hormone (GH)	Most tissues in the body	Stimulates growth by promoting protein synthesis
	Thyroid-stimulating hormone (TSH)	Thyroid gland	Increases secretion of thyroid hormone; increases the size of the thyroid gland
	Adrenocorticotropic hormone (ACTH)	Adrenal cortex	Increases secretion of adrenocortical hormones, especially glucocorticoids such as cortisol
	Follicle-stimulating hormone (FSH)	Ovarian follicles in the female; seminiferous tubules of testis in male	Follicle maturation and estrogen secretion in the female; spermatogenesis in the male
	Luteinizing hormone (LH); also called interstitial cell-stimulating hormone (ICSH) in males	Ovary in females, testis in males	Ovulation; progesterone production in female; testosterone production in male
	Prolactin	Mammary gland	Stimulates milk production
Posterior lobe of pituitary	Antidiuretic hormone (ADH)	Kidney	Increases water reabsorption (decreases water lost in urine)
	Oxytocin	Uterus; mammary gland	Increases uterine contractions; stimulates ejection of milk from mammary gland
Thyroid gland	Thyroxine and triiodothyronine	Most body cells	Increases metabolic rate; essential for normal growth and development
	Calcitonin	Primarily bone	Decreases blood calcium by inhibiting bone breakdown and release of calcium; antagonistic to parathyroid hormone
Parathyroid gland	Parathyroid hormone (PTH) or parathormone	Bone, kidney, digestive tract	Increases blood calcium by stimulating bone breakdown and release of calcium; increases calcium absorption in the digestive tract; decreases calcium lost in urine
Adrenal cortex	Mineralocorticoids (aldosterone)	Kidney	Increases sodium reabsorption and potassium excretion in kidney tubules; secondarily increases water retention
	Glucocorticoids (cortisol)	Most body tissues	Increases blood glucose levels; inhibits inflammation and immune response
	Androgens and estrogens	Most body tissues	Secreted in small amounts so that effect is generally masked by the hormones from the ovaries and testes
Adrenal medulla	Epinephrine, norepinephrine	Heart, blood vessels, liver, adipose	Helps cope with stress; increases heart rate and blood pressure; increases blood flow to skeletal muscle; increases blood glucose level
Pancreas (islets of Langerhans)	Glucagon	Liver	Increases breakdown of glycogen to increase blood glucose levels
	Insulin	General, but especially liver, skeletal muscle, adipose	Decreases blood glucose levels by facilitating uptake and utilization of glucose by cells; stimulates glucose storage as glycogen and production of adipose
Testes	Testosterone	Most body cells	Maturation and maintenance of male reproductive organs and secondary sex characteristics

Continued on following page

Table 10–1	**The Principal Endocrine Glands and Their Hormones** *continued*		
Gland	**Hormone**	**Target Tissue**	**Principal Actions**
Ovaries	Estrogens	Most body cells	Maturation and maintenance of female reproductive organs and secondary sex characteristics; menstrual cycle
	Progesterone	Uterus and breast	Prepares uterus for pregnancy; stimulates development of mammary gland; menstrual cycle
Pineal gland	Melatonin	Hypothalamus	Inhibits gonadotropin-releasing hormone, which consequently inhibits reproductive functions; regulates daily rhythms such as sleep and wakefulness
Thymus	Thymosin	Tissues involved in immune response	Immune system development and function

> The activity of the adenohypophysis is controlled by releasing hormones from the hypothalamus. The neurohypophysis is controlled by nerve stimulation.

Hormones of the Anterior Lobe (Adenohypophysis)

Growth Hormone. Growth hormone (GH) is a protein that stimulates the growth of bones, muscles, and other organs by promoting protein synthesis (Fig. 10–5). This hormone drastically affects the appearance of an individual because it influences height. If there is too little of the hormone in a child, that person may become a pituitary dwarf of normal proportions but small stature. An excess of the hormone in a child results in exaggerated bone growth, and the individual becomes exceptionally tall or a giant. After ossification is complete and an increase in bone length is no longer possible, excess GH causes an enlargement in the diameter of the bones. The result is a condition called acromegaly (ack-roh-MEG-ah-lee), in which the bones of the hands and face become abnormally large.

> GH promotes protein synthesis, which results in growth.

> Excessive secretion of a hormone is called **hypersecretion**. A deficiency of a hormone is called **hyposecretion**. Usually hyposecretion of GH in the adult poses no problems. However, in rare instances, the deficiency may be so drastic that body tissues atrophy and premature aging appears.

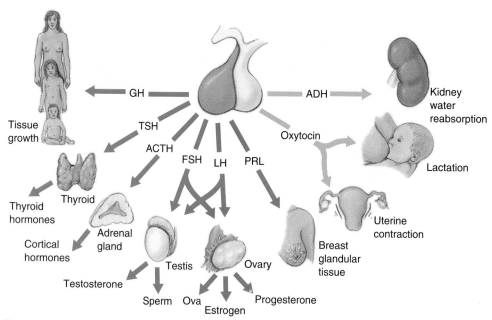

Figure 10–5 Effects of hormones from the pituitary gland.

Thyroid-Stimulating Hormone. Thyroid-stimulating hormone (TSH), or thyrotropin (thye-roh-TROH-pin), causes the glandular cells of the thyroid to secrete thyroid hormone (see Fig. 10–5). When there is a hypersecretion of TSH, the thyroid gland enlarges and secretes too much thyroid hormone. Hyposecretion of TSH results in atrophy of the thyroid gland and too little hormone.

> Thyrotropin affects the activity of the thyroid gland.

Adrenocorticotropic Hormone. Adrenocorticotropic (ah-dree-noh-kor-tih-koh-TROH-pik) hormone (ACTH) reacts with receptor sites in the cortex of the adrenal gland to stimulate the secretion of cortical hormones, particularly cortisol (see Fig. 10–5). ACTH also affects the melanocytes in the skin and increases pigmentation. Hypersecretion and hyposecretion of ACTH are reflected in the activity of the adrenal cortex.

> ACTH stimulates the secretion of cortisol from the adrenal cortex.

Gonadotropic Hormones. Gonadotropic (go-nad-oh-TROH-pik) hormones react with receptor sites in the gonads, or ovaries and testes, to regulate the development, growth, and function of these organs. Follicle-stimulating hormone (FSH) stimulates the development of eggs or ova in the ovaries and sperm in the testes (see Fig. 10–5). In addition, it stimulates estrogen production in the female. Luteinizing hormone (LH) causes ovulation and the production and secretion of the sex hormones, progesterone and estrogen, in the female. In the male, LH is sometimes called interstitial cell-stimulating hormone (ICSH) because it stimulates the interstitial cells of the testes to produce and secrete the male sex hormone testosterone (see Fig. 10–5). Without the gonadotropins FSH and LH, the ovaries and testes decrease in size, ova and sperm are not produced, and sex hormones are not secreted.

> FSH and LH are gonadotropic hormones, which regulate the development, growth, and function of the ovaries and testes.

Prolactin. Prolactin or lactogenic hormone promotes the development of glandular tissue in the female breast during pregnancy and stimulates milk production after the birth of the infant (see Fig. 10–5). This hormone does not cause the milk to be ejected from the breast. A hormone from the posterior pituitary and other neural influences are responsible for the ejection of the milk.

> Prolactin promotes development of glandular tissue in the breast and stimulates the production of milk.

Hyposecretion of prolactin presents no problem except in women who choose to breast feed their babies. Hypersecretion is more common and is usually the result of pituitary tumors. This causes inappropriate lactation and lack of menstruation in females. In males, it results in impotence.

Hormones of the Posterior Lobe (Neurohypophysis)

Antidiuretic Hormone. Antidiuretic (ant-eye-dye-yoo-RET-ik) hormone (ADH) promotes the reabsorption of water by the kidney tubules, with the result that less water is lost as urine (see Fig. 10–5). This mechanism conserves water for the body. Insufficient amounts of ADH cause excessive water loss in the urine. Large amounts of a very dilute urine are produced. This condition is called diabetes insipidus. ADH, especially in large amounts, also causes blood vessels to constrict, which increases blood pressure. For this reason, ADH is sometimes called vasopressin.

> ADH promotes the reabsorption of water in the kidney tubules.

Ingestion of alcoholic beverages inhibits ADH secretion and results in increased urine output.

Certain drugs, called diuretics, counteract the effects of ADH and result in fluid loss. These drugs are sometimes prescribed for patients with high blood pressure or those with edema due to congestive heart failure because the drugs have the effect of removing fluid from the body.

Oxytocin. Oxytocin (ahk-see-TOH-sin) causes contraction of the smooth muscle in the wall of the uterus. It also stimulates the ejection of milk from the lactating breast (see Fig. 10–5). A commercial preparation of this hormone, called Pitocin, is sometimes used to induce labor.

> Oxytocin causes uterine muscle contraction and ejection of milk from the lactating breast.

Oxytocin, or similar synthetic drugs, may be used to hasten the delivery of the placenta, to control bleeding after delivery, or to stimulate milk ejection.

● How do the mechanisms that regulate the anterior and posterior regions of the pituitary gland differ?

● Jerry has a severe case of the flu with excessive vomiting and diarrhea and is in a condition of dehydration. How does this affect the amount of ADH secreted by the posterior pituitary gland?

Thyroid Gland

The thyroid (THYE-royd) gland is a very vascular organ that is located in the neck (see Fig. 10–3). It consists of two lobes, one on each side of the trachea, just below the larynx or voice box. The two lobes are connected by a narrow band of tissue called the isthmus. Internally, the gland consists of follicles filled with a colloid and parafollicular cells interspersed between the follicles. The follicles, composed of simple cuboidal epithelium, secrete the hormones that contain iodine, such as thyroxine (thye-RAHK-sin) and triiodothyronine (trye-eye-oh-doh-THYE-roh-neen). Parafollicular cells secrete calcitonin (kal-sih-TOH-nin).

> The thyroid follicles produce thyroxine and triiodothyronine hormones, which contain iodine. Parafollicular cells produce calcitonin.

Thyroxine and Triiodothyronine

About 95 percent of the active thyroid hormone is thyroxine, and most of the remaining 5 percent is triiodothyronine. Both of these require iodine for their synthesis. The iodine is actively transported into the thyroid gland, where its concentration may become as much as 25 times that of the blood, and then it is incorporated into the hormone molecules. Thyroid hormone secretion is regulated by releasing hormones from the hypothalamus and by the circulating thyroid hormones that exert an inhibiting influence on the anterior pituitary and hypothalamus. This regulatory mechanism is illustrated in Figure 10–6.

> Thyroid hormone secretion is regulated by a negative feedback mechanism that involves the amount of circulating hormone, hypothalamus, and adenohypophysis.

If there is an iodine deficiency, the thyroid cannot make sufficient hormone. This stimulates the anterior pituitary to secrete TSH, which causes the thyroid gland to increase in size in a vain attempt to produce more hormone. But it cannot produce more hormone because it does not have the necessary raw materials, namely iodine. This type of thyroid enlargement is called simple goiter or iodine deficiency goiter.

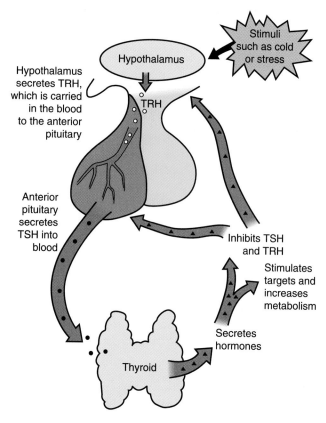

TRH = Thyrotropin-releasing hormone
TSH = Thyroid-stimulating hormone

Figure 10–6 Interaction of hypothalamus, anterior pituitary, and thyroid.

> A simple goiter is an enlarged thyroid gland resulting from a deficiency of iodine in the diet.

The thyroid hormones containing thyroxine and triiodothyronine help to regulate the metabolism of carbohydrates, proteins, and lipids in the body. They do not have a single target organ; instead they affect most of the cells in the body. They increase the rate at which cells release energy from carbohydrates, they enhance protein synthesis, they are necessary for normal growth and development, and they stimulate the nervous system.

In the infant, a deficiency or lack of thyroid hormone, hypothyroidism, results in a condition called cretinism (KREE-tin-izm). A cretin is a mentally retarded dwarf with abnormally developed skeletal features. If the condition is detected early enough, hormone therapy may stimulate growth, prevent the abnormal skeletal features, and increase the metabolic rate. However, therapy must be started within 2 months or less after birth to prevent severe mental retardation. Hypothyroidism in the adult results in a condition called myxedema (miks-eh-DEE-mah), which is characterized by lethargy, weight gain, loss of hair, decreased body temperature, low metabolic rate, and slow heart rate. Hormone therapy, in appropriate doses, usually alleviates these symptoms.

Hyperthyroidism results from an enlarged thyroid gland that produces too much hormone. This is characterized by a high metabolic rate, hyperactivity, insomnia, nervousness, irritability, and chronic fatigue. An individual with hyperthyroidism often has protruding eyes or exophthalmos (eks-off-THAL-mus) because there is swelling in the tissues behind the eyes. Removal, or destruction by radioactive iodine, of a portion of the thyroid may effectively reduce the symptoms of hyperthyroidism.

> Thyroxine and triiodothyronine affect the metabolism of carbohydrates, proteins, and lipids. Deficiency of the hormones leads to conditions related to decreased metabolism. Hyperthyroidism is characterized by a high metabolic rate.

When thyroxine and triiodothyronine, with their incorporated iodine, are released into the blood, more than **99** percent combines with plasma proteins. This iodine is called **protein-bound iodine (PBI)**. The amount of PBI can be measured by a laboratory procedure and is widely used as a test of thyroid function.

Calcitonin

Calcitonin is secreted by the parafollicular cells of the thyroid gland. This hormone opposes the action of the parathyroid glands by reducing the calcium level in the blood. If blood calcium becomes too high, calcitonin is secreted until calcium ion levels decrease to normal. Calcitonin reduces blood calcium levels by reducing the rate at which calcium is released from bone, by increasing the rate of calcium excretion by the kidneys, and by reducing calcium absorption in the intestines. A deficiency of calcitonin does not seem to increase blood calcium levels.

> Calcitonin, produced by thyroid parafollicular cells, "tones down," or reduces, calcium levels in the blood.

Parathyroid Glands

Four small masses of epithelial tissue are embedded in the connective tissue capsule on the posterior surface of the thyroid glands. These are the parathyroid glands, and they secrete **parathyroid hormone** (PTH, or parathormone). PTH is the most important regulator of blood calcium levels. The hormone is secreted in response to low blood calcium levels, and its effect is to increase those levels. It does this by increasing osteoclast activity in bones so that calcium is released from the bones into the blood, by increasing calcium reabsorption from the kidney tubules into the blood, which decreases the amount lost in the urine, and by increasing the absorption of dietary calcium in the intestines. Vitamin D is also necessary for dietary calcium to be absorbed in the intestines. PTH is antagonistic, or has the opposite effect, to calcitonin from the thyroid gland (Fig. 10–7).

> PTH increases blood calcium levels.

Hypoparathyroidism, or insufficient secretion of

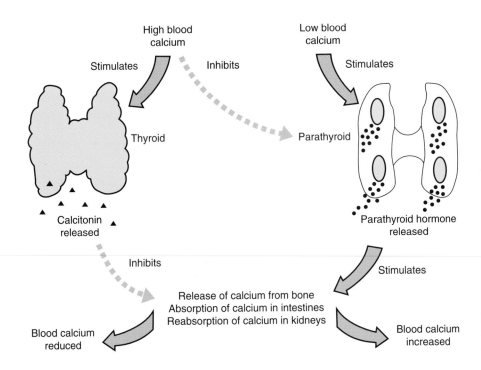

Figure 10-7 Effects of calcitonin and parathyroid hormone on blood calcium levels.

PTH, leads to increased nerve excitability. The low blood calcium levels trigger spontaneous and continuous nerve impulses, which then stimulate muscle contraction. Tumors of the parathyroid gland may cause excessive secretion of PTH or hyperparathyroidism. This leads to an increased osteoclast activity that removes calcium from the bones and increases the level in the blood. The excess calcium in the blood may precipitate in abnormal locations or cause kidney stones.

> Hypoparathyroidism reduces blood calcium levels, which may result in nerve irritability. Hypersecretion results in calcium loss from bones and precipitation in abnormal places.

Hypersecretion of parathyroid hormone sometimes causes a bone disease called **osteitis fibrosa cystica.** Bone mass decreases as a result of osteoclast activity, decalcification occurs, cystlike cavities appear in the bone, and spontaneous fractures result.

Adrenal (Suprarenal) Glands

The adrenal, or suprarenal (soo-prah-REE-null), glands are paired with one gland located near the upper portion of each kidney. The glands are embedded in the fat that surrounds the kidneys. Each gland is divided into an outer region, the adrenal cortex, and an inner region, the adrenal medulla (Fig. 10–8). The cortex and medulla of the adrenal gland, like the anterior and posterior lobes of the pituitary, develop from different embryonic tissues and secrete different hormones. The adrenal cortex is essential to life, but the medulla may be removed with no life-threatening effects because its functions are like those of the sympathetic nervous system.

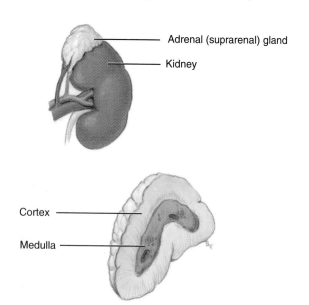

Figure 10–8 Adrenal gland.

> The adrenal gland is divided into an outer cortex and an inner medulla.

The hypothalamus of the brain influences both portions of the adrenal gland but by different mechanisms. The medulla receives direct stimulation from nerve impulses that originate in the hypothalamus and then travel through the brain stem, spinal cord, and sympathetic nerves (Fig. 10–9). The hypo-

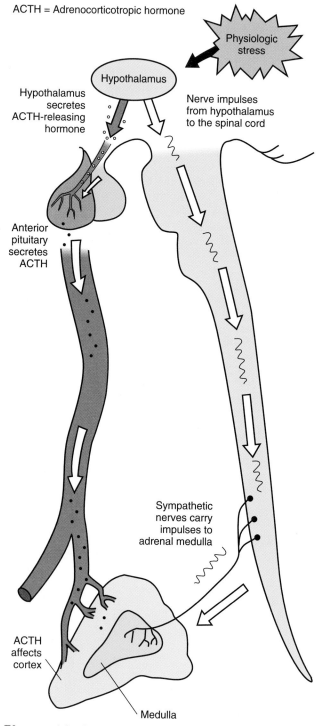

Figure 10–9 Hypothalamic control of the adrenal gland.

thalamus affects the cortex by secreting ACTH-releasing hormone, which stimulates the anterior pituitary to secrete ACTH, which then stimulates the adrenal cortex (see Fig. 10–9).

> The adrenal cortex is regulated by negative feedback involving the hypothalamus and ACTH; the medulla is regulated by nerve impulses from the hypothalamus.

Hormones of the Adrenal Cortex

The adrenal cortex consists of three different regions, with each region producing a different group or type of hormones. Chemically, all the cortical hormones are steroids.

> All hormones from the adrenal cortex are steroids.

Mineralocorticoids (min-er-al-oh-KOR-tih-koyds) are secreted by the outermost region of the adrenal cortex. As a group, these hormones help regulate blood volume and the concentration of mineral electrolytes in the blood. The principal mineralocorticoid is **aldosterone** (al-DAHS-ter-ohn). Although aldosterone primarily affects the kidneys, it also acts on the intestines, salivary glands, and sweat glands. In general, its effect is to conserve sodium ions and water in the body and to eliminate potassium ions. Sodium and potassium levels are important in maintaining blood pressure, nerve impulse conduction, and muscle contraction. When the kidney tubules reabsorb sodium ions and excrete potassium in response to aldosterone, they also conserve water and reduce urine output, which increases blood volume. Aldosterone is secreted in direct response to sodium and potassium ions. The rate of aldosterone secretion increases when there is an increase in blood potassium level or a decrease in blood sodium level. ACTH from the anterior pituitary has a minor effect on aldosterone secretion (Fig. 10–10).

> The principal mineralocorticoid is aldosterone, which acts to conserve sodium ions and water in the body.

A tumor of the adrenal cortex may lead to hypersecretion of mineralocorticoids. If this results in excessive potassium depletion, neurons and muscle fibers become less responsive to stimuli. Symptoms of this condition include paralysis, muscle weakness, and cramps.

Glucocorticoids (gloo-koh-KOR-tih-koyds) are secreted by the middle region of the adrenal cortex. As a group, these hormones help regulate nutrient levels in the blood. The principal glucocorticoid is **cortisol,** also called hydrocortisone. The overall effect of the glucocorticoids is to increase blood glucose levels. It does this by increasing the cellular utilization of proteins and fats as energy sources, thus conserving glucose. It also stimulates the liver cells to produce glucose from amino acids and fats. These actions help to maintain appropriate blood glucose levels between meals. In times of prolonged stress, cortisol is secreted in larger than normal amounts to help increase glucose levels to provide energy to respond to the stress. Glucocorticoid secretion is controlled by ACTH from the anterior pituitary gland under the influence of a releasing hormone from the hypothalamus (see Fig. 10–10). Cortisol also helps to counteract the inflammatory response. For this reason, it is used clinically to reduce the inflammation in certain allergic reactions, bursitis and arthritis, infections, and some types of cancer.

> The principal glucocorticoid is cortisol, which increases blood glucose levels.

Persons with inflamed joints often receive injections of a pharmaceutical glucocorticoid, cortisone, to relieve the pain and inflammation. Over-the-counter creams and ointments containing hydrocortisone are available to relieve the itching and inflammation of rashes.

The third group of steroids secreted by the adrenal cortex is the **gonadocorticoids** (go-nad-oh-KOR-tih-koyds), or sex hormones. These are secreted by the innermost region. Male hormones, **androgens,** and female hormones, **estrogens,** are secreted in minimal amounts in both sexes by the adrenal cortex, but their effect is usually masked by the hormones from the testes and ovaries. In females, the masculinization effect of androgen secretion may become evident after menopause, when estrogen levels from the ovaries decrease.

> Sex steroids from the adrenal cortex have minimal effect compared with the hormones from the ovaries and testes.

Tumors that result in hypersecretion of gonadocorticoids may have dramatic effects in prepubertal boys and girls. There is a rapid onset of puberty and sex drive in males. Females develop the masculine distribution of body hair, including a beard and the clitoris enlarges to become more like a penis.

Hyposecretion of the adrenal cortex leads to a condition known as Addison's disease. The lack of mineralocorticoids causes low blood sodium, high blood potassium, and dehydration, and the lack of glucocorticoids causes low blood glucose levels. In addition, there is increased pigmentation in the skin.

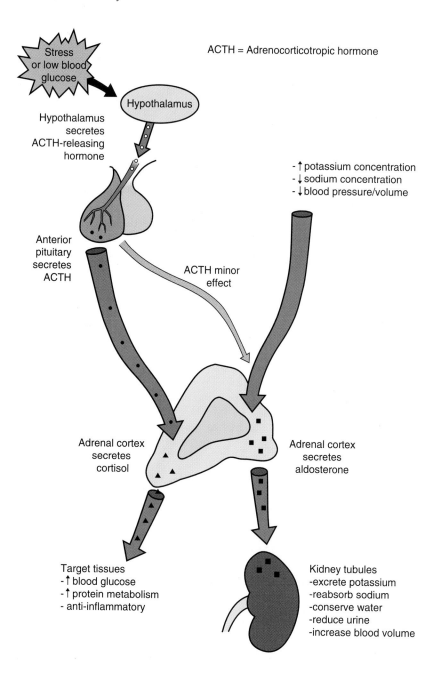

ACTH = Adrenocorticotropic hormone

Stress or low blood glucose

Hypothalamus

Hypothalamus secretes ACTH-releasing hormone

Anterior pituitary secretes ACTH

ACTH minor effect

- ↑ potassium concentration
- ↓ sodium concentration
- ↓ blood pressure/volume

Adrenal cortex secretes cortisol

Adrenal cortex secretes aldosterone

Target tissues
- ↑ blood glucose
- ↑ protein metabolism
- anti-inflammatory

Kidney tubules
-excrete potassium
-reabsorb sodium
-conserve water
-reduce urine
-increase blood volume

Figure 10–10 Regulation of aldosterone and cortisol secretion.

If untreated, hyposecretion of the adrenal cortex leads to death in a few days.

Hypersecretion of the adrenal cortex, whether from a tumor or excessive ACTH, causes Cushing's syndrome. This is characterized by elevated blood glucose levels, retention of sodium ions and water with subsequent puffiness or edema, loss of potassium ions, and, in females, masculinization. These effects are directly related to the actions of the three groups of hormones secreted by the cortex.

The effects of hypersecretion and hyposecretion of adrenocortical hormones are directly related to the actions of the three groups of steroids.

Hormones of the Adrenal Medulla

The adrenal medulla develops from neural tissue and secretes two hormones, **epinephrine** (adrenaline) and **norepinephrine** (noradrenaline). About 80 percent of the medullary secretion is epinephrine. These two hormones are secreted in response to stimulation by sympathetic nerves, particularly during stressful situations (Fig. 10–11). Epinephrine, a cardiac stimulator, and norepinephrine, a vasoconstrictor, together cause increases in heart rate, in the force of cardiac muscle contraction, and in blood pressure. They divert blood supply to the skeletal muscles and decrease the activity of the digestive tract, dilate the bronchioles and increase the breathing rate, and increase the rate of metabolism

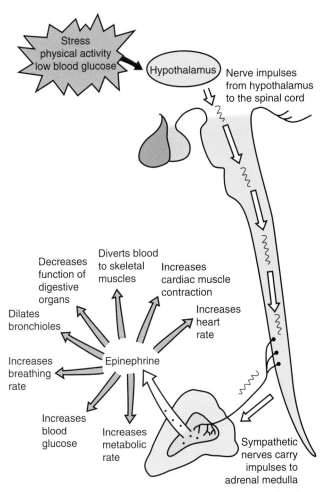

Figure 10-11 Epinephrine—its effects and control of its secretion.

to provide energy. They prepare the body for strenuous activity and are sometimes called the fight-or-flight hormones. Their effect on the body is similar to the sympathetic nervous system, but the effect lasts up to 10 times longer because the hormones are removed from the tissues slowly. The effects of epinephrine are summarized in Figure 10-11. A lack of hormones from the adrenal medulla produces no significant effects. Hypersecretion, usually from a tumor, causes prolonged or continual sympathetic responses.

> Epinephrine and norepinephrine, from the adrenal medulla, have effects similar to the sympathetic nervous system.

✓ QuickCheck

- How does iodine deficiency affect secretions from the anterior pituitary gland?

- What two hormones regulate calcium ion levels?

- What effect does aldosterone have on urine output? Explain.

Pancreas—Islets of Langerhans

The pancreas is a long, soft organ that lies transversely along the posterior abdominal wall, posterior to the stomach, and extends from the region of the duodenum to the spleen. This gland has an exocrine portion that secretes digestive enzymes that are carried through a duct to the duodenum and an endocrine portion that secretes hormones into the blood. The endocrine portion consists of over a million small groups of cells, called pancreatic islets or islets of Langerhans, that are interspersed throughout the exocrine tissue. The pancreatic islets contain alpha cells that secrete the hormone **glucagon** and beta cells that secrete the hormone **insulin.** Both of these hormones have a role in regulating blood glucose levels. It is important to maintain blood glucose levels within a normal range because this is the primary source of energy for the nervous system. If blood glucose levels fall too low, the nervous system does not function properly. If blood glucose levels become too high, the kidneys produce large quantities of urine, and dehydration may result.

> The endocrine portion of the pancreas consists of the pancreatic islets, which secrete glucagon and insulin.

Glucagon

Alpha cells in the pancreatic islets secrete the hormone glucagon in response to a low concentration of glucose in the blood. Glucagon's principal action is to raise blood glucose levels (Fig. 10-12). It does this by mobilizing glucose and fatty acids from their storage forms. It also stimulates the liver to break down glycogen into glucose and to manufacture glucose from noncarbohydrate sources such as proteins and fats. These mechanisms prevent hypoglycemia from occurring between meals or when glucose is being used rapidly.

> The principal action of glucagon, from the alpha cells, is to raise blood glucose levels.

Insulin

Beta cells in the pancreatic islets secrete the hormone insulin in response to a high concentration of glucose in the blood. The action of insulin is opposite or antagonistic to glucagon. It promotes cellular uptake and utilization of glucose for energy. It stimulates the liver and muscle to remove glucose from the blood and to store it as glycogen. When the liver has stored all the glycogen possible, glucose is converted to fat or adipose. Insulin inhibits the manufacture of glucose from noncarbohydrate sources. As a result of these actions, insulin decreases the blood glucose concentration (see Fig. 10-12). Hypoactivity of insulin may be caused by insufficient insulin se-

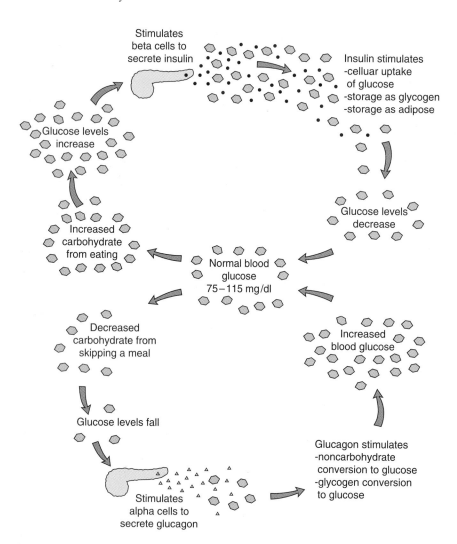

Figure 10–12   Effects of insulin and glucagon.

cretion, insufficient receptor sites on target cell membranes, or defective receptor sites that do not recognize insulin. These dysfunctions lead to diabetes mellitus, which is characterized by abnormally high blood glucose levels.

> The principal action of insulin, which is secreted by the beta cells, is to decrease blood glucose levels.

Hyperinsulinism is usually caused by an overdose of insulin, rarely by islet cell tumors. The result is **hypoglycemia,** or low blood sugar level. The low blood sugar stimulates the secretion of glucagon, epinephrine, and growth hormone, which causes anxiety, nervousness, tremors, and a feeling of weakness. Insufficient glucose to the brain leads to disorientation, convulsions, and unconsciousness. Death can occur quickly unless the blood glucose level is raised. The early symptoms can be treated easily by eating sugar.

Gonads (Testes and Ovaries)

The gonads, the primary reproductive organs, are the testes in the male and the ovaries in the female. These organs are responsible for producing the sperm and ova, but they also secrete hormones and are considered to be endocrine glands. A brief description of their endocrine functions is given here. Reproductive functions and a more thorough discussion of the hormones appear in Chapter 19.

Testes

Male sex hormones, as a group, are called **androgens** (AN-droh-jenz). The principal androgen is **testosterone** (tess-TAHS-ter-ohn), which is secreted by the testes. A small amount is also produced by the adrenal cortex. Production of testosterone begins during fetal development, continues for a short time after birth, nearly ceases during childhood, then resumes at puberty. This steroid hormone is responsible for the following:

- The growth and development of the male reproductive structures
- Increased skeletal and muscular growth
- Enlargement of the larynx accompanied by voice changes
- Growth and distribution of body hair
- Increased male sexual drive

Testosterone secretion is regulated by a negative feedback system that involves releasing hormones from the hypothalamus and gonadotropins from the anterior pituitary (Fig. 10–13).

> The testes produce androgens, primarily testosterone, which are responsible for the development and maintenance of male secondary sex characteristics.

Ovaries

Two groups of female sex hormones are produced in the ovaries, the **estrogens** (ESS-troh-jenz) and **progesterone** (proh-JESS-ter-ohn). These steroid hormones contribute to the development and function of the female reproductive organs and sex characteristics. At the onset of puberty, estrogens promote:

- The development of the breasts
- Distribution of fat evidenced in the hips, legs, and breasts
- Maturation of reproductive organs such as the uterus and vagina

Progesterone causes the uterine lining to thicken in preparation for pregnancy. Together, progesterone and estrogens are responsible for the changes that occur in the uterus during the female menstrual cycle. Like testosterone in the male, estrogen and progesterone activity is controlled by a negative feedback mechanism involving releasing hormones from the hypothalamus and the gonadotropins FSH and LH from the anterior pituitary.

> The ovaries produce estrogens and progesterone. Estrogens are responsible for the development and maintenance of female secondary sex characteristics. Progesterone maintains the uterine lining for pregnancy.

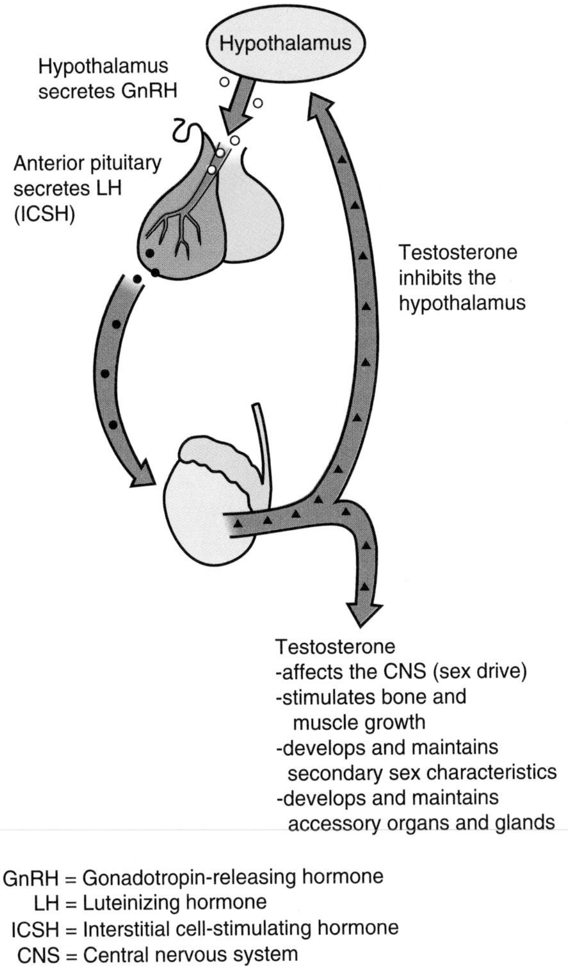

Pineal Gland

The **pineal** (PIE-nee-al) gland, also called pineal body or **epiphysis cerebri,** is a small cone-shaped structure that extends posteriorly from the third ventricle of the brain. The gland is often visible on radiographs because it becomes infiltrated with calcium deposits after puberty. It was once believed that this indicated an atrophy of the gland; however, this does not seem to be the case. Recent evidence indicates that the gland is active throughout the life of an individual. The presence of calcium suggests high metabolic activity.

The pineal gland consists of portions of neurons, neuroglial cells, and specialized secretory cells called **pinealocytes** (PIE-nee-al-oh-cytes). The pinealocytes synthesize the hormone **melatonin** (mell-ah-TOH-nihn) and secrete it directly into the cerebrospinal fluid, which takes it into the blood. Melatonin secretion is rhythmic in nature, with high levels secreted at night and low levels secreted during the day.

The function of the pineal gland and melatonin in humans has been the subject of controversy and speculation for centuries. Even the ancient Greeks wrote about it. Evidence accumulated during the 1980s indicates that melatonin has a regulatory role in sexual and reproductive development. Melatonin acts on the hypothalamus to inhibit gonadotropin-releasing hormone (GnRH), which then inhibits gonad development.

Another function of melatonin involves the organization and regulation of circadian rhythms, or daily changes, in physiologic processes that follow a regular pattern. An example of this is the sleepiness/wakefulness cycle. Increased plasma melatonin levels, which occur at night, are associated with

Hypothalamus secretes GnRH

Anterior pituitary secretes LH (ICSH)

Hypothalamus

Testosterone inhibits the hypothalamus

Testosterone
-affects the CNS (sex drive)
-stimulates bone and
   muscle growth
-develops and maintains
   secondary sex characteristics
-develops and maintains
   accessory organs and glands

GnRH = Gonadotropin-releasing hormone
   LH = Luteinizing hormone
ICSH = Interstitial cell-stimulating hormone
 CNS = Central nervous system

Figure 10–13   Relationship of the hypothalamus, anterior pituitary, and testes in testosterone production.

sleepiness. The hormone also seems to play a role in hunger/satiety cycles, mood changes, and jet lag. The high nighttime level of melatonin seems to be a mechanism to daily "reset" the biological clock.

> The pineal gland secretes melatonin, which affects reproductive development and daily physiologic cycles.

Melatonin production appears to be related to the amount of light that enters through the eye. People who work at night and sleep during the day have a reversed cycle of melatonin production. The high levels occur during the day while they are asleep and the low levels are at night when they are working and light is entering the eye.

Other Endocrine Glands

In addition to the major endocrine glands, other organs have some hormonal activity as part of their function. These include the thymus, stomach, small intestines, heart, and placenta.

The **thymus** gland is located near the midline in the anterior portion of the thoracic cavity. It is posterior to the sternum and a little superior to the heart. Through the production of the hormone **thymosin** (THYE-mohsin), the thymus gland assists in the development of certain white blood cells, called lymphocytes, which help protect the body against foreign organisms. In this way, the thymus plays an important role in the body's immune mechanism. If an infant is born without a thymus, the immune system does not develop properly and the body is highly susceptible to infections. The thymus is most active just before birth and during early childhood. It is relatively large in young children, then gradually diminishes in size with age as an individual reaches adulthood.

> Thymosin, produced by the thymus gland, plays an important role in the development of the body's immune system.

The lining of the stomach, the **gastric mucosa,** produces a hormone, called **gastrin,** in response to the presence of food in the stomach. This hormone stimulates the production of hydrochloric acid and the enzyme pepsin, which are used in the digestion of food. In this case, the stomach produces the hormone and is also the target organ.

The mucosa of the **small intestine** secretes the hormones **secretin** and **cholecystokinin.** Secretin stimulates the pancreas to produce a bicarbonate-rich fluid that neutralizes the stomach acid. Cholecystokinin stimulates contraction of the gallbladder, which releases bile. It also stimulates the pancreas to secrete digestive enzymes.

Surprisingly, the heart acts as an endocrine organ in addition to its major role of pumping blood. Special cells in the wall of the upper chambers of the heart, called atria, produce a hormone called **atrial natriuretic hormone,** or **atriopeptin.** The primary effect of this hormone is the loss of sodium and water in the urine. The result of this action is a decrease in blood volume and blood pressure.

The **placenta** develops in the pregnant female as a source of nourishment and gas exchange for the developing fetus. It also serves as a temporary endocrine gland. One of the hormones it secretes is **human chorionic gonadotropin** (hCG), which signals the mother's ovaries to secrete hormones to maintain the uterine lining so that it does not degenerate and slough off in menstruation. hCG reaches high levels early in pregnancy, then decreases. The placenta also produces **estrogen** and **progesterone** during pregnancy.

> Certain cells in the thymus, stomach, small intestines, heart, and placenta produce hormones.

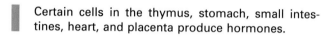
✓ QuickCheck

● What hormone is secreted in response to elevated blood glucose levels?

● What effect will injections of testosterone have on gonadotropins from the anterior pituitary gland?

● What gland secretes melatonin?

Prostaglandins

Prostaglandins (prahs-tih-GLAN-dins) are potent chemical regulators that are produced in minute amounts and are found widely distributed in cells throughout the body. They are similar to hormones but different enough that they are not classified as hormones. These hormonelike substances are derivatives of arachidonic acid, one of the essential fatty acids, and a dietary deficiency of this fatty acid results in an inability to synthesize prostaglandins. Whereas hormones are produced by specialized cells grouped together in structures called endocrine glands, prostaglandins are produced by cells widely distributed throughout the entire body. In contrast to a hormone, which is transported in the blood and may have an effect far distant from its point of origin, a prostaglandin has a localized effect on or near the cell in which it is made. For this reason it is sometimes called a local hormone. In addition to being localized, the effect is immediate and short term. These compounds cannot be stored in the body but must be synthesized "on demand" and are readily inactivated.

> Prostaglandins are produced in minute amounts and have an immediate, short-term, localized effect.

Numerous and varied effects are attributed to prostaglandins. These are often confusing because the same substance may have opposite effects on different tissues. Some modulate hormone action; others affect smooth muscle contraction; still others are involved in blood clotting mechanisms—some promote clotting and others inhibit the process. Prostaglandins foster many aspects of the inflammatory process, including the development of fever and pain. They also appear to inhibit the gastric secretion of hydrochloric acid. Some of the symptoms of premenstrual syndrome, severe menstrual cramps and pain, and premature labor are attributed to elevated levels of prostaglandins.

> Prostaglandins are responsible for many different tissue responses.

Nonsteroidal anti-inflammatory drugs, such as aspirin, ibuprofen, and acetaminophen (Tylenol), inhibit or block the synthesis of prostaglandins. Because prostaglandins promote the inflammatory response, inhibiting their production will reduce the inflammation of rheumatoid arthritis, bursitis, tennis elbow, and a wide variety of other inflammatory disorders.

In the stomach, prostaglandins inhibit hydrochloric acid secretion. Drugs that inhibit prostaglandin synthesis may make an individual susceptible to peptic ulcers by increasing hydrochloric acid secretion.

FOCUS ON AGING

With age, most endocrine glands show some degree of glandular atrophy, with increased amounts of fibrous tissue and fat deposits. However, the glands remain responsive to stimulation and secrete adequate amounts of hormones. Exceptions to this generalization are the gonads, which are discussed in Chapter 19. There is some evidence of a decline in the rate of hormone secretion, but this may be due to changes in the target tissues that decrease the cellular need for the hormone.

There is also evidence of a reduction in target-tissue receptor sites or in their sensitivity. Whatever the reason for the decline in hormone secretion, it is accompanied by a decreased rate of metabolic destruction so that the blood levels of circulating hormones remain relatively constant throughout senescence. There is no evidence that age-related structural changes in endocrine glands have functional significance or contribute to the overall aging process.

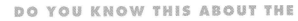

DO YOU KNOW THIS ABOUT THE

Endocrine System?

Diabetes Mellitus

Diabetes mellitus is one of the most common metabolic disorders in the United States, affecting about 4 percent of the American population at some time in their lives. The universal symptom is a chronic elevation in blood sugar levels, or **hyperglycemia,** because body cells are unable to utilize glucose and it remains in the blood. With normal blood sugar levels, all of the glucose that enters the kidney tubules when blood is filtered is later reabsorbed back into the blood and no glucose remains in the urine. In diabetes mellitus, however, the blood glucose levels exceed the renal threshold for reabsorption and the excess glucose appears in the urine. The presence

of glucose in the urine is called **glycosuria,** or sometimes glucosuria.

The hyperglycemia of diabetes mellitus also leads to three "poly" symptoms. Elevated glucose levels in the blood and glucose in the urine result in increased urine production because additional water is needed to carry the sugar load. Increased urine production is called **polyuria.** When large quantities of water are lost in the urine, the body dehydrates. In addition, the high concentration of sugar in the blood tends to pull water out of the cells by osmosis, which leads to further cellular dehydration. This cellular dehydration results in a sense of excessive thirst,

Continued on following page

called **polydipsia,** and a tendency to drink large quantities of water. Even though there is plenty of glucose in the blood, the body cells of diabetics are unable to use it and are starving to death. This leads to feelings of intense and continual hunger, called **polyphagia.** Hyperglycemia and these three "polys" are good indicators in screening for diabetes mellitus.

Insulin, produced by the beta cells in the pancreatic islets, enables glucose to pass through the cell membrane from the blood into the cell. Inside the cells, glucose is used to provide energy (adenosine triphosphate) for the body. In diabetics, insulin is ineffective and glucose remains in the blood. In some cases, the problem is in the beta cells and they do not produce insulin. In other types of diabetes, insulin is produced but a loss of receptor sites on the target cell membranes reduces the uptake of glucose. These two mechanisms of pathogenesis result in two different types of the disease.

Type I diabetes accounts for about 10 percent of all diabetes cases. It is sometimes referred to as **juvenile-onset diabetes** because it usually strikes during the teenage years. In this form, the beta cells are nonfunctional and there is an absolute deficiency of insulin. Type I diabetes is believed to be an autoimmune disease in which the body's own immune system attacks and destroys the beta cells in the pancreas. Without insulin, the body cannot utilize glucose and relies on fatty acids to produce adenosine triphosphate. As a result of fatty acid catabolism, organic acids, called ketones, accumulate in the blood and lower the pH. This is called ketoacidosis and can result in death. Daily injections of insulin are required to prevent death, so this type is called **insulin-dependent diabetes mellitus (IDDM).**

Type II diabetes mellitus is more common than type I and accounts for about 90 percent of all cases. Because this type most often occurs in people who are older than the age of 40, it is sometimes called **maturity-onset diabetes.** People who are overweight have an increased risk for developing type II diabetes. In this form, beta cells produce insulin, but it may be in reduced amounts. Sometimes antidiabetic drugs that stimulate the beta cells to produce more insulin are prescribed for this type and are able to maintain appropriate glucose metabolism. Many type II diabetics have adequate insulin but are less responsive to it because of a loss of insulin receptor sites on the target cells. Clinical symptoms for type II are usually mild and frequently respond well to changes in lifestyle that result in a balanced diet, adequate exercise, and maintenance of body weight within normal limits. Type II diabetes is called **non–insulin-dependent diabetes mellitus (NIDDM).** However, some patients may need insulin injections to control the symptoms.

The symptoms of type I diabetes are dramatic, and patients seek medical care soon after onset. The symptoms of type II are more subtle, and the American Diabetes Association estimates that over 7 million Americans have type II diabetes and are not aware of it. Long-term complications of untreated diabetes include atherosclerosis, heart disease, stroke, reduced circulation and gangrene in the extremities, blindness, and kidney disease. Authorities agree that careful regulation of blood sugar levels is the most important factor in reducing the long-term complications of the disease.

Representative Disorders of the Endocrine System

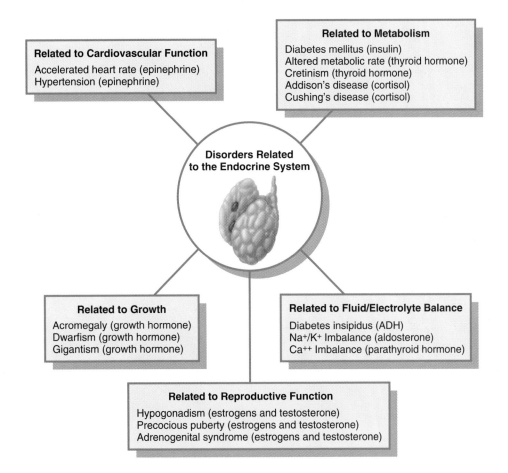

Related to Cardiovascular Function

Accelerated heart rate (epinephrine)
Hypertension (epinephrine)

Related to Metabolism

Diabetes mellitus (insulin)
Altered metabolic rate (thyroid hormone)
Cretinism (thyroid hormone)
Addison's disease (cortisol)
Cushing's disease (cortisol)

**Disorders Related
to the Endocrine System**

Related to Growth

Acromegaly (growth hormone)
Dwarfism (growth hormone)
Gigantism (growth hormone)

Related to Fluid/Electrolyte Balance

Diabetes insipidus (ADH)
Na+/K+ Imbalance (aldosterone)
Ca++ Imbalance (parathyroid hormone)

Related to Reproductive Function

Hypogonadism (estrogens and testosterone)
Precocious puberty (estrogens and testosterone)
Adrenogenital syndrome (estrogens and testosterone)

CHAPTER QUIZ

RECALL

Match the definitions on the left with the appropriate term on the right.

1. Product of an endocrine gland

2. Cells that have receptors for a given hormone

3. Lipid-soluble hormones

4. Produced by the adenohypophysis

5. Produced by the thyroid gland

6. Effect is to conserve sodium and water

7. Secreted by the adrenal medulla

8. Lowers blood glucose levels

9. Has short-term, localized, immediate effect

10. Source of melatonin

A. Aldosterone

B. Calcitonin

C. Epinephrine

D. Growth hormone

E. Hormone

F. Insulin

G. Pineal gland

H. Prostaglandin

I. Steroid

J. Target tissue

THOUGHT

1. Steroid hormones

    a. react with receptors on the surface of the cell membrane

    b. trigger the release of a "second messenger," usually adenosine triphosphate

    c. diffuse through the cell membrane to react with receptors

    d. include the tropic hormones from the adenohypophysis

2. Which of the following hormones is **NOT** produced by the anterior lobe of the pituitary gland?

    a. thyroid-stimulating hormone

    b. antidiuretic hormone

    c. prolactin

    d. luteinizing hormone

3. Which of the following hormones is released in response to a releasing hormone from the hypothalamus?

    a. oxytocin

    b. thyroxine

    c. aldosterone

    d. follicle-stimulating hormone

4. The hormone that is antagonistic (has the opposite effect) to calcitonin is

    a. triiodothyronine

    b. produced by the parathyroid gland

    c. thymosin

    d. produced by the pancreas

5. Susan has eaten a meal that is high in carbohydrates and finished the meal with a large banana split. As a result, her blood glucose level tends to increase. Which of the following will help maintain glucose homeostasis in this instance?

    a. glucagon is released to lower blood glucose

    b. cortisol mobilizes glucose to remove it from the blood

    c. glucagon is released to stimulate the liver to break down glycogen

    d. insulin is released to promote cellular uptake of glucose

APPLICATION

Candy, a high school senior, is pregnant. Also, she really doesn't pay much attention to what she eats—mostly fast foods, potato chips, and candy bars. She never drinks milk; instead, she usually has soft drinks, particularly colas. Under these circumstances, what is likely to happen to the amount of parathyroid hormone released from the gland. Explain.

Joe Cool is studying endocrinology and wants to compare two hormones—insulin and estrogen. Based on your knowledge of the chemical nature of hormones, their receptors, and mechanisms of action, predict which of the two hormones will cause a quicker metabolic response from their target cells. Explain.

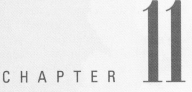

CHAPTER **11**

Blood

Outline/Objectives

Functions and Characteristics of the Blood 226
- Describe the physical characteristics and functions of blood.

Composition of the Blood 227
- Describe the composition of blood plasma.
- Identify the formed elements of the blood and state at least one function for each formed element.
- Discuss the life cycle of erythrocytes.
- Differentiate between five types of leukocytes on the basis of their structure.

Hemostasis 233
- Describe the mechanisms that reduce blood loss after trauma.

Blood Typing and Transfusions 235
- Characterize the different blood types and explain why some are incompatible for transfusions.

Key Terms

Agglutinin
Agglutinogen
Coagulation
Diapedesis
Erythrocyte
Erythropoietin
Hemocytoblast
Hematopoiesis
Leukocyte
Thrombocyte

Building Vocabulary

WORD PART	MEANING
agglutin-	clumping, sticking together
anti-	against
coagul-	clotting
-emia	blood condition
erythr-	red
fibr-	fiber
glob-	ball, globe
hem-	blood
kary-	nucleus
leuk-	white
-lysis	destruction
mon-	single, one
-penia	deficiency, lack of
-phil	love, affinity for
-poiesis	formation of
-rrhage	burst forth, flow
-stasis	control
thromb-	clot

he body consists of metabolically active cells that need a continuous supply of nutrients and oxygen. Metabolic waste products need to be removed from the cells to maintain a stable cellular environment. Blood is the primary transport medium that is responsible for meeting these cellular demands. A central pump, the heart, provides the force to move the blood through a system of vessels that extend throughout the body. The blood, heart, and blood vessels make up the cardiovascular system. This chapter focuses on the blood and how it supports cellular activities.

Functions and Characteristics of the Blood

Blood is one of the connective tissues. As a connective tissue, it consists of cells and cell fragments **(formed elements)** suspended in an intercellular matrix **(plasma).** Blood is the only liquid tissue in the body. The total blood volume in an average adult is 4 to 5 liters in the female and 5 to 6 liters in the male. It accounts for approximately 8 percent of the total body weight. Blood is slightly heavier and four to five times more viscous than water. It is slightly alkaline with a normal pH range between 7.35 and 7.45.

> Blood is a liquid connective tissue that measures about 5 liters in the adult human and accounts for 8 percent of the body weight. Its normal pH range is 7.35 to 7.45.

The activities of the blood may be categorized as **transportation, regulation,** and **protection.** These functional categories overlap and interact as the blood carries out its role in providing suitable conditions for cellular functions. The following activities of blood are transport functions:

- It carries oxygen and nutrients to the cells.
- It transports carbon dioxide and nitrogenous wastes from the tissues to the lungs and kidneys where these wastes can be removed from the body.
- It carries hormones from the endocrine glands to the target tissues.

The following activities of blood are in the regulation category:

- It helps regulate body temperature by removing heat from active areas, such as skeletal muscles, and transporting it to other regions or to the skin where it can be dissipated.
- It plays a significant role in fluid and electrolyte balance because the salts and plasma proteins contribute to the osmotic pressure.
- It functions in pH regulation through the action of buffers in the blood.

Functions of the blood that are in the protection category include the following:

- Its clotting mechanisms prevent fluid loss through hemorrhage when blood vessels are damaged.
- Certain cells in the blood, the phagocytic white blood cells, help to protect the body against micro-

CLINICAL TERMS

Anemia (ah-NEE-mee-ah) Deficiency in red blood cells or hemoglobin; most common form is iron deficiency anemia caused by a lack of iron to make hemoglobin; other types are aplastic anemia, hemolytic anemia, pernicious anemia, sickle cell anemia, and thalassemia

Ecchymosis (eck-ih-MOH-sis) A blue or purplish patch in the skin caused by intradermal hemorrhage; larger than a petechia; a bruise; plural, ecchymoses

Embolus (EMM-boh-lus) A moving clot or other plug; an object, often a blood clot, that moves in the blood until it obstructs a small vessel and blocks circulation

Erythrocytosis (ee-rith-roh-sye-TOH-sis) An increase in the number of red blood cells due to factors other than a disorder of the hematopoietic mechanism; secondary polycythemia

Hemophilia (hee-moh-FILL-ih-ah) Excessive bleeding caused by a congenital lack of one or more of the factors necessary for blood clotting

Leukocytosis (loo-koh-sye-TOH-sis) An increase in the number of white blood cells in the blood, which may result from hemorrhage, fever, infection, inflammation, or other factors

Leukopenia (loo-koh-PEE-nee-ah) A decrease in the number of white blood cells in the blood

Multiple myeloma (MULL-tih-pull my-eh-LOH-mah) Malignant tumor of the bone marrow

Petechia (pee-TEE-kee-ah) A pinpoint, purplish red spot in the skin caused by intradermal hemorrhage; plural petechiae

Polycythemia (pahl-ee-sye-THEE-mee-ah) Any type of increase in the number of red blood cells

Purpura (PER-pyoo-rah) A group of disorders characterized by multiple pinpoint hemorrhages and accumulation of blood under the skin

Reticulocyte (reh-TICK-yoo-loh-syte) An immature red blood cell with a network of granules in its cytoplasm

Thrombocytopenia (thrahm-boh-syte-oh-PEE-nee-ah) A lower than normal number of thrombocytes, or platelets, in the blood

Thrombus (THRAHM-bus) A blood clot.

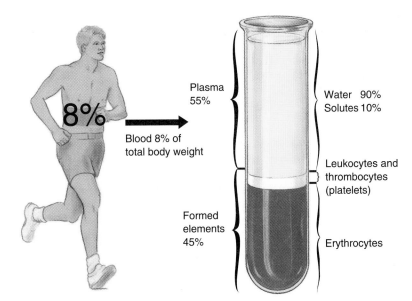

8%

Blood 8% of
total body weight

Plasma
55%

Water 90%
Solutes 10%

Leukocytes and
thrombocytes
(platelets)

Formed
elements
45%

Erythrocytes

Figure 11–1   Composition of the blood.

organisms that cause disease by engulfing and destroying the agent.

• Antibodies in the plasma help protect against disease by their reactions with offending agents.

> Blood functions as a transport medium. It also has roles in temperature regulation, fluid and electrolyte balance, pH regulation, prevention of fluid loss, and disease prevention.

Composition of the Blood

When a sample of blood is spun in a centrifuge, the cells and cell fragments are separated from the liquid intercellular matrix (Fig. 11–1). Because the **formed elements** are heavier than the liquid matrix, they are packed in the bottom of the tube by the centrifugal force. The straw-colored liquid on the top is the **plasma.** Figure 11–1 illustrates that the plasma accounts for about 55 percent of the blood volume and red blood cells make up the remaining 45 percent of the volume. The percentage attributed to the red blood cells is called the **hematocrit** (hee-MAT-oh-krit), or **packed cell volume (PCV).** The white blood cells and platelets form a thin white layer, called the "buffy coat," between the plasma and red blood cells.

> A given volume of blood is 55 percent plasma and 45 percent formed elements.

> **Anemia,** characterized by decreased numbers of red blood cells, results in a reduced hematocrit value. Conditions that have more red blood cells than normal, called polycythemia, show increased hematocrit values.

Plasma

Plasma, the liquid portion of the blood, is about 90 percent water. The remaining portion consists of more than 100 different organic and inorganic solutes dissolved in the water. Table 11–1 summarizes some of the major solutes in plasma. Because plasma is a transport medium, its solutes are continuously changing as substances are added or removed by the cells. With a healthy diet, the plasma is normally in a state of dynamic balance that is maintained by various homeostatic mechanisms.

> Plasma is the liquid portion of blood. It is 90 percent water and 10 percent solutes.

Plasma Proteins

Plasma proteins are the most abundant of the solutes in the plasma. These proteins normally remain in the blood and interstitial fluid and are not used for energy. The three major classes of plasma proteins are:

• Albumins
• Globulins
• Fibrinogen

Table 11–1 Major Solutes in Plasma		
Plasma Proteins	**Nitrogenous Molecules**	**Other**
Albumins—60%	Amino acids	Nutrients
Globulins—36%	Urea	Hormones
Fibrinogen— 4%	Uric acids	Oxygen
		Carbon dioxide
		Antibodies
		Electrolytes

Many of the plasma proteins are synthesized in the liver, and each one has a different function.

> Albumins, globulins, and fibrinogen are the major types of plasma proteins.

Albumins (al-BYOO-mins) account for about 60 percent of the plasma proteins. Albumin molecules are produced in the liver and are the smallest of the plasma protein molecules. Because they are so abundant, they contribute to the osmotic pressure of the blood and play an important role in maintaining fluid balance between the blood and interstitial fluid. If the osmotic pressure of the blood decreases, fluid moves from the blood into the interstitial spaces, which results in edema. This also decreases blood volume and, in severe cases, may reduce blood pressure. When blood osmotic pressure increases, fluid moves from the interstitial spaces into the blood and increases blood volume. This increases blood pressure and decreases the amount of water available to the cells.

> The most abundant plasma proteins are albumins, which maintain the osmotic pressure of the blood.

Globulins (GLOB-yoo-lins) account for about 36 percent of the plasma proteins. There are three types of globulins:

- Alpha
- Beta
- Gamma

Alpha and beta globulins are produced in the liver and function in transporting lipids and fat-soluble vitamins in the blood. Gamma globulins are the antibodies that function in immunity. These are produced in lymphoid tissue.

> Globulins function in lipid transport and in immune reactions.

The remaining 4 percent of the plasma proteins is **fibrinogen** (fye-BRIN-oh-jen), which is the largest of the plasma protein molecules. It is produced in the liver and functions in blood clotting. During the clotting process, a series of reactions converts the soluble fibrinogen into insoluble fibrin, which forms the foundation of a blood clot. When blood clots in a test tube, the liquid that remains is called **serum.** It is similar to plasma but has no fibrinogen because the fibrinogen is converted to fibrin.

> Fibrinogen makes up the smallest fraction of plasma proteins. It functions in the formation of blood clots.

Nonprotein Molecules That Contain Nitrogen

Along with the proteins, some other plasma solutes contain nitrogen. These include amino acids, urea, and uric acid. The amino acids are the products of protein digestion. They are absorbed into the blood and are transported to the cells that need them. Urea and uric acid are waste products of protein and nucleic acid catabolism. These molecules are transported to the kidneys for excretion.

Table 11–2 Formed Elements in the Blood			
Formed Element	**Description**	**Number**	**Function**
Erythrocytes	Biconcave disk; no nucleus; 7–8 μm in diameter	4.5–6.0 million/mm³	Transport oxygen and some carbon dioxide
Leukocytes	Nucleated cells	5,000–9,000/mm³	Part of the body's defense against disease
Neutrophil	Nucleus with 2 to 5 lobes; indistinct granules in the cytoplasm; 12–15 μm in diameter	60–70% of total WBCs	Phagocytosis
Eosinophils	Nucleus bilobed; red-staining granules in the cytoplasm; 10–12 μm in diameter	2–4% of total WBCs	Counteract histamine in allergic reactions; destroy parasitic worms
Basophils	Nucleus U-shaped or bilobed; granules in cytoplasm stain blue; 10–12 μm in diameter	Less than 1% of total WBCs	Release histamine and the anticoagulant heparin; called mast cells in the tissues
Lymphocytes	Agranulocyte; small cell with large round nucleus; 6–8 μm in diameter	20–25% of total WBCs	Produce antibodies; function in immunity
Monocytes	Agranulocyte; large cells with bean-shaped nucleus; may be 20 μm in diameter	3–8% of total WBCs	Phagocytosis; engulf relatively large particles; called macrophages in the tissues
Thrombocytes	Cell fragments of megakaryocytes; 2–5 μm in diameter	250,000–500,000/mm³	Help control blood loss by forming platelet plug and releasing factors necessary for blood clotting

Some of the solutes in plasma include derivatives of proteins and nucleic acids. These molecules add to the nitrogen content of the blood.

Nutrients and Gases

The simple nutrients that are the end products of digestion are transported in the blood so that they form a fraction of the plasma solutes. These nutrients include the amino acids from protein digestion, glucose and other simple sugars from carbohydrate digestion, and fatty acids from lipid digestion.

Oxygen and carbon dioxide are the main respiratory gases that are found as solutes in the plasma. About 3 percent of the oxygen and 7 to 10 percent of the carbon dioxide are transported as dissolved gases. Nitrogen is another gas that dissolves in the plasma, but it has little, if any, function in the human body.

Nutrients, oxygen, and carbon dioxide are transported as solutes in the plasma.

Electrolytes

Most of the electrolytes that are solutes in the plasma are inorganic ions, and they contribute to the osmotic pressure of the plasma. In addition, some are important in maintaining membrane potentials and others are significant in regulating the pH of body fluids. Common electrolytes found in the plasma include sodium (Na^+), potassium (K^+), calcium (Ca^{++}), chloride (Cl^-), bicarbonate (HCO_3^-), and phosphate (PO_4^{-3}).

Electrolytes contribute to the osmotic pressure of the blood, maintain membrane potentials, and regulate the pH of body fluids.

Formed Elements

The formed elements are cells and cell fragments suspended in the plasma. The three classes of formed elements are the **erythrocytes** (ee-RITH-roh-sytes), or red blood cells, the **leukocytes** (LOO-koh-sytes), or white blood cells, and the **thrombocytes** (THROM-boh-sytes), or platelets. Table 11–2 summarizes the formed elements in the blood.

Formed elements in the blood are erythrocytes, leukocytes, and thrombocytes.

The production of these formed elements, or blood cells, is called **hematopoiesis** (hemopoiesis). Before birth, hematopoiesis (hee-ma-to-poy-EE-sis) occurs primarily in the liver and spleen, but some cells develop in the thymus, lymph nodes, and red bone marrow. After birth, most production is limited to the red bone marrow in specific regions, but some white blood cells are produced in lymphoid tissue. All types of formed elements develop from a single cell type, as illustrated in Figure 11–2. The precursor cell, or stem cell, is called a **hemocytoblast** (hee-moh-SYTE-oh-blast). Seven different cell lines, each controlled by a specific growth factor, develop from the hemocytoblast.

All formed elements of the blood develop from a cell called a hemocytoblast. Hematopoiesis is the production of formed elements.

By the age of 25 years, a person's red bone marrow for **hematopoiesis** is limited to the flat bones of the skull, the iliac crests, ribs, sternum, vertebrae, and the proximal ends of the humerus and femur.

One area of current medical research involves developing viable options to bone marrow transplants. One such option is the harvesting of stem cells from umbilical cord blood. These cells develop into the different cell types that form bone marrow, make blood, and restore the immune system. Early results indicate a reduction in the number of difficulties commonly associated with other types of donor transplants. If found to be clinically successful, cord blood would be readily available because it is a painless, noninvasive donor procedure involving the umbilical cord and placenta, which are routinely discarded after births. As in all other transplant procedures, the highest ethical standards must be followed.

Erythrocytes

Characteristics and Functions. Erythrocytes (ee-RITH-roh-sytes), or red blood cells (RBCs), are the most numerous of the formed elements. Although the number varies, the normal range for a healthy adult male is 4.5 to 6 million RBCs per cubic millimeter (mm^3) of blood. The normal for females is slightly less. Erythrocytes are tiny **biconcave disks** about 7.5 micrometers (μm) in diameter. They are thin in the middle and thicker around the periphery. The shape of the RBC provides a combination of flexibility for moving through tiny capillaries with a maximum surface area for the diffusion of gases. Mature RBCs are **anucleate.** During development, the nucleus and most other organelles are lost from the cell, presumably to give more room for hemoglobin. Because the mature cells are anucleate, they cannot undergo mitosis, which means that replacement cells have to develop from the stem cells. Erythrocytes normally move from the bone marrow into the blood while they are still immature, but after they lose the nucleus. These immature erythrocytes that are circulating in the blood are called **reticulocytes.**

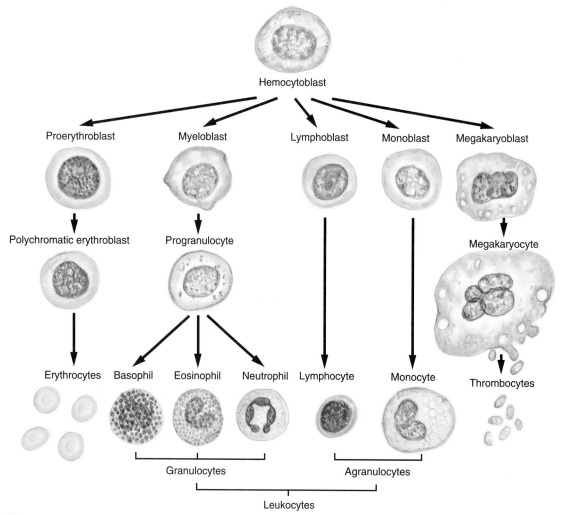

Figure 11-2   Development of the formed elements.

Erythrocytes, or red blood cells, are anucleate, biconcave disks, about 7.5 μm in diameter. There are 4.5 to 6 million RBCs/mm³ of blood.

The primary function of erythrocytes is to transport oxygen and, to a lesser extent, carbon dioxide. This function is directly related to the **hemoglobin** (hee-moh-GLOH-bin) within the RBC. About one third of each erythrocyte consists of hemoglobin. This molecule has two parts: **heme** and **globin.** The heme portion is formed from a pigment that contains iron. The globin portion is a protein. In the lungs, the heme portion combines with oxygen to form **oxyhemoglobin** (ok-see-hee-moh-GLOH-bin), which is bright red. About 97 percent of the oxygen used by the tissue cells is transported as oxyhemoglobin. In the tissues, the oxygen is released to diffuse into the tissue cells. This produces a reduced form, called **deoxyhemoglobin** (dee-ok-see-hee-moh-GLOH-bin), which has a darker color.

The main function of erythrocytes is to transport oxygen, which is usually combined with hemoglobin.

About 20 percent of a cigarette smoker's hemoglobin is nonfunctional for transporting oxygen because it is bound to carbon monoxide from the cigarette smoke.

Production of Erythrocytes. Erythrocyte production is regulated by a negative feedback mechanism that uses the hormone **erythropoietin** (ee-rith-roh-POY-ee-tin) to stimulate erythrocyte production (Fig. 11–3). The liver produces erythropoietin in an inactive form and secretes it into the blood. The kidneys produce a **renal erythropoietic factor** (REF), which activates the erythropoietin. When blood oxygen concentration is low, the kidneys release REF into

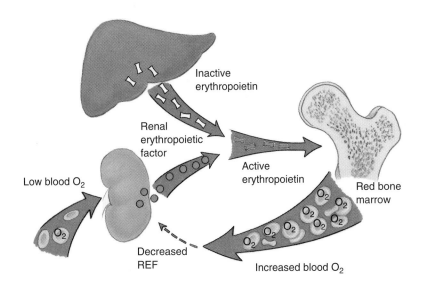

Figure 11–3   Regulation of erythrocyte production.

the blood, which activates the erythropoietin, which then stimulates the red bone marrow to produce RBCs. The additional RBCs combine with oxygen to increase the blood oxygen concentration. As blood oxygen concentration increases, REF decreases, active erythropoietin decreases, and RBC production decreases.

> The formation of red blood cells is regulated by erythropoietin.

> The **reticulocyte count** in circulating blood gives information about the rate of hematopoiesis. Normally 0.5 to 1.5 percent of the RBCs in normal blood are reticulocytes. A number below 0.5 percent indicates a slowdown in production. Values above 1.5 percent indicate a greater than normal rate of RBC formation.

Iron, vitamin B_{12}, and folic acid are essential to normal RBC production. The iron is necessary for the synthesis of normal hemoglobin. Iron deficiency anemia results when there is a lack of iron in the diet. This results in a reduced amount of hemoglobin, which decreases the blood's oxygen carrying capacity. All cells in the body require vitamins B_{12} and folic acid for normal formation. This is especially significant in erythrocytes because of the large numbers produced every day. Certain cells in the stomach produce **intrinsic factor,** a factor necessary for the absorption of vitamin B_{12} in the intestines. Without intrinsic factor, vitamin B_{12}, even though present in the diet, is not absorbed and the cells are defective. This condition is called **pernicious anemia.**

> Iron, vitamin B_{12}, and folic acid are essential to normal RBC production.

Destruction of Erythrocytes. Normal erythrocytes live for about 120 days. During this time they travel thousands of miles as they circulate through the body. Normally the erythrocytes have a flexible cell membrane that allows them to bend and squeeze through the capillaries. As they age, their membrane loses its elasticity and becomes fragile. When they are defective or worn out, macrophages, which are phagocytic cells in the spleen and liver, remove them from circulation and they are replaced by an equal number of new cells. Under typical conditions, over 2 million erythrocytes are destroyed and replaced every second!

> Erythrocytes usually function for about 120 days, then are destroyed by the spleen and liver.

When RBCs are destroyed, the hemoglobin is separated into its heme and globin components (Fig 11–4). The protein portion of the hemoglobin in the erythrocyte is broken down into its constituent amino acids, which are added to the supply of amino acids available in the body. The heme portion of the molecule is broken down into an iron compound and bilirubin, a yellow bile pigment. The liver recycles the iron and sends it to the bone marrow for new hemoglobin. Bilirubin becomes part of the bile, which is secreted by the liver, and is carried in the bile duct to the small intestine.

> When RBCs are destroyed, the body reuses the iron and protein in the hemoglobin. The pigment portion is converted to bilirubin and secreted in the bile.

> **Hemolytic anemia** is a reduction in erythrocytes due to excessive destruction. The excessive destruction leads to jaundice because of the accumulation of bilirubin in the blood.

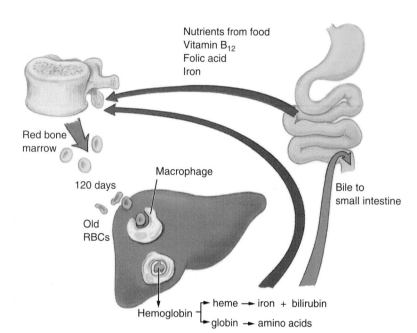

Nutrients from food
Vitamin B$_{12}$
Folic acid
Iron

Red bone marrow

120 days

Macrophage

Old RBCs

Bile to small intestine

Hemoglobin $\left\{\begin{array}{l} \text{heme} \rightarrow \text{iron + bilirubin} \\ \text{globin} \rightarrow \text{amino acids} \end{array}\right.$

Figure 11-4 Life cycle of red blood cells and breakdown of hemoglobin.

Leukocytes

Characteristics and Functions. Leukocytes (LOO-koh-sytes), or white blood cells (WBCs), are generally larger than erythrocytes, but they are fewer. An average leukocyte count ranges between 5,000 and 9,000 per cubic millimeter. All leukocytes are derived from hemocytoblast stem cells (see Fig. 11-2), but they do not lose their nuclei or accumulate hemoglobin during development. The lack of hemoglobin makes them appear whitish.

Even though they are considered to be blood cells, leukocytes do most of their work in the tissues. They use the blood as a transport medium. Some are phagocytic, others produce antibodies, some secrete histamine and heparin, and others neutralize histamine. Leukocytes are able to move through the capillary walls into the tissue spaces, a process called **diapedesis** (dye-ah-peh-DEE-sis). In the tissue spaces they provide a defense against organisms that cause disease and either promote or inhibit inflammatory responses.

> Leukocytes are WBCs. They have a nucleus, do not have hemoglobin, average between 5,000/mm^3 and 6,000/mm^3, and move through capillary walls by diapedesis.

Types of Leukocytes. There are two main groups of leukocytes in the blood. The cells that develop granules in the cytoplasm are called **granulocytes** and those that do not have granules are called **agranulocytes. Neutrophils, eosinophils,** and **basophils** are granulocytes. **Monocytes** and **lymphocytes** are agranulocytes.

> Granulocytes have cytoplasmic granules that stain with certain dyes. Agranulocytes do not have granules.

Neutrophils (NOO-troh-fills) are the most common type of leukocyte. These granulocytes make up 60 to 70 percent of the total number of WBCs. They are characterized by a multilobed nucleus (usually three to five lobes), and inconspicuous granules in the cytoplasm that stain pink with a neutral stain. Neutrophils are the first leukocytes to respond to tissue damage where they engulf bacteria by phagocytosis. The number of neutrophils increases significantly in acute infections.

> Neutrophils, the most numerous leukocytes, are phagocytic and have light-colored granules.

Eosinophils (ee-oh-SIN-oh-fills), which make up 2 to 4 percent of the WBCs, are characterized by a nucleus with two lobes and large granules in the cytoplasm that stain red with acid stains. These granulocytes neutralize histamine and their number increases during allergic reactions. They also destroy parasitic worms.

> Eosinophils have red granules and help counteract the effects of histamine.

Basophils (BAY-soh-fills), the least numerous of the leukocytes, usually account for less than 1 percent of the total WBCs. These granulocytes are about the same size as an eosinophil and have a nucleus that has two lobes or is U-shaped. The cytoplasm has large granules that stain dark blue with basic stains. Basophils that leave the blood and enter the tissues are called **mast cells.** In the tissues, mast cells secrete histamine and heparin. Histamine dilates blood vessels to increase blood flow to damaged tissues. It also dilates blood vessels in allergic reactions. Heparin is an anticoagulant; it inhibits blood clot formation.

> Basophils secrete histamine and heparin and have blue granules. In the tissues, they are called mast cells.

Lymphocytes (LIM-foh-sytes) account for 20 to 25 percent of the WBCs in the blood. These agranulocytes have a large spherical nucleus that is surrounded by a small amount of cytoplasm. They are especially abundant in lymphoid tissue and have an important role in the body's defense against disease. One group, the T lymphocytes, directly attacks invading microorganisms such as bacteria and viruses. Another group, the B lymphocytes, responds by producing antibodies that react with microorganisms or with bacterial toxins.

> Lymphocytes are agranulocytes that have a special role in immune processes. Some attack bacteria directly; others produce antibodies.

Monocytes (MON-oh-sytes), the largest of the WBCs, make up 3 to 8 percent of the leukocytes in the blood. These agranulocytes have a U- or bean-shaped nucleus surrounded by abundant cytoplasm. When monocytes leave the blood and enter the tissues they are called **macrophages** (MACK-roh-fahj-es). In damaged tissues, the macrophages engulf bacteria and cellular debris to finish the cleanup process started by the neutrophils.

> Monocytes are large phagocytic agranulocytes. In the tissues they are called macrophages.

A **differential count** determines the number of each of the different types of leukocytes. The cells are stained and a minimum of 100 cells are counted under a microscope. The numbers of neutrophils, lymphocytes, monocytes, basophils, and eosinophils are given as percentages.

Thrombocytes

Thrombocytes (THROM-boh-sytes), or **platelets,** are not complete cells, but are small fragments of very large cells called **megakaryocytes.** Megakaryocytes (meg-ah-KAIR-ee-oh-sytes) develop from hemocytoblasts in the red bone marrow. Platelets are one-third to one-half the size of an erythrocyte, and an average platelet count ranges from 250,000 to 500,000 platelets/mm³ of blood. Thrombocytes become sticky and clump together to form platelet plugs that close breaks and tears in blood vessels. They also initiate the formation of blood clots.

> Thrombocytes are fragments of megakaryocytes that function in blood clotting.

 QuickCheck

- Liver disease may lead to a decrease in plasma proteins. How would this affect the functions of the blood?

- How does an increase in oxygen delivery to the kidneys affect the level of active erythropoietin in the blood?

- WBCs circulate in the blood, but their effective work is in the tissue spaces. How do the cells get from the blood to the tissue spaces?

Hemostasis

Blood vessels that are torn or cut permit blood to escape into the surrounding tissues or to the outside of the body. This has damaging effects on the tissues and, in cases of excessive blood loss, may result in death. Whenever blood vessels are injured, several reactions occur that attempt to minimize blood loss and tissue damage. The stoppage of bleeding is called **hemostasis** (hee-moh-STAY-sis). It includes three separate but interrelated processes:

- Vascular constriction
- Platelet plug formation
- Coagulation

> Hemostasis, the stoppage of bleeding, includes vascular constriction, formation of a platelet plug, and coagulation.

Vascular Constriction

The first response to blood vessel injury is contraction of the smooth muscle in the vessel walls. This creates a **vascular constriction,** or **spasm,** that restricts the flow of blood through the opening in the vessel. The initial vascular spasm lasts for only a few minutes but allows enough time for the other aspects of hemostasis to begin. As platelets accumulate at the site of the injury, they secrete **serotonin,** a chemical that stimulates smooth muscle contraction and that prolongs the vascular spasm.

> Vascular constriction is the initial reaction that reduces the flow of blood through the opening in a torn or severed vessel.

Platelet Plug Formation

Normally platelets do not stick to each other or to the endothelium that lines blood vessel walls. When the lining of the blood vessel breaks, the underlying connective tissue is exposed. Collagen in the connective tissue attracts the platelets and they accumulate in the damaged region, where they adhere to the connective tissue and to each other. This creates a mass of platelets, a **platelet plug,** that obstructs the tear in the vessel. Normal daily activities create numerous tears in minute blood vessels, and these are closed by platelet plugs so that there is no blood loss or damage to surrounding tissues.

> Collagen in damaged vessels attracts platelets, which form a platelet plug to fill the gap in a broken vessel. This reduces blood loss.

Coagulation

The third and most effective mechanism in hemostasis is the formation of a blood clot, or **coagulation** (koh-ag-yoo-LAY-shun). The blood contains factors, called **procoagulants,** that promote clotting. It also contains **anticoagulants** that inhibit clotting. Normally the anticoagulants predominate and override the procoagulants so that the blood remains fluid and does not clot. When vessels are damaged, the procoagulants increase their activity, which results in the formation of a clot.

The formation of a blood clot involves a complex series of chemical reactions and includes numerous clotting factors that are present in the plasma. Even though it is a complex process, it can be summarized in three main steps, as illustrated in Figure 11–5.

1. Platelets and damaged tissues release chemicals that initiate a series of reactions that result in the formation of **prothrombin activator.**

2. In the presence of calcium ions and prothrombin activator, **prothrombin** (pro-THROM-bin) in the plasma is converted from an inactive form to active **thrombin.**

3. Thrombin, in the presence of calcium ions, acts as an enzyme to convert inactive and soluble **fibrinogen** (fye-BRIN-oh-jen) into active and insoluble **fibrin.** The fibrin threads form a mesh that adheres to the damaged tissue and traps blood cells and platelets to form the clot.

Platelets and all the necessary clotting factors must be available for successful clot formation. The liver produces most of the clotting factors, and many of them require vitamin K for their synthesis. Numerous reactions in the clotting process also require calcium ions. A low platelet count (thrombocytopenia), deficiency of vitamin K or calcium, and liver dysfunction can impair the clotting process.

> Coagulation is a multistep process that starts with the formation of prothrombin activator, continues with the conversion of prothrombin to thrombin, and ends with fibrinogen changing to fibrin. Calcium and vitamin K are necessary for successful clot formation.

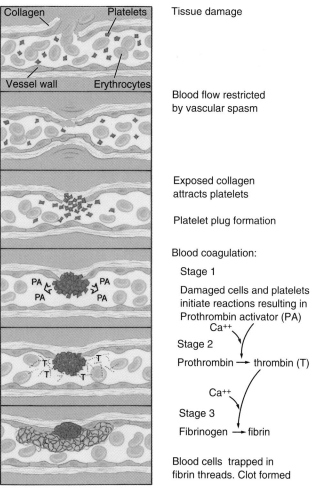

Figure 11–5 Hemostasis.

> The K in vitamin K is for "Koagulation," the German word for clotting. In other words, vitamin K is the "Koagulation" vitamin. Although this vitamin is necessary in the diet, it is also produced by bacteria in the large intestine and absorbed into the blood.

After a clot has formed, the fibrin strands contract. This process, called clot retraction, causes the clot to condense or shrink. Clot retraction pulls the edges of the damaged tissue closer together, reduces the flow of blood, reduces the probability of infection, and enhances healing. Fibroblasts migrate into the clot and form fibrous connective tissue that repairs the damaged area. As healing occurs, the clot is dissolved by a process called **fibrinolysis** (fye-brin-AHL-ih-sis).

> After a clot forms, it condenses or retracts to pull the edges of the wound together. As healing takes place, the clot dissolves by fibrinolysis.

One way to prevent excessive bleeding is to speed up the clotting process. This may be done by applying a rough surface such as gauze, by applying heat, or by pinching the area around the wound. Each of these causes platelets to disintegrate. In severe cases, purified thrombin or fibrin may be applied.

Blood Typing and Transfusions

When an individual loses a quantity of blood, the volume must be restored to prevent shock and death. Sometimes it is sufficient to replace the volume with plasma or a special preparation of solutes. Other times, erythrocytes must also be replaced to restore the oxygen carrying capacity of the blood. A **transfusion** is the transfer of blood, plasma, or other solution into the blood of another individual.

Early transfusion attempts produced varied results. Some transfusions were successful and the recipient benefitted from the procedure. Other transfusions resulted in reactions that were detrimental to the recipient, frequently causing death. In these cases, the RBCs clumped together and obstructed blood vessels and damaged the kidneys. The reactions also caused hemolysis (hee-MAHL-ih-sis), or rupture of the RBCs. These unsuccessful attempts led to the discovery of blood types and procedures for accurately typing blood for safe transfusions.

Agglutinogens and Agglutinins

The clumping of RBCs in unsuccessful transfusions is caused by interactions between antigens and antibodies. Antigens are molecules, usually proteins, that elicit a response from antibodies. Antibodies are protein molecules usually found in gamma globulin that are produced by certain lymphocytes in response to a foreign antigen. Antibodies are very specific, which means that a particular antibody will combine with only one certain type of antigen and no others. There are thousands of different antigens and antibodies in the body, but blood types are based on those specifically related to the RBCs.

> Blood types are based on specific antigens and antibodies related to RBCs.

Specific blood type antigens, called **agglutinogens** (ah-gloo-TIN-oh-jens), are found in the cell membrane of erythrocytes. Antibodies, called **agglutinins** (ah-GLOO-tih-nins), are in the plasma and are formed after birth. When agglutinins in the plasma combine with agglutinogens on the surface of the RBC, the result is **agglutination** (ah-GLOO-tih-nay-shun), a clumping of the RBCs. The agglutinogens on the red blood cells are organized into blood groups. Although many blood groups are recognized, the ABO and Rh groups are the most important.

> Blood type antigens, on the surface of RBCs, are agglutinogens. The antibodies in the plasma are called agglutinins.

ABO Blood Groups

The ABO blood groups are based on the presence or absence of certain agglutinogens (antigens) on the surface of the RBC membrane. These agglutinogens, A and B, are inherited; consequently blood types are also inherited. Type A blood has type A agglutinogens; type B blood has type B agglutinogens; type AB blood has both type A and type B agglutinogens; and type O blood has neither type A nor type B agglutinogens (Fig. 11–6). Certain agglutinins develop in the plasma shortly after birth. Specifically, a person with type A agglutinogens (type A blood) develops anti-B agglutinins; a person with type B agglutinogens (type B blood) develops anti-A agglutinins; a person with both type A and type B agglutinogens (type AB blood) develops neither anti-A nor anti-B agglutinins; and a person with neither type A nor type B agglutinogens (type O blood) develops both anti-A and anti-B agglutinins (see Fig. 11–6). Table 11–3 summarizes the agglutinogens and agglutinins of the ABO blood groups.

> Type A blood has A agglutinogens, type B blood has B agglutinogens, type AB blood has both A and B agglutinogens, and type O has neither agglutinogen.

A **donor** is a person who gives blood, and a **recipient** is the person who receives blood. Because agglutinins of one type will react with the same type agglutinogen, anti-A agglutinins react with type A agglutinogens, and anti-B agglutinins react with type B agglutinogens, these combinations must be avoided. The major concern in blood transfusions is that the agglutinins in the plasma of the recipient's blood not react with, or agglutinate, the cells of the donor's blood. A person (recipient) with type A blood should not receive type B blood (donor) because the anti-B agglutinins in the type A recipient will agglutinate the type B agglutinogens in the donor's blood (Fig. 11–7). Similar conditions exist when the recipient has type B blood and the donor has type A blood.

> In transfusion reactions involving mismatched blood, the recipient's agglutinins react with the donor's agglutinogens.

Because type AB blood has neither anti-A nor anti-B agglutinins to react with donor agglutinogens, it appears that a person with this type can receive blood of any type. For this reason, type AB blood is called the **universal recipient.** Type O blood has neither type A nor type B agglutinogen on the RBC so it is called the **universal donor.** The terms universal recipient and universal donor are misleading

Type A 40%

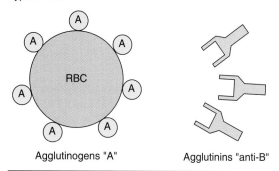

Agglutinogens "A"   Agglutinins "anti-B"

Type B 10%

Agglutinogens "B"   Agglutinins "anti-A"

Type AB 4%

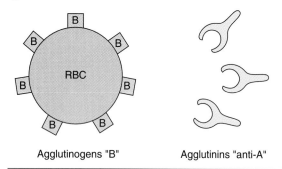

Agglutinogens "A" & "B"   No agglutinins

Type O 46%

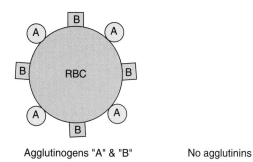

No agglutinogens   Agglutinins "anti-A" & "anti-B"

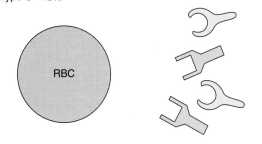

Figure 11-6 Agglutinogens (antigens) and agglutinins (antibodies) involved in the ABO blood groups.

because the agglutinins of the donor may react with agglutinogens of the recipient. Usually these reactions are not serious because the donor's agglutinins are diluted in the recipient's blood. In emergency, life-or-death situations, type O blood may be given

Table 11-3 Agglutinogens and Agglutinins in ABO Blood Types		
Blood Type	Agglutinogens on the Red Blood Cell	Agglutinins in the Plasma
A	A	anti-B
B	B	anti-A
AB	Both A and B	Neither anti-A nor anti-B
O	Neither A nor B	Both anti-A and anti-B

to a person with another type or a person with type AB blood may receive other types because the alternative is death. It is always best to use donor blood of the same type as the recipient blood, including the same Rh factor, which is discussed in the next section. Table 11-4 indicates the preferred and permissible donor types for each recipient type.

Type O blood is called the universal donor, and type AB is called the universal recipient.

Blood doping is a practice reportedly used by some athletes to improve their endurance for aerobic activities such as running, swimming, and cycling. A few weeks before the competition, blood is drawn from the athlete and the RBCs are separated and frozen. Normal hematopoiesis replaces the lost RBCs and brings the blood cell count back to normal. Then, just before the competition, the frozen RBCs are thawed and injected into the athlete. This creates an artificial polycythemia. The idea is that the additional RBCs are able to deliver more oxygen to the muscles and improve aerobic endurance. Whether this occurs is questionable and the practice is not without danger. All blood transfusions carry some risk. Furthermore, the additional cells increase the viscosity of the blood and put a strain on the heart.

Table 11-4 Preferred and Permissible Blood Types for Transfusions		
Recipient Blood Type	Preferred Donor Blood Type	Additional Types Acceptable
A+	A+	A−, O+, O−
A−	A−	O−
B+	B+	B−, O+, O−
B−	B−	O−
AB+	AB+	AB−, A+, A−, B+, B−, O+, O−
AB−	AB−	A−, B−, O−
O+	O+	O−
O−	O−	None

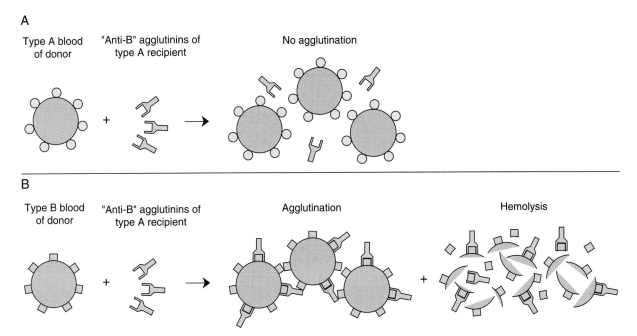

Figure 11-7 Agglutination reactions.

RH Blood Groups

Even after the ABO blood groups were well established and accurate blood typing procedures were developed, there were still unexplained cases of transfusion reactions. This led to more research, which led to the discovery of the Rh factor. It is called Rh because it was first studied in the rhesus monkey.

People are Rh positive (Rh+) if they have Rh agglutinogens on the surface of their red blood cells. About 85 percent of the population are Rh+. The other 15 percent do not have the Rh agglutinogens and they are Rh negative (Rh−). The presence or absence of Rh agglutinogens is an inherited trait. Normally, neither Rh+ nor Rh− individuals have anti-Rh agglutinins. If an Rh− person is exposed to Rh+ blood, either through a blood transfusion or by transfer of blood between a mother and fetus, the Rh− individual develops anti-Rh agglutinins. If that individual is exposed to Rh+ blood a second time, a transfusion reaction results. When transfusions are given, it is necessary to match both the Rh type and the ABO type (see Table 11-4).

> Rh+ blood has Rh agglutinogens on the RBCs; Rh− blood does not have these agglutinogens. Normally, neither has anti-Rh agglutinins in the plasma.

Hemolytic disease of the newborn (formerly called erythroblastosis fetalis) is a special problem associated with the Rh blood groups. This occurs in some pregnancies when the mother is Rh− and the fetus is Rh+ (Fig. 11-8). If some of the fetal Rh+ blood mixes with the maternal Rh− blood, usually through ruptured blood vessels in the placenta during birth, the mother is sensitized and develops anti-Rh agglutinins over a period of time. In a subsequent pregnancy with an Rh+ fetus, the anti-Rh agglutinins from the mother pass through the placenta and react with the Rh agglutinogens on the fetal RBCs. The reaction causes agglutination and hemolysis of fetal RBCs, which reduces the oxygen-carrying capacity of the blood. Clumps of RBCs may obstruct blood vessels and cause damage, especially in the kidney. Excessive destruction of the fetal blood causes increased bilirubin, which produces jaundice. Oxygen deficiency and high bilirubin concentrations may cause brain damage.

> Hemolytic disease of the newborn may develop when an Rh− mother has an Rh+ fetus.

If hemolytic disease of the newborn develops, the Rh+ blood of the fetus or newborn is slowly removed and replaced with Rh− blood. This provides RBCs that will not be affected by the anti-Rh agglutinins, increases the oxygen-carrying capacity of the infant's blood, and reduces the bilirubin level. Gradually, the transfused Rh− blood is destroyed by normal physiologic processes. Remember, the life span of an RBC is 120 days. Hematopoiesis in the infant's red bone marrow replaces it with Rh+ cells, but by this time the maternal agglutinins have disappeared.

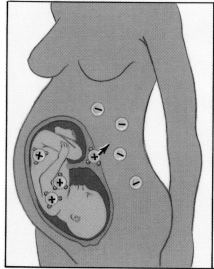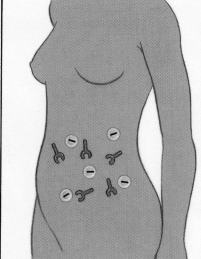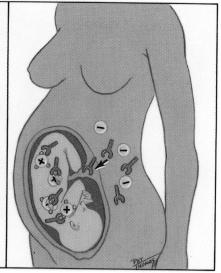

First pregnancy Rh⁻ mother exposed to Rh+ agglutinogens.

After exposure, Rh⁻ mother produces anti-Rh agglutinins.

Second pregnancy with Rh+ fetus. Anti-Rh agglutinins cause agglutination of fetal red blood cells.

Figure 11–8   Development of hemolytic disease in the newborn.

If hemolytic disease of the newborn develops, the fetal blood is temporarily replaced with Rh− blood.

Hemolytic disease of the newborn often may be prevented by treating the Rh− mother with a special preparation of anti-Rh gamma globulin (RhoGAM) during pregnancy or immediately after each delivery of an Rh+ baby. This inactivates any Rh+ agglutinogens that may enter the mother's blood, preventing the development of anti-Rh agglutinins. The agglutinins in the RhoGAM soon disappear and present no problem for future pregnancies.

 QuickCheck

- A sample of bone marrow has fewer than normal megakaryocytes. How will this affect blood clotting?
- A person with liver disease bruises easily. Why?
- A person with type A+ blood wants to donate blood to a friend who is AB+. Theoretically, is this transfusion permissible? Why?

● FOCUS ON AGING

The blood appears to be rather resistant to the aging process and under normal conditions blood values remain normal. The volume and composition remain consistent. Blood cells retain their normal size, shape, and structure. The amount of red bone marrow decreases with age so the capability for blood cell formation decreases, but the hematopoietic mechanisms are still adequate for normal replacement so that blood cell counts and hemoglobin levels stay within normal ranges. Unusual circumstances, such as hemorrhage, may put a strain on the hematopoietic mechanism so it takes longer to rebuild after a hemorrhagic event.

There is an increase in blood-related disorders with age, but these are secondary to other etiologic factors and are not primary disorders in the blood. For example, there is an increased incidence of anemia in the elderly, but this is often due to nutritional deficiencies rather than to a problem within the blood itself. There appears to be an increase in the incidence of leukemia, but this is caused by a breakdown in the immune system. Abnormal thrombus and embolus formation in the elderly is usually due to atherosclerosis in the blood vessels and is not a problem of the clotting factors within the blood. These examples illustrate that increases in the incidence of blood-related disorders in the elderly are usually secondary to disease processes elsewhere in the body.

Blood?

Bloodborne Pathogens

The reported incidence of diseases transmitted by pathogens that are carried in the blood (bloodborne pathogens) has increased alarmingly within the past decade. This has become a major concern in health care institutions where employees are likely to come in contact with blood and other potentially infectious materials. In December 1991, the Occupational Safety and Health Administration (OSHA) issued their bloodborne pathogens standard, "Occupational Exposure to Bloodborne Pathogens: Final Rule." This standard requires health care institutions to initiate practices aimed at protecting their employees from occupational exposure to **all** bloodborne pathogens. The main thrust of the initiative is directed toward the **hepatitis B virus (HBV)** and the **human immunodeficiency virus (HIV)** because these are the most common and well-known pathogens transmitted through occupational exposure to blood and body fluids.

Worldwide, it is estimated that 300 million people are infected with HBV. More than a million of these are in the United States. Among health care workers, the number of new infections ranges from 6,000 to 12,000 per year.

The virus is found in blood, saliva, and semen. Mothers who are infected with HBV can transmit the virus to their children before, during, or after birth. Because it is present in blood, it is also transmitted through needlesticks. The virus can remain active in dried blood for at least a week, but it is inactivated by heat and chemical sterilization procedures.

Hepatitis B has a long incubation period, ranging from 45 to 160 days. Many infected people never exhibit overt symptoms, but they can still transmit the virus. Others develop acute hepatitis with symptoms of abdominal pain, nausea, and jaundice after the incubation period, and liver damage may result. Most people recover completely from the acute form, but others become chronically infected and show symptoms ranging from fatigue to cirrhosis of the liver. Occasionally, a massive infection that destroys a large portion of the liver develops and is fatal. The most serious consequence of HBV is hepatocellular carcinoma. The virus is a known human carcinogen, and the carriers of the virus are 100 times more likely to develop this form of cancer than the noninfected population. The best protection against HBV is immunization, which is 90 to 95 percent effective in healthy people.

HIV is the agent that causes **acquired immunodeficiency syndrome (AIDS).** This is relatively new in the list of human diseases because it was first recognized as a discrete disease in 1981, and the virus was first isolated in 1983. The initial response to HIV invasion is a moderate decrease in the number of **helper T cells** in the immune system. At this time, people usually experience a brief flulike illness with nausea, weakness, and fever. The immune system quickly responds by making antibodies against HIV and the number of helper T cells returns to nearly normal. These infected individuals test positive for HIV antibodies but typically have few, if any, clinical signs or symptoms, and do not yet have AIDS.

After a latent period of 2 to 10 years, the virus becomes reactivated by some mechanism that is not understood, and the helper T cell population declines. At this point, the individual is diagnosed as having AIDS. As the immune responses weaken, the individual becomes increasingly susceptible to other pathogens, particularly pneumonia. Two diseases that are rare in the general population but common in AIDS patients are *Pneumocystis carinii* pneumonia, probably caused by a fungus, and Kaposi's sarcoma, an aggressive and rapidly fatal cancer.

Documented transmission of HIV is through infected blood, semen, or vaginal secretions and by way of breast milk from a nursing mother. The virus can penetrate the placental barrier to infect offspring in utero. Outside the body, HIV is fragile and is inactivated relatively easily. It is eliminated by drying, heat, and chemicals. At this time, there are no drugs against the virus and there are no vaccines. The only way to prevent AIDS is to block transmission of the virus. No cases have been reported of the reversal of AIDS or HIV infection, and all carriers of the virus are assumed to be infected for life and are capable of transmitting the virus to others.

There are still many unanswered questions about HIV and AIDS. How does the virus destroy T cells? Why and how does it reactivate? Why is the latent period longer in some people than in others? Why do some HIV-positive people develop AIDS whereas others do not? Is there a cofactor involved in the progression of the disease? Until these and other questions are answered, controversy, speculation, and myths will continue. Questions about the nature of the virus, how it works, and the pathogenesis of the disease must be answered through research before there is much chance of finding a cure.

CHAPTER QUIZ

RECALL

Match the definitions on the left with the appropriate term on the right.

1. Most abundant plasma protein

2. Plasma protein that functions in blood clotting

3. Precursor, or stem cell, from which blood cells develop

4. Red blood cell

5. Process by which WBCs move through the capillary wall

6. Found on the cell membrane of RBCs

7. Hormone that stimulates RBC production

8. Pigmented protein that binds with oxygen

9. 45% of blood volume

10. Granular leukocyte

A. Agglutinogen

B. Albumin

C. Basophil

D. Diapedesis

E. Erythrocyte

F. Erythropoietin

G. Fibrinogen

H. Formed elements

I. Hemocytoblast

J. Hemoglobin

THOUGHT

1. The plasma protein most responsible for maintaining blood osmotic pressure is

   a. gamma globulin

   b. prothrombin

   c. fibrinogen

   d. albumin

2. Immature erythrocytes are called

   a. hemocytes

   b. reticulocytes

   c. thrombocytes

   d. leukocytes

3. When oxygen delivery to the kidneys decreases,

   a. the liver increases production of albumins

   b. the kidneys decrease production of prothrombin

   c. the liver decreases production of erythropoietin

   d. the kidneys increase production of renal erythropoietic factor

4. Theoretically, a person with type A blood should be able to receive

   a. type AB blood and type A blood

   b. type B blood and type AB blood

   c. type O blood and type B blood

   d. type A blood and type O blood

5. Blood clotting is a multistep process. Which of the following represents the correct sequence of the steps in blood clotting?

   a. formation of prothrombin activator, formation of thrombin, formation of fibrin

   b. formation of thrombin, formation of fibrin, formation of prothrombin activator

   c. formation of fibrin, formation of prothrombin activator, formation of thrombin

   d. formation of prothrombin activator, formation of fibrin, formation of thrombin

APPLICATION

Why do individuals with advanced kidney disease often have a low hematocrit?

Why do individuals with advanced liver disease often bruise easily, bleed freely, and have a slow clotting time?

CHAPTER 12

Heart

Outline/Objectives

Overview of the Heart 243
- Describe the size and location of the heart.

Structure of the Heart 244
- Identify the layers of the heart wall and state the type of tissue in each layer.
- Label a diagram of the heart, identifying the chambers, valves, and associated vessels.
- Trace the pathway of blood flow through the heart, including chambers, valves, and pulmonary circulation.
- Identify the major vessels that supply blood to the myocardium and return the deoxygenated blood to the right atrium.

Physiology of the Heart 249
- Describe the components and function of the conduction system of the heart.
- Summarize the events of a complete cardiac cycle and correlate the heart sounds heard with a stethoscope with these events.
- Explain what is meant by stroke volume and cardiac output and describe the factors that affect these values.

Key Terms

Atrioventricular valve
Cardiac cycle
Cardiac output
Conduction myofibers
Diastole
Semilunar valve
Stroke volume
Systole

Building Vocabulary

WORD PART	MEANING
aort-	lift up
atri-	entrance room
brady-	slow
cardi-	heart
cusp-	point
diastol-	expand, separate
lun-	moon shaped
meg-	large
sphygm-	pulse
sten-	narrowing
systol-	contraction
tachy-	fast, rapid
valvu-	valve

Functional Relationships of the
Cardiovascular System

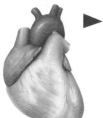

▶ Delivers oxygen and nutrients; removes carbon dioxide and other metabolic wastes; dissipates heat.

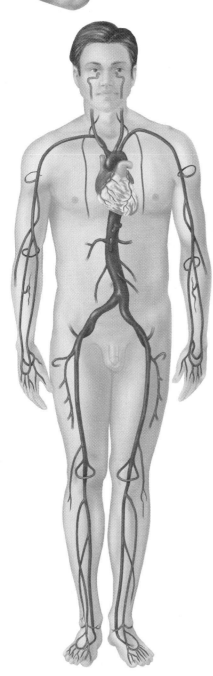

Integument

◀ Provides barrier against entry of pathogens; provides mechanical protection of superficial blood vessels; radiates heat for thermoregulation.

▶ Transports clotting factors and phagocytic cells to sites of skin wounds; hemoglobin in blood contributes to skin color.

Skeletal
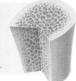

◀ Protects heart and thoracic vessels; produces blood cells in bone marrow; supplies calcium for cardiac muscle contraction and blood clotting.

▶ Delivers oxygen and nutrients and removes metabolic wastes; delivers erythropoietin to bone marrow; delivers hormones that regulate skeletal growth to osetoclasts and osteoblasts.

Muscular

◀ Skeletal muscle contraction assists venous return, promotes growth of new vessels; smooth and cardiac muscle contraction contributes to vessel and heart function.

▶ Removes heat and other waste products generated by muscle contraction; delivers oxygen for metabolism to sustain energy for muscle contraction.

Nervous

◀ Adjusts heart rate to maintain adequate cardiac output; regulates blood pressure; controls blood flow patterns in systemic circulation.

▶ Endothelial cells of capillaries help maintain blood-brain barrier and generate CSF.

Endocrine

◀ Hormones adjust heart rate, contraction strength, blood volume, blood pressure, and red blood cell production.

▶ Delivers oxygen and nutrients to endocrine glands; removes carbon dioxide and heat; transports hormones from glands to target tissue; heart secretes natriuretic hormone.

Lymphatic/Immune
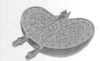

◀ Defends against pathogens and toxins in the blood; fights infections in the heart; returns interstitial fluid to the blood.

▶ Transports the agents of the immune response.

Respiratory

◀ Helps maintain blood pH; provides oxygen and removes wastes for cardiac tissue; breathing movements assist in venous return.

▶ Transports oxygen and carbon dioxide between lungs and tissues.

Digestive
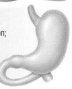

◀ Absorbs nutrients for blood cell formation; absorption of nutrients affects plasma composition; liver metabolism affects blood glucose content.

▶ Delivers hormones that affect the motility and glandular activity of the digestive tract; transports absorbed nutrients to liver.

Urinary

◀ Helps maintain blood pH and electrolyte composition; adjusts blood volume and pressure; initiates renin-angiotensin-aldosterone mechanism.

▶ Delivers wastes to be excreted in the urine; adjusts blood flow to maintain kidney function; transports hormones that regulate reabsorption in the kidneys.

Reproductive
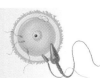

◀ Gonads produce hormones that help maintain healthy blood vessels; testosterone stimulates erythropoiesis.

▶ Transports reproductive hormones; provides nutrients for developing fetus and removes wastes; vasodilation responsible for erection in penis and clitoris.

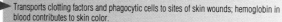

he heart is a muscular pump that provides the force necessary to circulate the blood to all the tissues in the body. Its function is vital because, to survive, the tissues need a continuous supply of oxygen and nutrients and metabolic waste products have to be removed from them. Deprived of these necessities, cells soon undergo irreversible changes that lead to death. Although blood is the transport medium, the heart is the organ that keeps the blood moving through the vessels. The normal adult heart pumps about 5 liters of blood every minute throughout life. If it loses its pumping effectiveness for even a few minutes, the individual's life is jeopadized.

Overview of the Heart

Form, Size, and Location of the Heart

Knowledge of the heart's position in the thoracic cavity is important in hearing heart sounds, in doing electrocardiograms (ECGs), and in performing cardiopulmonary resuscitation (CPR). The heart, illustrated in Figure 12–1, is located in the middle mediastinal region of the thoracic cavity between the two lungs. It is posterior to the sternum and anterior to the vertebral column, and it rests on the diaphragm. About two thirds of the heart mass is to the left of the midline and one third is on the right. The **apex,** or pointed end of the heart, is directed inferiorly, anteriorly, and to the left. It extends downward to the level of the fifth intercostal space. The opposite end, the **base,** is larger and less pointed than the apex and has several large vessels attached to it. The base is directed superiorly, posteriorly, and to the right. Its most superior portion is at the level of the second rib. The size of the heart varies with the size of the individual. On the average, it is about 9 cm wide and 12 cm long, about the size of a closed fist.

> The heart is about the size of a closed fist, with two thirds of the mass to the left of midline.

Coverings of the Heart

The heart and the proximal portions of the vessels attached to its base are enclosed by a loose-fitting, double-layered sac called the **pericardium** (pair-ih-KAR-dee-um), or pericardial sac. The outer layer of the pericardium is formed of tough, white fibrous connective tissue and is called the **fibrous pericardium.** It is attached to the diaphragm, the posterior portion of the sternum, the vertebrae, and the large vessels at the base of the heart. The fibrous pericardium is lined with a layer of serous membrane called the **parietal pericardium.** Where the pericardium is attached to the vessels at the base of the heart, the parietal pericardium reflects onto the surface of the heart to form the **visceral pericardium,** or **epicardium.** The small potential space between the parietal and visceral layers of the pericardium is the **pericardial cavity.** It contains a thin layer of serous fluid that reduces friction between the membranes as they rub against each other during heart contractions.

CLINICAL TERMS

Artifical pacemaker (ahr-tih-FISH-al PAYSE-may-ker) An electronic device that stimulates the initiation of an impulse within the heart

Auscultation (ahs-kool-TAY-shun) A physical assessment procedure using a stethoscope to listen to sounds within the chest, abdomen, and other parts of the body

Cardiac arrest (KAR-dee-ack ah-REST) Cessation of an effective heartbeat; heart may be completely stopped or quivering ineffectively in fibrillation

Cardiac catheterization (KAR-dee-ack kath-eh-ter-ih-ZAY-shun) The process of inserting a thin, flexible tube, called a catheter, into a vein or artery and guiding it into the heart for the purpose of detecting pressures and patterns of blood flow

Cardiomegaly (kar-dee-oh-MEG-ah-lee) Enlargement of the heart

Coronary artery bypass grafting (CABG) A surgical procedure in which a blood vessel from another part of the body is used to bypass the blocked region of a coronary artery

Cor pulmonale (kor pul-moh-NAY-lee) Hypertrophy of the right ventricle caused by hypertension in the pulmonary circulation

Defibrillation (dee-fib-rih-LAY-shun) A procedure in which an electric shock is applied to the heart with a defibrillator to stop an abnormal heart rhythm

Echocardiography (eck-oh-kar-dee-AHG-rah-fee) A noninvasive clinical procedure using pulses of high-frequency sound waves (ultrasound) that are transmitted into the chest, and echoes returning from the valves, chambers, and surfaces of the heart are plotted and recorded; provides information about valvular or structural defects and coronary artery disease

Fibrillation (fib-rih-LAY-shun) Rapid, random, ineffectual, and irregular contractions of the heart at 350 or more beats per minute

Mitral valve prolapse (MY-tral valve PRO-laps) Improper closure of the mitral valve when the heart is pumping blood; also called floppy valve syndrome

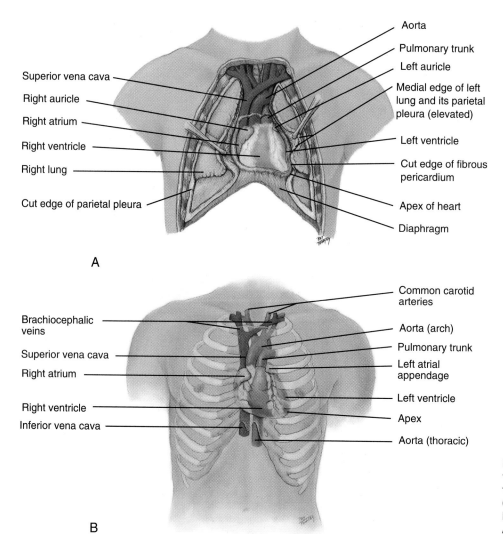

Superior vena cava
Right auricle
Right atrium
Right ventricle
Right lung
Cut edge of parietal pleura

Aorta
Pulmonary trunk
Left auricle
Medial edge of left lung and its parietal pleura (elevated)
Left ventricle
Cut edge of fibrous pericardium
Apex of heart
Diaphragm

A

Brachiocephalic veins
Superior vena cava
Right atrium
Right ventricle
Inferior vena cava

Common carotid arteries
Aorta (arch)
Pulmonary trunk
Left atrial appendage
Left ventricle
Apex
Aorta (thoracic)

B

Figure 12-1 *A*, Frontal view of the mediastinum, showing the position of the heart (*B*). (From Jarvis C: Physical Examination and Health Assessment. Philadelphia, WB Saunders, 1992.)

The heart is enclosed in a pericardial sac that is lined with the parietal layer of a serous membrane. The visceral layer of the serous membrane forms the epicardium.

Pericarditis is an inflammation of the pericardium. This may interfere with production of the serous fluid that lubricates the surfaces of the parietal and visceral layers. Painful adhesions may form that interfere with contraction of the heart.

Structure of the Heart

Layers of the Heart Wall

The heart wall is formed by three layers of tissue: an outer epicardium, a middle myocardium, and an inner endocardium. The **epicardium** (eh-pih-KAR-dee-um), which is the same as the visceral pericardium, is a serous membrane that consists of connective tissue covered by simple squamous epithelium. It is a thin protective layer that is firmly anchored to the underlying muscle. Blood vessels that nourish the heart wall are located in the epicardium.

The thick middle layer is the **myocardium** (my-oh-KAR-dee-um). It forms the bulk of the heart wall and is composed of cardiac muscle tissue. Refer to Chapter 4 for a review of the different types of muscle tissue. Cardiac muscle cells are elongated and branching with one or two nuclei per cell. The arrangement of myofilaments makes the fibers appear striated. The cells are connected together by **intercalated** (in-TER-kuh-lay-ted) disks and wrapped around the heart in a spiral fashion to make up the myocardium. Contractions of the myocardium provide the force that ejects blood from the heart and moves it through the vessels.

The smooth inner lining of the heart wall is **endocardium** (en-doh-KAR-dee-um), a layer of simple squamous epithelium overlying connective tissue. Its smooth surface permits blood to move easily through the heart. The endocardium also forms the valves of the heart and is continuous with the lining of the blood vessels. The heart wall is illustrated in Figure 12–2.

> The outer layer of the heart wall is the epicardium, the middle layer is the myocardium, and the inner layer is the endocardium.

Chambers of the Heart

The internal cavity of the heart is divided into four chambers (Fig. 12–3):

- Right atrium
- Right ventricle
- Left atrium
- Left ventricle

The two atria are thin-walled chambers that receive blood from the veins. The two ventricles are thick-walled chambers that forcefully pump blood out of the heart. Differences in thickness of the heart chamber walls are due to variations in the amount of myocardium present, which reflects the amount of force each chamber is required to generate.

> The two atria are thin-walled chambers that receive blood from the veins; the ventricles are thick-walled chambers that pump blood out of the heart.

The **right atrium** (A-tree-um) receives deoxygenated blood from the superior vena cava, the inferior vena cava, and the coronary sinus. The superior

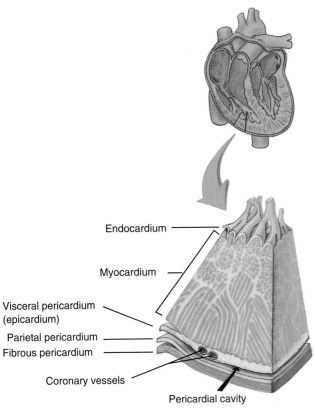

Endocardium

Myocardium

Visceral pericardium (epicardium)

Parietal pericardium

Fibrous pericardium

Coronary vessels

Pericardial cavity

Figure 12–2   Layers of the heart wall.

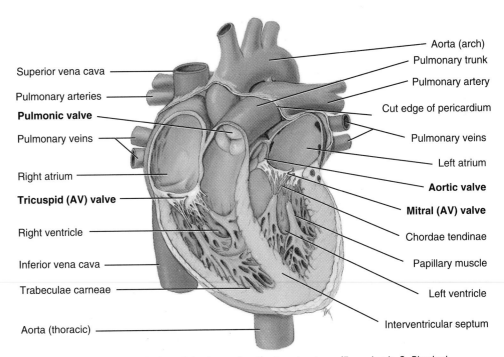

Superior vena cava

Pulmonary arteries

Pulmonic valve

Pulmonary veins

Right atrium

Tricuspid (AV) valve

Right ventricle

Inferior vena cava

Trabeculae carneae

Aorta (thoracic)

Aorta (arch)

Pulmonary trunk

Pulmonary artery

Cut edge of pericardium

Pulmonary veins

Left atrium

Aortic valve

Mitral (AV) valve

Chordae tendinae

Papillary muscle

Left ventricle

Interventricular septum

Figure 12–3   Internal view of the heart showing the chambers. (From Jarvis C: Physical Examination and Health Assessment. Philadelphia, WB Saunders, 1992.)

vena cava returns blood to the heart from the head, neck, and upper extremities. The inferior vena cava returns blood to the heart from the thorax, abdomen, pelvis, and lower extremities. The coronary sinus is a small venous structure on the posterior surface of the heart that returns blood to the right atrium from the myocardium of the heart wall. The **left atrium** receives oxygenated blood from the lungs through four pulmonary veins, two on the right and two on the left. Because the atria are "receiving" chambers rather than "pumping" chambers, their myocardium is relatively thin, which is reflected in their thin walls. Both atria have small extensions, called **auricles,** that protrude anteriorly. The right and left atria are separated by a partition called the **interatrial septum.** There is a thin region, called the **fossa ovalis,** in the interatrial septum. This represents an opening, the foramen ovale, that is present between the atria in the fetal heart.

> The right atrium receives deoxygenated blood from systemic veins; the left atrium receives oxygenated blood from the pulmonary veins.

The **right ventricle** (VEN-trih-kull) receives blood from the right atrium and pumps it out to the lungs where it picks up a new supply of oxygen. The **left ventricle,** which forms the apex of the heart, receives blood from the left atrium and pumps it out to the tissues of the whole body where the oxygen transported by the blood is used in metabolic activities. The ventricles are "pumping" chambers, and this is reflected by a thick myocardium. Because the left ventricle pumps blood to the whole body and the right ventricle only sends it to the lungs, the left ventricle has to generate a lot more pumping force than the right ventricle. This is reflected in the fact that the left ventricular wall has a thicker myocardium than the right. Both ventricles hold about the same volume of blood. In both ventricles, the myocardium is marked by ridges called **trabeculae carneae** (trah-BEK-yoo-lee KAR-nee-ee). Two or three fingerlike masses of myocardium, called **papillary** (PAP-ih-lair-ee) **muscles,** project from the wall of the ventricle into the chamber (see Fig. 12–3). The thick, muscular partition between the right and left ventricles is the **interventricular septum.**

> The right ventricle pumps blood to the lungs; the left ventricle pumps blood to the tissues of the whole body.

Valves of the Heart

Pumps need a set of valves to keep the fluid flowing in one direction, and the heart is no exception. The heart has two types of valves that keep the blood flowing in the correct direction. The valves between the atria and ventricles are called **atrioventricular (AV)** (ay-tree-oh-ven-TRIK-yoo-lar) valves, whereas those at the bases of the large vessels leaving the ventricles are called **semilunar (SL)** (seh-mee-LOO-nar) valves (see Fig. 12–3).

> There are two types of valves associated with the heart: AV and SL valves.

Atrioventricular Valves

The AV valves permit the flow of blood from the atria into the corresponding ventricle but prevent the backflow of blood from the ventricles into the atria. Each valve consists of a fibrous connective tissue ring, which reinforces the junction between the atrium and ventricle, and double folds of endocardium that form the **cusps** of the valve (Fig. 12–4). The valve cusps are attached to the papillary muscles in the ventricles by connective tissue strings called **chordae tendineae** (KOR-dee ten-DIN-ee) (see Fig. 12–3). As blood returns to the atria, it pushes the valve cusps open and the blood flows into the ventricles. When the ventricles contract, the force of the blood against the cusps causes them to close and prevents the backward flow of blood into the atria. With myocardial contraction, the papillary muscles exert tension on the chordae tendineae attached to the cusps and prevent the valve from opening back into the atria.

> AV valves are located between the atria and ventricles. When the ventricles contract, these valves close to prevent blood from flowing back into the atria.

The AV valve between the right atrium and right ventricle, located at the fourth intercostal space, has three cusps and is called the **tricuspid valve.** The valve between the left atrium and left ventricle has only two cusps, is at the level of the fourth costal cartilage, and is called the **bicuspid,** or **mitral, valve** (Fig. 12–5).

> The right AV valve is the tricuspid valve. The left AV valve is the bicuspid, or mitral, valve.

Semilunar Valves

SL valves are located at the bases of the large vessels that carry blood from the ventricles (see Fig. 12–3). Each valve consists of three cuplike cusps of fibrous connective tissue and endothelium. Contraction of the ventricular myocardium increases the pressure of the blood so that it pushes the valves open and the blood leaves the heart. As the ventricles relax and pressure decreases, the blood starts to flow back down the large vessels toward the ventricles. When the blood flows toward the ventricles, it enters the "cups" of the valve cusps and causes them to meet in the center of the vessel. This closes

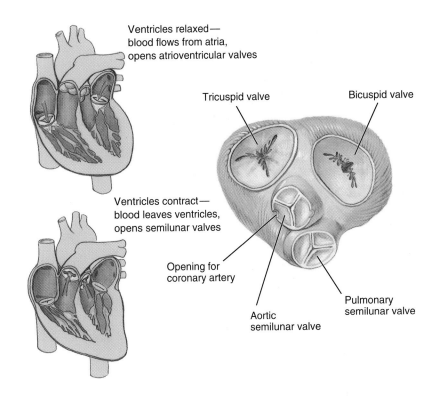

Ventricles relaxed—
blood flows from atria,
opens atrioventricular valves

Tricuspid valve

Bicuspid valve

Ventricles contract—
blood leaves ventricles,
opens semilunar valves

Opening for
coronary artery

Aortic
semilunar valve

Pulmonary
semilunar valve

Figure 12–4 Valves of the heart as
viewed from above.

the opening and prevents the flow of blood back
into the ventricles (see Fig. 12–4).

> The SL valves are at the exits of the ventricles.
> When the ventricles relax, these valves close to
> prevent blood from flowing back into the ventri-
> cles.

The valve at the exit of the right ventricle is in
the base of the pulmonary trunk and is called the
pulmonary semilunar valve. It is at the level of the
third costal cartilage. The valve at the exit of the left
ventricle is in the base of the ascending aorta. It is
called the **aortic semilunar valve** and is at the level
of the third intercostal space (see Fig. 12–5).

> The valve between the right ventricle and pulmo-
> nary trunk is the pulmonary semilunar valve. The
> valve between the left ventricle and the aorta is the
> aortic semilunar valve.

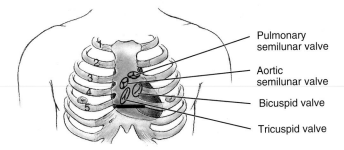

Pulmonary
semilunar valve

Aortic
semilunar valve

Bicuspid valve

Tricuspid valve

Figure 12–5 Surface projection of the heart valves.

> Sometimes disease processes damage the heart
> valves so that they are unable to function properly.
> Incompetent valves permit a "backflow" of blood
> and the heart has to pump that same blood over
> and over to get it into the vessels. In valvular steno-
> sis, the valves are stiff and have narrow openings.
> The heart has to work harder to pump blood out
> through the small opening.

Pathway of Blood Through the Heart

Although it is convenient to describe the flow of
blood through the right side of the heart and then
through the left side, it is important to realize that
both atria contract at the same time and that both
ventricles contract at the same time. The heart works
as two pumps, one on the right and one on the left,
that work simultaneously. The "right pump" pumps
the blood to the lungs (pulmonary circulation) at the
same time that the "left pump" pumps blood to the
rest of the body (systemic circulation). The sequence
in which the chambers contract is described in more
detail with the cardiac cycle.

The arrows in Figure 12–6 depict the direction
that blood flows through the heart. Venous blood
from systemic circulation, which is relatively low in
oxygen and high in carbon dioxide content, enters
the **right atrium** through the superior vena cava and
inferior vena cava. This blood flows through the
tricuspid valve and into the **right ventricle.** From
the right ventricle it passes through the **pulmonary**

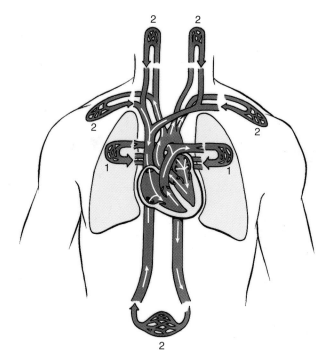

Red = oxygenated blood

Blue = deoxygenated blood

1 = capillary beds of lungs
   where gas exchange occurs

2 = capillary beds of body tissues
   where gas exchange occurs

Figure 12–6 Pathway of the blood through the heart.

semilunar valve into the **pulmonary trunk,** then into the **pulmonary arteries,** which carry the blood to the **lungs.** In the lungs, the blood releases carbon dioxide and picks up a new supply of oxygen; then **pulmonary veins** carry the blood to the **left atrium.** From the left atrium, it flows through the **bicuspid valve** into the **left ventricle,** and then through the **aortic semilunar valve** into the **ascending aorta.** Oxygen-rich blood flowing into the aorta is distributed to all parts of the body through systemic circulation.

> Blood flows from the right atrium to the right ventricle, and then is pumped to the lungs to receive oxygen. From the lungs, the blood flows to the left atrium, then to the left ventricle. From there it is pumped to the systemic circulation.

Blood Supply to the Myocardium

The myocardium of the heart wall is working muscle that needs a continuous supply of oxygen and nutrients to function with efficiency. Unlike skeletal muscle, cardiac muscle cannot build up an oxygen debt to be repaid at a later time. It needs a continuous oxygen supply or it dies. For this reason, car-

diac muscle has an extensive network of blood vessels to bring oxygen to the contracting cells and to remove waste products.

> **Angina pectoris** is chest pain that results when the heart muscle demand for oxygen exceeds the oxygen supply. Nitroglycerin is sometimes used in the treatment of angina pectoris because it dilates blood vessels, so the patient is less likely to develop a myocardial oxygen deficit.

Two main coronary arteries branch from the ascending aorta just distal to the aortic SL valve. The **right coronary artery** extends to the right from the ascending aorta and continues in the right AV sulcus to the posterior surface of the heart. Its branches supply blood to most of the myocardium in the right ventricle. The **left coronary artery,** which extends to the left from the ascending aorta, continues for about 2 cm, then divides into two major branches. The **anterior interventricular (descending) artery** descends in the anterior interventricular sulcus. The **circumflex artery** continues in the left atrioventricular sulcus to the posterior surface. The left coronary artery and its branches supply blood to most of the myocardium in the left ventricle. The arteries have numerous branches and they anastomose freely to provide alternative pathways for blood flow to the myocardium. Blood flow through the coronary arteries is greatest when the myocardium is relaxed. When the ventricles contract, they compress the arteries, which reduces the flow.

> The right and left coronary arteries, branches of the ascending aorta, supply blood to the walls of the myocardium.

> If a branch of coronary artery becomes blocked, blood supply to that region of the heart is cut off and the muscle cells in that area die of lack of oxygen. This is a **myocardial infarction (MI),** also called a coronary or a heart attack. The extent of the damage and chances of recovery depend on the location of the blockage and the length of time that elapses before medical intervention occurs.

> When heart muscle is damaged, the dying cells release enzymes into the bloodstream. These enzymes can be measured and are useful in confirming an MI. The enzymes assayed are creatine kinase (CK) and lactic acid dehydrogenase (LDH).

After blood passes through the capillaries in the myocardium, it enters a system of **cardiac (coronary)**

veins. The cardiac veins lie next to the coronary arteries, and the vessels are usually surrounded by deposits of fat. Most of the cardiac veins drain into the coronary sinus, which opens into the right atrium. The coronary arteries and cardiac veins are illustrated in Figure 12–7.

> Blood from the capillaries in the myocardium enters the cardiac veins, which drain into the coronary sinus. From there, it enters the right atrium.

✓ QuickCheck

- Certain bacterial diseases may damage heart valves. Damage to the left semilunar valve interferes with blood flow into what chamber or vessel?

- What structures prevent AV valves from opening back into the atria?

- Which two heart chambers contain oxygen-rich blood?

Physiology of the Heart

The work of the heart is to pump blood to the lungs through pulmonary circulation and to the rest of the body through systemic circulation. This is accomplished by systematic contraction and relaxation of the cardiac muscle in the myocardium. The intercalated disks permit impulses to travel rapidly between adjacent cells so that they function together as a single electrical unit instead of as individual cells. Effective contractions of the heart depend on this characteristic, and they are coordinated by the conduction system of the heart.

Conduction System

An effective cycle for productive pumping of blood requires that the heart be synchronized accurately. Both atria need to contract simultaneously, followed by contraction of both ventricles. Contraction of the chambers is coordinated by specialized cardiac muscle cells that make up the **conduction system** of the heart. These cells contain only a few myofibrils and instead of contracting, they act somewhat like neural tissue by initiating and distributing impulses throughout the myocardium to coordinate the events of the cardiac cycle.

> The conduction system of the heart consists of specialized cardiac muscle cells.

Components of the Conduction System

Sinoatrial Node. The conduction system includes several components (Fig. 12–8). The first part of the conduction system is the **sinoatrial (SA) node** (sye-noh-AY-tree-al node), which is located in the posterior wall of the right atrium, near the entrance of the superior vena cava. Without any neural stimulation, the SA node rhythmically initiates impulses (action potentials) 70 to 80 times per minute. Because it establishes the basic rhythm of the heartbeat, it is called the **pacemaker** of the heart. The impulses from the SA node rapidly travel throughout the atrial myocardium and cause the two atria to contract simultaneously. At the same time, the impulses reach the second part of the conduction system.

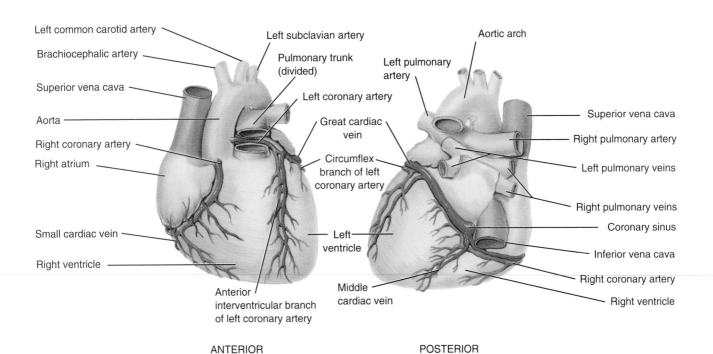

ANTERIOR   POSTERIOR

Figure 12-7 Blood supply to the myocardium.

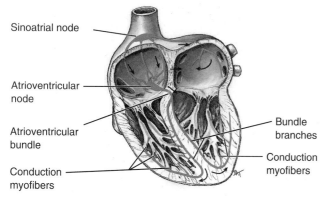

Sinoatrial node

Atrioventricular node

Atrioventricular bundle

Conduction myofibers

Bundle branches

Conduction myofibers

Figure 12-8 Conduction system.

■ **The SA node is the pacemaker of the heart.**

Atrioventricular Node. The **AV node,** the second part of the conduction system, is located in the floor of the right atrium, near the interatrial septum. The cells in the AV node conduct impulses more slowly than do other parts of the conduction system so there is a brief time delay as the impulses travel through the node. This allows time for the atria to finish their contraction phase before the ventricles begin contracting.

Atrioventricular Bundle, Bundle Branches, and Conduction Myofibers. From the AV node, the impulses rapidly travel through the **atrioventricular bundle** (bundle of His) to the **right** and **left bundle branches.** The bundle branches extend along the right and left sides of the interventricular septum to the apex. These branch profusely to form **conduction myofibers** (Purkinje fibers) that transmit the impulses to the myocardium. The AV bundle, bundle branches, and conduction myofibers rapidly transmit impulses throughout all the ventricular myocardium so that both ventricles contract at the same time. As the ventricles contract, blood is forced out through the SL valves into the pulmonary trunk and the ascending aorta. After the ventricles complete their contraction phase, they relax and the SA node initiates another impulse to start another cardiac cycle.

All parts of the conduction system and cardiac muscle cells are capable of initiating impulses to start a cardiac cycle. The SA node is called the pacemaker because impulses spontaneously originate in the SA node faster than in any other part. If the SA node is unable to function, another area such as the AV node becomes the pacemaker. The resulting heart rate is slower than normal.

■ The components of the conduction system of the heart are the SA node, AV node, AV bundle, bundle branches, and conduction myofibers. These coordinate the contraction and relaxation of the heart chambers.

Variations in normal contraction patterns are called arrhythmias. One type of arrhythmia occurs when a conduction myofiber or a heart muscle cell independently depolarizes to threshold and triggers a **premature heart contraction**. The cell responsible for the premature contraction is called an **ectopic focus**. Sometimes ectopic foci form feedback loops within the conduction system causing myocardial contractions to occur at a rapid rate. If not treated properly, this often leads to ventricular tachycardia, fibrillation, and death.

Electrocardiogram

Impulses conducted through the heart during a cardiac cycle produce electric currents that can be detected and measured on the surface of the body. A recording of this electrical activity is called an **electrocardiogram (ECG or EKG)**.

A normal electrocardiogram consists of waves or deflections that correlate with the depolarization and repolarization events of the cardiac cycle (Fig. 12–9). The **P wave** is a small upward deflection produced by depolarization of the atrial myocardium as the impulses travel through the myocardium just before contraction. The **QRS complex** is a large upward deflection produced by depolarization of the ventricular myocardium immediately preceding contraction of the ventricles. The greater magnitude of the QRS complex is due to the greater muscle mass in the ventricles. The third deflection, the **T wave,** is due to the repolarization of the ventricles that occurs just before the ventricles relax. A deflection that corresponds to atrial repolarization is not evident because it occurs at the same time as the QRS complex.

■ An electrocardiogram is a recording of the electrical activity of the heart.

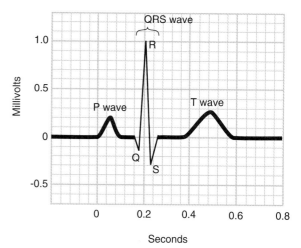

Figure 12-9 Electrocardiogram.

An electrocardiogram is useful in evaluating heart function. For example, a heightened P wave may indicate an enlarged atrium. A heightened QRS complex indicate an enlarged ventricle.

Cardiac Cycle

The cardiac cycle refers to the alternating contraction and relaxation of the myocardium in the walls of the heart chambers, coordinated by the conduction system, during one heartbeat (Fig. 12–10). The two atria contract at the same time, then they relax while the two ventricles simultaneously contract. The contraction phase of the chambers is called **systole** (SIS-toh-lee); the relaxation phase is called **diastole** (dye-AS-toh-lee). When the terms systole and diastole are used alone, they refer to action of the ventricles.

Systole is the contraction phase of the cardiac cycle, and diastole is the relaxation phase.

With a heart rate of 75 beats per minute, one cardiac cycle lasts 0.8 second. The cycle begins with **atrial systole,** when both atria contract (see Fig. 12–10). During this time, the AV valves are open, the ventricles are in diastole, and blood is forced into the ventricles. Atrial systole lasts for 0.1 second, then the atria relax (**atrial diastole**) for the remainder of the cycle, 0.7 second.

At a normal heart rate, one cardiac cycle lasts for 0.8 second. Atrial systole lasts for 0.1 second.

When the atria finish their contraction phase, the ventricles begin contracting. **Ventricular systole** lasts for 0.3 second. Pressure in the ventricles increases as they contract. This closes the AV valves and opens the SL valves, and blood is forced into the pulmonary trunk and ascending aorta that carry blood away from the heart. During this time, the atria are in diastole and are filling with blood returned through the venae cavae. After ventricular systole, when the ventricles relax, the SL valves close, the AV valves open, and blood flows from the atria into the ventricles. All chambers are in simultaneous diastole for 0.4 second, and about 70 percent of ventricular filling occurs during this period. The remaining blood enters the ventricles during atrial systole.

Ventricular systole lasts for 0.3 second. After this, all chambers are relaxed for the remainder of the cycle. Most ventricular filling occurs while all chambers are relaxed.

Heart Sounds

The sounds associated with the heartbeat are due to vibrations in the tissues and blood caused by closure of the valves. A **stethoscope** is used to listen to these sounds, usually described as lubb-dupp. The **first heart sound,** the lubb, is caused by closure of the AV valves at the beginning of ventricular systole. The **second heart sound,** the dupp, is caused by closure of the semilunar valves at the beginning of ventricular diastole. It has a higher pitch than the first heart sound. The time between the first and second heart sounds represents the period of ventricular systole. The time between the second heart

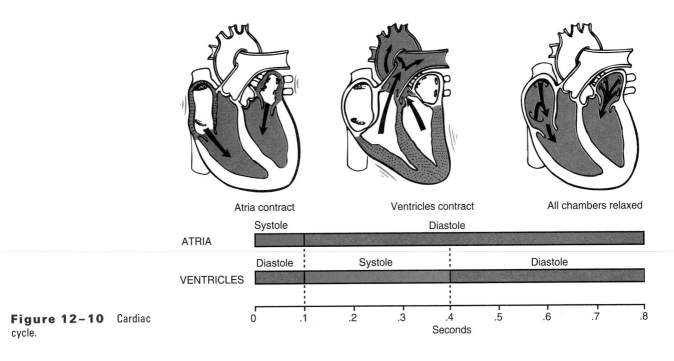

Figure 12–10 Cardiac cycle.

		Atria contract		Ventricles contract		All chambers relaxed
ATRIA		Systole		Diastole		
VENTRICLES		Diastole	Systole		Diastole	

0   .1   .2   .3   .4   .5   .6   .7   .8
Seconds

sound and the first heart sound of the next beat represents the period of ventricular diastole. Because diastole lasts longer than systole, there is a pause between the dupp of the first beat and the lubb of the second beat so that the sequence is lubb-dupp, pause, lubb-dupp, pause, lubb-dupp, pause, etc. Abnormal heart sounds, called **murmurs,** are caused by faulty valves.

> Heart sounds are due to vibrations in the blood caused by the valves closing. Abnormal heart sounds are called murmurs.

> Defective heart valves may result in abnormal heart sounds. For example, if the AV valves are faulty, a hissing sound may be heard between the first and second heart sounds.

Cardiac Output

Cardiac output is the volume of blood pumped by a ventricle in 1 minute. Because the primary function of the heart is to pump blood, this is a measure of its effectiveness. Cardiac output is calculated by multiplying the volume pumped out in one cardiac cycle (stroke volume) times the number of cycles or heartbeats in 1 minute (heart rate).

$$\underset{\text{(mL/min)}}{\text{cardiac output}} = \underset{\text{(mL/cycle)}}{\text{stroke volume}} \times \underset{\text{(cycles/min)}}{\text{heart rate}}$$

In a normal resting adult, stroke volume averages about 70 milliliters and heart rate averages about 72 beats per minute. Cardiac output is calculated as follows:

$$\begin{aligned} \text{cardiac output} &= 70 \text{ mL/beat} \times 72 \text{ beats/min} \\ &= 5040 \text{ mL/min} \end{aligned}$$

This is approximately equal to the total volume of blood in the body. This means that when the body is at rest, the heart pumps the body's total blood volume out to systemic circulation every minute. When the needs of the body cells change, the cardiac output must change also. For example, with

strenuous activity the skeletal muscles need more oxygen. In response, the heart rate increases to provide additional cardiac output so that more oxygen is delivered to the muscle cells. Anything that affects either the stroke volume or the heart rate changes the cardiac output. Various control mechanisms operate on the stroke volume and the heart rate to adjust the cardiac output as the needs of the body change.

> Cardiac output equals heart rate times stroke volume. Anything that affects either the rate or the volume affects the cardiac output.

Stroke Volume

Stroke volume is the amount of blood pumped from a ventricle each time the ventricle contracts. Stroke volume depends on the amount of blood in the ventricle when it contracts (end-diastolic volume) and the strength of the contraction (Fig. 12–11). The end-diastolic volume, the amount of blood in the ventricle at the end of diastole (or beginning of systole), is directly related to venous return. The more blood returned by the veins, the greater the volume in the ventricle to be pumped out again. In this way, increased venous return increases end-diastolic volume, which increases stroke volume.

The amount of blood in the ventricle also affects contraction strength. There is a direct relationship between venous return, end-diastolic volume, and contraction strength. This relationship is known as **Starling's law of the heart.** As blood fills the ventricles, the cardiac muscle fibers stretch to accommodate the increasing volume. In response to stretch, the fibers contract with a greater force, which increases the amount of blood ejected from the ventricle (stroke volume). Conversely, if venous return decreases, end-diastolic volume decreases, there is less stretch in the muscle fibers, and contraction strength decreases.

The autonomic nervous system also affects stroke volume by altering the contraction strength. Sympathetic stimulation increases the contraction strength of the ventricular myocardium. When sympathetic

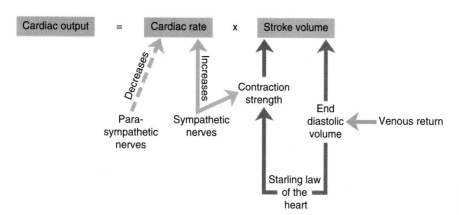

Figure 12–11 Factors that affect cardiac output.

stimulation is removed, the contraction strength decreases.

| Stroke volume is influenced by end-diastolic volume and contraction strength.

Digitalis is a drug that increases the strength and regularity of heart contractions.

Heart Rate

The SA node, acting alone, produces a constant rhythmic heart rate. Regulating factors act on the SA node to increase or decrease the heart rate to adjust cardiac output to meet the changing needs of the body. Most changes in the heart rate are mediated through the **cardiac center** in the medulla oblongata of the brain. This center has both sympathetic and parasympathetic components to regulate the action of the heart. Factors such as blood pressure levels and the relative need for oxygen determine which component is active. Generally, the sympathetic impulses increase the heart rate and cardiac output whereas parasympathetic impulses decrease the heart rate.

| The cardiac center in the medulla oblongata has both sympathetic and parasympathetic components that adjust the heart rate to meet the changing needs of the body.

Baroreceptors are stretch receptors in the wall of the aorta and in the wall of the internal carotid arteries, which deliver blood to the brain. As blood pressure increases, the vessels are stretched, which increases the frequency of impulses going from the receptors to the medulla oblongata. This prompts the cardiac center to increase parasympathetic stimulation and to decrease sympathetic stimulation so heart rate, cardiac output, and blood pressure decrease. As blood pressure decreases, the frequency of impulses also decrease. In response, the cardiac center increases sympathetic impulses and decreases parasympathetic impulses to increase the pressure.

Other factors also influence heart rate. Emotions such as excitement, anxiety, fear, or anger cause increased sympathetic stimulation, which results in increased heart rate. Depression influences the parasympathetic system and decreases the heart rate. Epinephrine, secreted from the adrenal medulla in response to stress, increases heart rate. Increased carbon dioxide concentration and decreased pH of the blood, detected by chemoreceptors, increase the heart rate to deliver more blood to the tissues. Correct concentrations of potassium, calcium, and sodium ions are important to maintaining a regular heartbeat. Body temperature affects the metabolic rate of all cells, including cardiac muscle. Elevated body temperature increases the heart rate whereas decreased temperature reduces the rate. Body temperature sometimes is deliberately decreased below normal (hypothermia) to reduce heart action during surgery.

| Peripheral factors such as emotions, ion concentrations, and body temperature may affect heart rate. These are usually mediated through the cardiac center.

 QuickCheck

- What will be the effect on heart rate if the SA node is not functioning?
- What happens in the atria during ventricular systole?
- Identify two factors that increase stroke volume by increasing contraction strength.

 FOCUS ON AGING

There are numerous "age-related" changes in the heart. How many of these are due to an actual aging process and how many are due to other factors are questions worth considering. Is it possible to lessen the effects of aging by adjusting lifestyle? Cardiac changes that were once thought to be the result of aging are now believed to be the consequence of a sedentary lifestyle that many consider their "reward" after retirement. Others are due to a lifetime of habits that, while seemingly enjoyable at the time, take their toll later in life. It is difficult to isolate the aging process of the heart because it is so closely related to diet, exercise, and disease processes, but even when these factors are excluded, a clinical pattern of cardiac aging emerges.

In the absence of cardiovascular disease, the heart, particularly the left ventricle, tends to become slightly smaller in elderly people. This is partially due to a decrease in the number and size of cardiac muscle cells and partially due to the reduced demands placed on it by decreasing physical activity. However, because of cardiovascular disease, the heart is often enlarged.

There is a general thickening of the endocardium and valves of the heart as part of the aging process.

Continued on following page

The valves tend to become more rigid and incompetent. Thus, heart murmurs are detected more frequently in the elderly. Structural changes also occur throughout the conduction system as conducting myofibers are replaced with fibrous tissue. Usually, this does not alter the resting pulse, but there is a greater than normal increase in heart rate in response to activity. Arrhythmias also are more frequent.

There appears to be no significant change in resting heart rate or stroke volume; thus, cardiac output remains about the same in the elderly. However, there is a decline in cardiac reserve. There is decreasing ability for the heart to respond to stress, either sudden or prolonged. Sympathetic controls of the heart are less effective, and the aging heart rate becomes more variable. Physically active people have less change in this respect than the sedentary elderly.

Numerous disease processes that occur more frequently in the aging individual have an effect on the heart. Most notable of these is arteriosclerosis, or hardening of the arteries. This puts additional stress on the heart and aggravates the normal age-related changes. Prevention is better and less expensive than cure. Adopt a "healthy heart" lifestyle.

DO YOU KNOW THIS ABOUT THE
Heart?
Myocardial Infarctions, ECGs, and Enzymes

In a **myocardial infarction,** commonly called a heart attack, cardiac muscle cells die of lack of oxygen, usually caused by an occlusion in one of the coronary arteries. The affected tissue degenerates and creates a nonfunctional area known as an **infarct.** Although an infarction may occur in any region of the heart, the left ventricle is the chamber most frequently affected.

The area of cardiac muscle damaged by a myocardial infarction forms three zones based on electrical activity. The **zone of infarction** is at the center of the damaged area. This is the area of cell death where the heart muscle is destroyed so that polarization of the cell membranes is not possible. The zone of infarction is surrounded by a **zone of injury,** where the cells are damaged but not to the extent that they die. Injury usually results from a deficient arterial blood supply. The cell membranes in this zone are capable of polarization to some extent but are unable to reach full polarization. The third and outermost region is the **zone of ischemia,** in which repolarization is impaired. Ischemia is often due to a lack of blood supply but may have other causes. Minor degrees of cardiac disturbances, which may not be sufficient to cause infarction, may produce ischemic changes.

Each of the three zones of cardiac muscle damage produces a different effect in an ECG. The zone of infarction causes abnormal Q waves in the ECG. The Q wave, which is normally small, is the first deflection after the P wave and is the beginning of the QRS complex. An electrode placed directly over an acute myocardial infarct receives no signal from the dead muscle tissue but "looks through" the dead area and records impulses from the opposite side of the heart. These impulses cause a significant Q wave, which is at least one third the height of the QRS complex and 0.04 second in duration. This is the electrocardiographic evidence of myocardial infarction. Because muscle cells do not reproduce, the dead cells cannot be replaced, and the significant Q wave appears on subsequent ECGs.

Electrodes placed over the zone of injury, surrounding the zone of infarction, record shifts in the ST segment of the ECG. After the QRS deflection, which represents depolarization of the ventricles, the ECG tracing normally returns to the base line, or isoelectric line, before the T wave begins. Recordings of impulses from the zone of injury show the ST segment shifted away from the isoelectric line. Shifts in the ST segments caused by acute infarctions usually last only a few days and disappear when the injured tissue heals. Electrodes placed over the zone of ischemia produce only T wave changes. Recordings of a normal heart show the T wave, which represents repolarization of the ventricles, as a deflection from the isoelectric line. Inverted T waves are often recorded from the zone of ischemia because the diminished blood supply impairs repolarization. The T waves return to normal when adequate blood supply is restored.

With an acute attack of angina pectoris, injury and ischemia of the heart occur, but there is no infarct. As a consequence, the Q wave remains normal but changes in the ST segments and T waves develop during the attack. Characteristically, the changes disappear with the cessation of pain.

A diagnosis of MI is sometimes impossible from an ECG because of the location of the infarct. For example, an infarct that is located within the wall of the heart and that does not involve the epicardium or endocardium cannot be detected by electrocardiography. Enzyme studies may provide useful information in these cases. When heart muscle is damaged, the cells accumulate enzymes involved with anaerobic metabolism. As their cell membranes deteriorate, the dying cells release these enzymes into the surrounding intercellular fluids and from there they enter the bloodstream. These enzymes can be measured and are useful in confirming a myocardial infarction. The enzymes that are tested for include creatine kinase and lactic acid dehydrogenase.

Time is of major importance when dealing with a suspected MI. Most often, the attack is the result of a blot clot in one of the coronary arteries. As soon as blood flow is restricted, damage to the heart muscle begins. The longer the process goes on without intervention, the greater the extent of the damage and the less chance there is for a full recovery. Therapy to dissolve the clot, called thrombolytic therapy, works in most cases if given quickly enough. Prompt evaluation is also important because muscle damage may result in arrhythmias. Some arrhythmias are not serious but others can initiate ventricular fibrillation. When this happens, the heart stops beating effectively and death follows within minutes unless medical personnel are available to restore a normal heartbeat. Remember that in a heart attack, time is muscle—cardiac muscle.

REPRESENTATIVE DISORDERS OF THE CARDIOVASCULAR SYSTEM

Related to Heart

Conduction: Arrhythmia
Blocks
Infection: Bacterial endocarditis
Rheumatic heart disease
Ischemia: Coronary artery disease
Infarction
Angina pectoris
Congenital: Septal defects
Tetralogy of Fallot
Patent foramen ovale

Disorders Related to the Cardiovascular System

Related to Blood

Clotting: Hemophilia
RBCs: Anemia
Polycythemia
WBCs: Leukemia
Volume: Hypovolemia
Hemorrhage

Related to Vessels

Occlusion: Thrombus
Atherosclerosis
Distortion: Aneurysm
Varicose veins

CHAPTER QUIZ

RECALL

Match the definitions on the left with the appropriate term on the right.

1. Contraction phase of cardiac cycle

2. Phase of cardiac cycle when most ventricular filling occurs

3. Cardiac muscle

4. Valve between right atrium and right ventricle

5. Valve at the exit of the left ventricle

6. Heart chamber with thickest walls

7. Heart chamber with oxygen-poor blood

8. Volume of blood pumped by left ventricle in 1 minute

9. Location of cardiac center in the brain

10. Pacemaker of the heart

A. Aortic semilunar valve

B. Cardiac output

C. Diastole

D. Left ventricle

E. Medulla oblongata

F. Myocardium

G. Right ventricle

H. Sinoatrial node

I. Systole

J. Tricuspid valve

THOUGHT

1. The atrioventricular valve on the same side of the heart as the pulmonary semilunar valve is the
   a. tricuspid valve
   b. bicuspid valve
   c. mitral valve
   d. aortic valve

2. The chamber that receives oxygen-rich blood through the pulmonary veins is the
   a. right atrium
   b. right ventricle
   c. left atrium
   d. left ventricle

3. In a cardiac cycle that lasts for 0.8 second, the ventricles are in systole for
   a. 0.1 second
   b. 0.2 second
   c. 0.3 second
   d. 0.4 second

4. If an individual has a heart rate of 70 beats per minute and a stroke volume of 70 milliliters, what is the cardiac output?
   a. 70 mL/min
   b. 140 mL/min
   c. 1400 mL/min
   d. 4900 mL/min

5. Increased venous return
   a. increases both end-diastolic volume and contraction strength
   b. increases both cardiac rate and stroke volume
   c. increases end-diastolic volume, but decreases contraction strength
   d. increases both cardiac rate and contraction strength

APPLICATION

Which of the following occur when the semilunar valves are open?

a. coronary arteries fill

b. blood enters the aorta

c. AV valves are closed

d. blood enters the ventricles

e. blood enters the pulmonary trunk

f. atria contract

g. ventricles are in systole

A heart rate of 45 beats per minute and an absence of P waves on the ECG suggests damage to which component of the conduction system?

CHAPTER 13

Blood Vessels

Outline/Objectives

Classification and Structure of Blood Vessels 260

- Describe the structure and function of arteries, capillaries, and veins.

Physiology of Circulation 263

- Discuss how oxygen, carbon dioxide, glucose, and water move across capillary walls.
- Discuss the factors that affect blood flow through arteries, capillaries, and veins.
- Describe the mechanisms and pressures that move gases and fluids across capillary walls.
- Discuss four primary factors that affect blood pressure and how blood pressure is regulated.

Circulatory Pathways 269

- Trace blood through the pulmonary circuit from the right atrium to the left atrium.
- Identify the major systemic arteries and veins.
- Describe the blood supply to the brain.
- Describe five features of fetal circulation that make it different from adult circulation.

Key Terms

Diastolic pressure
Korotkoff sounds
Peripheral resistance
Pulse
Systolic pressure
Vasoconstriction
Vasodilation

Building Vocabulary

WORD PART	MEANING
angi-	vessel
arter-	artery
ather-	yellow fatty plaque
brachi-	arm
carotid	put to sleep
cephal-	head
edem-	to swell
embol-	stopper, wedge
isch-	deficiency
phleb-	vein
scler-	hard
sten-	narrowing
-tripsy	crushing
vas-	vessel

Blood vessels are the channels or conduits through which blood is distributed to body tissues. The vessels make up two closed systems of tubes that begin and end at the heart (Fig. 13–1). One system, the **pulmonary vessels,** transports blood from the right ventricle to the lungs and back to the left atrium. The other system, the **systemic vessels,** carries blood from the left ventricle to the tissues in all parts of the body and then returns the blood to the right atrium. Based on their structure and function, blood vessels are classified as either arteries, capillaries, or veins.

Classification and Structure of Blood Vessels

Arteries

Arteries carry blood away from the heart. Pulmonary arteries transport blood that has a low oxygen content from the right ventricle to the lungs. Systemic arteries transport oxygenated blood from the left ventricle to the body tissues. Blood is pumped from the ventricles into large elastic arteries that branch repeatedly into smaller and smaller arteries until the branching results in microscopic arteries called **arterioles** (ar-TEER-ee-ohlz). The arterioles play a key role in regulating blood flow into the tissue capillaries. About 10 percent of the total blood volume is in the systemic arterial system at any given time.

> Arteries carry blood away from the heart. In systemic arteries, the blood is oxygenated. In pulmonary arteries, the blood has a low oxygen content.

The wall of an artery consists of three layers (Fig. 13–2). The innermost layer, the **tunica intima** (also called **tunica interna**), is simple squamous epithelium surrounded by a connective tissue basement membrane with elastic fibers. The middle layer, the

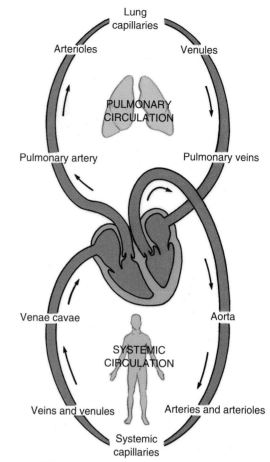

Figure 13–1 Scheme of circulation.

tunica media, is primarily smooth muscle and is usually the thickest layer. It not only provides support for the vessel but also changes vessel diameter to regulate blood flow and blood pressure. The outermost layer, which attaches the vessel to the sur-

---

CLINICAL TERMS

Angiography (an-jih-AHG-rah-fee) A procedure in which a radiopaque substance is injected into the bloodstream and then radiographs are taken; used to determine the condition of blood vessels

Angioplasty (AN-jih-oh-plas-tee) Surgical repair of a blood vessel or vessels

Arterectomy (ahr-teh-RECK-toh-mee) Surgical removal of an artery

Arteriosclerosis (ahr-tee-rih-oh-skleh-ROH-sis) A condition of hardening of an artery; an artery becomes less elastic and does not expand under pressure

Atherosclerosis (ath-er-oh-skleh-ROH-sis) A form of arteriosclerosis characterized by the buildup of fatty plaques in the wall of the vessel

Hemangioma (hee-man-jee-OH-mah) A benign tumor of a blood vessel

Hemorrhoids (HEM-oh-royds) Varicose veins in the anal canal resulting from a persistent increase in venous pressure

Phlebitis (fleh-BYE-tis) Inflammation of veins, which may be caused by pooling and stagnation of blood; often leads to the formation of blood clots within the vessel

Phlebotomy (fleh-BAH-toh-mee) Incision into a vein

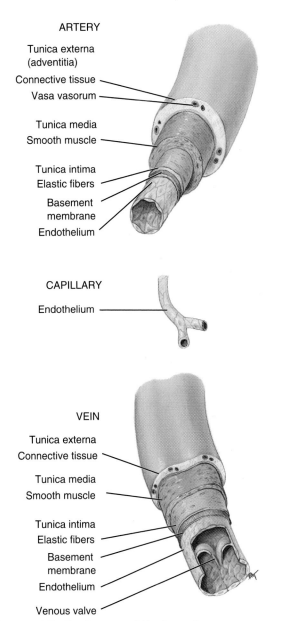

ARTERY

Tunica externa
(adventitia)
Connective tissue
Vasa vasorum

Tunica media
Smooth muscle

Tunica intima
Elastic fibers

Basement
membrane
Endothelium

CAPILLARY

Endothelium

VEIN

Tunica externa
Connective tissue

Tunica media
Smooth muscle

Tunica intima
Elastic fibers

Basement
membrane

Endothelium

Venous valve

Figure 13–2   Structure of blood vessels.

An **aneurysm** is a bulge, or bubble, that develops at a weakened region in the wall of an artery. This is especially dangerous if it is in the aorta or arteries of the brain. If diagnosed soon enough, the aneurysm sometimes may be removed and the vessel surgically repaired. Because the wall is weakened, an aneurysm is subject to rupture. Little can be done when this happens because the massive bleeding usually leads to death before medical care can be obtained.

Capillaries

Capillaries, the smallest and most numerous of the blood vessels, form the connection between the vessels that carry blood away from the heart (arteries) and the vessels that return blood to the heart (veins). They are the continuation of the smallest arterioles. Arterioles are the smallest vessels with three distinguishable layers in the wall. When the arterioles branch into capillaries, the middle and outer layers of the wall disappear so that the capillary wall is only a thin endothelium (simple squamous epithelium) with a basement membrane. The thin wall permits the exchange of materials between the blood in the capillary and the adjacent tissue cells. This exchange is the primary function of capillaries.

Capillaries are microscopic vessels that form a connection between arteries and veins. Their primary function is the exchange of materials between the blood and tissue cells.

The diameter of a capillary is so small that erythrocytes must pass through them in single file. This slows the blood flow to allow ample time for the transport of substances across the capillary endothelium.

It is estimated that if all the capillaries in the body were placed end to end, they would encircle the earth at the equator two and one-half times!

Capillary distribution varies with the metabolic activity of body tissues. Tissues such as skeletal muscle, liver, and kidney have extensive capillary networks because they are metabolically active and require an abundant supply of oxygen and nutrients. Other tissues, such as connective tissue, have a less abundant supply of capillaries. The epidermis of the skin and the lens and cornea of the eye completely lack a capillary network. About 5 percent of the total blood volume is in the systemic capillaries at any given time. Another 10 percent is in the lungs.

rounding tissues, is the **tunica externa** or **tunica adventitia.** This layer is connective tissue with varying amounts of elastic and collagenous fibers. The connective tissue in this layer is quite dense where it is adjacent to the tunica media, but it changes to loose connective tissue near the periphery of the vessel. The tunica externa of the larger arteries contains small blood vessels, called **vasa vasorum** (VAS-ah vah-SOR-um), that provide the blood supply for the tissues of the vessel wall.

The innermost layer of the arterial wall is simple squamous epithelium, the middle layer is smooth muscle, and the outer layer is connective tissue.

Metabolically active tissues have extensive capillary networks.

Blood flow from the arterioles into the capillaries is regulated by smooth muscle cells in the arterioles where they branch to form the capillaries. These **precapillary sphincters** constrict to reduce blood flow into the capillary bed and relax to increase the blood flow. When the precapillary sphincters contract, blood passes directly from small arterioles into small venules through **metarterioles** (met-ahr-TEER-ee-ohlz), or **arteriovenous anastomoses** (ar-teer-ee-oh-VAY-nus ah-NAS-toh-moh-ses) (Fig. 13–3). This arrangement allows blood to be diverted from one capillary bed to another for distribution to the regions that need it most at any given time.

The small arterioles and precapillary sphincters regulate blood flow into the capillaries.

Veins

Veins carry blood toward the heart. After blood passes through the capillaries, it enters the smallest veins, called **venules.** From the venules, it flows into progressively larger and larger veins until it reaches the heart. In the pulmonary circuit, the pulmonary veins transport blood from the lungs to the left atrium of the heart. This blood has a high oxygen content because it has just been oxygenated in the lungs. Systemic veins transport blood from the body tissues to the right atrium of the heart. This blood has a reduced oxygen content because the oxygen has been used for metabolic activities in the tissue cells.

Veins carry blood toward the heart.

The walls of veins have the same three layers as the arteries (see Fig. 13–2). Although all the layers are present, there is less smooth muscle and connective tissue. This makes the walls of veins thinner than those of arteries, which is related to the fact that blood in the veins has less pressure than in the arteries. Because the walls of the veins are thinner and less rigid than arteries, veins can hold more blood. Almost 70 percent of the total blood volume is in the veins at any given time. Medium and large veins have **venous valves,** similar to the semilunar valves associated with the heart, that help keep the blood flowing toward the heart. Venous valves are especially important in the arms and legs, where they prevent the backflow of blood in response to the pull of gravity.

Veins have thinner walls than arteries and have valves to prevent backflow of blood.

Varicose veins are veins that are twisted and dilated with accumulated blood. These frequently occur in the legs. Conditions that hinder venous return, such as pregnancy, obesity, and standing for long periods of time, allow blood to accumulate in the veins of the extremities. This stretches the veins so the valve flaps no longer overlap and they permit the backflow of blood. Superficial veins are more susceptible because they receive less support from surrounding tissue.

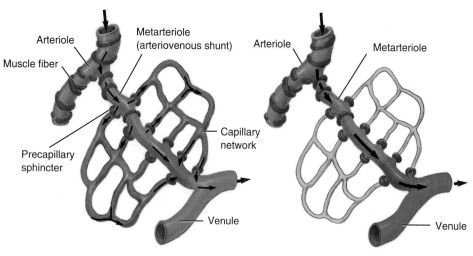

Precapillary sphincters open

Sphincters closed—blood shunted to venule

Figure 13–3
Organization of a capillary network.

☑ **Quick**Check

● At any given time, which type of vessel contains the greatest volume of blood?

● What is the purpose of valves in the veins?

● What happens to blood flow in a given capillary bed when the precapillary sphincter relaxes?

Physiology of Circulation

Role of the Capillaries

In addition to forming the connection between the arteries and veins, capillaries have a vital role in the exchange of gases, nutrients, and metabolic waste products between the blood and the tissue cells. Tissue cells are surrounded by a small amount of extracellular fluid, called **interstitial fluid** (in-ter-STISH-al FLOO-id). This fluid is formed from the fluids and solutes that leave the capillaries (Fig. 13–4). Substances that transfer between the blood and tissue cells must pass through the interstitial fluid, and therefore the interstitial fluid plays an intermediary role in the exchange.

Substances pass through the capillary wall by diffusion, filtration, and osmosis. Oxygen, carbon dioxide, and glucose move across the capillary wall, from higher concentrations to lower concentrations, by diffusion. Blood entering the capillary has higher oxygen and glucose concentrations than the interstitial fluid and tissue cells, thus the oxygen and glucose diffuse through the capillary wall and enter the interstitial fluid and then the tissue cells. Metabolically active tissue cells produce carbon dioxide as a waste product so there is a higher concentration inside the cells. The carbon dioxide diffuses down the concentration gradient from the tissue cells to the interstitial fluid and then into the capillary.

> Oxygen and carbon dioxide move across the capillary wall by diffusion.

Filtration involves hydrostatic pressure to force (push) water molecules and certain dissolved substances through the capillary wall. In capillaries, the hydrostatic pressure is blood pressure generated by ventricular contractions. Because blood pressure is higher at the arteriolar end of the capillary than it is at the venule end, more filtration occurs at the arteriolar end.

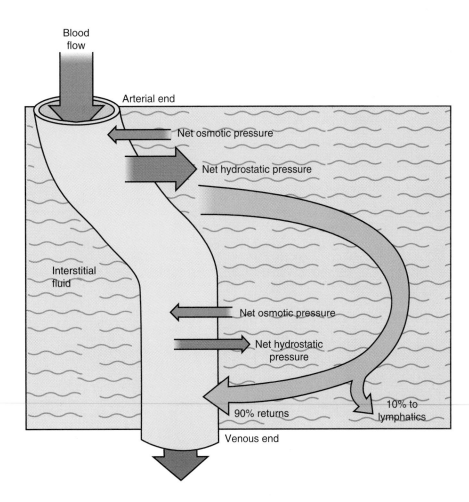

Figure 13–4   Capillary microcirculation.

Protein molecules are generally too large to pass through the capillary wall so they remain in the plasma and create an osmotic pressure in the blood. There are relatively few protein molecules in the interstitial fluid so its osmotic pressure is negligible. Osmotic pressure attracts (or pulls) water into the capillary. At the arteriolar end of the capillary, hydrostatic pressure is greater than the osmotic pressure, so fluid leaves the capillary. Hydrostatic (blood) pressure decreases as the blood moves through the capillary. At the venule end, the attraction produced by the osmotic pressure overcomes the hydrostatic pressure and draws fluid into the capillary (see Fig. 13–4).

> Fluid movement across a capillary wall is determined by a combination of hydrostatic and osmotic pressures.

The net result of the capillary microcirculation created by hydrostatic and osmotic pressures is that substances leave the blood at one end of the capillary and return at the other end. Normally, more fluid leaves the capillaries than is returned to them. About 90 percent of the fluid is returned at the venule end; the remaining 10 percent is collected by lymphatic vessels and is returned to the general circulation in venous blood. Because of the capillary microcirculation, the interstitial fluid is continually changing and nutrients, gases, and waste products are moved between the tissue cells and blood.

> Fluid moves out of the capillary at the arteriole end and returns at the venule end.

> **Edema** is an abnormal accumulation of interstitial fluid, or swelling. This may be caused by a disruption of normal capillary microcirculation. Factors that may lead to edema include an increase in capillary blood pressure, a decrease in the quantity of plasma proteins, and an increase in the permeability of the capillary wall so that proteins leak out.

Blood Flow

Relationship of Blood Flow to Pressure

Blood flow refers to the movement of blood through the vessels from arteries to the capillaries and then into the veins. Pressure is a measure of the force that the blood exerts against vessel walls. It moves the blood through the vessels. Like all fluids, blood flows from a high pressure area to a region with lower pressure. Because the contraction of the ventricles provides this force, or pressure, it is greatest during ventricular systole when the blood is pumped from the left ventricle into the aorta. Figure 13–5 illustrates the progressive decrease in pressure through the arteries, capillaries, and veins, so that it is lowest as the venae cavae enter the right atrium. The pressure in the right atrium is often called the **central venous pressure.** Blood flows in the same direction as the pressure gradient.

> Blood flows in the same direction as the decreasing pressure gradient: arteries to capillaries to veins.

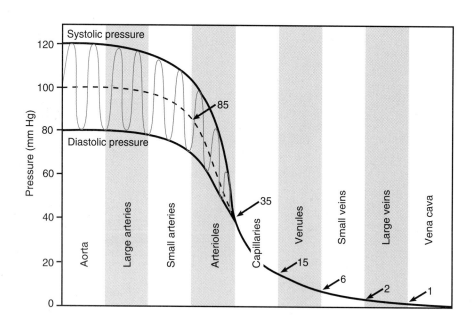

Figure 13–5 Blood pressure in various types of systemic vessels.

Velocity of Blood Flow

The rate, or velocity, of blood flow varies inversely with the total cross-sectional area of the blood vessels. As the total cross-sectional area of the vessels increases, the velocity of flow decreases (Fig. 13–6). Therefore, velocity is greatest in the aorta and progressively decreases as the blood flows through increasing numbers of smaller and smaller vessels. Blood flow is slowest in the capillaries, which have the largest total cross-sectional area. This allows time for the exchange of gases and nutrients. Velocity increases again as the blood enters decreasing numbers of progressively larger and larger veins during the return to the heart.

▌ Blood flow is slowest in the capillaries, which allows time for exchange of gases and nutrients.

Relationship of Blood Flow to Resistance

Resistance is a force that opposes the flow of a fluid. For example, it is more difficult to get a milkshake through a straw than water because the milkshake offers more resistance. It opposes the flow. In blood vessels, most of the resistance is due to vessel diameter. As vessel diameter decreases, the resistance increases and blood flow decreases. The autonomic nervous system plays a role in regulating blood flow by changing the vascular resistance through vasodilation and vasoconstriction. During exercise, autonomic control causes vasoconstriction in the viscera and skin (increases resistance) and vasodilation in the skeletal muscles (decreases resistance). As a result, blood flow to the viscera and skin decreases and blood flow to the skeletal muscles increases.

When you are in the sun for an extended period, the cutaneous blood vessels dilate to bring more blood to the surface for cooling. This decreases the amount of blood in other parts of the body and may diminish the blood supply to the brain. If you are sunbathing and stand up abruptly, you may feel dizzy. This is because the blood momentarily remains in the dilated cutaneous vessels instead of returning to the heart. This causes a decrease in blood pressure. The dizziness is a signal that the brain is not receiving enough oxygen.

Contraction and relaxation of the precapillary sphincters control the flow of blood into the capillaries by changing the vessel diameter to modify the resistance. When precapillary sphincters contract, the diameter of the vessel decreases and local resistance increases. Blood flow to that area decreases. When the sphincters relax, vessel diameter increases, resistance decreases, and blood flows through the capillaries. An increase in carbon dioxide, a decrease in pH, or a decrease in oxygen causes the precapillary sphincters to relax, which allows increased blood flow to deliver more oxygen to the tissues and to carry away the waste products.

▌ When resistance increases, blood flow decreases.

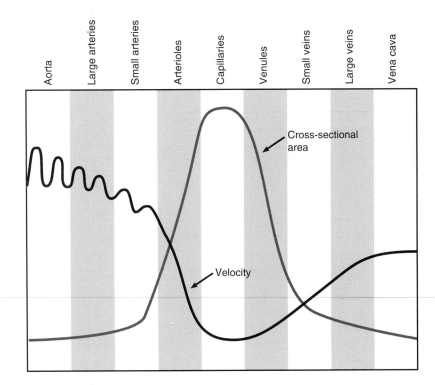

Figure 13–6 Relation of blood flow to total vessel cross-sectional area.

Venous Blood Flow

Very little pressure remains by the time blood leaves the capillaries and enters the venules. Blood flow through the veins is not the direct result of ventricular contraction. Instead, venous return depends on **skeletal muscle action** and **respiratory movements** and **constriction of the veins.**

When skeletal muscles contract, they thicken, which squeezes the veins adjacent to them. The squeezing, or milking, action creates a localized high pressure area and the blood flows from that high pressure region to an area with lower pressure. Figure 13–7 illustrates this action. Valves in the veins offer very little resistance to blood flowing toward the heart but they close to prevent blood from flowing in the opposite direction. Muscular contraction during exercise enhances venous return. A lack of

muscular movement allows blood to accumulate, or pool, in the extremities rather than to return to the heart for circulation.

Respiratory movements create pressure gradients that enhance the movement of venous blood. When the diaphragm contracts during inspiration, it exerts pressure in the abdomen and decreases the pressure in the thoracic cavity. Blood in the abdominal veins moves from the higher pressure in the abdomen to the lower pressure in the thorax. Valves prevent the blood from flowing in the opposite direction into the legs. During exercise, when the breathing rate increases, respiratory movements increase the rate at which blood is returned to the heart, which increases the cardiac output to meet the needs of the muscular activity.

Sympathetic reflexes cause contraction of the smooth muscle in the walls of the veins. This venous constriction along with valves to prevent backflow moves blood toward the heart. As mentioned previously, about 70 percent of the total blood volume is in the veins at any given time, which makes them an important blood reservoir. If there is blood loss for some reason, and blood pressure decreases, sympathetic reflexes stimulate venoconstriction. This moves blood out of the venous reservoir and helps restore blood pressure to normal.

> Venous blood flow depends on skeletal muscle action, respiratory movements, and contraction of smooth muscle in venous walls.

> The difference in blood pressure between arteries and veins is obvious when the vessels are cut. Blood flows smoothly and freely from a vein, but it spurts forcefully from an artery.

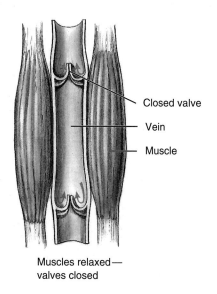

Muscles relaxed—
valves closed

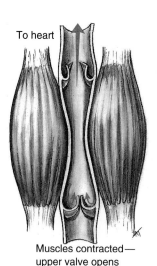

To heart

Muscles contracted—
upper valve opens

Figure 13–7 Effect of skeletal muscle contraction on venous blood flow.

Closed valve

Vein

Muscle

Pulse and Blood Pressure

Meaning of Pulse

Pulse is the alternating expansion and recoil of an artery in response to the surge of blood ejected from the left ventricle during contraction. This pulse can be felt in places where an artery is near the surface of the body and passes over something firm like a bone. Figure 13–8 illustrates the location of nine commonly used **pulse points** where the pulse may be detected by placing the fingers over a superficial artery. Taking a person's pulse provides information about the rate, strength, and rhythmicity of the heartbeat.

> Pulse refers to the rhythmic expansion of an artery that is caused by ejection of blood from the ventricle. It can be felt where an artery is close to the surface and rests on something firm.

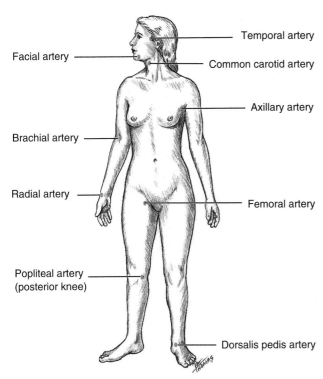

Facial artery

Brachial artery

Radial artery

Popliteal artery
(posterior knee)

Temporal artery

Common carotid artery

Axillary artery

Femoral artery

Dorsalis pedis artery

Figure 13-8 Pulse points.

Weak pulses usually indicate a decreased stroke volume or increased constriction of the arteries. The arteries do not expand as much so the pulse feels weaker.

Arterial Blood Pressure and its Determination

In common usage, the term **blood pressure** refers to arterial blood pressure, the pressure in the aorta and its branches. The pressure in the arteries is greatest during ventricular contraction (systole) when blood is forcefully ejected from the left ventricle into the aorta. This is called **systolic pressure.** Arterial pressure is lowest when the ventricles are in the relaxation phase (diastole) of the cardiac cycle just before the next contraction. This is called **diastolic pressure.** The difference between the systolic pressure and diastolic pressure is called **pulse pressure.** The standard units of measurement for blood pressure are millimeters of mercury (mm Hg). Each unit of pressure will lift a column of mercury 1 millimeter. A blood pressure of 110 mm Hg will lift a column of mercury 110 millimeters.

Systolic pressure is due to ventricular contraction. Diastolic pressure occurs during cardiac relaxation. Pulse pressure is the difference between systolic pressure and diastolic pressure.

In arteriosclerosis the arteries lose their elasticity and cannot expand when blood is pumped into them. This increases the systolic pressure, and then the pressure falls rapidly, resulting in a large pulse pressure. Increased stroke volume during exercise also increases pulse pressure.

In most clinical settings, a **sphygmomanometer** (sfig-moh-mah-NAHM-eh-ter) is used to measure blood pressure in the brachial artery (Fig. 13–9). An inflatable cuff, connected to the sphygmomanometer and an air supply, is wrapped around the patient's arm, just above the elbow. The cuff is inflated with sufficient air pressure to collapse the brachial artery. A sensor is placed over the brachial artery. While the examiner is listening through the stethoscope and watching the column of mercury on the sphygmomanometer, air is slowly released through the pressure valve on the cuff. As the pressure gradually decreases, sounds representing the first flow of blood through the collapsed artery are heard in the stethoscope. The sounds heard through the stethoscope as a result of blood flow are called **Korotkoff** (koh-ROT-kof) **sounds.**

The pressure at which the first Korotkoff sound is heard represents the systolic pressure, which normally averages about 120 mm Hg. As the pressure in the cuff continues to decline, the Korotkoff sounds change in tone and loudness until they completely stop. This represents the point at which the artery is completely open and blood flows freely and is recorded as diastolic pressure, which normally averages about 80 mm Hg. The blood pressure is recorded as systolic pressure over diastolic pressure, in this case 120/80. Pulse pressure in this instance is 40 mm Hg.

Blood pressure is measured with a sphygmomanometer and is recorded as the systolic pressure over the diastolic pressure.

Factors That Affect Blood Pressure

Four major factors interact to affect blood pressure. These are **cardiac output, blood volume, peripheral resistance,** and **viscosity.** Each one has a direct relationship to blood pressure.

Cardiac output is the amount of blood pumped by the heart in 1 minute (see Chapter 12). It is determined by multiplying the heart rate times the stroke volume. Anything that increases either the heart rate or the stroke volume will increase cardiac output and also increase blood pressure. When either heart rate or stroke volume decreases, cardiac output decreases, which decreases blood pressure.

The volume of blood in the body directly affects blood pressure. Although blood volume varies with age, body size, and gender, the normal average is about 5 liters for adults. Blood volume may be re-

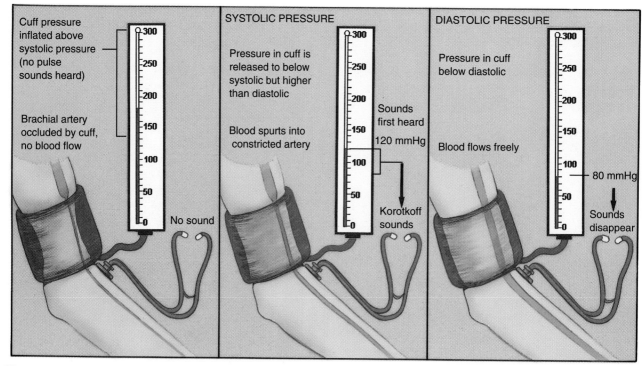

Figure 13-9 Measurement of blood pressure.

duced by severe hemorrhage, vomiting, diarrhea, or reduced fluid intake. Any changes in blood volume are accompanied by corresponding changes in blood pressure. When blood volume decreases, blood pressure also decreases. When the blood volume is restored by a transfusion or fluid intake, blood pressure returns to normal. If the body retains too much fluid, blood volume and blood pressure increase.

Circulatory shock is a condition in which blood cannot circulate normally because the vessels are not adequately filled. One type, called **hypovolemic shock,** occurs when there is a loss in blood volume from a severe hemorrhage. When blood volume drops rapidly, heart rate increases in an attempt to maintain cardiac output, and thus there is a rapid pulse. Fluid volume should be replaced as soon as possible.

Peripheral resistance is the opposition to blood flow caused by friction of the vessel walls. Increased peripheral resistance causes an increase in blood pressure. Vasoconstriction decreases the vessel diameter and increases resistance. This increases blood pressure. When blood vessels lose their elasticity, their resistance increases and so does blood pressure.

Viscosity is a physical property of blood that refers to the ease with which the molecules and cells slide across each other. Viscosity opposes the flow of a fluid. Syrup does not flow as easily as water so the syrup is said to be more viscous. Normally the

viscosity of blood remains fairly constant, but it changes when either the number of blood cells or concentration of plasma proteins changes. If the number of erythrocytes increases (polycythemia), the blood becomes more viscous and blood pressure increases.

When cardiac output, blood volume, peripheral resistance, or blood viscosity increases, blood pressure also increases.

Regulation of Arterial Blood Pressure

Arterial blood pressure is maintained within normal ranges by changes in cardiac output and peripheral resistance. Pressure receptors (baroreceptors) are located in the walls of the large arteries in the thorax and neck. They are abundant in the carotid sinus, located at the bifurcation of the common carotid arteries in the neck, and in the aortic arch. These receptors respond when the walls are stretched by sudden increases in pressure. The action potentials from the baroreceptors are transmitted to the cardiac and vasomotor centers in the medulla oblongata. The centers in the medulla respond by sending out signals that decrease heart rate (decrease cardiac output) and cause vasodilation (decrease peripheral resistance). These actions return blood pressure toward normal. Decreases in blood pressure reduce the frequency of action potentials from the receptors, which increases heart rate and causes vasoconstriction. Baroreceptors are important for moment-by-moment short-term pressure regulation.

Baroreceptors in the aortic arch and carotid sinus are important for short-term blood pressure regulation.

Sometimes there is a feeling of dizziness when rising rapidly from lying down to a standing position. This is because the baroreceptors have not had time to respond to the decrease in blood pressure caused by the downward pull of gravity on the blood. The dizziness is a signal that the brain is not receiving enough blood.

Chemoreceptors near the carotid sinus and aortic arch respond to changes in carbon dioxide concentration, hydrogen ion concentration (pH), and oxygen concentration. When carbon dioxide or hydrogen ion concentrations increase, or oxygen concentration decreases, these receptors send impulses to the medulla oblongata. The medulla oblongata responds by sending out impulses that increase heart rate and peripheral resistance to increase blood pressure. This increases blood flow to the lungs and to the tissues. Chemoreceptors have a significant role in blood pressure regulation only in emergency situations.

Certain hormones also have an effect on blood pressure. Epinephrine and norepinephrine from the adrenal medulla have an effect similar to the sympathetic nervous system to increase cardiac output and blood pressure. Antidiuretic hormone from the posterior pituitary gland reduces fluid loss through urine and increases body fluid volume. This increases blood volume, which increases blood pressure.

When blood pressure decreases, the kidneys secrete **renin,** an enzyme, into the blood. Renin acts on certain blood proteins to produce **angiotensin.**

Active angiotensin is a powerful vasoconstrictor, which increases blood pressure back toward normal. Angiotensin also promotes the secretion of **aldosterone** from the adrenal cortex. Aldosterone acts on the kidneys to conserve sodium ions and water so that blood volume increases, which increases blood pressure. The **renin/angiotensin/aldosterone** mechanism has a significant role in the long-term regulation of blood pressure.

Angiotensin causes vasoconstriction and promotes the release of aldosterone. Both actions result in increased blood pressure.

✓ QuickCheck

- What happens to fluid when blood pressure is greater than capillary osmotic pressure?
- In which type of vessel is the rate of blood flow the slowest?
- Why does exercise increase cardiac output?
- External pressure on the common carotid artery, just below the carotid sinus, decreases the blood pressure in the carotid sinus. How does this affect heart rate?

Circulatory Pathways

The blood vessels of the body are functionally divided into two distinct circuits:

- Pulmonary circuit
- Systemic circuit

The pump for the pulmonary circuit, which circulates blood through the lungs, is the right ventricle. The left ventricle is the pump for the systemic circuit, which provides the blood supply for the tissue cells of the body.

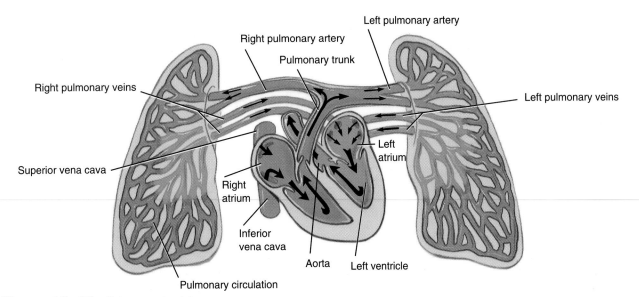

Figure 13–10 Pulmonary circulation.

Pulmonary Circuit

The pulmonary circuit takes blood from the right side of the heart to the lungs, then returns it to the left side of the heart (Fig. 13–10). Oxygen-poor blood, which has increased levels of carbon dioxide, is returned to the **right atrium** from the tissue cells of the body. It passes through the **tricuspid valve** into the **right ventricle.** During ventricular systole, the blood is ejected through the **pulmonary semilunar valve** into the **pulmonary trunk,** which divides into the right and left **pulmonary arteries.** Each pulmonary artery enters a lung and repeatedly divides into smaller and smaller vessels until they become capillaries. The **capillaries of the lungs** form networks that surround the air sacs, or alveoli, of the lungs. Here CO_2 diffuses from the capillary blood into the alveoli of the lungs, and O_2 diffuses from the alveoli into the blood. The newly oxygenated blood enters pulmonary venules, which form progressively larger veins, until two **pulmonary veins** emerge from each lung and carry the blood to the **left atrium.** In the pulmonary circuit, the arteries carry deoxygenated blood away from the heart, and the veins carry oxygenated blood to the heart.

> Pulmonary circulation transports oxygen-poor blood from the right ventricle to the lungs where the blood picks up a new oxygen supply. Then it returns the oxygen-rich blood to the left atrium.

Systemic Circuit

The systemic circulation provides the functional blood supply to all body tissues. It carries oxygen and nutrients to the cells and picks up carbon dioxide and waste products. Systemic circulation carries oxygenated blood from the left ventricle, through the arteries, to the capillaries in the tissues of the body. From the tissue capillaries, the deoxygenated blood returns through a system of veins to the right atrium of the heart. The major systemic arteries are illustrated in Figure 13–11 and are schematically represented in Figure 13–12.

Major Systemic Arteries

All systemic arteries are branches, either directly or indirectly, from the aorta. The aorta ascends from the left ventricle, curves posteriorly and to the left, then descends through the thorax and abdomen. This geography divides the aorta into three portions: **ascending aorta, aortic arch,** and **descending aorta.** The descending aorta is further subdivided into the **thoracic aorta** and **abdominal aorta.** Table 13–1 summarizes the divisions of the aorta, the major vessels that branch from each region, and the organs supplied by each branch. The major branches of the aorta are illustrated in Figure 13–13.

Ascending Aorta. The ascending aorta, which begins at the aortic semilunar valve, is the portion that ascends from the left ventricle. The **right and left coronary arteries** are the only tributaries that branch from this portion. The coronary arteries, which supply oxygenated blood to the myocardium, branch from the ascending aorta just distal to the semilunar valve. When the semilunar valve is open, while blood is forcefully ejected from the heart during ventricular systole, the valve cusps cover the openings into the coronary arteries. When the valve is closed during ventricular diastole, the openings into the coronary arteries are clear and blood flows into them.

> The coronary arteries are the only vessels that branch from the ascending aorta.

Aortic Arch. The aortic arch, which is a continuation of the ascending aorta, curves posteriorly and to the left. There are three main branches from this region of the aorta. The first and most anterior branch is the **brachiocephalic (bray-kee-oh-seh-FAL-ik) artery,** which supplies blood to the right side of the head and neck, right shoulder, and right upper extremity. This vessel divides into the **right subclavian (sub-KLAY-vee-an) artery** and the **right common carotid (kah-ROT-id) artery.** The middle branch from the aortic arch is the **left common carotid artery,** which supplies the left side of the head and neck. The third and most posterior branch is the **left subclavian artery,** which takes blood to the left shoulder and left upper extremity.

> The brachiocephalic, left common carotid, and left subclavian arteries branch from the aortic arch.

> The word "carotid" means to put to sleep. If the carotid arteries are blocked, the patient is "put to sleep," or becomes unconscious.

Descending Aorta. The descending aorta is a continuation of the aortic arch. It descends through the thoracic and abdominal regions immediately anterior to the vertebral column and slightly to the left of it. The descending aorta is subdivided into the **thoracic aorta** in the thoracic region and the **abdominal aorta** in the abdomen.

Small, paired **intercostal arteries** branch from the thoracic aorta. These vessels are found in the spaces between the ribs where they supply the intercostal muscles. Other small arteries supply the viscera in the thorax. After the descending aorta goes through the diaphragm, it is called the abdominal aorta. Major branches of the abdominal aorta are the **celiac (SEE-lee-ak) artery, superior mesenteric (MES-en-tair-ik) artery, renal (REE-nal) arteries, gonadal (go-NAD-al) arteries, inferior mesenteric artery,** and **lumbar arteries.** Approximately at the L4 vertebral

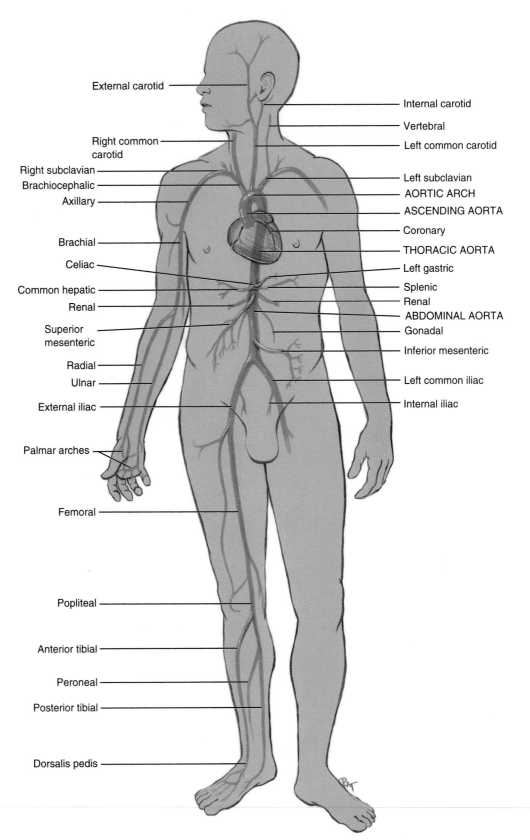

External carotid

Internal carotid

Vertebral

Right common carotid

Left common carotid

Right subclavian

Brachiocephalic

Axillary

Left subclavian

AORTIC ARCH

ASCENDING AORTA

Brachial

Coronary

THORACIC AORTA

Celiac

Left gastric

Common hepatic

Splenic

Renal

Renal

ABDOMINAL AORTA

Superior mesenteric

Gonadal

Inferior mesenteric

Radial

Ulnar

Left common iliac

External iliac

Internal iliac

Palmar arches

Femoral

Popliteal

Anterior tibial

Peroneal

Posterior tibial

Dorsalis pedis

Figure 13–11 Major systemic arteries.

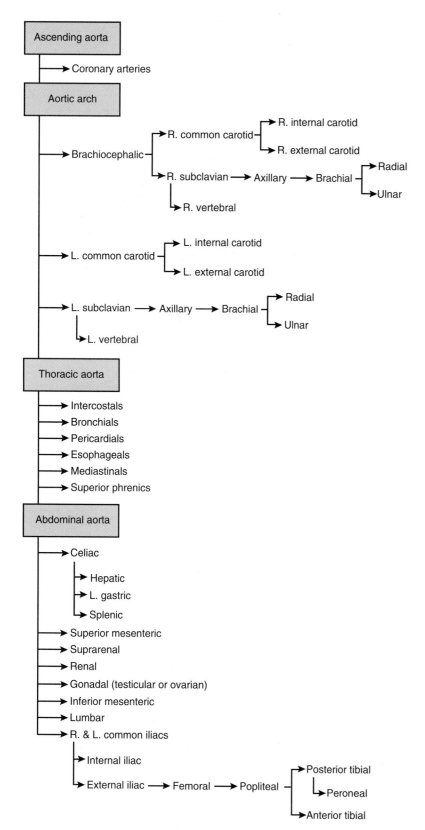

Figure 13–12 Schematic diagram of the major systemic arteries.

Table 13-1   Summary of Major Arteries and Regions They Supply

Artery	Region Supplied	Comments
From the Ascending Aorta		
Right & left coronary	Myocardium of heart wall	Branches of ascending aorta
From the Aortic Arch		
Brachiocephalic	Head and arm on right side	First branch of aortic arch; divides into right common carotid and right subclavian
Common carotid	Head and neck	The right is a branch of the brachiocephalic; the left comes directly from the aortic arch; divides into external and internal carotids
External carotid	Face, scalp, pharynx, larynx, superficial neck	
Internal carotid	Brain	Enters the cranium through the carotid canal
Subclavian	Shoulder and upper extremity	The right is a branch of the brachiocephalic; the left comes directly from the aortic arch
Vertebral	Brain	Branches from the subclavian; ascends neck in transverse foramina; enters cranium through foramen magnum
Axillary	Axilla or armpit	Continuation of the subclavian
Brachial	Arm	Continuation of the axillary
Radial	Lateral side of forearm and hand	Formed from the brachial at the elbow
Ulnar	Medial side of forearm and hand	Formed from the brachial at the elbow
Palmar arches	Hand and fingers	Formed by anastomosis of radial and ulnar arteries; branches extend into fingers
From the Thoracic Aorta		
Intercostals	Intercostal and other muscles of the thoracic wall	Numerous, paired vessels
Bronchials	Bronchi and other passageways of the respiratory tract	Numerous, paired vessels
Pericardials	Pericardium	
Esophageals	Esophagus	
Mediastinals	Structures in the mediastinum	
Superior phrenics	Diaphragm	
From the Abdominal Aorta		
Celiac	Liver, stomach, pancreas, spleen	Short trunk that branches into the hepatic, left gastric, and splenic
Hepatic	Liver	Branch of the celiac
Left gastric	Stomach	Branch of the celiac
Splenic	Spleen, pancreas, stomach	Branch of the celiac
Superior mesenteric	Small intestine and part of the large intestine	Numerous branches located between the layers of the mesentery
Suprarenal	Suprarenal (adrenal) glands	Paired, one right and one left
Renal	Kidneys	Paired, one right and one left
Gonadal	Gonads (ovaries/testes)	Paired, one right and one left
Inferior mesenteric	Distal portion of the large intestine	Single vessel with several branches
Lumbar	Spinal cord and lumbar region of the back	Four or five pairs branch from the aorta
Common iliac	Pelvis and lower extremities	Two vessels formed by bifurcation of the aorta
Internal iliac	Muscles of the pelvic wall and the urinary and reproductive organs in the pelvis	Branch of the common iliac
External iliac	Lower extremities	Branch of the common iliac; continues as femoral in the thigh
Femoral	Muscles of the thigh	Continuation of the external iliac; becomes popliteal in the knee region
Popliteal	Knee and leg	Continuation of the femoral
Anterior tibial	Anterior muscles of the leg	Formed from the popliteal
Posterior tibial	Posterior muscles of the leg	Formed from the popliteal
Peroneal	Lateral muscles of the leg	Branches from the posterior tibial
Dorsal pedis	Ankle and dorsal part of foot	Continuation of the anterior tibial

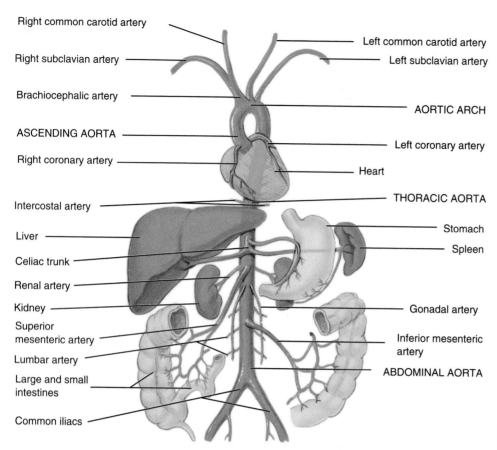

Right common carotid artery

Right subclavian artery

Brachiocephalic artery

ASCENDING AORTA

Right coronary artery

Intercostal artery

Liver

Celiac trunk

Renal artery

Kidney

Superior mesenteric artery

Lumbar artery

Large and small intestines

Common iliacs

Left common carotid artery

Left subclavian artery

AORTIC ARCH

Left coronary artery

Heart

THORACIC AORTA

Stomach

Spleen

Gonadal artery

Inferior mesenteric artery

ABDOMINAL AORTA

Figure 13–13 Branches of the aorta.

level, the abdominal aorta bifurcates to form the **right and left common iliac (ILL-ee-ak) arteries.**

Arteries of the Head and Neck. The arterial blood supply for the head and neck comes from branches of the aortic arch. Note from Figure 13–13 that one of the branches of the short brachiocephalic artery is the right common carotid artery. There is no brachiocephalic artery on the left side. The left common carotid artery branches directly from the aortic arch.

The common carotid arteries ascend along each side of the neck to the angle of the mandible where each one divides into an **external carotid artery** and an **internal carotid artery** (see Figs. 13–11 and 13–12). At the base of the internal carotid artery there is a slight enlargement called the **carotid sinus,** which contains baroreceptors and chemoreceptors to monitor pressure and chemical conditions of the blood. The external carotid arteries have numerous branches that carry blood to the skin and muscles of the neck, face, and scalp. The internal carotid arteries enter the cranial cavity through the carotid canals in the temporal bones and provide blood to the brain.

Another source of blood for the brain is through the **vertebral arteries,** which are branches of the subclavian arteries. The vertebral arteries ascend the neck through the foramina in the transverse processes of the cervical vertebrae and enter the cranial cavity through the foramen magnum. Inside the cra-

nial cavity, the right and left vertebral arteries join to form a single **basilar (BASE-ih-lar) artery,** which passes over the pons. Branches of the basilar artery supply the brain stem and cerebellum.

Branches of the basilar and internal carotid arteries join together, or anastomose, to form a system of vessels called the **circle of Willis** at the base of the brain (Fig. 13–14). Most of the arteries that supply blood to the brain branch from the circle of Willis. The internal carotid arteries provide most of the blood supply for the brain. The vertebral arteries are a secondary supply. Blood from the vertebral arteries is not sufficient to sustain life if the carotid supply is blocked.

Blood supply for the brain is provided by the internal carotid and vertebral arteries.

Arteries of the Upper Extremity (see Fig. 13–11). The blood supply to the shoulder and upper extremity is provided by the **subclavian arteries.** The right subclavian artery is a branch of the brachiocephalic artery, but the left subclavian artery branches directly from the aortic arch. After passing under the clavicle, the subclavian artery continues in the axilla as the **axillary (AK-sih-lair-ee) artery,** which then continues in the arm as the **brachial (BRAY-kee-al) artery.** At the elbow, the brachial divides to form the **ulnar artery** on the medial side of the forearm and

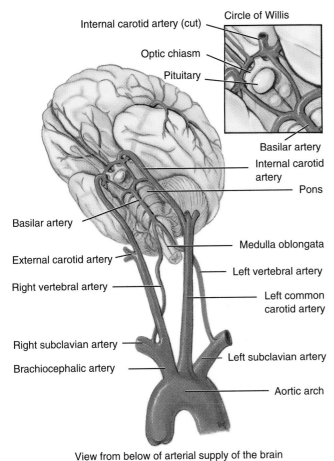

Internal carotid artery (cut)
Optic chiasm
Pituitary
Circle of Willis
Basilar artery
Internal carotid artery
Pons
Medulla oblongata
Left vertebral artery
Left common carotid artery
Left subclavian artery
Aortic arch
Basilar artery
External carotid artery
Right vertebral artery
Right subclavian artery
Brachiocephalic artery

View from below of arterial supply of the brain

Figure 13-14 Circle of Willis.

third of the large intestine. Several **lumbar arteries** arise from the abdominal aorta and provide the blood supply for the muscles and spinal cord in the lumbar region (see Figs. 13–11 and 13–13).

The celiac, superior mesenteric, suprarenal, renal, gonadal, and inferior mesenteric arteries branch from the abdominal aorta to supply the abdominal viscera. Lumbar arteries provide blood for the muscles and spinal cord.

Arteries of the Lower Extremity (see Fig. 13–11). At its termination, the aorta divides into the **right and left common iliac arteries.** Each common iliac artery branches to form a larger **external iliac artery** and a smaller internal iliac artery. The **internal iliac artery** enters the pelvis and has numerous branches that supply the urinary bladder, uterus, vagina, muscles of the pelvic floor and wall, and external genitalia. The external iliac arteries continue into the thigh as the **femoral** (FEM-or-al) **arteries,** which continue into the posterior knee region as the **popliteal** (pop-lih-TEE-al) **arteries.** The popliteal arteries branch to form the **anterior tibial arteries** and the **posterior tibial arteries.** The anterior tibial artery supplies the anterior portion of the leg, then continues as the **dorsal pedis artery** that supplies the ankle and foot. The posterior tibial artery supplies the posterior portion of the leg. A branch of the posterior tibial, the **peroneal** (pair-oh-NEE-al) **artery,** goes to the lateral portion of the leg.

Branches of the external iliac artery provide the blood supply for the lower extremity. The internal iliac artery supplies the pelvic viscera.

Pulse in the dorsal pedis artery is an indication of the integrity of circulation in the legs. If the dorsal pedis pulse is strong, circulation is probably good because this point is farthest from the heart.

the **radial artery** on the lateral side. Branches from the radial and ulnar arteries join to form a network of arteries, the **palmar arches,** that supply the hand. The radial artery is frequently used for taking a pulse.

The subclavian arteries provide the blood supply for the upper extremity.

Arteries of the Abdominal Viscera. The first major branch from the abdominal aorta, shown in Figures 13–11 and 13–13, is the **celiac** (SEE-lee-ak) **trunk** (artery). This short, unpaired vessel divides to form the **common hepatic artery,** which goes to the liver, the **left gastric artery,** which goes to the stomach, and the **splenic artery,** which supplies the pancreas and spleen.

The **superior mesenteric artery** is the second branch from the abdominal aorta. It supplies the small intestine and the proximal two thirds of the large intestine. Next there are three paired branches: the **suprarenal, renal,** and **gonadal arteries.** The suprarenal arteries go to the suprarenal, or adrenal, glands. The renal arteries supply the kidneys and the gonadal arteries supply the testes in the male and ovaries in the female. The final visceral branch from the abdominal aorta is the unpaired **inferior mesenteric artery,** which supplies the distal one

Major Systemic Veins

After blood delivers oxygen to the tissues and picks up carbon dioxide, it returns to the heart through a system of veins. The capillaries, where the gaseous exchange occurs, merge into venules and these converge to form larger and larger veins until the blood reaches either the **superior vena cava** or the **inferior vena cava,** both of which drain into the right atrium. The extremities have superficial veins that empty into deep veins. Venous tributaries that provide alternate pathways for blood flow form complex interconnecting networks between the superficial and deep veins. This makes it difficult to follow venous routes; however, the major deep veins usually follow the corresponding arteries and have the same name. The major systemic veins are illustrated in Figure 13–15 and are schematically represented

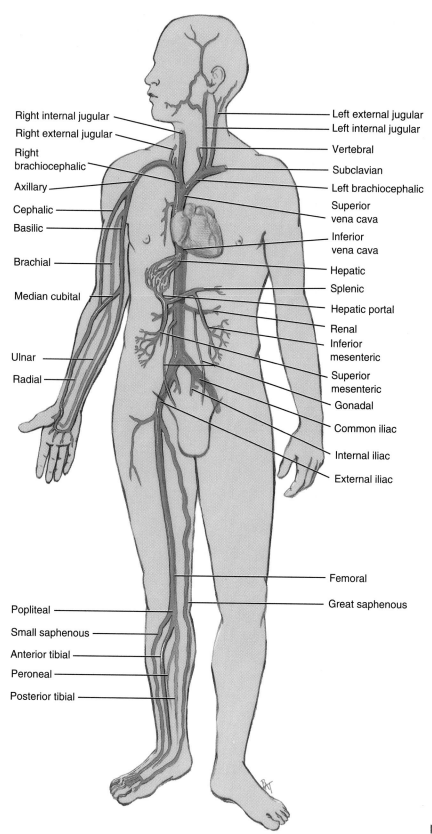

Right internal jugular

Right external jugular

Right brachiocephalic

Axillary

Cephalic

Basilic

Brachial

Median cubital

Ulnar

Radial

Left external jugular

Left internal jugular

Vertebral

Subclavian

Left brachiocephalic

Superior vena cava

Inferior vena cava

Hepatic

Splenic

Hepatic portal

Renal

Inferior mesenteric

Superior mesenteric

Gonadal

Common iliac

Internal iliac

External iliac

Femoral

Great saphenous

Popliteal

Small saphenous

Anterior tibial

Peroneal

Posterior tibial

Figure 13-15 Major systemic veins.

in Figure 13–16. They are summarized in Table 13–2.

> The superior vena cava and inferior vena cava are the two large veins that empty into the right atrium.

Veins of the Head and Neck. The **external jugular** (JUG-yoo-lar) **veins** are superficial vessels that drain blood from the skin and muscles of the face, scalp, and neck. The external jugular veins descend through the neck and empty into the **subclavian veins.** A small tributary may also drain into the internal jugular vein on each side.

The **internal jugular veins** receive blood from the veins and venous sinuses of the brain and from the deep regions of the face. The internal jugular veins are large vessels that descend through the neck and join the subclavian veins to form the **brachiocephalic veins.** The right and left brachiocephalic veins merge to form the **superior vena cava.**

> The internal jugular veins are the vessels visible in the neck when a person is angry or wearing a tight collar.

Vertebral veins also drain blood from the posterior regions of the brain. These vessels descend

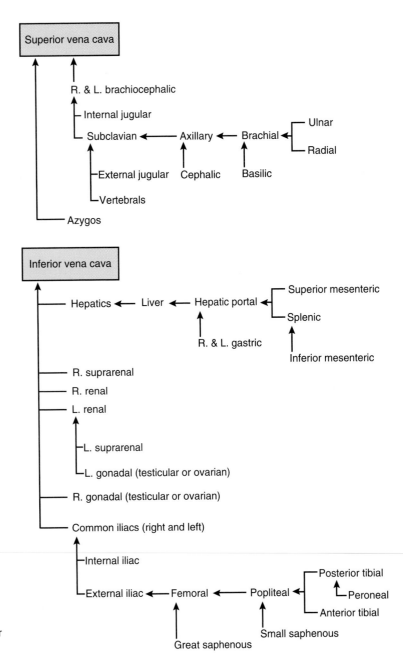

Figure 13–16   Schematic diagram of the major systemic veins.

Table 13-2   Summary of Major Veins and Regions They Drain

Vein	Region Drained	Comments
Blood Returned to Heart by Superior Vena Cava		
Brachiocephalic	Head, neck, upper extremity	Right and left brachiocephalics join to form superior vena cava
Internal jugular	Brain and portions of face and neck	Drains regions supplied by internal carotid artery; joins with subclavian to form brachiocephalic
Subclavian	Shoulder and upper extremity	Joins with internal jugular to form brachiocephalic; receives blood from axillary
Axillary	Axilla (armpit)	Receives blood from brachial and cephalic; drains into subclavian
Brachial	Deep vein of the arm	Receives blood from ulnar, radial, and basilic; drains into axillary
Radial	Deep vein on lateral side of forearm	Drains into brachial
Ulnar	Deep vein on medial side of forearm	Drains into brachial
Vertebral	Brain	Descends the neck in transverse foramina; drains into subclavian
External jugular	Face and scalp	Drains the region supplied by the external carotid artery; drains into subclavian and also has branches into internal jugular
Cephalic	Superficial vein on lateral side of forearm and arm	Drains into the axillary
Basilic	Superficial vein on medial side of forearm and arm	Drains into the brachial
Azygos	Thoracic and abdominal walls	Drains into the superior vena cava; receives blood from intercostal, internal thoracic, and lumbar veins
Blood Returned to Heart by Inferior Vena Cava		
Hepatic	Liver	Receives blood from venous sinusoids in liver
Hepatic portal	Digestive tract	Receives blood from gastric, splenic, and superior mesenteric veins and takes it to liver
Gastric	Stomach	Drains into the hepatic portal vein
Superior mesenteric	Small intestine and proximal portion of large intestine	Joins with splenic vein to form hepatic portal vein
Splenic	Spleen, pancreas, and portion of stomach	Joins with superior mesenteric vein to form hepatic portal vein
Inferior mesenteric	Distal portion of large intestine	Drains into the splenic vein
Suprarenal	Suprarenal (adrenal) glands	On the right, the vein empties into the inferior vena cava; on the left, it drains into the renal vein
Renal	Kidneys	Drains into the inferior vena cava; on the left, the renal vein receives blood from the left suprarenal and left gonadal veins
Gonadal	Gonads (ovaries/testes)	On the right, they drain into the inferior vena cava; on the left, they empty into the renal vein
Common iliac	Pelvis and lower extremities	Right and left join to form the inferior vena cava
Internal iliac	Muscles of the pelvic wall and the urinary and reproductive organs in the pelvis	Joins with the external iliac to form the common iliac vein
External iliac	Lower extremities	Joins with the internal iliac to form the common iliac vein; continuation of femoral vein from the thigh
Femoral	Deep region of thigh	Receives blood from the popliteal and great saphenous veins
Popliteal	Knee and leg	Receives blood from the anterior and posterior tibial veins and the small saphenous vein; continues in the thigh as the femoral vein
Anterior tibial	Anterior muscles of leg	Deep vein of the leg that joins with posterior tibial to form the popliteal vein
Posterior tibial	Posterior muscles of leg	Deep vein of the leg that joins with anterior tibial to form the popliteal vein; receives blood from peroneal vein
Peroneal	Lateral muscles of the leg	Drains into the posterior tibial vein
Small saphenous	Superficial tissues of posterior and lateral leg	Superficial vein that drains into the popliteal vein
Great saphenous	Superficial tissues of anterior and medial leg and thigh	Longest vein in the body; superficial vein that empties into the femoral vein

through the neck within the foramen in the transverse processes of the cervical vertebrae. The vertebral veins empty into the subclavian veins.

> The internal jugular and vertebral veins are the primary vessels that drain blood from the brain.

Veins of the Shoulder and Arms. The deep veins of the shoulder and arm follow a pattern similar to the arteries. The **radial vein,** on the lateral side of the forearm, and the **ulnar vein,** on the medial side, join in the region of the elbow to form the **brachial vein.** This vessel follows the path of the brachial artery and continues as the **axillary vein** and then as the **subclavian vein.**

The superficial veins of the upper extremity form complex networks just underneath the skin and drain into the deep veins mentioned in the previous paragraph. The major superficial veins are the **basilic** (bah-SILL-ik) and the **cephalic** (seh-FAL-ik). The basilic vein ascends the forearm and arm on the medial side. In the upper part of the arm, it then penetrates the tissues to join the brachial vein and form the axillary vein. The cephalic ascends the forearm and arm on the lateral side. In the shoulder region, the cephalic vein goes deep and joins the axillary vein to form the subclavian vein. A **median cubital** (KYOO-bih-tal) **vein** is usually prominent on the anterior surface of the arm at the bend of the elbow. This vessel ascends from the cephalic vein to the basilic vein and is frequently used as a site for drawing blood.

> The primary superficial veins of the upper extremity are the basilic on the medial side and the cephalic on the lateral side.

Veins of the Thoracic and Abdominal Wall. The **azygos** (AZ-ih-gus) **vein** drains blood from most of the muscle tissue of the thoracic and abdominal wall. This vessel begins in the dorsal abdominal wall, ascends along the right side of the vertebral column, and empties into the superior vena cava.

> The azygos vein drains blood from the thoracic and abdominal walls. It empties into the superior vena cava.

Veins of the Abdominal and Pelvic Organs (see Fig. 13–15). Blood from the abdominal organs, pelvic cavity, and lower extremities is returned to the right atrium by the **inferior vena cava.** The **hepatic** (liver), **right suprarenal** (adrenal glands), **renal** (kidneys), and **right gonadal** (ovaries or testes) **veins** empty directly into the inferior vena cava. On the left side the suprarenal and gonadal veins empty into the left renal vein, which carries the blood to the inferior vena cava.

Blood from the other abdominal organs enters the **hepatic portal system** and is carried to the liver before going to the inferior vena cava. The hepatic portal system begins with capillaries in the viscera and ends with capillaries in the liver (Fig. 13–17). The **splenic vein** and the **superior mesenteric vein** join to form the **hepatic portal vein,** which enters the liver. The superior mesenteric vein drains the

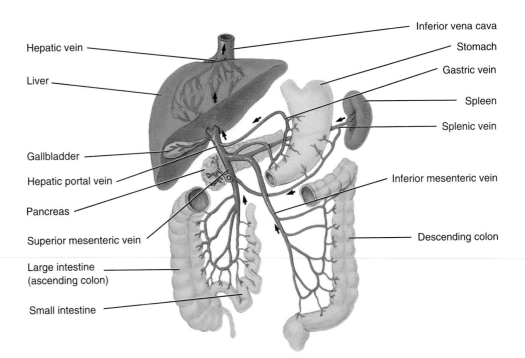

Figure 13–17   Hepatic portal circulation.

small intestine and proximal portion of the large intestine, and the splenic vein drains the spleen and pancreas. The **inferior mesenteric vein** drains blood from the distal portion of the large intestine, then empties into the splenic vein. The **right** and **left gastric arteries** are small vessels from the stomach that empty into the portal vein. Blood in the hepatic portal vein is rich in nutrients from the intestines, but it may also contain harmful substances that are toxic to the tissues. The liver removes the nutrients from the blood and either stores them or modifies them so that they can be used by the body cells. The liver also removes the toxic substances from the blood and either neutralizes them or alters them so that they are less harmful. Blood from the liver is collected into hepatic veins, which take it to the inferior vena cava.

> Blood from the digestive system enters the hepatic portal vein and goes through the liver before it enters the inferior vena cava.

The **internal iliac veins,** illustrated in Figure 13–15, drain blood from the pelvic viscera and pelvic wall. These vessels join the **external iliac veins** from the lower extremity to form the **common iliac veins.** The two common iliac veins merge to form the inferior vena cava, which empties into the right atrium.

Veins of the Lower Extremity (see Fig. 13–15). The arrangement of veins in the lower extremity is similar to that in the upper extremity. There is a deep set of veins that follows the pathway of the arteries. A superficial set of veins forms a complex network just underneath the skin, then penetrates the tissues to drain into the deep veins.

In the leg, the deep veins are the **anterior tibial vein,** which drains the dorsal foot and anterior muscles in the leg, and the **posterior tibial vein,** which drains the plantar region of the foot and posterior muscles in the leg. The **peroneal vein,** which drains the lateral muscles in the leg, empties into the posterior tibial vein. In the knee region, the anterior and posterior tibial veins join to form the single **popliteal vein,** which continues through the thigh as the **femoral vein.** The **external iliac vein** is a continuation of the femoral vein.

> Blood from the lower extremities returns to the external iliac veins. These join the internal iliac veins from the pelvis to form the common iliac veins. The right and left common iliac veins join to form the inferior vena cava.

The two major superficial veins of the lower extremity are the small and great **saphenous** (sah-FEE-nus) **veins.** The **small saphenous vein** ascends under the skin along the posterior leg. Near the knee, it penetrates the tissues to empty into the popliteal vein. The **great saphenous vein** is the longest vein in the body. It begins near the medial malleolus of the tibia and ascends through the leg and thigh un-

til it empties into the femoral vein. The saphenous veins have numerous interconnecting tributaries and also have many branches that connect with the deep veins. These provide alternate pathways by which blood can be returned to the inferior vena cava from the lower extremities.

> The great saphenous vein, a superficial vessel on the medial side of the lower extremity, is the longest vein in the body.

A portion of the great saphenous vein frequently is removed and used for grafts during coronary artery bypass surgery. This reduces the risk of tissue rejection by the immune system.

✓ **Quick**Check

- Damage to the celiac trunk interferes with blood flow to what organs?

- Blood from the superior mesenteric vein drains into what vessel?

- An embolism from a blood clot in the great saphenous vein circulates until it reaches a vessel smaller than the clot. What vessel is most likely to become blocked by the embolus?

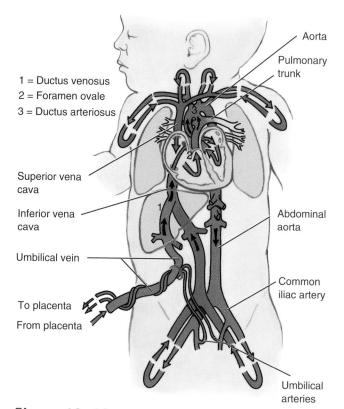

1 = Ductus venosus
2 = Foramen ovale
3 = Ductus arteriosus

Aorta
Pulmonary trunk
Superior vena cava
Inferior vena cava
Umbilical vein
Abdominal aorta
Common iliac artery
To placenta
From placenta
Umbilical arteries

Figure 13–18 Fetal circulation.

Fetal Circulation

Most circulatory pathways in a fetus are like those in the adult but there are some notable differences because the lungs, the gastrointestinal tract, and the kidneys are not functioning before birth. The fetus obtains its oxygen and nutrients from the mother and also depends on maternal circulation to carry away the carbon dioxide and waste products. Figure 13–18 illustrates the features of fetal circulation.

The exchange of gases, nutrients, and waste products occurs through the **placenta**, which is attached to the uterine wall of the mother and connected to the umbilicus (navel) of the fetus by the **umbilical cord.** The umbilical cord contains two **umbilical arteries** and one **umbilical vein.** Umbilical arteries, branches of the internal iliac arteries, carry blood that is loaded with carbon dioxide and waste products from the fetus to the placenta. In the placenta, the carbon dioxide and waste products diffuse from the fetal blood into the maternal blood. At the same time, oxygen and nutrients diffuse from the maternal blood in the placenta into the umbilical vein, which carries the oxygen- and nutrient-rich blood to fetal circulation. Diffusion normally takes place across capillary walls, and there is no mixing of fetal and maternal blood in the placenta.

> The umbilical cord contains two umbilical arteries to carry fetal blood to the placenta and one umbilical vein to carry oxygen- and nutrient-rich blood from the placenta to the fetus.

The umbilical vein carries blood to the fetal liver where it divides into two branches. One small branch supplies blood for nourishment of the liver cells. Most of the blood enters the other branch, the **ductus venosus** (DUK-tus veh-NO-sus), which by-passes the immature liver and goes directly to the inferior vena cava and then to the right atrium.

> The ductus venosus allows blood to bypass the immature liver in fetal circulation.

Because the fetal lungs are collapsed and non-functional, two structures permit most of the blood to circumvent the pulmonary circuit. An opening in the interatrial septum, the **foramen ovale**, allows some of the blood to go directly from the right atrium into the left atrium and into systemic circulation. The rest of the blood enters the right ventricle and is pumped into the pulmonary trunk. A short vessel, the **ductus arteriosus** (DUK-tus ar-teer-ee-OH-sus), connects the pulmonary trunk to the aorta. Because the fetal lungs are collapsed, most of the blood that enters the pulmonary trunk enters the systemic circulation by this route. A small amount of blood goes to the lungs to maintain their viability.

> The foramen ovale and ductus arteriosus are modifications that permit blood to bypass the lungs in fetal circulation.

When the foramen ovale between the two atria fails to close after birth, the result is an **interatrial septal defect**. Because pressure in the right atrium is lower than in the left, blood flows from the left atrium back into the right atrium without going through the systemic circulation. This defect overloads the pulmonary circulation and puts a strain on the heart as it attempts to pump enough blood to maintain adequate supplies to the body tissues.

Table 13–3   Summary of Special Structures in Fetal Circulation

Structure	Location	Function	Fate After Birth
Umbilical arteries	Two vessels in the umbilical cord	Transports blood from fetus to the placenta to pick up oxygen and nutrients and to get rid of carbon dioxide	Degenerates to become lateral umbilical ligaments
Umbilical vein	Single vessel in the umbilical cord	Transports oxygen- and nutrient-rich blood from placenta to the fetus	Becomes the round ligament (ligamentum teres) of the liver
Ductus venosus	Continuation of umbilical vein to the inferior vena cava	Carries blood directly from umbilical vein to the inferior vena cava; bypasses the liver	Becomes ligamentum venosum of the liver
Foramen ovale	In the septum between the right and left atria	Allows blood to go directly from the right atrium into the left atrium to bypass pulmonary circulation	Closes after birth to become the fossa ovalis
Ductus arteriosus	Between the pulmonary trunk and aorta	Permits blood in the pulmonary trunk to go directly into the descending aorta and to bypass pulmonary circulation	Becomes a fibrous cord, the ligamentum arteriosum

At or shortly after birth, when pulmonary, renal, and digestive functions are established, the special structures in the fetal circulatory pathway are no longer necessary. Changes occur that make the structures nonfunctional, and the circulatory pattern becomes like that of an adult. Table 13–3 summarizes the special features of fetal circulation and the changes that occur.

FOCUS ON AGING

Problems with blood vessels are relatively rare in childhood and youth. But signs of vascular aging begin to appear as early as age 40. One of the most common and significant changes is a decrease in the amount of elastic fibers and an increase in the amount of collagen. Furthermore, the collagen is altered and is less flexible than normal. The result is a decreased elasticity of the vessel walls called **arteriosclerosis,** or hardening of the arteries. The overall effect is an increased resistance to each surge of blood from ventricular contraction, which produces an increased systolic pressure. The vessels are less able to maintain diastolic pressure so pulse pressure increases. Increased peripheral resistance from the loss of vessel elasticity puts an extra load on the heart, which then has to work harder and it enlarges to compensate.

The internal diameter of blood vessels tends to decrease with age because lipids gradually accumulate in the wall. This condition in which fatty, cholesterol-filled deposits, called atheromas, develop in the vessel walls is called **atherosclerosis.** Atheromas are especially common in areas of high blood pressure or turbulence, such as the coronary arteries, aorta, iliac arteries, ca-

rotid arteries, and cerebral arteries. The decreased lumen caused by the atheromas contributes to increased peripheral resistance. The decreased blood flow that results may not be significant until a time when maximum flow is needed. Atherosclerosis is often the primary agent in cerebrovascular accident, myocardial infarction, thrombus formation, and embolisms.

The walls of veins may become thicker with age because of an increase in connective tissue and calcium deposits. The valves also tend to become stiff and incompetent. Varicose veins develop. Because of the low blood pressure in veins, these changes probably are not significant for cardiovascular function. They may be of concern because of the possibility of phlebitis and thrombus formation.

While some degree of arteriosclerosis probably is inevitable in the aging process, a lot of vascular disease can be prevented by a proper diet, regular walking or other aerobic exercise, and the elimination of cigarette smoking. In other words, lifestyle probably has more effect on the cardiovascular system than does aging.

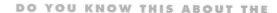

DO YOU KNOW THIS ABOUT THE

Blood Vessels?

Atherosclerosis, Coronary Artery Bypass Grafting, and Angioplasty

Arteriosclerosis, or hardening of the arteries, is a group of vascular disorders in which the blood vessel walls thicken and lose their elasticity. One common form of arteriosclerosis is **atherosclerosis,** in which fatty plaques, called **atheromas,** damage the vessels. Atheromas are localized lesions composed of smooth muscle cells, collagen, fibrin, platelets, and fatty substances such as cholesterol and triglycerides. The factors that cause the development of atheromas are unclear, but the first event in their formation appears to be damage to the endothelial lining (tunica intima) of the vessel wall. After this, cells proliferate and lipids build up within the cells and in the inter-

stitial spaces to form a fatty plaque that projects into the lumen of the vessel. The significance of atherosclerosis lies in its potential (1) to obstruct vessels, which reduces blood flow and decreases the oxygen supply; (2) to weaken the wall of a vessel, which makes it vulnerable to the formation of an aneurysm or rupture; and (3) to predispose a person to thrombus formation.

Atheromas may develop in any artery, but they most commonly form at sites of high pressure or turbulence in the blood, such as coronary arteries, the aorta, iliac arteries, carotids, and cerebral arteries. Atheromas in these vessels make atherosclerosis the chief cause of ischemia of the heart muscle (heart attacks), the brain (strokes), and the extremities (peripheral vascular disease). The formation of an atheroma in a blood vessel results in narrowing of the lumen, which obstructs blood flow. If the obstruction evolves gradually, collateral circulation often develops and even the complete occlusion of a vessel may not cause symptoms. If collateral circulation is not available or the demand is unusual and excessive, such as occurs when shoveling snow, the narrowing of the lumen due to the plaques may be sufficient to cause serious ischemia in the heart.

Several factors increase the chances of developing atherosclerosis. Significant risk factors include hypertension, obesity, cigarette smoking, high fat intake (particularly animal fat and cholesterol), coincidental diseases such as diabetes mellitus, stress, an intense "achiever" personality, and a sedentary lifestyle. Under the age of 40, atherosclerosis seems to be more severe in men than in women, but it apparently progresses more rapidly in women after menopause. Regular exercise may help reduce the risk. The good news is that atheromas are, to some extent, reversible. With a reduction of high blood cholesterol levels, atheromatous plaques tend to shrink.

One of the most common consequences of atherosclerosis is coronary artery disease, in which the plaques form in the coronary arteries. This causes coronary ischemia by reducing the blood supply to the myocardium and may lead to myocardial infarction. In the early stages, vasodilators such as nitroglycerin may be used to increase the blood supply to the heart. This is a common treatment for angina pectoris.

Coronary artery bypass grafting (CABG) is a surgical procedure for increasing blood supply to the heart. In CABG (pronounced cabbage), a portion of a vessel from some other part at the body is used to bypass the blockage. One end of the "new" vessel, frequently a segment of the great saphenous vein, is sutured to the aorta and the other end is sutured to the coronary artery, distal to the obstruction. If more than one artery is blocked, additional bypasses may be necessary.

A nonsurgical procedure used to open clogged arteries is **percutaneous transluminal coronary angioplasty (PTCA).** In this procedure, a balloon catheter is inserted into an artery of an arm or leg and under radiographic viewing is guided through the arterial system until it reaches the obstruction. At the blockage site, the balloonlike device at the end of the catheter is inflated. This compresses the obstructing plaque against the artery walls to increase blood flow. One problem with this procedure is that the obstruction frequently recurs because the plaque is only compressed and not destroyed.

A newly developing technique for opening coronary arteries blocked by atherosclerosis is **excimer laser angioplasty.** This procedure uses a type of angioplasty catheter to reach the obstruction, but instead of a balloon it uses laser energy delivered through fiberoptics. A prescribed mixture of gases produces a high-energy laser beam that vaporizes most types of plaque, including those that are moderately calcified. The microscopic particles of the destroyed plaque pass into the blood and are removed by the body's normal filtration system in the kidneys, without risk of clogging smaller vessels and capillaries. The advantage in this procedure is that it destroys the plaque so recurrences are less frequent. It is estimated that this new laser technique may benefit as many as 200,000 patients a year who currently undergo balloon angioplasty treatments or coronary bypass surgery.

CHAPTER QUIZ

RECALL

Match the definitions on the left with the appropriate term on the right.

1. Carry blood away from the heart

2. Smallest blood vessels

3. Primarily smooth muscle

4. Fluid between cells

5. Heard through the stethoscope

6. Fetal opening in the interatrial septum

7. Frequently used for drawing blood

8. First major branch from the abdominal aorta

9. Returns blood from the head, neck, and arms to the heart

10. Used to measure blood pressure

A. Arteries

B. Capillaries

C. Celiac trunk

D. Foramen ovale

E. Interstitial fluid

F. Korotkoff sounds

G. Median cubital vein

H. Sphygmomanometer

I. Superior vena cava

J. Tunica media

THOUGHT

1. The layer of the arteriole wall that provides contractility and elasticity for vasoconstriction and vasodilation is the

   a. tunica externa

   b. tunica adventitia

   c. tunica media

   d. tunica interna

2. At any given time, most of the blood in the body is found in the

   a. capillaries

   b. veins

   c. heart

   d. arteries

3. When a precapillary sphincter relaxes,

   a. blood flows into a capillary bed

   b. blood flows through the arteriovenous anastomoses

   c. blood flows into metarterioles

   d. blood backs up in the arterioles

4. Which of the following factors opposes the flow of blood?

   a. decreased blood viscosity

   b. increased diameter of blood vessels

   c. decreased total cross-sectional area of blood vessels

   d. increased resistance in blood vessels

5. A portion of a blood clot in the femoral vein breaks loose. In what vessel is this embolus likely to lodge?

   a. inferior vena cava

   b. capillary in the lungs

   c. capillary in the liver

   d. capillary in the brain

APPLICATION

Trace a drop of blood from the inferior vena cava to the muscles on the lateral side of the right forearm. List all vessels, heart chambers, and valves.

Briefly describe two ways in which angiotensin increases blood pressure.

CHAPTER 14

Lymphatic System and Body Defense

Outline/Objectives

Functions of the Lymphatic System 287

• State three functions of the lymphatic system.

Components of the Lymphatic System 287

• List the components of the lymphatic system, describe their structure, and explain their functions.
• Describe the origin of lymph and describe the mechanisms that move the fluid through lymphatic vessels.

Resistance to Disease 291

• List four nonspecific mechanisms that provide resistance to disease and explain how each functions.
• State the two characteristics of specific defense mechanisms and identify the two principal cells involved in specific resistance.
• Briefly describe the mechanism of cell-mediated immunity and list four subgroups of T cells.
• Briefly describe the mechanism of antibody-mediated immunity and list two subgroups of B cells.
• Distinguish between the primary response and the secondary response to a pathogen.
• List five classes of immunoglobulins and state the role each has in immunity.

• Give examples of active natural immunity, active artificial immunity, passive natural immunity, and passive artificial immunity.

Key Terms

Active immunity

Antibody

Antigen

Artificial immunity

Immunoglobulin

Natural immunity

Passive immunity

Primary response

Resistance

Secondary response

Susceptibility

Building Vocabulary

WORD PART	MEANING
aden-	gland
-ectomy	surgical removal
immun-	protection
lymph-	lymph
-megaly	large
-pexy	fixation
splen-	spleen
tox-	poison
thym-	thymus

Functional Relationships of the
Lymphatic/Immune System

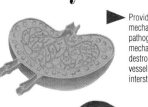

Provides specific defense mechanisms against pathogens; surveillance mechanisms detect and destroy cancer cells; lymph vessels remove excess interstitial fluid.

Integument

Provides mechanical barrier against entry of pathogens

Supplies antibodies to skin surface for specific defense.

Skeletal
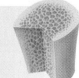

Leukocytes involved in immune response arise from stem cells in bone marrow; protects thymus and spleen.

Maintains interstitial fluid balance in bone tissue; assists in defense against pathogens and repair of bone tissue following trauma.

Muscular

Skeletal muscle contraction moves lymph within vessels; protects superficial lymph nodes.

Maintains interstitial fluid balance in muscle tissue; assists in defense against pathogens and repair of muscle tissue following trauma.

Nervous

Innervates lymphoid organs and helps regulate immune response.

Assists in defense against pathogens and repair of neural and sensory tissue following trauma; removes excess interstitial fluid from tissues surrounding nerves.

Endocrine

Hormones from thymus influence lymphocyte development; glucocorticoids suppress immune response.

Protects against infection in endocrine glands.

Cardiovascular
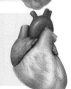

Provides oxygen and nutrients to lymphoid organs and removes wastes; transports agents involved in immune response.

Returns interstitial fluid to the blood to maintain blood volume; protects against infections; spleen disposes of old RBCs.

Respiratory
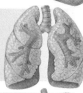

Provides lymphoid tissue and immune cells with oxygen and removes wastes; tonsils located in pharynx; breathing movements assist lymph flow.

Tonsils combat pathogens that enter through nasal passages; IgA protects respiratory mucosa.

Digestive
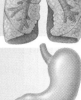

Absorbs nutrients needed by lymphoid tissue and immune cells; stomach acid provides nonspecific defense against ingested pathogens.

Lacteals absorb fats and fat soluble vitamins from the intestine.

Urinary

Helps maintain water, electrolyte, and pH balance of body fluids for effective immune cell function; acid pH of urine acts as barrier against urinary tract pathogens.

Immune cells provide specific defense against urinary tract pathogens.

Reproductive
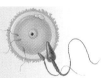

Acidic vaginal secretions provide barrier against reproductive tract infections; blood-testis barrier prevents immune destruction of sperm cells.

Provides specific defense against pathogens that enter the body through the reproductive tract; surveillance against cancer cells.

The lymphatic system sometimes is considered to be a part of the circulatory system because it transports a fluid through vessels and empties it into venous blood. Because it consists of organs that work together to perform certain functions, it may be treated as a separate system. The lymphatic system has a major role in the body's defense against disease, so that topic also is included in this chapter.

Functions of the Lymphatic System

The lymphatic system has three primary functions. First, it returns excess interstitial fluid to the blood. Chapter 13 described capillary microcirculation in which fluid leaves the capillary at the arteriole end and returns at the venous end. Of the fluid that leaves the capillary, about 90 percent is returned. The 10 percent that does not return becomes part of the interstitial fluid that surrounds the tissue cells. Small protein molecules may "leak" through the capillary wall and increase the osmotic pressure of the interstitial fluid. This further inhibits the return of fluid into the capillary, and fluid tends to accumulate in the tissue spaces. If this continues, blood volume and blood pressure decrease significantly and the volume of tissue fluid increases, which results in edema. Lymph capillaries pick up the excess interstitial fluid and proteins and return them to the venous blood.

The second function of the lymphatic system is the absorption of fats and fat-soluble vitamins from the digestive system and the subsequent transport of these substances to the venous circulation. The mucosa that lines the small intestine is covered with fingerlike projections called **villi.** There are blood capillaries and special lymph capillaries, called **lacteals** (lak-TEELS), in the center of each villus. Most nutrients are absorbed by the blood capillaries, but the fats and fat-soluble vitamins are absorbed by the lacteals. The lymph in the lacteals has a milky appearance due to its high fat content and is called **chyle** (KYL).

The third function of the lymphatic system is defense against invading microorganisms and disease. Lymph nodes and other lymphatic organs filter the lymph to remove microorganisms and other foreign particles. Lymphatic organs contain lymphocytes that destroy invading organisms.

> The lymphatic system returns excess interstitial fluid to the blood, absorbs fats and fat-soluble vitamins, and provides defense against disease.

Components of the Lymphatic System

The lymphatic system consists of a fluid (lymph), vessels that transport the lymph, and organs that contain lymphoid tissue.

Lymph

Lymph is a fluid similar in composition to blood plasma. It is derived from blood plasma as fluids pass through capillary walls at the arterial end. As the interstitial fluid begins to accumulate, it is picked up and removed by tiny lymphatic vessels and returned to the blood. As soon as the interstitial fluid enters the lymph capillaries, it is called **lymph.** Returning the fluid to the blood prevents edema and helps to maintain normal blood volume and pressure.

> Lymph is the fluid in the lymphatic vessels. It is picked up from the interstitial fluid and returned to the blood plasma.

CLINICAL TERMS

Allergen (AL-er-jen) A substance capable of causing a specific hypersensitivity in the body; a type of antigen

Anaphylaxis (an-ah-fill-AKS-is) An exaggerated or unusual hypersensitivity to foreign protein or other substances, characterized by a systemic vasodilation with a dramatic decrease in blood pressure that can be life threatening

Autoimmune disease (aw-toh-ih-MYOON dih-ZEEZ) A condition in which the body's immune system becomes defective and produces antibodies against itself

Interleukins (in-ter-LOO-kins) Proteins that stimulate the growth of T cell lymphocytes and activate immune responses

Lymphadenitis (lim-fad-en-EYE-tis) Inflammation of the lymph glands (nodes)

Lymphangiogram (lim-FAN-jee-oh-gram) A procedure in which a dye is injected into lymph vessels in the foot and radiographs are taken to show the path of lymph flow as it moves into the chest region

Lymphedema (lim-fah-DEE-mah) Swelling of tissues due to fluid accumulation resulting from obstruction of lymph vessels or disorders of the lymph nodes

Lymphoma (lim-FOH-mah) Malignant tumor of lymph nodes and lymph tissue

Metastasis (meh-TASS-tah-sis) Spread of a malignant tumor to a secondary site

Mononucleosis (mah-noh-noo-klee-OH-sis) An acute infectious disease, caused by the Epstein-Barr virus, with enlarged lymph nodes, increased numbers of agranulocytes in the bloodstream, fatigue, sore throat, and enlarged, tender lymph nodes

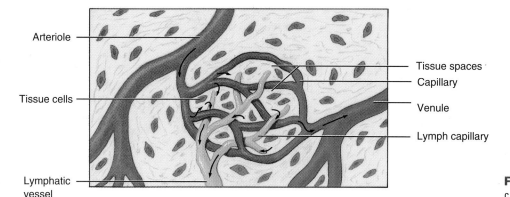

Figure 14–1 Lymph capillaries in the tissue spaces.

Lymphatic Vessels

Lymphatic vessels, unlike blood vessels, only carry fluid away from the tissues. The smallest lymphatic vessels are the **lymph capillaries,** which begin in the tissue spaces as blind-ended sacs (Fig. 14–1). Lymph capillaries are found in all regions of the body except the bone marrow, central nervous system, and tissues, such as the epidermis, that lack blood vessels. The wall of the lymph capillary is composed of endothelium in which the simple squamous cells overlap to form a simple one-way valve. This arrangement permits fluid to enter the capillary but prevents lymph from leaving the vessel.

> Lymphatic vessels carry fluid away from the tissues.

The microscopic lymph capillaries merge to form **lymphatic vessels.** These vessels are similar to veins in structure, but they have thinner walls and more valves than veins. Small lymphatic vessels join to form larger tributaries, called **lymphatic trunks,** which drain large regions. Lymphatic trunks merge until the lymph enters the two **lymphatic ducts.** The **right lymphatic duct** receives lymph from the vessels in the upper right quadrant of the body (Fig. 14–2). This includes the right side of the head and neck, the right upper extremity, and the right side of the thorax. The right lymphatic duct empties into the right subclavian vein. The **thoracic duct** collects the lymph from the remaining regions of the body (see Fig. 14–2). The thoracic duct begins in the upper abdomen and ascends through the thorax to empty into the left subclavian vein. The beginning of the thoracic duct is called the **cisterna chyli** (sis-TER-nah KY-lee). The cysterna chyli collects lymph from two lumbar trunks that drain the lower limbs and from the intestinal trunk that drains the digestive organs. **Lymph nodes** that filter the lymph are located along the various routes of the lymphatic system.

> The right lymphatic duct drains lymph from the upper right quadrant of the body. The thoracic duct drains all the rest.

Anything that interferes with the flow of lymph, such as an obstruction or surgical ligation, may cause tissue fluid to accumulate, resulting in edema. Because plasma proteins that have "leaked out" of the capillaries are returned to the bloodstream by means of the lymph, obstruction of lymph flow may cause a decrease in plasma protein concentration.

The development of breast cancer often necessitates the removal of part or all of the breast tissue, a surgical procedure called a **mastectomy.** There is an extensive network of lymphatic vessels associated with the breast, and the cancer cells from the breast can spread to surrounding lymph nodes through these vessels. For this reason, the axillary nodes may be removed with the breast tissue. Sometimes this procedure interferes with lymph drainage from the arm and the fluid accumulates, resulting in swelling, or **lymphedema.**

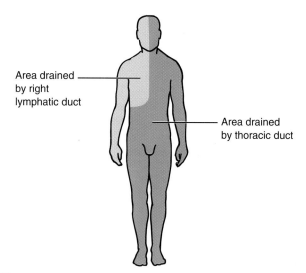

Figure 14–2 Regions drained by lymphatic ducts.

Like veins, the lymphatic tributaries have thin walls and have valves to prevent backflow of blood. There is no pump in the lymphatic system like the heart in the cardiovascular system. The pressure gradients to move lymph through the vessels have to come from external sources. These pressure gradients come from skeletal muscle contraction, from respiratory movements, and from contraction of the smooth muscle within the wall of the vessel. Because there is no rhythmic heart to pump it along, lymph transport is sporadic and much slower than the transport of blood in the veins.

> Pressure gradients that move fluid through the lymphatic vessels come from the skeletal muscle action, respiratory movements, and contraction of smooth muscle in vessel walls.

Lymphatic Organs

Lymphatic organs are characterized by clusters of **lymphocytes** and other cells, such as macrophages, enmeshed in a framework of short, branching connective tissue fibers. The lymphocytes originate in the red bone marrow with other types of blood cells and are carried in the blood from the bone marrow to the lymphatic organs. When the body is exposed to microorganisms and other foreign substances, the lymphocytes proliferate within the lymphatic organs and are sent in the blood to the site of the invasion. This is part of the immune response that attempts to destroy the invading agent. The lymph nodes, tonsils, spleen, and thymus are examples of lymphatic organs.

Lymph Nodes

Lymph nodes are small bean-shaped structures that are usually less than 2.5 cm in length. They are widely distributed throughout the body along the lymphatic pathways where they filter the lymph before it is returned to the blood. Lymph nodes are not present in the central nervous system. There are three superficial regions on each side of the body where lymph nodes tend to cluster. These areas are the inguinal nodes in the groin, the axillary nodes in the armpit, and the cervical nodes in the neck (Fig. 14–3).

> Lymph nodes are located along lymphatic vessels except in the nervous system. Superficial nodes are found in the groin, axilla, and neck.

The typical lymph node is surrounded by a connective tissue **capsule** and divided into compartments called **lymph nodules** (Fig. 14–4). The lymph nodules are dense masses of lymphocytes and macrophages and are separated by spaces called **lymph sinuses.** Several **afferent lymphatic vessels,** which carry lymph into the node, enter the node on the

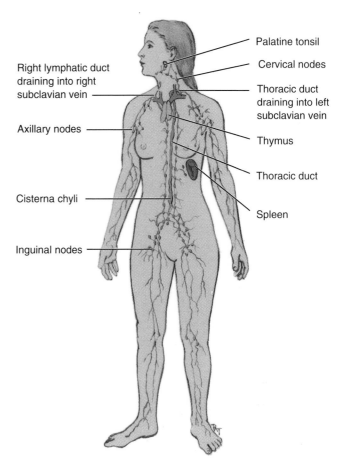

Figure 14–3   Location of the clusters of superficial lymph nodes.

convex side. The lymph moves through the lymph sinuses and enters an **efferent lymphatic vessel,** which carries the lymph away from the node. Because there are more afferent vessels than efferent vessels, the passage of lymph through the sinuses is slowed down, which allows time for the cleansing process. The efferent vessel leaves the node at an indented region called the **hilum.**

> Lymph enters a lymph node through afferent vessels, filters through the sinuses, and leaves through an efferent vessel.

The lymphatic system is one route by which cancer cells can spread from a primary tumor site to other areas of the body. As the cells travel with the lymph, they pass through the lymph nodes where the lymph is filtered. At first this traps the cancer cells within the lymph node, and the cells are destroyed. Eventually, the number of cancer cells may overwhelm the filtration ability of the lymph nodes, and some of the cells pass through the nodes to establish secondary tumors.

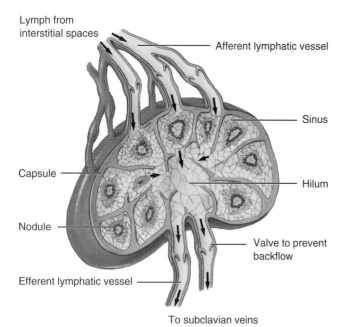

Lymph from interstitial spaces

Afferent lymphatic vessel

Sinus

Capsule

Hilum

Nodule

Valve to prevent backflow

Efferent lymphatic vessel

To subclavian veins

Figure 14–4   Structure of a lymph node.

Lymph nodes are the only structures that filter the lymph, and this is their primary function. As the lymph moves through the sinuses, infectious agents, damaged cells, cancerous cells, and cellular debris become trapped in the fibrous mesh so that the lymph is cleansed before it enters the blood. The lymphocytes react against the bacteria, viruses, and cancerous cells to destroy them. Macrophages, also present in the node, engulf the destroyed pathogens, the damaged cells, and the cellular debris.

> Lymph nodes filter and cleanse the lymph before it enters the blood.

Tonsils

Tonsils are clusters of lymphatic tissue just under the mucous membranes that line the nose, mouth, and throat (pharynx). There are three groups of tonsils. The **pharyngeal tonsils** are located near the opening of the nasal cavity into the pharynx. When these tonsils become enlarged they may interfere with breathing and are called **adenoids**. The **palatine tonsils** are the ones that are commonly called "the tonsils." These are located near the opening of the oral cavity into the pharynx. **Lingual tonsils** are located on the posterior surface of the tongue, which also places them near the opening of the oral cavity into the pharynx. Lymphocytes and macrophages in the tonsils provide protection against harmful substances and pathogens that may enter the body through the nose or mouth.

> Tonsils are clusters of lymphatic tissue associated with openings into the pharynx and provide protection against pathogens that may enter through the nose and mouth.

Tonsils usually function to prevent infection from the bacteria that attempt to enter the body through the nose and mouth. Sometimes, however, they become severely and repeatedly infected themselves and may need to be removed. The palatine tonsils are the ones removed in a **tonsillectomy**. If the pharyngeal tonsils are enlarged they may interfere with breathing. Removal of these tonsils is called an **adenoidectomy**.

Spleen

The **spleen** is located in the upper left abdominal cavity, just beneath the diaphragm, and posterior to the stomach. It is similar to a lymph node in shape and structure but it is much larger. The spleen is the largest lymphatic organ in the body. Surrounded by a connective tissue capsule, which extends inward to divide the organ into lobules, the spleen consists of two types of tissue called **white pulp** and **red pulp**. The white pulp is lymphatic tissue consisting mainly of lymphocytes around arteries. The red pulp consists of venous sinuses filled with blood and cords of lymphatic cells, such as lymphocytes and macrophages. Blood enters the spleen through the splenic artery, moves through the sinuses where it is filtered, then leaves through the splenic vein.

The spleen filters blood in much the same way that the lymph nodes filter lymph. Lymphocytes in the spleen react to pathogens in the blood and attempt to destroy them. Macrophages then engulf the resulting debris, the damaged cells, and the other large particles. The spleen, along with the liver, removes old and damaged erythrocytes from the circulating blood. Like other lymphatic tissue, it produces lymphocytes, especially in response to invading pathogens. The sinuses in the spleen are a reservoir for blood. In emergencies such as hemorrhage, smooth muscle in the vessel walls and in the capsule of the spleen contracts. This squeezes the blood out of the spleen into the general circulation. If the spleen must be removed (splenectomy), its functions will be performed by other lymphatic tissue and the liver.

> The spleen is a lymph organ that filters blood and also acts as a reservoir for blood.

The spleen is a rather soft and fragile organ, and, although it is somewhat protected by the ribs, it is often ruptured in abdominal injuries. Because the spleen is a reservoir for blood, this results in severe internal hemorrhage and shock, which may lead to death if is not stopped. A **splenectomy**, surgical removal of the spleen, may be necessary to stop the bleeding.

Thymus

The **thymus** is a soft organ with two lobes that is located anterior to the ascending aorta and posterior to the sternum. It is relatively large in infants and children but after puberty it begins to decrease in size so that in older adults it is quite small.

The primary function of the thymus is the processing and maturation of special lymphocytes called **T lymphocytes** or **T cells.** While in the thymus, the lymphocytes do not respond to pathogens and foreign agents. After the lymphocytes have matured, they enter the blood and go to other lymphatic organs where they help provide defense against disease. The thymus also produces a hormone, **thymosin,** that stimulates the maturation of lymphocytes in other lymphatic organs.

> The thymus is large in the infant and atrophies after puberty. T lymphocytes mature in the thymus.

✓ QuickCheck

- Because there is no "heart" to pump fluid through the lymphatic vessels, what provides the pressure gradients for lymph flow?

- Why do lymph nodes enlarge during infections?

- What is the "crisis" or danger when the spleen ruptures from an abdominal injury?

Resistance to Disease

The human body is continually exposed to disease-producing organisms, called **pathogens,** and other harmful substances. If these enter the body, they may disrupt normal homeostasis and cause disease. The body's ability to counteract the effects of pathogens and other harmful agents is called **resistance** and is dependent on a variety of defense mechanisms. **Susceptibility** is a lack of resistance. Some defense mechanisms, called **nonspecific mechanisms,** act against all harmful agents and provide **nonspecific resistance.** Other defense mechanisms only act against certain agents and are called **specific mechanisms.** These provide **specific resistance,** or **immunity** (Fig. 14–5). To maintain a state of health, all the body's defense mechanisms must act together to provide protection against invading pathogens, foreign cells that are transplanted into the body, and the body's own cells that have become cancerous.

> The ability to counteract pathogens is resistance. Susceptibility is a lack of resistance.

Nonspecific Defense Mechanisms

Nonspecific defense mechanisms are directed against all pathogens and foreign substances regardless of their nature. They present the initial defense against invading agents. The first line of defense is the barrier against entry into the body. If the foreign agent succeeds in passing the barrier and entering the body, then the second line of defense comes into action. This includes the chemical action of complement and interferon, and the processes of phagocytosis and inflammation.

Barriers

Intact, or unbroken, skin and mucous membranes form effective mechanical barriers against the entry of foreign substances. The cells of the skin are closely packed and full of keratin, which makes it difficult for pathogens to penetrate. Microorganisms that normally grow on the surface of the skin offer a barrier against pathogens because they inhibit the growth of other bacteria by competing for space and nutrients. Mucous membranes that line the respiratory and digestive tracts are not as tough as skin but the mucus produced by these membranes traps foreign particles before they gain entry. Some mucous membranes, especially those in the respiratory tract, have cilia that propel the mucus with the entrapped particles upward to be expelled or swallowed.

Fluids, such as tears flowing across the eyes, saliva that is swallowed, and urine passing through the urethra, are examples of mechanical barriers that flush pathogens out of the body before they have a chance to damage the tissues.

Lysozymes in the tears, saliva, and nasal secretions destroy bacteria. Sebaceous secretions and the salts in perspiration also have an antimicrobial action. Hydrochloric acid in the stomach inhibits the growth of bacteria that are swallowed. These are all examples of chemical barriers that deter microbial invasion.

> Barriers that deter microbial invasion may be mechanical (skin), fluid (tears), or chemical (lysozymes).

Chemical Action

Various body chemicals, including complement, stimulate phagocytosis and inflammation. Others, including interferon, are produced as a direct response to microbial invasion. These are part of the second line of defense that continues the battle against disease if microorganisms succeed in getting through the barriers of the first defense.

Complement is a group of proteins normally found in the plasma in an inactive form. Certain complement proteins become activated when they come in contact with a foreign substance. A series of reactions, similar to the cascade reactions in the clotting process, follows. The reactions proceed in an orderly sequential manner with step 1 necessary for step 2, then step 2 necessary for step 3, and so on. As each complement protein is activated, it activates

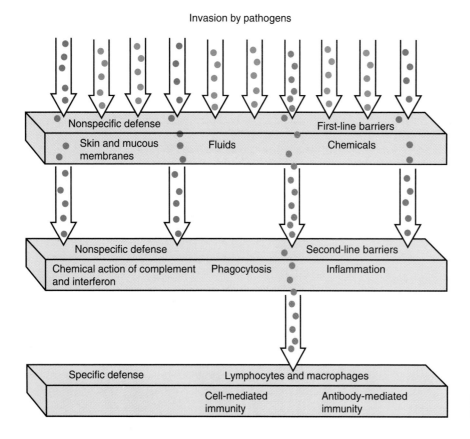

Invasion by pathogens

Nonspecific defense — First-line barriers

Skin and mucous membranes — Fluids — Chemicals

Nonspecific defense — Second-line barriers

Chemical action of complement and interferon — Phagocytosis — Inflammation

Specific defense — Lymphocytes and macrophages

Cell-mediated immunity — Antibody-mediated immunity

Figure 14-5 Overview of defense mechanisms.

the next complement protein, until the final protein is activated. The final activated complement enhances phagocytosis and inflammation. It also causes bacterial cells to rupture.

▌ Complement is a chemical defense that promotes phagocytosis and inflammation.

Interferon (in-ter-FEER-on) has particular significance because it offers protection against viruses. When a cell becomes infected with a virus, the cell usually stops its normal functions. The virus uses the cell's metabolic machinery for one goal—viral replication. When the cell is full of viruses, it ruptures and releases myriad viruses to infect new cells. In this way, the viral infection is established. When a virus infects a cell, that cell produces interferon, which diffuses into neighboring uninfected cells. Interferon stimulates the uninfected cells to produce a protein that blocks viral replication. In this way, the uninfected cells are protected from the virus. Interferon does not protect the cell in which it was produced or the cells in which the virus is already established, but it does protect the neighboring uninfected cells.

▌ Interferon is produced by virus-infected cells to provide protection for the neighboring cells.

Although interferon has not proved to be the great cancer cure that was hoped when it was discovered in the 1950s, some useful therapies have emerged. It is produced naturally in such small amounts that its harvest and use were impractical until researchers developed genetic engineering techniques that utilize bacteria to make it in sufficient quantities for clinical use. Interferon has been tested as an anticancer agent, as a treatment for devastating viral diseases, and in the treatment of AIDS patients. Results are mixed. Some are helped, others are not. Some have side effects, others do not. The research continues.

Phagocytosis

Phagocytosis is the ingestion and destruction of solid particles by certain cells. The cells are called **phagocytes,** and the particles may be microorganisms or their parts, foreign particles, an individual's own dead or damaged cells, or cell fragments. The primary phagocytic cells are **neutrophils** and **macrophages.**

Neutrophils, described in Chapter 11, are small granular leukocytes. They are usually the first cells to leave the blood and migrate to the site of an infection, where they phagocytize the invading bacteria. This is a "suicide mission" because the neutrophils die after engulfing only a few bacteria. Pus is primarily an accumulation of dead neutrophils, cellular debris, and bacteria. The number of neutrophils greatly increases in acute infections.

Macrophages are monocytes that have left the blood and entered the tissues. Monocytes, described in Chapter 11, are large agranular leukocytes. When they leave the blood, they become macrophages by increasing in size and developing additional lysosomes. Macrophages usually appear at the scene of an infection after the neutrophils and are responsible for clearing away cellular debris and dead neutrophils during the latter stages of an infection. Macrophages are also present in uninfected tissues where they may phagocytize the invading agents before there is tissue damage. For example, they are present in the lymph nodes where they cleanse the lymph as it filters through the node. They perform a similar cleansing action on the blood as it passes through the liver and spleen.

> Neutrophils and macrophages are the primary phagocytic cells. Neutrophils usually are first at the scene of tissue damage. Macrophages come later to clean up debris.

Inflammation

Inflammation, briefly discussed in Chapter 4, is a nonspecific defense mechanism that occurs in response to tissue damage from microorganisms or trauma. **Localized inflammation** is contained in a specific region. It is evidenced by **redness** (rubor), **warmth** (calor), **swelling** (tumor), and **pain** (dolor). A combination of these effects frequently causes loss of function, at least temporarily, and the irritation sometimes makes inflammation more harmful than beneficial. In spite of this, it usually is a worthwhile process because it is aimed at localizing the damage and destroying its source. Inflammation also sets the stage for tissue repair. The unpleasant signs and symptoms also have a protective function because they warn that tissue damage has occurred so that the source of the damage may be removed. Below are the steps of the inflammatory process.

1. Bacteria or foreign particles enter the body.
2. Tissues are damaged.
3. Damaged tissues release chemical mediators.
4. Chemical mediators have three effects:
   • Attract neutrophils and macrophages (chemotaxis)
   • Increase blood flow through vasodilation
   • Increase capillary permeability
5. Overall effect of chemical mediators is to bring additional phagocytes to damaged area.
6. Phagocytes are successful and destroy bacteria.
7. Area is cleansed of debris.
8. Tissues are repaired.
9. If phagocytes are not successful, steps 2 to 5 continue to result in chronic inflammation.

Figure 14–6 briefly describes the inflammatory process.

> Inflammation is characterized by redness, warmth, swelling, and pain.

Systemic inflammation is not contained in a localized region but is widespread throughout the body. The warmth, redness, swelling, pain, and loss of function associated with localized inflammation may be present at specific sites, but the systemic nature of the inflammation is evidenced by three additional responses.

• Bone marrow is stimulated to produce more white blood cells, especially neutrophils and monocytes, so there is a condition of leukocytosis.
• Chemical mediators include **pyrogens** (PYE-roh-jenz) that influence the hypothalamus and cause an increase body temperature or **fever.** The fever speeds up the metabolic reactions in the body, including those directed at destroying the invading pathogens.
• Vasodilation and increased capillary permeability may become so generalized that there is a drastic and dangerous decrease in blood pressure. Systemic inflammation is a medical crisis and needs immediate attention.

Figure 14–7 summarizes the components of nonspecific defense mechanisms.

> Systemic inflammation shows leukocytosis, fever, and decreased blood pressure.

☑ QuickCheck

● If pathogens succeed in passing through the first line barriers that inhibit their entry into the body, what other nonspecific defense mechanisms are available to prevent disease?

● What type of infection may result in elevated levels of interferon?

Specific Defense Mechanisms

In contrast to the nonspecific defense mechanisms that react against all types of foreign agents, the specific defense mechanisms are programmed to be selective. This characteristic is called **specificity.** Another characteristic of specific defense mechanisms is **memory.** Once the system has been exposed to a particular invading agent, components of the specific defense mechanisms "remember" that agent and launch a quicker attack if it enters the body again. Specific defense mechanisms provide the third line of defense against microbial invasion. This third line of defense is **specific resistance,** or **immunity.** The primary cells involved are **lymphocytes** and **macrophages.** Nonspecific mechanisms and immune responses take place at the same time, and

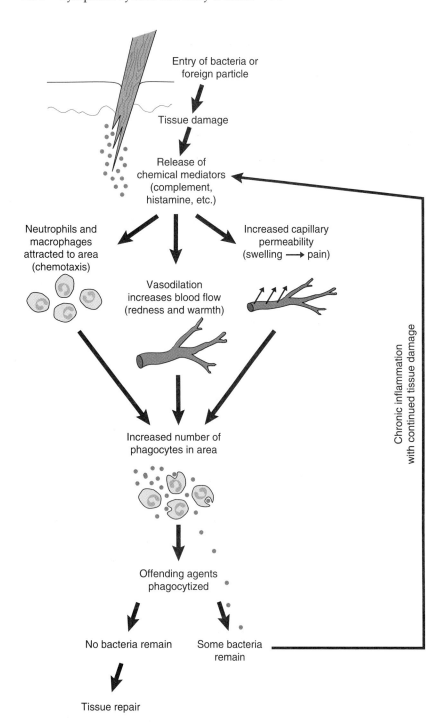

Entry of bacteria or foreign particle

Tissue damage

Release of chemical mediators (complement, histamine, etc.)

Neutrophils and macrophages attracted to area (chemotaxis)

Increased capillary permeability (swelling ⟶ pain)

Vasodilation increases blood flow (redness and warmth)

Increased number of phagocytes in area

Chronic inflammation with continued tissue damage

Offending agents phagocytized

No bacteria remain

Some bacteria remain

Tissue repair

Figure 14–6 Steps in inflammation.

resistance to disease depends on the interaction of all the mechanisms.

> Specificity and memory are two characteristics of specific defense mechanisms. The two primary cells that are involved are lymphocytes and macrophages.

Recognition of Self Versus Nonself

For the immune system to function properly, lymphocytes have to distinguish between self and non-self. During their development and maturation process, the lymphocytes learn to recognize the proteins and other large molecules that belong to the body. They interpret these as "self." Molecules that are not recognized as self are interpreted as "nonself," and defense mechanisms are set in motion to destroy them. A molecule that is interpreted as nonself and that triggers an immune response is called a foreign **antigen.** Antigens are usually some form of protein or large polysaccharide molecules on the surface of cell membranes. Normally, antigens that cause problems are foreign molecules that enter the body, but

Component	Mechanism			Action

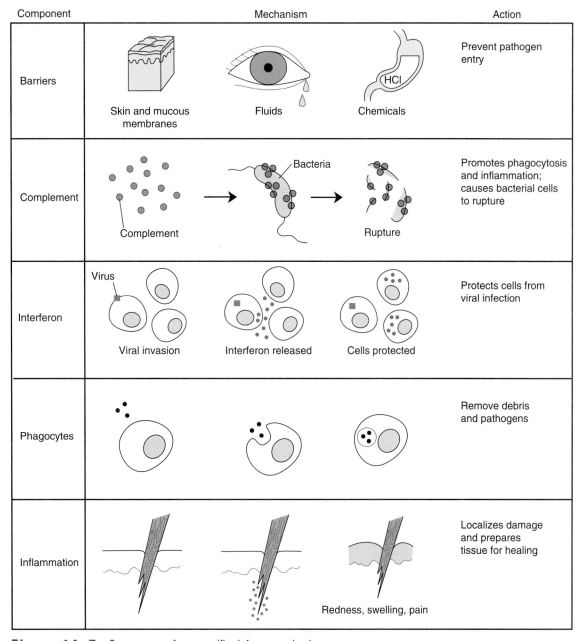

Figure 14-7   Components of nonspecific defense mechanisms.

sometimes the body fails to recognize its own molecules and triggers an immune reaction against self. This damages normal body tissue and is the basis of **autoimmune diseases** such as rheumatoid arthritis.

Antigens are molecules that trigger an immune response.

Development of Lymphocytes

Like all other blood cells, lymphocytes develop from stem cells in the bone marrow (Fig. 14–8). During fetal development, the bone marrow releases immature and undifferentiated (unspecialized) lymphocytes into the blood. Some of these go to the thymus gland where they acquire the ability to distinguish between self and nonself molecules. These lymphocytes differentiate to become **T lymphocytes,** or **T cells,** in the thymus gland. For several months after birth the thymus gland continues to process the T lymphocytes for specific activities in immune reactions. Differentiated T cells leave the thymus, enter the blood, and are distributed to lymphoid tissue, especially the lymph nodes. About 70 percent of the circulating lymphocytes are T cells.

Lymphocytes that do not go to the thymus travel in the blood to some other area, probably the fetal liver, where they differentiate into **B lymphocytes,**

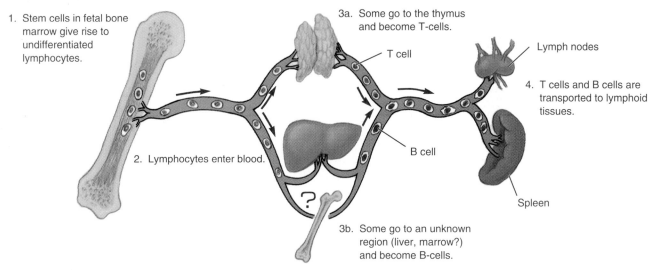

1. Stem cells in fetal bone marrow give rise to undifferentiated lymphocytes.

2. Lymphocytes enter blood.

3a. Some go to the thymus and become T-cells.

T cell

B cell

3b. Some go to an unknown region (liver, marrow?) and become B-cells.

Lymph nodes

4. T cells and B cells are transported to lymphoid tissues.

Spleen

Figure 14–8   Development of lymphocytes.

or **B cells.** After they acquire the ability to distinguish between self and nonself and are prepared for their special roles in immune responses, B cells enter the blood and are also distributed to lymphoid tissues. B cells account for about 30 percent of the circulating lymphocytes.

> Lymphocytes that mature in the thymus are called T cells. Those that mature elsewhere are called B cells.

In the differentiation and maturation process, thousands of different types of T cells and B cells are produced. Each type has receptor sites that fit with specific antigens. Thus they provide specific resistance. There has to be an exact match between the receptor site on the lymphocyte and the antigen of the invader before an immune reaction occurs.

Cell-Mediated Immunity

T cells are responsible for **cell-mediated immunity** in which the T cells directly attack the invading antigen. Cell-mediated immunity is most effective against virus-infected cells, cancer cells, foreign tissue cells (transplant rejection), fungi, and protozoan parasites.

> Cell-mediated immunity is the result of T cell action.

When the antigen is introduced into the body, it is phagocytized by a macrophage, which then presents the antigen to the T cell population (Fig. 14–9). T cells that have receptor sites for that specific antigen recognize it and become activated. Both the macrophage and the activated T cells secrete chemicals that stimulate division of the activated T cells.

This results in large numbers of cells that are all alike, a clone of activated T cells. There are four subgroups within the **clone** of activated T cells, and each group has a specific function. **Killer T cells** directly destroy the cells with the offending antigen. **Helper T cells** secrete substances that stimulate B cells and promote the immune response. **Suppressor T cells** have the opposite effect; they inhibit B cells and the immune response. The helper and suppressor T cells are regulatory cells that control the immune response. Normally, in a correctly operating immune system, there are twice as many helper cells as suppressor cells. The fourth group of cells is the population of **memory T cells.** These cells "remember" the specific antigen and stimulate a faster and more intense response if the same antigen is introduced another time.

> Activated T cells produce clones of killer T cells, helper T cells, suppressor T cells, and memory T cells.

Antibody-Mediated Immunity (Humoral Immunity)

B cells are responsible for **antibody-mediated immunity.** Like T cells, each type of B cell can respond to only one specific type of antigen. There must be a match between the receptor on the B cell and the antigen. Unlike T cells, B cells do not directly assault the antigen. Instead, they are responsible for the production of antibodies that react with the antigen or substances produced by the antigen. Because the antibodies are found in body fluids, it is sometimes called humoral immunity. Antibody-mediated immunity is most effective against bacteria, viruses that are outside body cells, and toxins. It is also involved in allergic reactions.

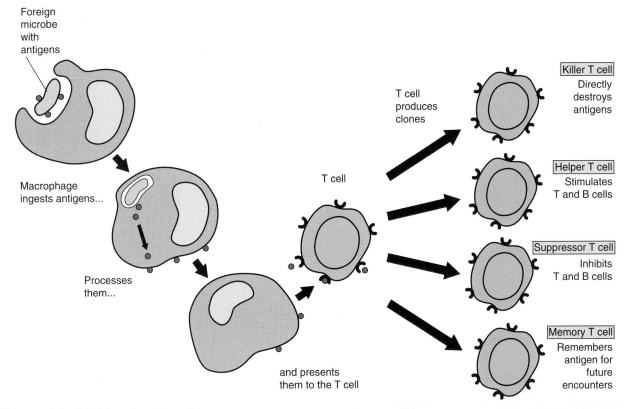

Foreign microbe with antigens

Macrophage ingests antigens...

Processes them...

and presents them to the T cell

T cell

T cell produces clones

Killer T cell
Directly destroys antigens

Helper T cell
Stimulates T and B cells

Suppressor T cell
Inhibits T and B cells

Memory T cell
Remembers antigen for future encounters

Figure 14–9 Cell-mediated immunity.

> Antibody-mediated immunity is also called humoral immunity. It is the result of B-cell action.

When an antigen enters the body, a macrophage engulfs and processes it, then presents it to B cells and helper T cells (Fig. 14–10). The B cells and helper T cells that have receptors for that specific antigen are activated. The activated helper T cells secrete substances that stimulate the activated B cells to rapidly divide and to form a clone of cells consisting of **plasma cells** and **memory B cells.**

> Activated B cells produce clones of plasma cells and memory cells.

One of the substances secreted by activated T cells is **interleukin-2,** which stimulates production of both T cells and B cells. Researchers are using interleukin-2 made by genetic engineering techniques to stimulate the immune system. The converse of this is that decreasing the activity of interleukin-2 can suppress the immune system. **Cyclosporine,** a drug that inhibits the production of interleukin-2, is used to prevent the rejection of transplanted organs.

Plasma cells rapidly produce large quantities of protein molecules, called **antibodies,** that are transported in the blood and lymph to the site of the infection where they inactivate the invading antigens. This initial action is the **primary response.** When the antigens are destroyed, macrophages clean up the debris, and suppressor T cells decrease the immune response. Memory B cells remain dormant in lymphatic tissue until the same antigen again enters the system. The memory cells recognize the antigen and launch a rapid and intense response against it. This is called a **secondary response** (Fig. 14–11). The purpose of vaccinations is to provide an initial exposure so memory cells are available for a rapid and intense reaction against subsequent exposure to the antigen.

> Plasma cells produce antibodies that react with specific antigens.

All antibodies have a similar structure but one portion of the molecule differs so that each antibody is capable of reacting with only a specific antigen. They belong to the class of proteins called **globu-**

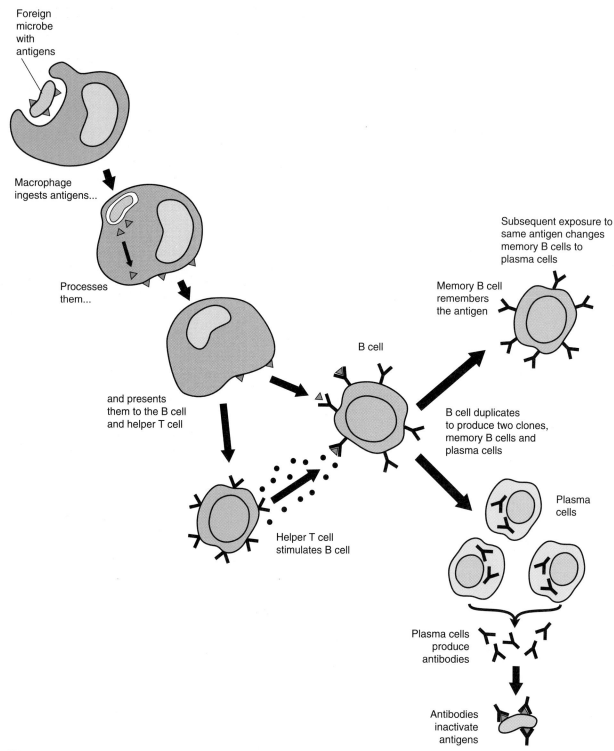

Foreign microbe with antigens

Macrophage ingests antigens...

Processes them...

and presents them to the B cell and helper T cell

Helper T cell stimulates B cell

B cell

Subsequent exposure to same antigen changes memory B cells to plasma cells

Memory B cell remembers the antigen

B cell duplicates to produce two clones, memory B cells and plasma cells

Plasma cells

Plasma cells produce antibodies

Antibodies inactivate antigens

Figure 14–10 Antibody-mediated immunity.

lins, and because they are involved in immune reactions, they are called **immunoglobulins** (ih-myoo-noh-GLOB-yoo-lins), abbreviated **Ig.** There are several classes of antibodies or immunoglobulins, designated as *IgA, IgG, IgM, IgE,* and *IgD.* Immunoglobulins of the IgG class are called gamma globulins. Each class has a specific role in immunity, which is summarized in Table 14–1.

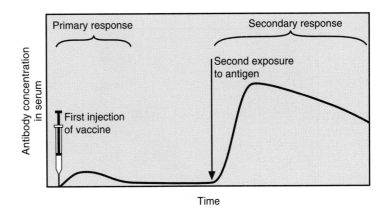

Figure 14-11 Comparison of primary and secondary responses.

Hypersensitivity reactions, commonly known as allergies, are conditions in which the body reacts with an exaggerated immune response and produces tissue damage and disordered function rather than immunity. These reactions vary in intensity from the rhinitis familiar to hayfever sufferers to systemic anaphylaxis, which may be life threatening. An **allergen,** the agent that sets off an allergic response, initiates a series of reactions that release histamine into the systems. Histamine increases capillary permeability, which results in edema. Antihistamines are preparations that counteract the effects of histamine.

Acquired Immunity

There are four ways to acquire specific resistance, or immunity. The terms **active** and **passive** refer to whose immune system reacts to the antigen. Active immunity occurs when the individual's own body produces memory T cells and B cells in response to a harmful antigen. Active immunity takes several days to develop and lasts for a long time because

memory cells are produced. Passive immunity results when the immune agents develop in another person (or animal) and are transferred to an individual who was not previously immune. Passive immunity provides immediate protection but is effective for only a short time because no memory cells are produced in the individual.

> Active immunity takes several days to develop but lasts a long time. Passive immunity is immediately effective but doesn't last long.

The terms **natural** and **artificial** refer to how the immunity is obtained. Natural immunity occurs when the immunity is acquired through normal, everyday living, without any deliberate action. Artificial immunity results when some type of deliberate action is taken to acquire the immunity, such as getting a vaccination. Combining the terms gives the four types of acquired immunity (Fig. 14-12):

- Active natural immunity
- Active artificial immunity
- Passive natural immunity
- Passive artificial immunity

Table 14-1   Classes of Antibodies

Class	Percent of Total	Location	Function
IgG	75–85	Blood plasma	Major antibody in primary and secondary immune responses; inactivates antigen; neutralizes toxins; crosses placenta to provide immunity for newborn; responsible for Rh reactions
IgA	5–15	Saliva, mucus, tears, breast milk	Protects mucous membranes on body surfaces; provides immunity for newborn
IgM	5–10	Attached to B cells; released into plasma during immune response	Causes antigens to clump together; responsible for transfusion reactions in the ABO blood typing system
IgD	0.2	Attached to B cells	Receptor sites for antigens on B cells; binding with antigen results in B cell activation
IgE	0.5	Produced by plasma cells in mucous membranes and tonsils	Binds to mast cells and basophils, causing release of histamine; responsible for allergic reactions

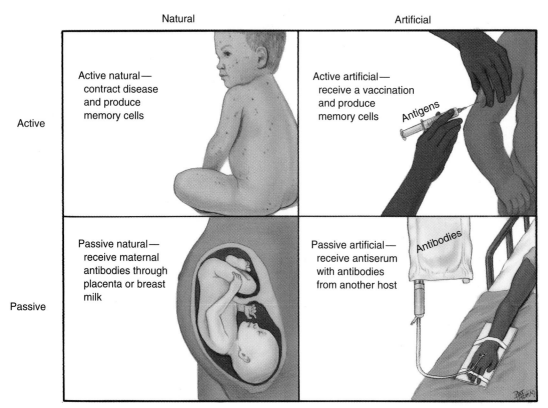

Figure 14–12 Acquired immunity.

Natural immunity is acquired through normal activities. Artificial immunity requires some deliberate action.

Active Natural Immunity

Active natural immunity results when a person is exposed to a harmful antigen, contracts the disease, and recovers. Exposure to the pathogen stimulates production of memory cells. In subsequent exposures, the memory cells recognize the pathogen and launch a rapid assault before the disease develops. An example of this is the child who gets chickenpox, recovers, and never contracts it again although exposed many times.

Active Artificial Immunity

Active artificial immunity develops when a specially prepared antigen is deliberately introduced into an individual's system. This is called **vaccination.** The prepared antigen, called a **vaccine** (vak-SEEN), usually consists of weakened (attenuated), inactivated, or dead pathogens or their toxins. The antigens stimulate the immune system but are altered so they do not produce the symptoms of the disease. Nearly everyone is familiar with the vaccines, for example, for mumps, diphtheria, whooping cough, and tetanus.

Passive Natural Immunity

Passive natural immunity results when antibodies are transferred from one person to another through natural means. This occurs only in the prenatal and postnatal relationship between mother and child. Some antibodies (IgG) can cross the placenta and enter fetal blood. This provides protection for the child for a short time after birth, but eventually the antibodies deteriorate and the infant must rely on its own immune system. IgA antibodies are transferred from mother to infant through the mother's milk. This accounts for less than 1 percent of an infant's immunity, but offers some intestinal protection not available through the placenta.

Passive Artificial Immunity

Passive artificial immunity results when antibodies that developed in another person (or animal) are injected into an individual. **Antiserum** is the general term used for the preparation that contains the antibodies. Antisera may contain antibodies that act against microorganisms (e.g., hepatitis and rabies); bacterial toxins (e.g., tetanus and botulism); or venoms (e.g., poisonous snakes and spiders). Passive artificial immunity provides immediate but short-term protection.

The four types of acquired immunity are active natural immunity, active artificial immunity, passive natural immunity, and passive artificial immunity.

After a period of time, the number of antibodies against a particular antigen may decrease. A **booster** is an additional dose of vaccine given to increase the number of antibodies.

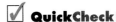

☑ **QuickCheck**

- How do helper T cells influence humoral immunity?
- What class of immunoglobulins is responsible for most primary and secondary immune responses?
- Gamma globulins from the female cross the placenta to provide some protection for the newborn. What type of immunity is this?

● FOCUS ON AGING

Most lymphoid tissues, such as the spleen, thymus, tonsils, and lymph nodes, undergo structural changes with age. They reach their maximum development at the time of puberty, then slowly regress after that period. There is reduced bone marrow, but enough stem cells remain to produce adequate blood cells for replacement of old cells. There does not appear to be a significant decrease in the number of lymphocytes in the elderly.

The thymus progressively degenerates after puberty so that most of the adult gland is connective tissue. Structural changes in the gland are accompanied by a decreased production of the hormone thymosin, which affects the differentiation and functional activity of T lymphocytes. Consequently, there is an increase in immature T cells and a decrease in the number and/or activity of mature T cells.

The number of B lymphocytes does not appear to change significantly with age; however, there is a decrease in antigen–antibody reactions. This indicates that the B cells are less responsive to the antigens and do not form plasma-cell clones to produce antibodies. However, this may be because the helper T cells are less active and do not stimulate the B cells as they normally do.

In general, in older people there is a decrease in immune sensitivity and an increase in autoimmune reactions in which the immune system fails to recognize the body's own cells. Older people are more susceptible to infectious diseases and autoimmune disorders than are younger people. The declining immune system also accounts, in part, for the increased incidence of cancer in the elderly.

DO YOU KNOW THIS ABOUT

Immunology?

Hypersensitivities

Hypersensitivity reactions, commonly known as **allergies,** are conditions in which the body reacts with an exaggerated immune response and produces tissue damage and disordered function rather than immunity. The agent, or antigen, that produces an allergic reaction is termed an **allergen.** Hypersensitivity is a multistep process that involves an initial exposure to an allergen, a dormant period during which an individual becomes sensitized, and a reaction to a subsequent exposure to the same allergen. Historically, these reactions have been classified into two categories according to the time that elapses between exposure to the allergen and the appearance of clini-

cal symptoms. If clinical symptoms appear within 48 hours, it is called **immediate hypersensitivity.** If the symptoms appear after 48 hours, it is called **delayed hypersensitivity.** More recently, however, it has been determined that the fundamental difference between the two categories is not time but the mechanism of reaction. Immediate hypersensitivity primarily involves the reaction of antibodies with antigens, or humoral immunity. Delayed hypersensitivity involves the T lymphocytes of cellular immunity.

Immediate hypersensitivity reactions, sometimes called anaphylactic hypersensitivities, vary in intensity from the rhinitis familiar to hayfever

Continued on following page

sufferers to a general systemic anaphylaxis, which may be life threatening. This type of allergy begins with the entry of an allergen into the body. Allergens include a wide variety of substances such as dust, pollen, bee venom, and penicillin. The immune system responds to the allergen by producing antibodies, specifically IgE. The IgE antibodies have a high infinity for mast cells and attach to the surface of these cells. Mast cells are connective tissue cells that contain granules of histamine and are abundant in the respiratory tract, digestive tract, and near blood vessels. An individual becomes **sensitized** when IgE antibodies are attached to the mast cells. Multiple exposures to the allergen may be required to sensitize a person fully.

If a sensitized individual is exposed to the allergen again, symptoms occur rapidly. The allergen molecules combine with the antibodies that are attached to the mast cells. This antigen–antibody interaction results in the rupture of the mast cell and the release of its granules into the extracellular fluid. Although the granules contain many chemical mediators, two significant ones are **histamine** and **serotonin.** The principal activities of these mediators is to cause contraction of smooth muscles in the body and to increase capillary permeability. Smooth muscle contraction in the respiratory tract leads to difficulty in breathing. In the digestive tract, smooth muscle contraction results in painful cramps. Increased capillary permeability is manifest in edema as the fluids leave the vessels and enter the interstitial space. If the sensitized mast cells are widely distributed throughout the body, widespread systemic anaphylaxis may result. Blood pressure falls drastically as fluids leave the blood and as contraction of muscles in the respiratory passages blocks air flow. Because death may follow within minutes, the key to survival is fast action. Individuals known to have hypersensitivities of this type may be advised to carry an injection kit of epinephrine with them. Epinephrine, quickly administered, stabilizes the mast cells to prevent further release of histamine, dilates the air passages, and constricts the capillaries to keep the fluid in circulation.

Fortunately, the vast majority of immediate hypersensitivity reactions lead to sensitization in localized areas of the body. These are the common allergies. An example of this is hay fever in which sensitization occurs in the eyes, nose, and upper respiratory tract. Subsequent exposures cause reddened teary eyes, sneezing, and swollen mucous membranes. Antihistamines, preparations that counteract the effects of histamine, usually are sufficient to relieve the symptoms.

Delayed hypersensitivity is sometimes called cellular hypersensitivity because it is an exaggeration of the process of cellular immunity. It involves sensitized T lymphocytes and monocytes instead of B cells and antibodies. The effect of the "delayed" reactions develops slowly and is not evident until 48 to 72 hours after exposure. Two major forms of delayed hypersensitivity are **infection allergy** and **contact dermatitis.**

An important application of infection allergy is the skin test for tuberculosis. A purified protein derivative (PPD) of the bacterium that causes tuberculosis is applied to the skin by intradermal injection. If an individual has been previously sensitized by exposure to tuberculosis, a hypersensitivity reaction takes place. The injection site becomes red, a vesicle appears, and the skin around the site becomes thick and dry. Because this is a screening test and a positive test is not conclusive, the individual is referred for more extensive diagnostic tests.

Contact dermatitis develops after exposure to a wide variety of materials such as metals, extracts of certain plants, insecticides, and cosmetics. Earrings worn in pierced ears frequently are a cause of contact dermatitis. Body tissues are in constant contact with some part of the earring, either a metal post or hook. After a few weeks or months, the point of contact becomes red and swollen. Continued exposure increases the severity of the allergic reaction and infection may occur. Clinical symptoms disappear a few weeks after use is discontinued. Another example of contact dermatitis is poison ivy. In this case the symptoms include redness and watery blisters in the area of contact with the plant allergen. This may spread by scratching and then touching another site. Although uncomfortable, the symptoms usually are not severe, but secondary infections may lead to serious complications.

Representative Disorders of the Lymphatic/Immune System

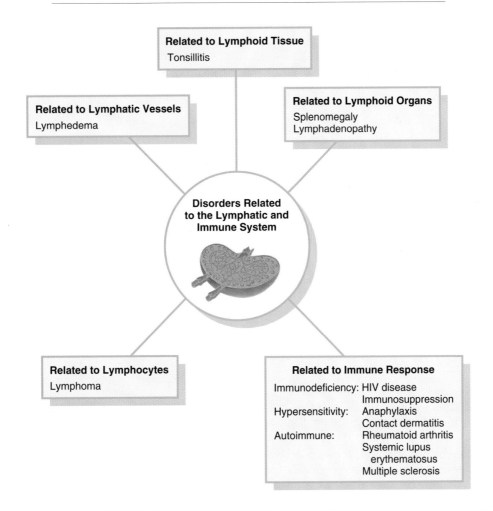

Related to Lymphoid Tissue
Tonsillitis

Related to Lymphatic Vessels
Lymphedema

Related to Lymphoid Organs
Splenomegaly
Lymphadenopathy

Disorders Related to the Lymphatic and Immune System

Related to Lymphocytes
Lymphoma

Related to Immune Response
Immunodeficiency: HIV disease
Immunosuppression
Hypersensitivity: Anaphylaxis
Contact dermatitis
Autoimmune: Rheumatoid arthritis
Systemic lupus
erythematosus
Multiple sclerosis

CHAPTER QUIZ

RECALL

Match the definitions on the left with the appropriate term on the right.

1. Lymph capillaries

2. Collects lymph from three fourths of the body

3. Enlarged pharyngeal tonsils

4. Lack of resistance

5. Provides localized protection against viruses

6. Cause an increase in body temperature

7. Principal cell involved in cell-mediated immunity

8. Protein that triggers an immune response

9. Produce antibodies

10. Rapid, intense reaction against an antigen

A. Adenoids

B. Antigen

C. Interferon

D. Lacteal

E. Plasma cells

F. Pyrogens

G. Secondary response

H. Susceptibility

I. T cells

J. Thoracic duct

THOUGHT

1. Lymphatic vessels carry lymph away from the tissues and eventually return it to the blood in the

   a. inferior vena cava

   b. superior vena cava

   c. subclavian arteries

   d. subclavian veins

2. Lymph is filtered by the

   a. spleen

   b. lymph nodes

   c. liver

   d. tonsils

3. Which of the following describes, or is a characteristic of, nonspecific defense mechanisms?

   a. phagocytosis

   b. memory

   c. B cells

   d. immunoglobulins

4. Which of the following statements about T lymphocytes is false?

   a. are responsible for humoral immunity

   b. some are regulatory cells that control the immune response

   c. some directly destroy antigens

   d. some stimulate B cells

5. Active immunity is produced when

   a. an individual receives an injection of gamma globulin

   b. an infant receives antibodies through the placenta or breast milk

   c. an individual receives an injection of vaccine

   d. an individual is injected with an antiserum

APPLICATION

In treating a woman for breast cancer, the surgeon removed some of the axillary lymph nodes on the right side. After surgery, she experiences edema in the right upper extremity. Explain why this side effect occurred?.

Booster shots may be given as part of a vaccination regimen. A booster shot is a second dose of the same vaccine given sometime after the original vaccination. Why are booster shots given if they are just a repeat of the same vaccine?

CHAPTER 15

Respiratory System

Outline/Objectives

Functions and Overview of Respiration 307

- Define five activities or functions of the respiratory process.

Ventilation 307

- Describe the structures and features of the upper respiratory tract and the lower respiratory tract.
- Describe the structure of the lungs including shape, lobes, tissue, and membranes.
- Name and define three pressures involved in pulmonary ventilation and relate these pressures to the sequence of events that results in inspiration and expiration.
- Define four respiratory volumes and four respiratory capacities, state their average normal values, and describe factors that influence them.

Basic Gas Laws and Respiration 315

- Discuss factors that govern the diffusion of gases into and out of the blood.
- Distinguish between external respiration and internal respiration.

Transport of Gases 317

- Describe how oxygen and carbon dioxide are transported in the blood.

Regulation of Respiration 320

- Name two regions in the brain that make up the respiratory center and two nerves that carry impulses from the center.
- Describe the role of chemoreceptors, stretch receptors, higher brain centers, and temperature in regulating breathing.

Key Terms

Alveolus

Bronchial tree

Bronchopulmonary segment

External respiration

Internal respiration

Respiratory membrane

Surfactant

Ventilation

Building Vocabulary

WORD PART	MEANING
-a	lack of
alveol-	tiny cavity
anthrac-	coal
bronchi-	bronchi
-coni-	dust
cric-	ring
dys-	difficult
-ectasis	dilation
eu-	good
phon-	voice
-pnea	breathing
pneum-	lung, air
-ptysis	spitting
pulmon-	lung
-rrhea	flow or discharge
rhin-	nose
spir-	breath
thyr-	shield
-tion	act of, process of
ventilat-	to fan or blow

Functional Relationships of the
Respiratory System

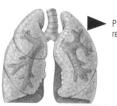

Provides oxygen and removes carbon dioxide.

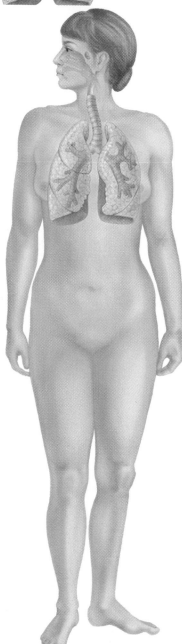

Integument

Helps maintain body temperature for metabolism; hairs of nasal cavity filter particles that may damage the upper respiratory tract.

Furnishes oxygen and removes carbon dioxide by gaseous exchange with blood.

Skeletal

Encases the lungs for protection; provides passageways for air through the nasal cavity.

Supplies oxygen for bone tissue metabolism and removes carbon dioxide.

Muscular

Muscle contractions control airflow through respiratory passages and create pressure changes necessary for ventilation.

Supplies oxygen for muscle metabolism and removes carbon dioxide.

Nervous

Innervates muscles involved in breathing; controls rate and depth of breathing.

Supplies oxygen for brain, spinal cord, and sensory tissue; removes carbon dioxide; helps maintain pH for neural function.

Endocrine

Thyroxine and epinephrine promote cell respiration; epinephrine stimulates bronchodilation.

Supplies oxygen, removes carbon dioxide, and helps maintain pH for metabolism in endocrine glands; converts angiotensin I into angiotensin II.

Cardiovascular
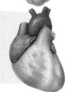
Transports oxygen and carbon dioxide between lungs and tissues.

Breathing movements assist in venous return; helps maintain blood pH; supplies oxygen and removes carbon dioxide for cardiac tissue.

Lymphatic/Immune

Tonsils combat pathogens that enter through respiratory passageways; IgA protects respiratory mucosa.

Provides lymphoid tissue and immune cells with oxygen and removes carbon dioxide; pharynx contains the tonsils; breathing movements assist in flow of lymph.

Digestive
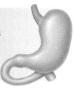
Absorbs nutrients that are necessary for maintenance of cells in the lungs and other tissues of the respiratory tract.

Provides oxygen for metabolism of cells in digestive system; removes carbon dioxide; helps maintain pH of body fluids for effective enzyme function.

Urinary

Helps maintain water, electrolyte, and pH balance of body fluids for effective respiratory function; eliminates waste products generated by respiratory organs.

Assists in the regulation of pH by removing carbon dioxide.

Reproductive
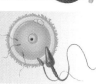
Sexual arousal stimulates changes in rate and depth of breathing.

Supplies oxygen and removes carbon dioxide to maintain metabolism in tissues of reproductive system; helps maintain pH for gonadal hormone function.

When the respiratory system is mentioned, people generally think of breathing, but this is only one of the activities of the respiratory system. The body cells need a continuous supply of oxygen for the metabolic processes that are necessary to maintain life. The respiratory system works with the circulatory system to provide this oxygen and to remove the waste products of metabolism. It also helps to regulate the pH of the blood.

Functions and Overview of Respiration

Respiration is the sequence of events that results in the exchange of oxygen and carbon dioxide between the atmosphere and the body cells. Every 3 to 5 seconds nerve impulses stimulate the breathing process, or **ventilation,** which moves air through a series of passages into and out of the lungs. After this, there is an exchange of gases between the lungs and the blood. This is called **external respiration.** The blood **transports** the gases to and from the tissue cells. The exchange of gases between the blood and tissue cells is **internal respiration.** Finally, the cells utilize the oxygen for their specific activities. This is cellular metabolism, or **cellular respiration,** which is discussed in Chapter 17. Together these activities constitute respiration.

> The entire process of respiration includes ventilation, external respiration, transport of gases, internal respiration, and cellular respiration.

Ventilation

Ventilation, or breathing, is the movement of air through the conducting passages between the atmosphere and the lungs. The air moves through the passages because of pressure gradients that are produced by contraction of the diaphragm and thoracic muscles.

Conducting Passages

The conducting passages are divided into the **upper respiratory tract** and the **lower respiratory tract** (Fig. 15–1). The upper respiratory tract includes the nose, pharynx, and larynx. The lower respiratory tract consists of the trachea, bronchial tree, and lungs. These passageways open to the outside and are lined with mucous membrane. In some regions, the membrane has hairs that help filter the air. Other regions may have cilia to propel mucus.

Nose and Nasal Cavities

The framework of the **nose** consists of bone and cartilage. Two small nasal bones and extensions of the maxillae form the bridge of the nose, which is the bony portion. The remainder of the framework is cartilage. This is the flexible portion. Connective tissue and skin cover the framework.

The interior chamber of the nose is the **nasal cavity.** It is divided into two parts by the **nasal septum,** a vertical partition formed by the vomer and the perpendicular plate of the ethmoid bone. Air enters

CLINICAL TERMS

Aspiration (as-pih-RAY-shun) The process of removing substances by means of suction

Atelectasis (at-eh-LECK-tah-sis) Collapse of the alveoli; the lung is airless

Bronchogenic carcinoma (brong-koh-JEN-ik kar-sin-OH-mah) Cancerous tumors arising from a bronchus; lung cancer; smoking is the primary etiologic agent; spreads readily to the liver, brain, and bones

Chronic obstructive pulmonary disease (COPD) (KRAHN-ik ob-STRUCK-tiv PULL-mon-air-ee dih-ZEEZ) A chronic condition of obstructed air flow through the bronchial tubes and lungs, usually accompanied by dyspnea; includes emphysema and chronic bronchitis

Coryza (koh-RYE-zah) The common cold, characterized by sneezing, nasal discharge, coughing, and malaise; caused by a rhinovirus

Croup (KROOP) Acute respiratory syndrome in infants and children, characterized by obstruction of the larynx, barking cough, and strained, high-pitched, noisy breathing

Pertussis (per-TUSS-is) Whooping cough; a highly contagious bacterial infection of the pharynx, larynx, and trachea; characterized by explosive coughing spasms ending in a "whooping" sound

Pneumoconiosis (new-moh-koh-nee-OH-sis) General term for lung pathology that occurs after long-term inhalation of pollutants, characterized by chronic inflammation, infection, and bronchitis

Pneumonectomy (new-moh-NECK-toh-mee) Surgical removal of all or part of a lung, such as a lobe; removal of a lobe is also called lobectomy

Pulmonary edema (PULL-mon-air-ee eh-DEE-mah) Swelling and fluid in the air sacs and bronchioles; often caused by inability of the heart to pump blood, the blood then backs up in the pulmonary blood vessels and fluid seeps out into the alveoli and bronchioles

Rhinoplasty (RYE-noh-plas-tee) Plastic surgery on the nose; medical term for a "nose job"

Thoracocentesis (thor-ah-koh-sen-TEE-sis) A surgical procedure through the chest wall into the pleural cavity to remove fluid

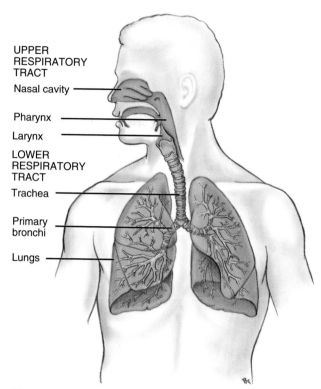

UPPER RESPIRATORY TRACT
Nasal cavity
Pharynx
Larynx
LOWER RESPIRATORY TRACT
Trachea
Primary bronchi
Lungs

Figure 15–1 Conducting passages of the respiratory system.

and swollen. The swelling may block the passages and cause the mucus to accumulate in the sinuses. As the mucus accumulates, pressure within the sinuses increases, resulting in a sinus headache.

> The frontal, maxillary, ethmoidal, and sphenoidal sinuses are air-filled cavities that open into the nasal cavity.

As air passes through the nasal cavity, it is filtered, warmed, and moistened. The mucous membrane that lines most of the nasal cavity is ciliated pseudostratified columnar epithelium, which filters the air. Goblet cells in the mucous membrane produce mucus that traps microorganisms, dust, and other foreign particles. Cilia propel the mucus with the trapped particles toward the pharynx where it is swallowed. Acid in the gastric juice destroys most of the microorganisms that are swallowed. Extensive capillary networks under the mucous membrane warm and moisten the air before it reaches the rest of the respiratory tract.

> **Rhinitis** is an inflammation of the nasal mucosa accompanied by excessive mucus production. It can be caused by cold viruses, certain bacteria and allergens.

the nasal cavity from the outside through two openings, the **nostrils,** or **external nares** (NAY-reez). The openings from the nasal cavity into the pharynx are the **internal nares.** The **palate** forms the floor of the nasal cavity and separates the nasal cavity from the oral cavity. The anterior portion of the palate is called the **hard palate** because it is supported by bone. The posterior portion has no bony support, so it is the **soft palate.** The soft palate terminates in a projection called the **uvula** (YOO-vyoo-lah), which helps direct food into the oropharynx. Three **nasal conchae** (KONG-kee), bony ridges that project medially into the nasal cavity from each lateral wall, increase the surface area of the cavity to warm and moisten the air and also to help direct air flow. Dust and other nongaseous particles in the air tend to become trapped in the mucous membrane around the conchae. Figure 15–2 illustrates the features of the nasal cavity.

Paranasal sinuses are air-filled cavities in the frontal, maxillae, ethmoid, and sphenoid bones. These sinuses, which have the same names as the bones in which they are located, surround the nasal cavity and open into it. They function to reduce the weight of the skull, to produce mucus, and to influence voice quality by acting as resonating chambers. The sinuses are lined with mucous membrane that produces mucus, which drains into the nasal cavity. During infections and allergies, the membranes in the passages that drain the sinuses become inflamed

Pharynx

The **pharynx** (FAIR-inks), commonly called the throat, is a passageway, about 13 cm long, that extends from the base of the skull to the level of the sixth cervical vertebra. It serves both the respiratory and digestive systems by receiving air from the nasal cavity and air, food, and water from the oral cavity. Inferiorly, it opens into the larynx and esophagus. The pharynx is divided into three regions according to location (see Fig. 15–2).

The **nasopharynx** (nay-zoh-FAIR-inks) is the portion of the pharynx that is posterior to the nasal cavity and extends inferiorly to the uvula. Air enters this region from the nasal cavity through the internal nares. The mucous membrane in the nasopharynx is similar to the lining of the nasal cavity. The **auditory** (eustachian) **tubes** from the two middle ear cavities open into the nasopharynx. The auditory tubes help to equalize the air pressure on both sides of the tympanic membrane (eardrum). Collections of lymphoid tissue, called **pharyngeal tonsils,** or **adenoids,** are located in the posterior wall of the nasopharynx.

The **oropharynx** (ohr-oh-FAIR-inks) is the portion of the pharynx that is posterior to the oral cavity. It extends from the uvula down to the level of the hyoid bone and receives air, food, and water from the oral cavity. During swallowing, the soft palate and uvula move upward to prevent the material

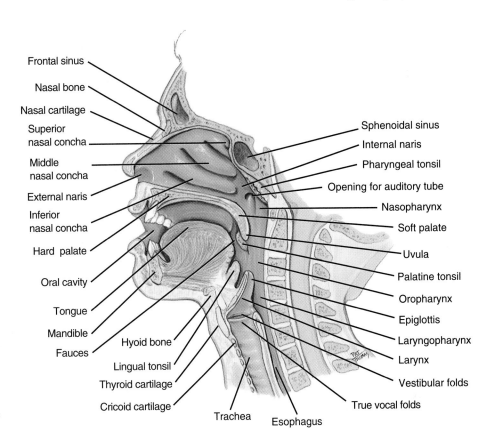

Figure 15-2 Features of the upper respiratory tract.

Labels (clockwise from top left):
Frontal sinus
Nasal bone
Nasal cartilage
Superior nasal concha
Middle nasal concha
External naris
Inferior nasal concha
Hard palate
Oral cavity
Tongue
Mandible
Fauces
Hyoid bone
Lingual tonsil
Thyroid cartilage
Cricoid cartilage
Trachea
Esophagus
True vocal folds
Vestibular folds
Larynx
Laryngopharynx
Epiglottis
Oropharynx
Palatine tonsil
Uvula
Soft palate
Nasopharynx
Opening for auditory tube
Pharyngeal tonsil
Internal naris
Sphenoidal sinus

from going into the nasopharynx. The opening between the oral cavity and oropharynx is called the **fauces** (FAW-seez), and it is bordered by masses of lymphoid tissue called **tonsils.** The **palatine tonsils** are in the lateral walls of the oropharynx, adjacent to the fauces, and the **lingual tonsils** are located on the surface of the posterior portion of the tongue, also in the region of the fauces. Because they are lymphoid tissue, all of the tonsils in the pharynx function in immune responses and help prevent infections.

The most inferior portion of the pharynx is the **laryngopharynx** (lah-ring-goh-FAIR-inks) that extends from the hyoid bone down to the lower margin of the larynx. Both the oropharynx and laryngopharynx are lined with a mucous membrane of stratified squamous epithelium.

> The pharyngeal, palatine, and lingual tonsils are located in the pharynx.

> Inflammation of the pharynx, or a sore throat, is **pharyngitis.**

Larynx

The **larynx** (LAIR-inks), commonly called the voice box, is the passageway for air between the pharynx

above and the trachea below. It is about 5 cm long and extends from the fourth to the sixth vertebral levels. It is formed by nine cartilages that are connected to each other by muscles and ligaments. Six of the cartilages are grouped into three pairs. These are the **arytenoid, corniculate,** and **cuneiform.** The other three, the **thyroid, cricoid,** and **epiglottis,** are single cartilages. All of the cartilages are hyaline cartilage, except the epiglottis, which is elastic cartilage. The larynx is also supported by ligaments that attach to the hyoid bone.

The three largest cartilages of the larynx are the **thyroid cartilage,** the **cricoid** (KRY-koyd) **cartilage,** and the **epiglottis** (eh-pih-GLOT-is) (see Fig. 15–2). The thyroid cartilage, consisting of two shield-shaped plates, is the most superior of the cartilages. It forms an anterior projection in the neck called the Adam's apple. This is more pronounced in males than in females. The cricoid cartilage is the most inferior of the laryngeal cartilages. It forms the base of the larynx and is attached to the trachea. The epiglottis is a long leaf-shaped structure. Its inferior margin is attached to the thyroid cartilage but the upper portion is a movable flap that projects superiorly. During swallowing, the epiglottis covers the opening into the larynx to prevent food and water from entering.

> The thyroid cartilage is the Adam's apple. The epiglottis acts like a trap door to keep food and other particles from entering the larynx.

Inside the larynx, two pairs of ligaments, covered by mucous membrane, extend from the **arytenoid cartilages** to the posterior surface of the thyroid cartilage. The upper pair are the **vestibular folds,** or **false vocal cords.** They work with the epiglottis to prevent particles from entering the lower respiratory tract. The lower pair are the **true vocal cords,** which function in sound production. Muscles control the length and tension of the true vocal cords. They are relaxed during normal breathing; but when they are under tension, exhaled air moving by them causes them to vibrate and produce sound. The length of the vocal cords determines the pitch of the sound, and the force of the moving air regulates the loudness. The opening between the true vocal cords is the **glottis,** which leads to the trachea.

> There are two pairs of folds in the larynx. The lower pair are the true vocal cords, and the opening between the vocal cords is the glottis.

> Inflammation of the vocal cords is called **laryngitis.** The inflammation may be caused by overuse of the voice, bacteria, viruses, or inhalation of irritating particles. Laryngitis results in hoarseness or an inability to speak above a whisper.

Trachea

The **trachea,** commonly called the windpipe, is a tube that extends from the cricoid cartilage of the larynx, at the level of the sixth cervical vertebra, into the mediastinum where it divides into the right and left bronchi at the level of the fifth thoracic vertebra (Fig. 15–3). It is about 12 to 15 cm long. The anterior and lateral walls of the trachea are supported by 15 to 20 C-shaped pieces of hyaline cartilage that hold the trachea open despite the pressure changes that occur during breathing. The posterior open part of the C-shaped cartilages is closed by smooth muscle and connective tissue and is next to the esophagus. During swallowing, the esophagus bulges into the soft part of the trachea.

> The hyaline cartilage in the tracheal wall provides support and keeps the trachea from collapsing. The posterior soft tissue allows for expansion of the esophagus, which is immediately posterior to the trachea.

> A **tracheotomy** is the creation of an opening into the trachea through the neck and insertion of a tube to facilitate passage of air or removal of secretions.

The mucous membrane that lines the trachea is ciliated pseudostratified columnar epithelium similar to that in the nasal cavity and nasopharynx. Goblet cells produce mucus that traps airborne particles and microorganisms; and the cilia propel the mucus upward, where it is either swallowed or expelled. Continued irritation from cigarette smoke and other air pollutants damages the cilia, and the mucus with

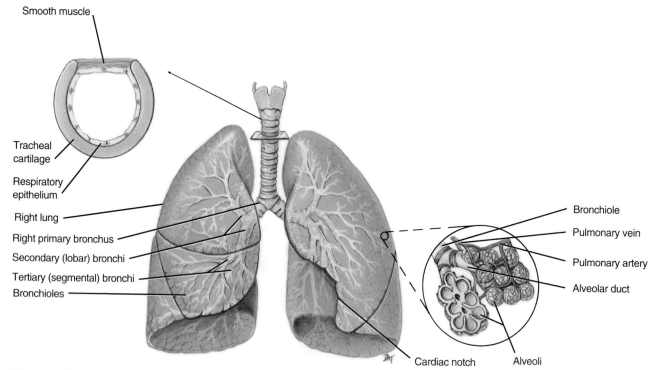

Figure 15-3 Features of the lower respiratory tract.

the trapped particles is not removed. Microorganisms thrive in the accumulated mucus, which results in respiratory infections. Irritation and inflammation of the mucous membrane stimulates the cough reflex.

> Cigarette smoke and other air pollutants inhibit the cleansing action of the cilia in the trachea.

Foreign objects that become lodged in the larynx or trachea are usually expelled by coughing. If a person cannot speak or make a sound because of the obstruction, it means that the airway is completely blocked. This is a life-threatening situation. The Heimlich maneuver is a procedure in which the air in the person's own lungs is used to forcefully expel the object.

Bronchi and Bronchial Tree

In the mediastinum, at the level of the fifth thoracic vertebra, the trachea divides into the **right** and **left primary bronchi.** In the region of the tracheal bifurcation, the hyaline cartilage forms a ridge called the **carina** (kah-RYE-nah). The right primary bronchus is shorter, more vertical, and wider in diameter than the left bronchus. Because the right bronchus is wider and more vertical than the left, foreign particles tend to enter it more frequently.

After the bronchi enter the lungs, they branch several times into smaller and smaller passages to form the **bronchial tree** (see Fig. 15–3). The primary bronchi divide to form **secondary (lobar) bronchi,** then the secondary bronchi branch into **tertiary (segmental) bronchi.** There are three secondary and 10 tertiary bronchi on the right side but only two secondary and eight tertiary bronchi on the left side. The branching continues, finally giving rise to the **bronchioles.** The terminal bronchioles branch into smaller respiratory bronchioles, which lead into microscopic **alveolar ducts.** Alveolar ducts terminate in clusters of tiny air sacs called **alveoli.**

> The bronchi branch into smaller and smaller passageways until they terminate in tiny air sacs called alveoli.

Bronchoscopy is a procedure in which a fiberoptic bundle is inserted into the trachea and directed along the conducting passageways to the smaller bronchi. This allows direct visualization of the inside of the bronchi and collection of specimens for cytologic and bacterial studies.

The cartilage and mucous membrane of the primary bronchi are similar to that in the trachea. As the branching continues through the bronchial tree, the amount of hyaline cartilage in the walls decreases until it is absent in the smallest bronchioles. As the cartilage decreases, the amount of smooth muscle increases. The mucous membrane also undergoes a transition from ciliated pseudostratified columnar epithelium to simple cuboidal epithelium to simple squamous epithelium. Because there is abundant smooth muscle and no cartilage in the walls of the bronchioles, they can constrict to a very small size when the smooth muscle contracts, which happens during an asthma attack. This restricts the flow of air and makes breathing difficult.

There are several different forms of **asthma,** but they all have sensitive conducting passages. In many cases the agent that triggers the attack is an allergen in the air. The most obvious and dangerous symptom involves the constriction of the smooth muscle around the bronchial tree. The airways become narrow and breathing difficult. Treatment includes the use of bronchodilators to dilate the respiratory passages and to permit air to flow through.

The alveolar ducts and alveoli consist primarily of simple squamous epithelium, which permits rapid diffusion of oxygen and carbon dioxide. Exchange of gases between the air in the lungs and the blood in the capillaries occurs across the walls of the alveolar ducts and alveoli.

> The alveoli consist of simple squamous epithelium. This thin tissue permits rapid diffusion of oxygen and carbon dioxide.

Lungs

The two **lungs,** which contain all the components of the bronchial tree beyond the primary bronchi, occupy most of the space in the thoracic cavity (Fig. 15–4). The lungs are soft and spongy because they

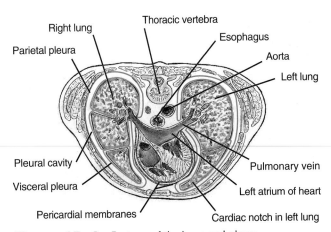

Figure 15–4   Features of the lungs and pleura.

are mostly air spaces surrounded by the alveolar cells and elastic connective tissue. They are separated from each other by the mediastinum, which contains the heart. Each lung is roughly cone shaped, rests on the diaphragm, and extends upward just above the midpoint of the clavicle. The only point of attachment for each lung is at the **hilum,** or **root,** on the medial side. This is where the bronchi, blood vessels, lymphatics, and nerves enter the lungs.

The **right lung** is shorter, is broader, and has a greater volume than the left lung. It is divided into three lobes (superior, middle, and inferior) by two fissures. Each lobe is supplied by one of the secondary (lobar) bronchi. The lobes are further subdivided into **bronchopulmonary** (brong-koh-PUL-moh-nair-ee) **segments (lobules)** by connective tissue septa that are not visible on the surface. Because each segment has its own bronchus and blood supply, which do not cross the septa, a segment can be surgically removed with relatively little damage to the rest of the lung.

The **left lung** is longer and narrower than the right lung. It has an indentation, called the **cardiac notch,** on its medial surface for the apex of the heart. The left lung is divided into two lobes by a single fissure.

> The right lung is divided into three lobes; the left lung has two lobes.

Each lung is enclosed by a double layered **serous membrane,** called the **pleura** (see Fig. 15–4). The **visceral pleura** is firmly attached to the surface of the lung. At the hilum, the visceral pleura is continuous with the **parietal pleura** that lines the wall of the thorax. The small space between the visceral and parietal pleurae is the **pleural cavity.** It contains a thin film of serous fluid that is produced by the pleura. The fluid acts as a lubricant to reduce friction as the two layers slide against each other, and it helps to hold the two layers together as the lungs inflate and deflate.

> **Pleuritis,** or **pleurisy,** is an inflammation of the pleura and is often painful because the sensory nerves in the parietal pleura are irritated. As the condition progresses, the permeability of the membranes changes, which results in an accumulation of fluid in the pleural cavity, making breathing difficult.

✓ **QuickCheck**

● How many secondary (lobar) bronchi are associated with the right lung?

● What is the serous membrane that encloses the lungs?

Mechanics of Ventilation

Pulmonary ventilation is commonly referred to as breathing. It is the process of air flowing into the lungs during inspiration (inhalation) and out of the lungs during expiration (exhalation). Air flows because of pressure differences between the atmosphere and the gases inside the lungs.

One of the fundamental properties of gases, called Boyle's law, is that with a constant temperature, when the volume increases the pressure decreases, and when volume decreases the pressure increases. This is stated in equation form as $P_1V_1 = P_2V_2$. A gas expands to fill a given container and when it expands (volume increases), the pressure of the gas decreases. In ventilation, the containers are the atmosphere, the lungs, and the pleural cavity. Ventilation depends on changes in pressures and volumes within the containers.

Pressures in Pulmonary Ventilation

Air, like other gases, flows from a region with higher pressure to a region with lower pressure. Muscular breathing movements and recoil of elastic tissues create the changes in pressure that result in ventilation. Pulmonary ventilation involves three different pressures (Fig. 15–5A):

- Atmospheric pressure
- Intra-alveolar (intrapulmonary) pressure
- Intrapleural pressure

Atmospheric pressure is the pressure of the air outside the body. At sea level this pressure is normally 760 mm Hg. **Intra-alveolar** (in-trah-al-VEE-oh-lar) **pressure,** also called **intrapulmonary** (in-trah-PUL-mon-air-ee) **pressure,** is the pressure inside the alveoli of the lungs. When the lungs are at rest, between breaths, this pressure equals atmospheric pressure. The intrapulmonary pressure varies as the thoracic cavity changes size with each breath, and it is responsible for air moving into and out of the lungs. When intra-alveolar pressure is less than atmospheric pressure, air flows into the lungs. When it is greater than atmospheric pressure, air flows out of the lungs.

Intrapleural (in-trah-PLOO-ral) **pressure** is the pressure within the pleural cavity, between the visceral and parietal pleura (see Fig. 15–5A). This pressure also changes with each breath, but under normal conditions it is slightly less than both the atmospheric pressure and the intra-alveolar pressure. It represents a partial vacuum or negative pressure and is an important factor in keeping the lungs inflated. Because the pressure inside the lungs is greater than the intrapleural pressure, the lungs always expand to fill the space and press against the thoracic wall. If the intrapleural pressure becomes greater than the intra-alveolar pressure, the lungs collapse and are nonfunctional.

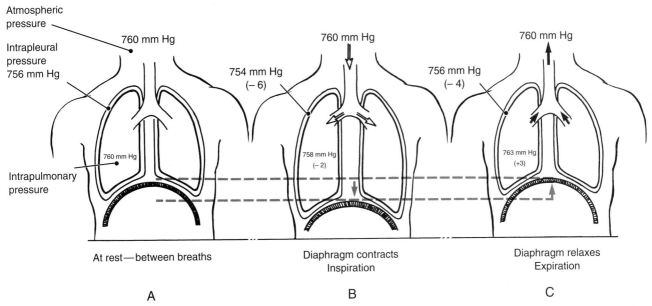

Atmospheric
pressure

760 mm Hg   760 mm Hg   760 mm Hg

Intrapleural
pressure
756 mm Hg

754 mm Hg   756 mm Hg
(– 6)   (– 4)

760 mm Hg   758 mm Hg   763 mm Hg
                   (– 2)   (+3)

Intrapulmonary
pressure

At rest—between breaths   Diaphragm contracts   Diaphragm relaxes
                          Inspiration   Expiration

A   B   C

Figure 15–5   Pressures in pulmonary ventilation.

> The three pressures responsible for pulmonary ventilation are atmospheric pressure, intra-alveolar pressure, and intrapleural pressure.

The accumulation of air in the pleural cavity is called **pneumothorax.** This condition can occur in pulmonary disease, such as emphysema, carcinoma, tuberculosis, or lung abscesses, when rupture of a lesion allows air to escape from the alveoli into the pleural cavity. It also may follow trauma in which the chest wall is perforated and atmospheric air enters the cavity.

Inspiration

Inspiration, also called inhalation, is the process of taking air into the lungs. It is the active phase of ventilation because it is the result of muscle contraction. In normal, quiet breathing, the primary muscle involved in inspiration is the **diaphragm,** a dome-shaped muscle that separates the thoracic cavity from the abdominal cavity. When the diaphragm contracts, it drops, or becomes flatter, and increases the size (volume) of the thoracic cavity. When it relaxes, the volume of the cavity decreases.

The parietal and visceral layers of the pleura tend to adhere to each other because there is an attraction between the water molecules in the serous fluid between the two layers. Because the two layers of pleura stick together, increasing the volume of the thoracic cavity causes the lungs to expand, or to increase in volume. The fact that the intrapleural pressure is less than the pressure within the lungs also contributes to lung expansion because

the lungs enlarge (inflate) into the lower pressure region.

Between breathing cycles, when the lungs are at rest, the intra-alveolar pressure within the lungs is equal to the atmospheric pressure outside the body. Contraction of the diaphragm causes the thoracic volume to increase and the intra-alveolar pressure decreases below atmospheric pressure (Boyle's law). Air flows from the region of higher atmospheric pressure outside the body into the region of lower intra-alveolar pressure within the lungs (Fig. 15–5B). Air continues to flow into the alveoli until intra-alveolar pressure equals atmospheric pressure.

During labored breathing, the **external intercostal muscles** and other muscles of respiration work with the diaphragm to create a greater increase in the volume of the thoracic cavity. This results in a greater lung expansion and allows more air to flow into the lungs.

> During inspiration, the diaphragm contracts and the thoracic cavity increases in volume. This decreases the intra-alveolar pressure so that air flows into the lungs. Inspiration draws air into the lungs.

Expiration

Expiration, or **exhalation,** is the process of letting air out of the lungs during the breathing cycle. In normal quiet breathing it is a passive process involving the relaxation of respiratory muscles and the elastic recoil of tissues. Forceful expiration requires the active contraction of the **internal intercostal muscles.**

When the diaphragm and other muscles used in inspiration relax, the volume of the thoracic cavity decreases to its normal resting size. Following

Boyle's law, this decreases lung volume and increases the intra-alveolar pressure (Fig. 15-5C). Air now flows from the region of higher intra-alveolar pressure within the lungs to the region of lower atmospheric pressure outside the body until the two pressures are equal.

> During expiration, the relaxation of the diaphragm and elastic recoil of tissue decrease the thoracic volume and increase the intra-alveolar pressure. Air flows out of the lungs.

As air leaves the lungs during expiration, the alveoli become smaller. The interior surfaces of the alveoli are coated with a thin layer of fluid. The fluid molecules are attracted to each other (surface tension), which tends to cause the surfaces to adhere to each other. This makes it harder to inflate the lungs during inspiration and creates a tendency for the lungs to collapse. Normally this is prevented by a substance called **surfactant** (sir-FAK-tant), a lipoprotein substance that is produced by certain cells within the lung tissue and that reduces the attraction between the fluid molecules. Without surfactant, the alveoli collapse and become nonfunctional.

> Surfactant reduces the surface tension inside the alveoli so they do not adhere to each other and collapse.

Surfactant is not produced until the late stages of fetal life. Newborns that are born prematurely may not have enough surfactant, and the forces of surface tension collapse the alveoli. The newborn must reinflate the alveoli with each breath, which requires tremendous energy. The lack of surfactant accounts for many of the signs and symptoms of infant respiratory distress syndrome (IRDS). The condition is treated by using positive-pressure respirators that maintain pressure within the alveoli to keep them inflated.

Respiratory Volumes and Capacities

Under normal conditions, the average adult takes 12 to 15 breaths per minute. A breath is one complete respiratory cycle that consists of one inspiration and one expiration. The amount of air that is exchanged during one cycle varies with age, sex, size, and physical condition.

An instrument called a **spirometer** (spy-ROM-eh-ter) is used to measure the volume of air that moves into and out of the lungs, and the process of taking the measurements is called **spirometry.** Figure 15-6 illustrates a graphic record, called a **spirogram,** produced by a spirometer. Respiratory (pulmonary) volumes are an important aspect of pulmonary function testing because they can provide information about the physical condition of the lungs. The four respiratory volumes measured by spirometry are the **tidal volume, inspiratory reserve volume, expiratory reserve volume,** and **residual volume.** These are described, with their normal values, in Table 15-1 and are illustrated by the spirogram in Figure 15-6.

Respiratory capacity (pulmonary capacity) is the sum of two or more volumes. Four respiratory capacities that are measured are the **vital capacity, inspiratory capacity, functional residual capacity,** and **total lung capacity** (see Table 15-1 and Fig. 15-6). In normal, healthy lungs, vital capacity equals about 80 percent of the total lung capacity.

Factors such as age, sex, body build, and physical conditioning have an influence on lung volumes and capacities. Lungs usually reach their maximum in early adulthood and decline with age after that. Females generally have 20 to 25 percent less lung volume than males. Tall people tend to have greater lung capacity than short individuals. Slender people have greater capacity than do obese people. Physical conditioning can increase lung capacity as much as 40 percent. Muscular diseases and factors that reduce the elasticity of the lungs reduce the capacity.

> A spirometer is used to measure respiratory volumes and capacities. These measurements provide useful information about the condition of the lungs.

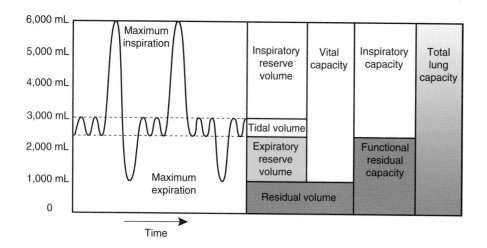

Figure 15-6 Respiratory volumes and capacities.

Table 15–1 Respiratory Volumes and Capacities

Term	Abbreviation	Normal Value	Description
Lung Volumes			The four separate components of total lung capacity
Tidal volume	TV	500 mL	Amount of air that is inhaled and exhaled in a normal quiet breathing cycle
Inspiratory reserve volume	IRV	3100 mL	Maximum amount of air that can be forcefully inhaled after a tidal inspiration
Expiratory reserve volume	ERV	1200 mL	Maximum amount of air that can be forcefully exhaled after a tidal expiration
Residual volume	RV	1200 mL	Amount of air that remains in the lungs after a maximum expiration
Lung Capacities			Measurements that are the sum of two or more lung volumes
Vital capacity	VC	4800 mL	Maximum amount of air that can be exhaled after a maximum inspiration; equals TV + IRV + ERV
Inspiratory capacity	IC	3600 mL	Maximum amount of air that can be inhaled; equals TV + IRV
Functional residual capacity	FRC	2400 mL	Amount of air remaining in the lungs after a tidal expiration; equals RV + ERV
Total lung capacity	TLC	6000 mL	Amount of air in the lungs after a maximum inspiration; equals RV + TV + IRV + ERV

✓ QuickCheck

● Why does the lung often collapse when air enters the pleural cavity?

● What is the significance of surfactant in the lungs?

● During a recent episode of pneumonia, Marie had fluid accumulate in her alveoli. Explain how this affected her vital capacity.

Basic Gas Laws and Respiration

The diffusion of gases from the alveoli to the blood (external respiration) and from the blood to the tissues (internal respiration) depends on two fundamental properties of gases. These are known as **Dalton's law of partial pressures** and **Henry's law.**

Properties of Gases

Dalton's Law of Partial Pressures

Dalton's law of partial pressures, or simply Dalton's law, states that the total pressure exerted by a mixture of gases is equal to the sum of the pressures exerted by each gas independently. If P stands for pressure, then

$$P_{gas\ 1} + P_{gas\ 2} + P_{gas\ 3} + P_{gas\ 4} = P_{Total}.$$

Further, the pressure exerted by each individual gas, its **partial pressure,** is proportional to its percentage in the total mixture. For example, if a gas mixture contains 75 percent nitrogen and 25 percent oxygen, and the total pressure is 160 mm Hg, then the partial pressure due to nitrogen is 120 mm Hg (75 percent of 160) and the partial pressure due to oxygen is 40 mm Hg (25 percent of 160). Air is a mixture of gases, namely, nitrogen, oxygen, carbon dioxide, and water vapor. At sea level the total pressure is 760 mm Hg. Because the air is about 21 percent oxygen, the partial pressure of oxygen in the air is 159.6 mm Hg. Table 15–2 compares the composition of atmospheric air and alveolar air.

Henry's Law

According to Henry's law, when a mixture of gases is in contact with a liquid, each gas dissolves in the liquid in proportion to its own solubility and partial pressure. The higher the solubility, the more gas will dissolve in the liquid. Of the gases, carbon dioxide is the most soluble, oxygen is intermediate, and nitrogen is the least soluble.

More gas dissolves in a liquid if the partial pressure of the gas is greater. Nearly everyone is familiar with what happens to a can of soda if it is left open. It goes "flat." When the soda was made, carbon dioxide, under high pressure, dissolved in the liquid. When the can is opened, the pressure is reduced and the carbon dioxide "undissolves" and escapes.

Henry's law is familiar to deep-sea divers. As they descend, the total pressure around them increases, consequently the total pressure of nitrogen increases. Normally, very little nitrogen dissolves in the blood, but the increased partial pressure makes more of it dissolve. If the diver ascends too rapidly, nitrogen gas comes out of solution and forms bubbles in body fluids. At first, the bubbles escape into the joints, which causes severe pain but is not particularly damaging. This condition is called the **bends** because the person bends over in pain. A serious situation arises when the nitrogen bubbles travel in the bloodstream where they may cause infarctions and cerebral damage.

Table 15–2 Partial Pressures (PP) of Gases in the Atmosphere and Alveolar Air*

Gas	Atmosphere			Alveolar Air		
	Percent	PP (mm Hg) (sea level)	PP (mm Hg) (6,000 ft)	Percent	PP (mm Hg) (sea level)	PP (mm Hg) (6,000 ft)
Nitrogen	78.60	597.0	479.0	74.9	569	456
Oxygen	20.90	159.0	127.0	13.7	104	83
Carbon dioxide	0.04	0.3	0.2	5.2	40	32
Water vapor	0.46	3.7	2.8	6.2	47	38
Total	100%	760 mm Hg	609 mm Hg	100%	760 mm Hg	609 mm Hg

*These values are approximate and vary with the weather.

External Respiration

External respiration is the exchange of oxygen and carbon dioxide between the air in the lungs and the blood in the surrounding capillaries. Oxygen diffuses from the alveoli of the lungs into the blood, and carbon dioxide diffuses from the blood into the air in the alveoli. The surfaces in the lungs where diffusion occurs constitute the **respiratory membrane.** Some diffusion takes place in the respiratory bronchioles so these passages do contribute a small amount of surface area to the respiratory membrane.

The respiratory membrane consists of the layers that the gases must travel through to get into or out of the alveoli (Fig. 15–7). These layers are:

- Thin layer of fluid that lines the alveolus
- Simple squamous epithelium in the alveolar wall
- Basement membrane of the epithelium
- Small interstitial space
- Basement membrane of capillary epithelium
- Simple squamous epithelium (endothelium) of the capillary wall

Carbon dioxide and oxygen pass through the respiratory membrane in the lungs during external respiration.

The rate of gaseous exchange across the respiratory membrane depends on the surface area of the membrane, the thickness of the membrane, the solubility of the gas, and the difference in partial pressure of the gas on the two sides of the membrane. Most of the approximately 70 square meters of surface area included in the respiratory membrane comes from the more than 300 million alveoli in healthy adult lungs. Diseases such as emphysema destroy alveolar walls and reduce the surface area of

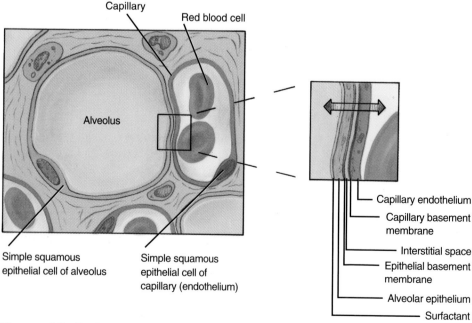

Figure 15–7 Components of the respiratory membrane.

the respiratory membrane. This adversely affects the diffusion of oxygen and carbon dioxide. Normally, the membrane is very thin, but in patients with pulmonary edema fluids accumulate in the alveoli and the gases must diffuse through a fluid lining that is thicker than normal. The diffusion rate decreases because the respiratory membrane is thicker. Increasing the breathing rate or increasing the volume of air exchanged with each breath increases the amount of oxygen in the alveoli and decreases the amount of carbon dioxide. This increases the differences in partial pressures on the two sides of the membrane and increases the rate of diffusion. Conversely, anything that reduces either the breathing rate or volume also reduces the diffusion rate.

> The rate at which external respiration occurs varies with the surface area and thickness of the membrane, the solubility, and the difference in partial pressures on the two sides of the membrane.

Internal Respiration

Internal respiration is the exchange of gases between the tissue cells and the blood in the tissue capillaries. After oxygen diffuses into the blood and carbon dioxide diffuses out of the blood in external respiration, the blood returns to the left side of the heart, which pumps it to the tissue capillaries. This blood has a higher concentration of oxygen and a lower concentration of carbon dioxide than the body tissue cells. The tissue cells use oxygen for metabolism and produce carbon dioxide in the process. This creates a lower oxygen content and a higher carbon dioxide content in the cells than in the capillaries. The concentration gradients that exist drive the oxygen from the capillaries into the tissue cells and the carbon dioxide from the tissue cells into the capillaries. Between the tissue cells and the capillaries, both gases pass through the interstitial fluid. External and internal respiration are illustrated in Figure 15–8.

> Oxygen diffuses from the blood into the tissue cells, and carbon dioxide diffuses from the tissue cells into the blood during internal respiration.

Transport of Gases

The blood transports the respiratory gases, oxygen and carbon dioxide, between the lungs and tissue cells. Erythrocytes (red blood cells) have the major role in transporting oxygen. Plasma has the major role in transporting carbon dioxide.

Oxygen Transport

After oxygen diffuses across the respiratory membrane from the alveolus into the capillary, it first dissolves in the plasma. About 3 percent of the oxygen remains in the plasma as a dissolved gas and is transported this way. The remainder quickly diffuses from the plasma into the red blood cells where it combines with the heme portion of the hemoglobin molecules to form a compound called **oxyhemoglobin** (ahk-see-HEE-moh-gloh-bin). Because the oxygen is bound to hemoglobin, this increases the amount of oxygen in a given amount of blood without increasing the partial pressure of oxygen. About 97 percent of the oxygen is transported as oxyhemoglobin.

> Approximately 3 percent of the oxygen is transported as a dissolved gas in the plasma. The remaining 97 percent is carried by hemoglobin molecules.

The reaction between oxygen and hemoglobin, which occurs in the lungs where oxygen content (partial pressure) is high, is called **loading** (Fig. 15–9A).

$$\text{Hemoglobin} + \text{Oxygen} \longrightarrow \text{Oxyhemoglobin}$$
$$\text{Hb} \qquad\qquad \text{O}_2 \qquad\qquad \text{HbO}_2$$

The bonds between oxygen and hemoglobin are relatively unstable and are reversible. When the blood reaches the tissue capillaries, where the oxygen content (partial pressure) is low, the bonds break and oxygen is released to the tissues. This is called **unloading** (Fig. 15–9B).

$$\text{Oxyhemoglobin} \longrightarrow \text{Hemoglobin} + \text{Oxygen}$$
$$\text{HbO}_2 \qquad\qquad \text{Hb} \qquad\qquad \text{O}_2$$

Not all the oxygen is released to the tissue cells in unloading. Only about 25 percent of the oxygen in the blood is delivered to the tissue cells. The other 75 percent remains attached to hemoglobin. This means that oxygen-poor, or deoxygenated, blood is carrying 75 percent of its maximum oxygen load on the return trip from the tissue cells to the lungs.

> Loading occurs in the lungs when oxygen combines with hemoglobin. Unloading occurs in the tissues when hemoglobin releases oxygen.

Several factors influence the unloading of oxygen in the tissues. More oxygen is released from oxyhemoglobin when oxygen levels (partial pressure) are low, carbon dioxide levels (partial pressure) are increased, temperature is increased, and pH is more acidic. Cells use oxygen for metabolism. They produce carbon dioxide and heat as by-products of metabolism. The carbon dioxide reacts with water to form carbonic acid, which makes the cellular environment more acidic. Cells that are metabolically active, such as skeletal muscle, create an environment that favors the unloading of oxygen from oxyhemoglobin.

> Oxygen and carbon dioxide levels, temperature, and pH affect loading and unloading.

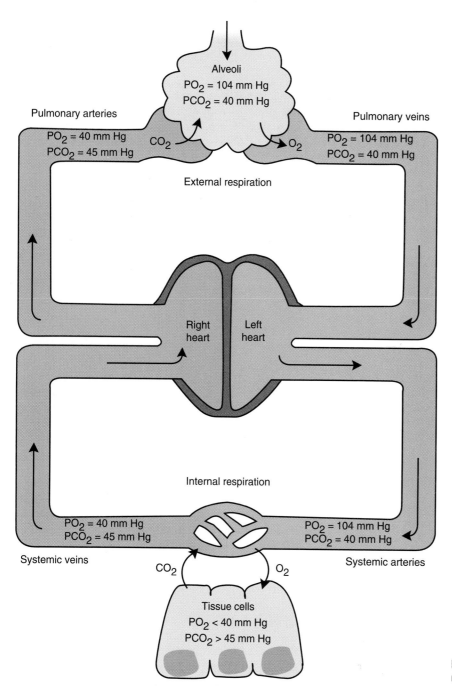

Figure 15–8   External and internal respiration.

Carbon Dioxide Transport

Carbon dioxide, which is a byproduct of cellular metabolism, diffuses from the tissue cells into the blood in the capillaries. The blood transports the carbon dioxide to the lungs by three mechanisms (Fig. 15–10):

- Dissolved in the plasma
- Combined with hemoglobin
- As part of bicarbonate ions

When carbon dioxide diffuses from the tissue cells into the blood, about 7 percent of it dissolves in the plasma. In the lungs, where carbon dioxide levels are low, the carbon dioxide leaves the plasma and diffuses into the alveoli. It is removed from the body in the exhaled air.

Approximately 23 percent of the carbon dioxide passes through the plasma, diffuses into the red blood cells, and combines with hemoglobin. Carbon dioxide combines with the protein portion of the hemoglobin molecule to form **carbaminohemoglobin** (kar-bah-meen-oh-HEE-moh-gloh-bin).

$$\text{Carbon dioxide} + \text{Hemoglobin} \longrightarrow \text{Carbaminohemoglobin}$$
$$CO_2 \qquad\qquad Hb \qquad\qquad\qquad HbCO_2$$

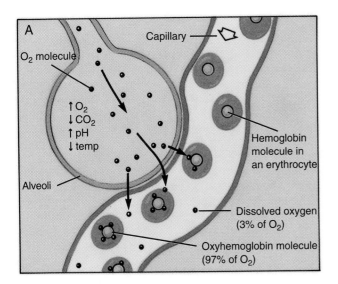

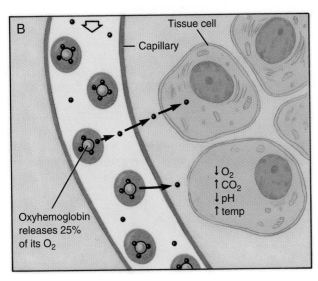

Figure 15–9   Loading (*A*) and unloading (*B*) of oxygen.

Because oxygen and carbon dioxide react with different parts of the molecule, hemoglobin can carry both at the same time. In the lungs, this reaction reverses and carbon dioxide detaches from the hemoglobin.

Carbaminohemoglobin $\longrightarrow$ Hemoglobin + Carbon dioxide
$\quad$ HbCO$_2$ $\qquad\qquad$ Hb $\qquad\qquad$ CO$_2$

The carbon dioxide diffuses out of the red blood cell into the plasma and then diffuses from the plasma into the alveoli and is exhaled.

Most of the carbon dioxide, approximately 70 percent, is transported in the form of **bicarbonate ions.** The carbon dioxide diffuses into the red blood cell where it combines with water to form **carbonic acid.** An enzyme inside the red blood cell, **carbonic anhydrase,** speeds up this reaction so that it happens quite rapidly. The carbonic acid dissociates into hydrogen ions and bicarbonate ions. The carbon dioxide is contained within the bicarbonate ions.

Carbon dioxide + Water $\longrightarrow$ Carbonic acid $\longrightarrow$
$\quad$ CO$_2$ $\qquad\qquad$ H$_2$O $\qquad\qquad$ H$_2$CO$_3$

$\qquad\qquad$ Hydrogen ions + Bicarbonate ions
$\qquad\qquad\qquad$ H$^+$ $\qquad\qquad$ HCO$_3^-$

Most of the hydrogen ions combine with hemoglobin so they do not cause a dramatic and potentially dangerous drop in the pH of the blood. The bicarbonate ions diffuse out of the red blood cell into the plasma where they are transported to the lungs.

In the lungs, where the carbon dioxide content is relatively low, the above reactions reverse. The bicarbonate ions reenter the red blood cell and combine with hydrogen ions to form carbonic acid, which dissociates into water and carbon dioxide.

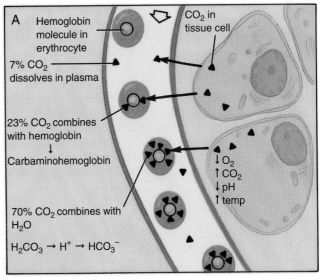

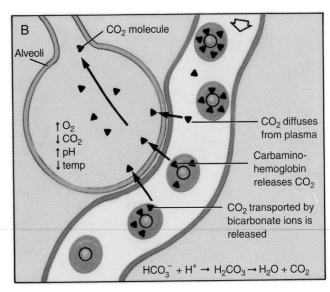

Figure 15–10   Carbon dioxide transport. (*A*) CO$_2$ diffuses from tissue cells into blood for transport. (*B*) CO$_2$ is released from blood components and diffuses into alveoli.

The carbon dioxide diffuses into the alveoli and is exhaled.

Bicarbonate ions + Hydrogen ions $\longrightarrow$
$$HCO_3^- \qquad\qquad H^+$$

Carbonic acid $\longrightarrow$ Water + Carbon dioxide
$$H_2CO_3 \qquad H_2O \qquad CO_2$$

An increase in carbon dioxide in the blood causes an increase in the number of hydrogen ions, which reduces the pH. Conversely, a decrease in carbon dioxide in the blood causes a decrease in the number of hydrogen ions, which makes the blood more alkaline and increases the pH.

> Carbon dioxide is transported by three mechanisms. Approximately 7 percent is transported as a gas dissolved in plasma. Another 23 percent combines with hemoglobin to form carbaminohemoglobin. The remaining 70 percent is transported as bicarbonate ions in the plasma.

Regulation of Respiration

Normal breathing rate in adults averages between 12 and 20 times per minute. The rate is higher, up to 40 times per minute, in children. The basic rate is established by the respiratory center in the brain stem but environmental conditions, both external and internal, and emotions induce variations in the rate.

Respiratory Center

Groups of neurons in the pons and medulla oblongata, regions of the brain stem, collectively make up the **respiratory center** (Fig. 15–11). This center, which contains both **inspiratory** and **expiratory areas,** controls the rate and depth of breathing. The inspiratory area sends impulses along the **phrenic nerve** to the diaphragm and, for deeper breathing, along the **intercostal nerves** to the external intercostal muscles. When the respiratory center sends out impulses, the muscles contract and inspiration results. The inspiratory neurons fatigue quickly and quit sending impulses to the muscles. When the impulses cease, the muscles relax and expiration occurs. When more forceful expirations are necessary, the expiratory area sends impulses to the internal intercostal muscles. If the respiratory center in the brain stem is damaged, the impulses cease and breathing stops. Figure 15–12 illustrates the sequence of events in quiet respiration and in forced respiration.

> The respiratory center includes groups of neurons in the medulla oblongata and pons.

Factors That Influence Breathing

Even though the respiratory center establishes the basic rhythm of breathing, it is influenced by factors that cause variations in the rate and depth of

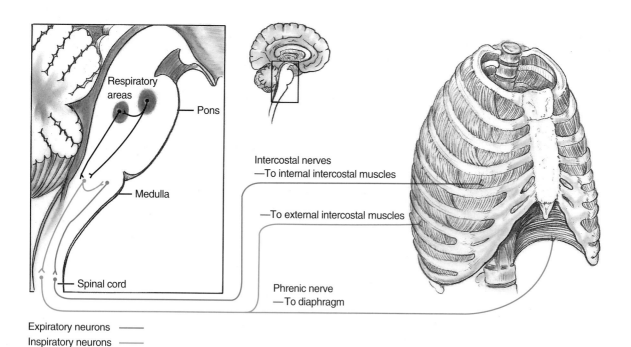

Expiratory neurons ——
Inspiratory neurons ——

Figure 15–11 Respiratory center in the brain stem.

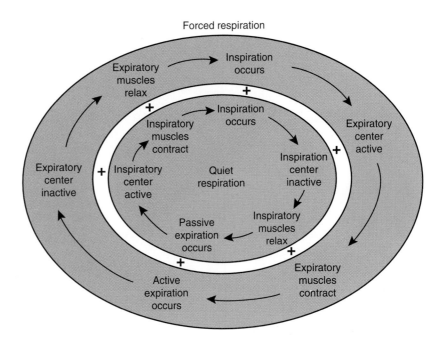

Figure 15–12 Events in respiratory center regulation of breathing. Inner region represents quiet respiration. Outer region represents events that are added for forced respiration.

breathing (Fig. 15–13). Some conditions are detected by receptors that relay the information to the respiratory center. Other factors act on the respiratory center drectly.

Chemoreceptors

Chemoreceptors in the medulla oblongata respiratory center are sensitive to changes in carbon dioxide and hydrogen ion concentrations in the blood and cerebrospinal fluid. They are not sensitive to changes in oxygen levels. If carbon dioxide and hydrogen ion concentrations increase, the receptors stimulate the respiratory center to increase the rate and depth of breathing. This decreases the concentrations back to normal. In contrast, low carbon dioxide and hydrogen ion levels decrease the rate and depth of breathing. Breathing may even stop for brief periods of time until concentrations increase to normal.

Receptors that are sensitive to changes in oxygen levels are located in the aortic and carotid bodies. These receptors send sensory impulses to the respiratory center, which responds by altering the rate and depth of breathing. A decrease in oxygen level is usually not a strong stimulus for breathing. The primary effect seems to be to make the receptors in the respiratory center more sensitive to changes in carbon dioxide levels. Blood oxygen levels become an important stimulus under conditions, such as those created by emphysema, that result in chronic high carbon dioxide concentrations. Oxygen deficiency may also become a stimulus for breathing when oxygen levels decrease but carbon dioxide levels are also low or unchanged. Examples of this are sudden exposure to high altitudes and cases of shock when blood pressure is alarmingly low.

Central chemoreceptors in the medulla oblongata are sensitive to increases in carbon dioxide and hydrogen ion levels. Peripheral chemoreceptors in the aortic and carotid bodies detect decreases in oxygen levels, but this is not a strong stimulus for breathing.

Patients with severe chronic lung disease often have elevated carbon dioxide in the blood and the respiratory drive comes from the receptors for low arterial oxygen. If these patients are given too much oxygen, they may literally stop breathing because the stimulus to breathe (low oxygen) has been removed.

Stretch Receptors and the Hering-Breuer Reflex

Stretch receptors in the lungs initiate the Hering-Breuer reflex that prevents overinflation of the lungs. As the alveoli expand during inspiration, stretch receptors in the lungs are stimulated. Impulses from the stretch receptors travel to the medulla oblongata, where they inhibit the inspiratory neurons and cause expiration. This reflex supports the rhythm of breathing by inhibiting extended inspiration.

Stimulus from Higher Brain Centers

Impulses from higher brain centers may override the respiratory center temporarily. These impulses may be either voluntary or involuntary; however, the voluntary controls are limited. If you try to voluntarily hold your breath, you can do so for only a

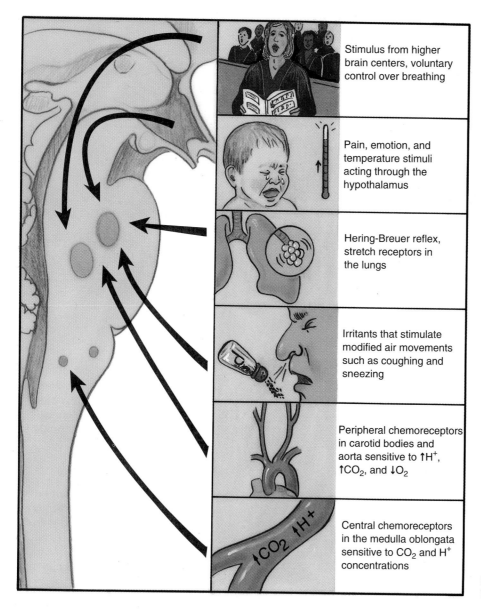

Stimulus from higher brain centers, voluntary control over breathing

Pain, emotion, and temperature stimuli acting through the hypothalamus

Hering-Breuer reflex, stretch receptors in the lungs

Irritants that stimulate modified air movements such as coughing and sneezing

Peripheral chemoreceptors in carotid bodies and aorta sensitive to $\uparrow H^+$, $\uparrow CO_2$, and $\downarrow O_2$

Central chemoreceptors in the medulla oblongata sensitive to CO_2 and H^+ concentrations

Figure 15-13 Factors that influence breathing.

limited time. When CO_2 levels reach a certain critical point, the impulses from the higher brain centers are ignored and the respiratory center resumes regular breathing.

Involuntary impulses from higher brain centers may stimulate rapid breathing in response to emotions such as anxiety or excitement. Chronic pain also may result in involuntary stimulation from the higher brain centers. In contrast, sudden pain or sudden cold may cause a gasp or a momentary cessation of breathing.

Temperature

An increase in body temperature, such as occurs during a fever or strenuous exercise, increases breathing rate. The increased body temperature is associated with increased metabolism, which uses more oxygen and gives off more carbon dioxide. When body temperature decreases, metabolic rate diminishes and breathing rate also decreases.

The Hering-Breuer reflex inhibits inspiration to prevent overinflation of the lungs. Limited voluntary control of breathing from the higher brain centers is possible.

Nonrespiratory Air Movements

In addition to the normal air movements that occur during breathing and that result in pulmonary ventilation, there are a number of modifications called **nonrespiratory air movements.** Some of these are reflexes that clear air passages, others are voluntary, and some express emotions (Table 15–3).

Table 15–3   Nonrespiratory Air Movements

Movement	Description
Sneezing	Spasmodic contraction of the expiratory muscles that forces air through the nose and mouth
Coughing	Long inspiration followed by closure of the glottis; then a strong expiration forces the glottis open and sends a blast of air through the upper respiratory tract
Sighing	Long inspiration followed by a shorter but forceful expiration
Hiccuping	Spasmodic contraction of the diaphragm followed by sudden closure of the glottis to produce a sharp sound
Crying	An inspiration followed by many short expirations; the glottis remains open and the vocal cords vibrate; usually accompanied by tears and characteristic facial expressions
Laughing	Same basic movements as crying but facial expressions differ; may be indistinguishable from crying
Yawning	A deep inspiration through a widely opened mouth

 QuickCheck

● Emphysema, characterized by shortness of breath and inability to tolerate physical exertion, destroys alveolar walls. How does this affect external respiration?

● Why does anemia with reduced hemoglobin result in less oxygen being delivered to the tissues?

● Patients with severe chronic lung disease often have elevated carbon dioxide levels in the blood. How does this affect the body's pH?

● What effect does an elevated hydrogen ion concentration have on the medullary respiratory centers?

● What nerve carries impulses from the medullary respiratory center to the diaphragm?

 ## FOCUS ON AGING

Various harmful substances, including cigarette smoke, air pollution, and pathogens, continually bombard the respiratory system and take their toll. There is no way to avoid all of these irritants except to stop breathing! Some, like cigarette smoke, can be decreased, but others are inescapable. Because of the continual contact between the respiratory system and the environment, it is difficult to distinguish between the changes in the tissues of the breathing apparatus, including the lungs, that are due to aging and those that are the result of disease or other factors outside the body. Modifications in the lining of the respiratory tract probably are due to environmental, rather than solely aging, factors. Long-term exposure to irritants results in deterioration of the cilia, which hinders their cleansing action and movement of mucus. As a consequence, the incidence of emphysema and chronic bronchitis increases with age. Diminishing effectiveness of the immune system makes the elderly more susceptible to pneumonia and other microbial diseases. However, excluding external influences, there are changes that take place as a result of "normal" aging.

One of the most common signs of respiratory aging, in general, is when a person is unable to maintain the same level of physical activity that was experienced in younger years. This is a gradual decline and may not be noticeable until phrases such as, "I used to be able to . . ." become part of the conversation. The cardiovascular and muscular systems have an effect on endurance, and the skeletal system has an effect on thoracic volume, but the major change is a decreased ability of the respiratory system to acquire and deliver oxygen to the arterial blood.

The functional impairment in oxygen delivery is the result of structural changes that take place in the respiratory tissues. One type of structural change is a loss of elasticity. The cartilage in the walls of the trachea and bronchi undergo a progressive calcification. Smooth muscle fibers in the bronchioles are replaced by fibrous tissue so that they are less able to stretch and contract. Modifications in lung tissue cause the alveoli to lose some of their elastic recoil. The cumulative effect of these changes is a gradual decrease in tidal volume and vital capacity and an increase in the volume of residual air in the lungs. Another type of structural change is a deterioration of the walls between adjacent alveoli. This increases the size of each individual alveolus but reduces the total surface area of the respiratory membrane for diffusion of gases. A lower percentage of the oxygen in alveolar air is able to diffuse into the lung capillaries. These two types of structural changes result in the functional change of decreased ability to acquire and deliver oxygen to the arterial blood, which reduces the capacity for physical activity.

Respiratory System?

Sleep Apnea

Do you snore and snort while sleeping? Do you wake up tired every morning? Are you overweight? What do these three questions have in common? They are all related to sleep disorders.

Sleep disorders, often the subject of jokes and wisecracks, are much more common than most people think. For the person who is affected, however, a sleep disorder is no joke. It can cause problems ranging from just being tired all the time to actual functional impairment at work. Because the individual is continually fatigued, both physically and mentally, job performance and social relationships tend to suffer. As a result, chronic depression may set in and this, together with the physical symptoms, can lead to serious consequences.

The most common sleep disorder is **obstructive sleep apnea,** or the cessation of breathing during sleep caused by an obstruction. The obstruction in the breathing passages, which occurs when muscles in the airway relax during sleep, may be due to an enlarged soft palate, uvula, tonsils, or adenoids, a deviated nasal septum, or excess fatty tissue. Breathing may stop for a period lasting from several seconds to 2 minutes. During these episodes, the brain detects increases in carbon dioxide and decreases in oxygen levels. Finally, the brain sends a signal to arouse the person so breathing starts again. During periods of arousal, the person often snorts and thrashes about. The brain is "awake" even though the person may not wake up and be alert. The individual feels tired during the daytime because normal sleep patterns are disturbed by these arousals.

Five or more episodes of sleep apnea per hour represent a significant sleep disruption. Twenty or more apneas per hour is considered severe, and some people may have as many as 100 to 500 apneas in one night. These individuals are chronically tired because they never experience an extended period of deep sleep that results in rest and renewal. The brain repeatedly

arouses them so that they will breathe. Severe sleep apnea can result in cardiac arrhythmias, hypertension, and enlargement of the heart. It is especially dangerous for people who already have cardiovascular disease.

How does a person know if he or she has sleep apnea or some other sleep disorder? Obstructive sleep apnea can affect people of any age or sex. Studies indicate, however, that the incidence is nine times greater in males than in females and that it is most common in middle-aged, overweight males. The extra fatty tissue in the throat of an overweight individual can relax during sleep and block the airway. Loud snoring is an indication of sleep apnea. Morning headaches, another possible symptom of sleep apnea, may be caused by the decreased blood oxygen levels that occur during the pauses in breathing.

Clinics and centers that specialize in the diagnosis and treatment of sleep disorders are available for people with symptoms of these problems. The person undergoes a sleep study evaluation that monitors blood pressure, heart, and respiration rates during sleep. The evaluation determines the number and degree of apneas that the person experiences and serves as the basis for a treatment plan.

Because many people who experience sleep apnea are overweight, treatment often begins with a weight loss program, but this is a slow process. Immediate relief is available through nasal **continuous positive airway pressure** (CPAP). This nonsurgical treatment involves a nose mask, tubing, and a small air compressor. It works by directing air through the nose to keep the airway open as muscles relax during sleep. The mask is worn during sleep, and the amount of air pressure required depends on the severity of the obstruction. In severe cases, surgical intervention may be necessary. The procedure, called **pharyngoplasty,** involves removing the soft tissue that obstructs the breathing passage.

Representative Disorders of the Respiratory System

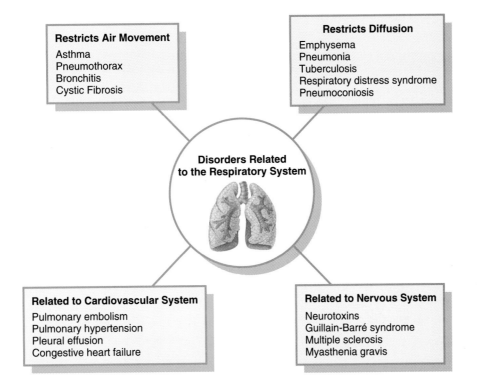

Restricts Air Movement
Asthma
Pneumothorax
Bronchitis
Cystic Fibrosis

Restricts Diffusion
Emphysema
Pneumonia
Tuberculosis
Respiratory distress syndrome
Pneumoconiosis

Disorders Related to the Respiratory System

Related to Cardiovascular System
Pulmonary embolism
Pulmonary hypertension
Pleural effusion
Congestive heart failure

Related to Nervous System
Neurotoxins
Guillain-Barré syndrome
Multiple sclerosis
Myasthenia gravis

CHAPTER QUIZ

RECALL

Match the definitions on the left with the appropriate term on the right.

1. Tiny air sacs in the lungs

2. Exchange of gases between air and blood

3. Reduces surface tension inside alveoli

4. Supported by C-shaped hyaline cartilage

5. Serous membrane around the lungs

6. Primary muscle of inspiration

7. Air exchanged in normal quiet breathing

8. Form in which most oxygen is transported

9. Form in which most carbon dioxide is transported

10. Initiate the Hering-Breuer reflex

A. Alveoli

B. Bicarbonate ions

C. Diaphragm

D. External respiration

E. Oxyhemoglobin

F. Pleura

G. Stretch receptors

H. Surfactant

I. Tidal volume

J. Trachea

THOUGHT

1. The most superior portion of the pharynx

   a. is called the laryngopharynx

   b. contains the palatine tonsils

   c. has openings for the auditory (eustachian) tubes

   d. opens into the oral cavity through the fauces

2. Which of the following does NOT pertain to the left lung?

   a. surrounded by a serous membrane

   b. has three lobes

   c. has a cardiac notch for the apex of the heart

   d. is longer and narrower than the right lung

3. When intra-alveolar pressure exceeds atmospheric pressure,

   a. the lung collapses

   b. air is forced into the lungs

   c. intrapleural pressure also becomes greater than atmospheric pressure

   d. expiration occurs

4. Vital capacity is the

   a. sum of tidal volume, inspiratory reserve volume, and expiratory reserve volume

   b. maximum amount of air that can be inhaled

   c. sum of reserve volume, tidal volume, inspiratory reserve volume, and expiratory reserve volume

   d. amount of air that remains in the lungs after a maximum expiration

5. Which of the following statements is true about the partial pressure of carbon dioxide?

   a. it is higher in the pulmonary veins than in the systemic arteries

   b. it is higher in systemic arteries than in systemic veins

   c. it is higher in systemic veins than in pulmonary arteries

   d. it is higher in pulmonary arteries than in pulmonary veins

APPLICATION

Why does a person who hyperventilates for several seconds experience a period of apnea before normal breathing resumes? Explain.

As a result of a street fight, Jason was rushed to the emergency department with a deep stab wound in the left thorax. Examination revealed pneumothorax and a collapsed lung on the left side. Explain why the lung collapsed and why only the left lung was affected.

CHAPTER 16

Digestive System

Outline/Objectives

Introduction 329
- List the components of the digestive tract and the accessory organs.

Functions of the Digestive System 329
- List six functions of the digestive system.

General Structure of the Digestive Tract 330
- Describe the general histology of the four layers, or tunics, in the digestive tract wall.

Components of the Digestive Tract 331
- Describe the features and functions of the oral cavity, teeth, pharynx, and esophagus.
- Name and describe the location of the three major types of salivary glands and describe the functions of the saliva they produce.
- Describe the structure and histologic features of the stomach and its role in digestion.
- Describe the structure and histologic features of the small intestine and its role in digestion and absorption.
- Describe the structure, histologic features, and functions of the large intestine.

Accessory Organs of Digestion 341
- Describe the structure and functions of the liver, gallbladder, and pancreas.

Chemical Digestion 345
- Summarize carbohydrate, protein, and lipid digestion by writing equations that show the intermediate and final products and the enzymes that facilitate the digestive process.

Absorption 346
- Compare the absorption of simple sugars and amino acids with that of lipid-related molecules.

Key Terms

Absorption

Chylomicrons

Chyme

Mesentery

Peristalsis

Plicae circulares

Rugae

Building Vocabulary

WORD PART	MEANING
-algia	pain
amyl-	starch
-ary	pertaining to
-ase	enzyme
bili-	bile, gall
chole-	gall, bile
cyst-	bladder
dent-	tooth
-emesis	vomit
enter-	intestine
gastr-	stomach
gingiv-	gums
hepat-	liver
lingu-	tongue
-orexia	appetite
prandi-	meal
proct-	rectum, anus
-rrhea	flow or discharge
sial-	saliva
verm-	worm

Functional Relationships of the
Digestive System

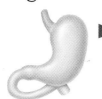

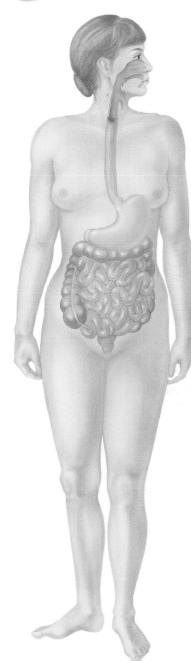

Absorbs nutrients and ions required by body cells.

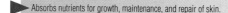

Integument

Provides vitamin D for intestinal absorption of calcium; stores fat in subcutaneous tissue.

Absorbs nutrients for growth, maintenance, and repair of skin.

Skeletal

Supports and protects organs of the digestive system; provides attachment for muscles of mastication.

Absorbs calcium and phosphate ions for bone growth, maintenance, and repair.

Muscular

Supports and protects organs of the digestive system; smooth muscle contraction functions in peristalsis and defecation; muscles function in chewing and swallowing.

Absorbs calcium ions necessary for muscle contraction; absorbs nutrients necessary for muscle growth, maintenance, and repair; liver metabolizes lactic acid from muscle metabolism.

Nervous

Autonomic nervous system controls motility and glandular activity of the digestive tract.

Absorbs nutrients necessary for neural growth, maintenance, and repair; provides nutrients for synthesis of neurotransmitters and energy for impulse conduction; liver maintains glucose levels for neural function.

Endocrine

Hormones influence glandular secretion in the digestive tract, gallbladder secretion, and pancreatic secretion of enzymes; insulin and glucagon adjust glucose metabolism in the liver.

Absorbs nutrients necessary for hormone synthesis and metabolism of endocrine cells.

Cardiovascular

Transports nutrients from digestive tract to liver; delivers hormones that affect motility and glandular secretion of the digestive tract.

Provides nutrients for blood cell formation; absorbs vitamin K for blood clotting; liver metabolism affects blood glucose concentration, liver synthesizes plasma proteins.

Lymphatic/Immune

Lacteals absorb fats and fat-soluble vitamins from the digestive tract; lymphoid tissue along the digestive tract provides defense against pathogens.

Acids and enzymes along the digestive tract aid the immune system by providing nonspecific defense against pathogens; absorb nutrients needed by lymphoid tissue.

Respiratory
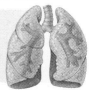

Provides oxygen for metabolism of cells in digestive system; removes carbon dioxide; helps maintain pH of body fluids for effective enzyme action; contraction of respiratory muscles aids in defecation; pharynx provides passageway for food.

Absorbs nutrients needed by cells in lungs and other tissues in the respiratory tract.

Urinary

Excretes toxins absorbed by the digestive system; excretes metabolic wastes produced by the liver.

Liver synthesizes urea, which is excreted by kidneys; liver metabolizes hormones, toxins, and drugs to forms that can be excreted in urine; absorbs nutrients for urinary tissues.

Reproductive
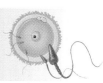

During pregnancy, expanding uterus may crowd intestines causing constipation and heartburn; gonadal steroids have an effect on metabolic rate.

Provides nutrients for growth, maintenance, and repair of reproductive tissues; provides nutrients for repair of endometrium following menstruation.

The digestive system includes the **digestive tract** and its **accessory organs,** which process food into molecules that can be absorbed and utilized by the cells of the body (Fig. 16–1). Food is broken down, bit by bit, until the molecules are small enough to be absorbed and the waste products are eliminated. The digestive tract, also called the **alimentary canal** or **gastrointestinal (GI) tract,** consists of a long continuous tube that extends from the mouth to the anus. It includes the mouth, pharynx, esophagus, stomach, small intestine, and large intestine. The tongue and teeth are accessory structures located in the mouth. The salivary glands, liver, gallbladder, and pancreas are not part of the digestive tract but are major accessory organs that have a role in digestion. These secrete fluids into the digestive tract.

> The digestive tract includes the mouth with tongue and teeth, pharynx, esophagus, stomach, small intestine, and large intestine. The salivary glands, liver, gallbladder, and pancreas are accessory organs.

Functions of the Digestive System

Food undergoes three types of processes in the body:

- Digestion
- Absorption
- Metabolism

Digestion and absorption occur in the digestive tract. After the nutrients are absorbed, they are available to all cells in the body and are utilized by the body cells in metabolism. The process of metabolism is discussed in Chapter 17.

The digestive system prepares nutrients for utilization by body cells through six activities, or functions.

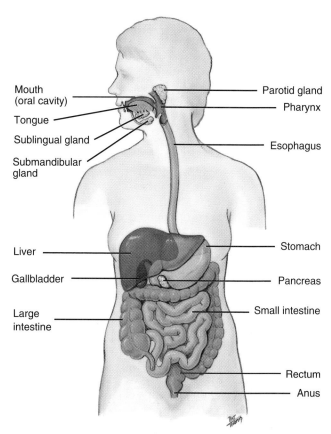

Figure 16–1 Organs of the digestive system.

- **Ingestion**—The first activity of the digestive system is to take in food. This process, called ingestion, has to take place before anything else can happen.

CLINICAL TERMS

Aphagia (ah-FAY-jee-ah) Inability to swallow

Ascites (ah-SYE-teez) An accumulation of serous fluid in the peritoneal cavity

Borborygmus (bor-boh-RIG-mus) Rumbling noise caused by propulsion of gas through the intestines

Cholecystitis (kohl-ee-sis-TYE-tis) Inflammation of the gallbladder; sometimes caused by obstruction of the cystic duct with gallstones

Cholelithiasis (kohl-ee-lith-EYE-ah-sis) Formation of gallstones

Colostomy (koh-LAHS-toh-mee) Surgical procedure in which an opening from the colon is created through the abdominal wall; the opening serves as a substitute anus

Diarrhea (dye-ah-REE-ah) Frequent passage of unformed watery feces

Dysphagia (dis-FAY-jee-ah) Difficulty in swallowing because of inflammation, paralysis, or obstruction

Emesis (EM-eh-sis) Vomiting

Eructation (ee-ruck-TAY-shun) Belching or burping; the expulsion of gas through the mouth

Flatus (FLAY-tus) Gas in the stomach or intestines, which may result from gas released during the breakdown of foods, from swallowing air, or from drinking carbonated beverages

Gavage (gah-VAHJ) Procedure in which liquid or semiliquid food is fed through a tube

Hematemesis (hee-mat-EM-eh-sis) Blood in the vomit

Laparoscopy (lap-ah-RAHS-koh-pee) Procedure in which the inside of the abdomen is viewed with a lighted instrument, or a surgical procedure performed through the instrument

Volvulus (VAHL-vyoo-lus) A twisting of the bowel on itself that causes an obstruction

- **Mechanical digestion**—The large pieces of food that are ingested have to be broken into smaller particles that can be acted upon by various enzymes. This is mechanical digestion, which begins in the mouth with chewing or **mastication** (mas-tih-KAY-shun) and continues with churning and mixing actions in the stomach.
- **Chemical digestion**—The complex molecules of carbohydrates, proteins, and fats are transformed by chemical digestion into smaller molecules that can be absorbed and utilized by the cells. Chemical digestion, through a process called **hydrolysis,** uses water to break down the complex molecules. **Digestive enzymes** speed up the hydrolysis process, which is otherwise very slow. The following equation summarizes chemical digestion.

$$\text{Complex nonabsorbable molecules} + \text{Water} \xrightarrow[\text{Hydrolysis}]{\text{(digestive enzymes)}} \text{Simple usable molecules}$$

- **Movements**—After ingestion and mastication, the food particles move from the mouth into the pharynx, then into the esophagus. This movement is **deglutition** (dee-gloo-TISH-un), or swallowing. **Mixing movements** occur in the stomach as a result of smooth muscle contraction. These repetitive contractions usually occur in small segments of the tube and mix the food particles with enzymes and other fluids. The movements that propel the food particles through the digestive tract are called **peristalsis.** These are rhythmic waves of contractions that move the food particles through the various regions in which mechanical and chemical digestion takes place.
- **Absorption**—The simple molecules that result from chemical digestion pass through cell membranes of the lining in the small intestine into the blood or lymph capillaries. This process is called absorption.
- **Elimination**—The food molecules that cannot be digested need to be eliminated from the body. The removal of indigestible wastes through the anus, in the form of feces, is **defecation** (def-eh-KAY-shun).

General Structure of the Digestive Tract

The long continuous tube that is the digestive tract is about 9 meters in length. It opens to the outside at both ends, through the mouth at one end and through the anus at the other. Although there are variations in each region, the basic structure of the wall is the same throughout the entire length of the tube.

The wall of the digestive tract has four layers or **tunics** (Fig. 16–2):

- Mucosa
- Submucosa

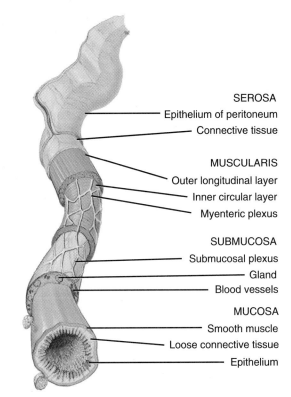

SEROSA
- Epithelium of peritoneum
- Connective tissue

MUSCULARIS
- Outer longitudinal layer
- Inner circular layer
- Myenteric plexus

SUBMUCOSA
- Submucosal plexus
- Gland
- Blood vessels

MUCOSA
- Smooth muscle
- Loose connective tissue
- Epithelium

Figure 16–2   Basic histology of the digestive tract.

- Muscular layer
- Serous layer or serosa

The **mucosa,** or mucous membrane layer, is the innermost tunic of the wall. It lines the lumen of the digestive tract. The mucosa consists of epithelium, an underlying loose connective tissue layer called the lamina propria, and a thin layer of smooth muscle called the muscularis mucosa. In certain regions, the mucosa develops folds that increase the surface area. Certain cells in the mucosa secrete mucus, digestive enzymes, and hormones. Ducts from other glands pass through the mucosa to the lumen. In the mouth and anus, where thickness for protection against abrasion is needed, the epithelium is stratified squamous. The stomach and intestines have a thin simple columnar epithelial layer for secretion and absorption.

The lining, or mucosa, of the digestive tract consists of epithelium, loose connective tissue, and smooth muscle.

The **submucosa** is a thick layer of loose connective tissue that surrounds the mucosa. This layer also contains blood and lymphatic vessels, nerves, and some glands. Abundant blood vessels supply necessary nourishment to the surrounding tissues. Blood and lymph carry away absorbed nutrients that are the end products of digestion. The nerves in the submucosa form a network called the **submuco-**

sal plexus (Meissner's plexus) that provides autonomic nerve impulses to the muscle layers of the digestive tract.

> The submucosa is loose connective tissue with blood vessels, lymphatic vessels, and nerves. Glands may be embedded in this layer.

The **muscular layer,** which is outside the submucosa, consists of two layers of smooth muscle. The **inner circular layer** has fibers arranged in a circular manner around the circumference of the tube. When these muscles contract, the diameter of the tube is decreased. In the **outer longitudinal layer** the fibers run lengthwise along the long axis of the tube. When these fibers contract, the length decreases and the tube shortens. There is a network of autonomic nerve fibers, called the **myenteric (mye-en-TAIR-ik) plexus** (Auerbach's plexus), between the circular and longitudinal muscle layers. The myenteric plexus, with the submucosal plexus, is important for controlling the movements and secretions of the digestive tract. In general, parasympathetic impulses stimulate movement and secretion in the gastrointestinal tract and sympathetic impulses inhibit these activities.

> The smooth muscle responsible for movements of the digestive tract is arranged in two layers, an inner circular layer and an outer longitudinal layer. The myenteric plexus is between the two muscle layers.

The fourth and outermost layer in the wall of the digestive tract is called the **adventitia** if it is above the diaphragm and the **serosa** if it is below the diaphragm. The adventitia is composed of connective tissue. The serosa, which is below the diaphragm, has a layer of epithelium covering the connective tissue. It is actually the **visceral peritoneum** and secretes serous fluid for lubrication so that the abdominal organs move smoothly against each other without friction.

> Above the diaphragm, the outermost layer of the digestive tract is a connective tissue adventitia. Below the diaphragm, it is serosa.

Components of the Digestive Tract

Mouth

The mouth, or **oral cavity,** is the first part of the digestive tract. It is adapted to receive food by ingestion, break it into small particles by mastication, and mix it with saliva. The lips, cheeks, and palate form the boundaries. The oral cavity contains the teeth and tongue and receives the secretions from the salivary glands (Fig. 16–3).

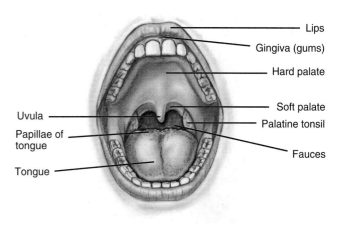

Figure 16–3   Features of the oral cavity.

Lips and Cheeks

The lips and cheeks help hold food in the mouth and keep it in place for chewing. They are also used in the formation of words for speech.

The lips are folds of skeletal muscle covered with a thin transparent epithelium. Their reddish color is due to the many blood vessels underlying the epithelium. The lips contain numerous sensory receptors that are useful for judging the temperature and texture of foods.

> **Cold sores,** or fever blisters, are small fluid-filled blisters that itch and are painful, usually appearing around the lips and in the mouth. They are caused by recurring infections with the herpes simplex virus. After the initial infection, the virus remains dormant in a cutaneous nerve until it is activated by stress, fever, or ultraviolet radiation.

The cheeks form the lateral boundaries of the oral cavity. The main substance of the cheeks is the **buccinator muscle** and other muscles of facial expression. On the outside, the muscles are covered by skin and subcutaneous tissue. Inside the oral cavity, the muscles are lined with a moist mucous membrane of stratified squamous epithelium. The multiple layers of epithelium provide protection against abrasion from food particles.

Palate

The **palate** is the root of the oral cavity. It separates the oral cavity from the nasal cavity. The anterior portion, the **hard palate,** is supported by bone. The posterior portion, the **soft palate,** is skeletal muscle and connective tissue. Posteriorly, the soft palate ends in a projection called the **uvula.** During swallowing, the soft palate and uvula move upward to direct food away from the nasal cavity and into the oropharynx.

Cleft palate is a condition in which the bones in the hard palate do not fuse completely during prenatal development. This leaves an opening between the nasal and oral cavities. An infant with this problem has difficulty creating enough suction for proper feeding. Cleft palate usually can be corrected surgically.

A person with a short lingual frenulum is "tongue tied." The movement of the tongue is abnormally limited, which causes difficulties in speech. Surgically cutting the frenulum corrects this problem.

Tongue

The largest and most movable organ in the oral cavity is the **tongue.** Most of the tongue's substance is skeletal muscle. The major attachment for the tongue is the posterior region, or **root,** which is anchored to the hyoid bone. The anterior portion is relatively free but is connected to the floor of the mouth, in the midline, by a membranous fold of tissue called the **frenulum** (FREN-yoo-lum). The dorsal surface of the tongue is covered by tiny projections called **papillae.** In addition to providing friction for manipulating food in the mouth, the papillae contain the taste buds (see Chapter 9). Masses of lymphoid tissue, the **lingual tonsils,** are embedded in the posterior dorsal surface. These provide defense against bacteria that enter the mouth.

The muscles in the tongue allow it to manipulate the food in the mouth for mastication, move the food around to mix it with saliva, shape it into a ball-like mass called a bolus, and direct it toward the pharynx for swallowing. It is a major sensory organ for taste and is one of the major organs used in speech.

> The tongue manipulates food in the mouth and is used in speech. The surface is covered with papillae that provide friction and contain the taste buds.

Teeth

Two different sets of teeth develop in the mouth. The first set begins to appear at approximately 6 months of age and continues to develop until about 2½ years of age. This set, called the **primary** or **deciduous teeth,** contains 5 teeth in each quadrant (10 in each jaw) for a total of 20 teeth. Figure 16–4*A* illustrates the types of primary teeth. Starting at 6 years of age, the primary teeth begin to fall out and they are replaced by the **secondary** or **permanent teeth.** This set contains 8 teeth in each quadrant (16 in each jaw) for a total of 32 teeth. These teeth are illustrated in Figure 16–4*B*.

The third molars are the last teeth to erupt. These are sometimes called "wisdom teeth" because they usually erupt between the ages of 17 and 25 years, when one is supposed to be wise. These teeth may remain embedded in the jawbone. If this happens, they are said to be impacted. In some cases, wisdom teeth are absent altogether.

Different teeth are shaped to handle food in different ways. The **incisors** are chisel shaped and have sharp edges for biting food; **cuspids (canines)** are conical and have points for grasping and tearing food, **bicuspids (premolars)** and **molars** have flat surfaces with rounded projections for crushing and grinding. Note the location of each type of teeth in

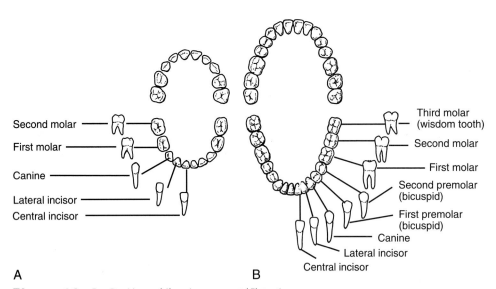

Second molar
First molar
Canine
Lateral incisor
Central incisor

Third molar (wisdom tooth)
Second molar
First molar
Second premolar (bicuspid)
First premolar (bicuspid)
Canine
Lateral incisor
Central incisor

A   B

Figure 16-4 Deciduous (*A*) and permanent (*B*) teeth.

Table 16–1	Ages at Which Teeth Erupt and Are Shed	
Tooth Type	**Age at Eruption**	**Age at Shedding**
Deciduous Teeth		
Central incisors	6–8 months	5–7 years
Lateral incisors	8–10 months	6–8 years
First molars	12–16 months	9–11 years
Canines	16–20 months	8–11 years
Second molars	20–30 months	9–11 years
Permanent Teeth		
First molars	6–7 years	
Central incisors	6–8 years	
Lateral incisors	7–9 years	
Canines	9–10 years	
First premolars	9–11 years	
Second premolars	10–12 years	
Second molars	11–13 years	
Third molars	15–25 years	

Figure 16–4. Table 16–1 summarizes the number and types of teeth in the primary and secondary sets. They are listed in the sequence in which they erupt. There is considerable variation in the ages at which teeth erupt and when the deciduous teeth are shed. The times listed represent an average range and there may be exceptions.

> A complete set of deciduous teeth contains 20 teeth. There are 32 teeth in a complete permanent set. The shape of each tooth type corresponds to the way it handles food.

Although the different types of teeth have different shapes, each one has three parts:

- A crown
- A neck
- A root

The **crown** is the visible portion of the tooth, covered by **enamel,** and the **root** is the portion that is embedded in the alveolar processes (sockets) of the mandible and maxilla. The **neck,** a small region in which the crown and root meet, is adjacent to the **gingiva,** or **gum.**

> **Gingivitis** is an inflammation of the gingiva, or gum. The gums become sore and red and may bleed. This condition is reversible if it is not neglected and corrective action is taken. Periodontal disease results when gingivitis is neglected and bacteria invade the bone around the tooth. This is a major cause of tooth loss in adults.

The central core of a tooth is the **pulp cavity.** It contains the **pulp,** which consists of connective tis-

sue, blood vessels, and nerves. In the root, the pulp cavity is called the **root canal.** Nerves and blood vessels enter the root through an **apical foramen.** The pulp cavity is surrounded by **dentin,** which forms the bulk of the tooth. Dentin is a living cellular substance similar to bone. In the root, the dentin is surrounded by a thin layer of calcified connective tissue called **cementum,** which attaches the root to the **periodontal ligaments.** The ligaments have fibers that firmly anchor the root in the alveolar process. **Enamel,** the hardest substance in the body, surrounds the dentin in the crown of the tooth. Figure 16–5 shows a longitudinal section of a tooth and illustrates the major features.

> A tooth is divided into a crown, neck, and root. The central core is the pulp cavity and this is surrounded by dentin. Enamel, the hardest substance in the body, covers the crown, or visible portion, of the tooth.

> **Caries,** or dental cavities, are caused by the demineralization of the teeth due to the action of bacteria that live in the mouth. The bacteria metabolize sugars in the mouth, producing acids that dissolve the calcium salts of the tooth. If the bacteria reach the pulp cavity, it is necessary to perform a **root canal** procedure. In this procedure, the pulp cavity with its nerve is destroyed and the cavity is completely filled with a solid filling material.

Salivary Glands

Three pairs of major **salivary glands** and numerous smaller ones secrete saliva into the oral cavity,

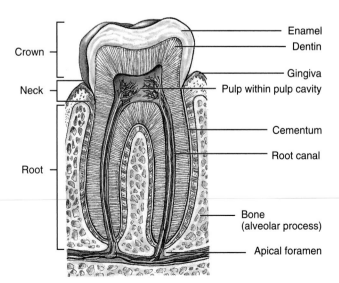

Figure 16–5 Longitudinal section of a tooth.

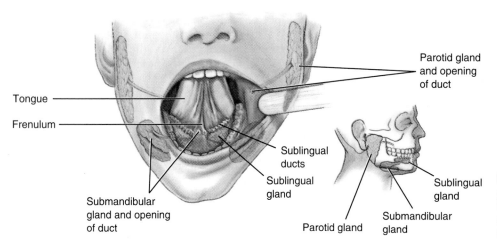

Figure 16-6 Salivary glands. (From Jarvis C: Physical Examination and Health Assessment. Philadelphia, WB Saunders, 1992.)

where it is mixed with food during mastication (Fig. 16-6). The **parotid glands** are the largest of the salivary glands. One gland is located on each side, between the skin and masseter muscle, just anterior and inferior to the ear. The duct from each parotid gland (parotid duct) opens into the oral cavity next to the second upper molar. **Submandibular glands** are located on the floor of the mouth along the medial surface of the mandible. The submandibular ducts open into the oral cavity by the lingual frenulum. Small **sublingual glands** are in the floor of the mouth, anterior to the submandibular glands, and under the tongue. They have numerous small ducts that open into the cavity along the frenulum.

Mumps is a viral infection of the parotid glands. The infection causes inflammation in the gland, which makes opening the mouth and chewing difficult. If the disease occurs in postadolescent males, the infection may spread to the testes, which, in severe cases, may result in sterility.

Saliva contains water, mucus, and the enzyme **amylase.** Functions of saliva include the following:

• It has a cleansing action on the teeth
• It moistens and lubricates food during mastication and swallowing.
• It dissolves certain molecules so that foods can be tasted.
• It begins the chemical digestion of starches through the action of amylase, which breaks down polysaccharides into disaccharides.

The parotid, submandibular, and sublingual glands secrete saliva, which contains the enzyme amylase.

Halitosis, commonly called bad breath, results from an overabundance of bacteria in the mouth. In some cases it may be due to poor oral hygiene. In others, it may be caused by a disease process that reduces the secretion of saliva for cleansing the mouth and moving food particles to the pharynx for swallowing. As a result, some food particles remain in the mouth and decompose, which provides a wonderful growth medium for the bacteria.

Pharynx

The **pharynx** is a fibromuscular passageway that connects the nasal and oral cavities to the larynx and esophagus (see Fig. 15-2). It serves both the respiratory and digestive systems as a channel for air and food. The upper region, the **nasopharynx,** is posterior to the nasal cavity. It contains the pharyngeal tonsils, or adenoids, functions as a passageway for air, and has no function in the digestive system. The middle region posterior to the oral cavity is the **oropharynx.** This is the first region food enters when it is swallowed. The opening from the oral cavity into the oropharynx is called the **fauces.** Masses of lymphoid tissue, the **palatine tonsils,** are near the fauces. The lower region, posterior to the larynx, is the **laryngopharynx,** or hypopharynx. The laryngopharynx opens into both the esophagus and the larynx.

Food is forced into the pharynx by the tongue. When food reaches the opening, sensory receptors around the fauces respond and initiate an involuntary swallowing reflex. This reflex action has several parts. The uvula is elevated to prevent food from entering the nasopharynx. The epiglottis drops downward to prevent food from entering the larynx and to direct the food into the esophagus. Peristaltic movements propel the food from the pharynx into the esophagus.

> The pharynx is a passageway that transports food to the esophagus. The region posterior to the oral cavity is the oropharynx, and the opening from the oral cavity into this region is the fauces.

Esophagus

The **esophagus** is a collapsible muscular tube, about 25 cm long, that serves as a passageway for food between the pharynx and stomach. As it descends, it is posterior to the trachea and anterior to the vertebral column. It passes through an opening in the diaphragm, called the esophageal hiatus, and then empties into the stomach. The mucosa has glands that secrete mucus to keep the lining moist and well lubricated to ease the passage of food. The lower esophageal sphincter, sometimes called the cardiac sphincter, controls the movement of food between the esophagus and the stomach.

☑ QuickCheck

- What portion of a tooth is covered by enamel?
- The trachea is supported by C-shaped cartilages with the open part of the C directed posteriorly. Why is this important for swallowing?
- What keeps food from going back into the esophagus from the stomach?

Stomach

The **stomach,** which receives food from the esophagus, is located in the upper left quadrant of the abdomen. Its capacity varies, but in the adult it averages about 1.5 liters, although in some individuals it may hold up to 4 liters.

Structure

The stomach is divided into the cardiac, fundic, body, and pyloric regions (Fig. 16–7). The **cardiac region** is a small region around the opening from the esophagus. The **fundus,** the most superior region, balloons above the cardiac region to form a temporary storage area. The **body** is the main portion of the stomach, which curves to the right and creates two curvatures. The **lesser curvature** is concave and is directed superiorly and to the right. On the opposite side, the convex **greater curvature** is directed inferiorly and to the left. As the body approaches the exit from the stomach, it narrows into the **pyloric region.** A circular band of smooth muscle forms the **pyloric sphincter,** which acts as a valve between the stomach and small intestine.

> The stomach is divided into the fundus, cardiac, body, and pyloric regions. The lesser and greater curvatures are on the right and left sides, respectively, of the stomach.

The muscular layer in the wall of the stomach has three layers, instead of two as found in other parts of the digestive tract. The additional third layer is innermost, located just under the submucosa, and is formed of oblique muscle fibers. The next muscle layer is the circular layer and the outermost one is the longitudinal layer. The oblique layer adds another dimension to the mixing action of the stomach. When the stomach is empty, the mucosa and submucosa show longitudinal folds, called **rugae** (ROO-jee). These folds allow the stomach to expand and as it fills the rugae become less apparent.

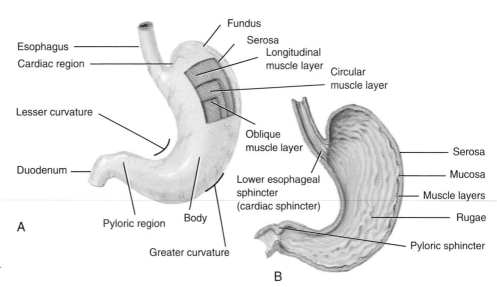

Figure 16–7 Features of the stomach. (*A*) External view. (*B*) Internal view.

The stomach wall has three smooth muscle layers. The innermost is oblique, the middle is circular, and the outermost is longitudinal. Rugae are longitudinal folds that permit expansion of the stomach.

A **hiatal hernia** occurs when the stomach protrudes into the thoracic cavity through a weakened area of the diaphragm. Frequently, it develops when a small region of the fundus balloons backward through the esophageal hiatus. Symptoms of this condition include pain in the upper abdomen and "heart burn" due to the reflux of stomach acid into the esophagus, especially when the person is lying down.

Gastric Secretions

The mucosal lining of the stomach is simple columnar epithelium with numerous tubular **gastric glands.** The gastric glands open to the surface of the mucosa through tiny holes called **gastric pits.** Four different types of cells make up the gastric glands:

- Mucous cells
- Parietal cells
- Chief cells
- Endocrine cells

The secretions of the exocrine gastric glands—composed of the mucous, parietal, and chief cells—make up the gastric juice. Approximately 2 to 3 liters of gastric juice are produced every day. The products of the endocrine cells are secreted directly into the bloodstream and are not a part of the gastric juice.

Mucous cells produce two types of **mucus** in the stomach. One type is thick and alkaline and forms a protective coating for the stomach lining. The other type is thin and watery. It mixes with the food and creates a fluid medium for chemical reactions. **Parietal cells** secrete **hydrochloric acid** and **intrinsic factor.** The hydrochloric acid kills bacteria and provides an acid environment for the action of enzymes in the stomach. Intrinsic factor aids in the absorption of vitamin B_{12}. **Chief cells** secrete **pepsinogen,** an inactive form of the enzyme pepsin. Hydrochloric acid converts the inactive pepsinogen into the active enzyme pepsin, which begins the chemical digestion of proteins. The **endocrine cells** secrete the hormone **gastrin,** which functions in the regulation of gastric activity. Table 16–2 summarizes the various cells and secretions of the gastric glands.

Exocrine gastric glands secrete mucus, hydrochloric acid, pepsinogen, and intrinsic factor. The endocrine cells secrete gastrin.

The churning actions of the muscles in the stomach wall break the food particles of the bolus that

Table 16–2 Secretions of Gastric Glands

Cell Type	Secretion	Function
Mucous cells	Mucus (thick alkaline)	Protects stomach lining
	Mucus (thin, watery)	Medium for chemical reactions
Parietal cells	Hydrochloric acid	Kills bacteria; activates pepsinogen
	Intrinsic factor	Absorption of vitamin B_{12}
Chief cells	Pepsinogen (active form is pepsin)	Begins digestion of proteins into polypeptides
Endocrine cells	Gastrin (a hormone)	Stimulates gastric gland secretion

was swallowed into smaller sizes and mix them with the gastric juice. This produces a semifluid mixture called **chyme** (KYME), which leaves the stomach through the pyloric sphincter and enters the small intestine.

Regulation of Gastric Secretions

The regulation of gastric secretions is accomplished through neural and hormonal mechanisms. Gastric juice is produced all the time, but the amount varies subject to the regulatory factors. Regulation of gastric secretions may be divided into cephalic, gastric, and intestinal phases (Fig. 16–8).

The **cephalic phase** begins when an individual thinks pleasant thoughts about food or sees, smells, or tastes food. This phase anticipates food and prepares the stomach to receive it. The sensory input stimulates centers in the medulla oblongata, which sends impulses along the parasympathetic neurons in the vagus nerve (cranial nerve X) to the stomach. These impulses cause an increase in secretion of gastric juice. The impulses also increase the secretion of the hormone gastrin, which enters the blood and circulates back to the stomach to increase activity of the gastric glands.

The **gastric phase,** which accounts for more than two thirds of the gastric juice secretion, begins when food reaches the stomach. The presence of food in the stomach and the distention of the stomach wall both stimulate local reflexes that result in gastrin secretion. Gastrin, in turn, stimulates the secretion of gastric juice, which contains hydrochloric acid and pepsinogen. The hydrochloric acid acidifies the stomach contents and activates the pepsinogen into pepsin, which breaks down proteins into peptides. Stomach distention also sends signals to the brain, which responds by transmitting impulses back to the gastric glands along the vagus nerve.

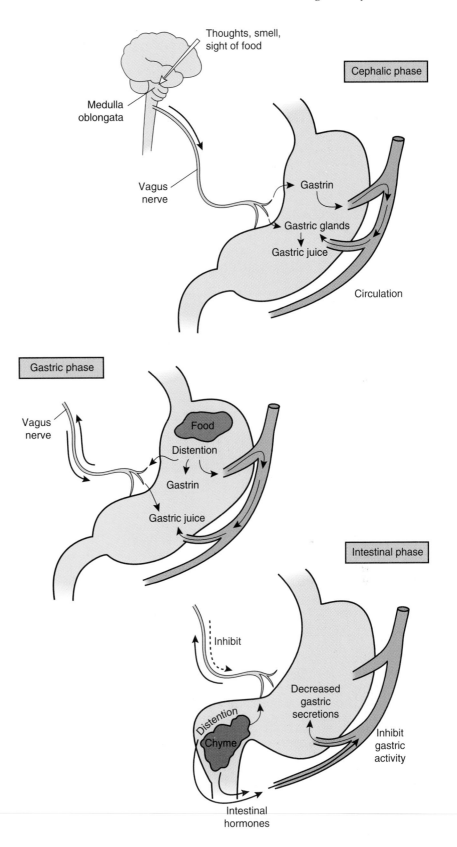

Figure 16-8   Regulation of gastric secretions.

The passage of chyme through the pyloric sphincter into the first part (duodenum) of the small intestine triggers the **intestinal phase** of regulation. Distention and the presence of acid chyme in the duodenum stimulate the secretion of intestinal hormones, which in turn inhibit gastric secretions. These factors also initiate responses in the medulla oblongata that inhibit gastric secretions. These hormonal and neural inhibitory responses help prevent excess acid chyme from entering the small intestine. When the chyme is neutralized and moves away from the duodenum, the inhibitory responses stop and gastric secretion is again stimulated. The intestinal phase regulates the entry of chyme into the small intestine.

> Thought and smell of food start the cephalic phase of gastric secretions; the presence of food in the stomach initiates the gastric phase; and the presence of acid chyme in the small intestine begins the intestinal phase.

Stomach Emptying

Peristalsis in the stomach pushes chyme toward the pyloric region. As the chyme accumulates, the pyloric sphincter relaxes and a small amount of chyme is pumped into the small intestine. The rate at which the stomach empties depends on the nature of the contents and the receptivity of the small intestine. The stomach is usually empty within 4 hours after a meal. Liquids tend to pass through the stomach quickly. Solids stay in the stomach until they are well mixed with gastric juice. Carbohydrates move through rather quickly, proteins take a little longer, and fatty foods may stay in the stomach as long as 4 to 6 hours. The presence of chyme in the first part of the small intestine decreases the receptivity and slows the emptying process.

If the stomach empties too slowly, the rate at which nutrients are digested and absorbed is diminished. There is also danger that the highly acid chyme will damage the stomach lining. On the other hand, if the stomach empties too quickly, before particles are thoroughly mixed with the gastric juice, the efficiency of digestion is reduced and the acid chyme may damage the intestinal mucosa. The neural and hormonal mechanisms that control gastric secretions also regulate stomach emptying.

> Relaxation of the pyloric sphincter allows chyme to pass from the stomach into the small intestine. The rate at which this occurs depends on the nature of the chyme and the receptivity of the small intestine.

> Vomiting is the forceful ejection of the stomach contents through the mouth. It can be initiated by extreme stretching of the stomach or by the presence of irritants such as bacterial toxins, alcohol, spicy foods, and certain drugs. The vomiting action is a coordinated reflex controlled by the vomiting center of the medulla oblongata.

Small Intestine

The small intestine is about 2.5 centimeters in diameter and 6 meters long. It extends from the pyloric sphincter to the ileocecal valve, where it empties into the large intestine. The small intestine finishes the process of digestion, absorbs the nutrients, and passes the residue on to the large intestine. The liver, gallbladder, and pancreas are accessory organs of the digestive system that are closely associated with the small intestine. These are described later in this chapter.

Structure

The small intestine follows the general structure of the digestive tract in that the wall has a mucosa with simple columnar epithelium, submucosa, smooth muscle with inner circular and outer longitudinal layers, and serosa. The mucosa and submucosa show circular folds, called **plicae circulares** (PLY-kee sir-kyoo-LAIR-eez), which increase the surface area for absorption (Fig. 16–9). Fingerlike extensions of the mucosa, called **villi,** project from the circular folds, and this further increases the surface area. Each villus surrounds a blood capillary network and a lymph capillary, or **lacteal.** These function in the absorption of nutrients. **Intestinal glands** extend downward between adjacent villi. The surface epithelium on the villi has tiny hairlike cytoplasmic extensions, called **microvilli,** that form a **brush border,** which again increases surface area.

> The absorptive surface area of the small intestine is increased by plicae circulares, villi, and microvilli.

Although the structure is similar throughout, the length of the small intestine is divided into three regions:

• Duodenum
• Jejunum
• Ileum

The **duodenum** is the first part and is about 25 centimeters long. It begins at the pyloric sphincter and continues in a C-shaped curve to the jejunum. The duodenum is behind the parietal peritoneum and is the most fixed portion of the small intestine. It receives the chyme from the stomach and secretions from the liver and pancreas. A distinguishing feature of the duodenum is the presence of

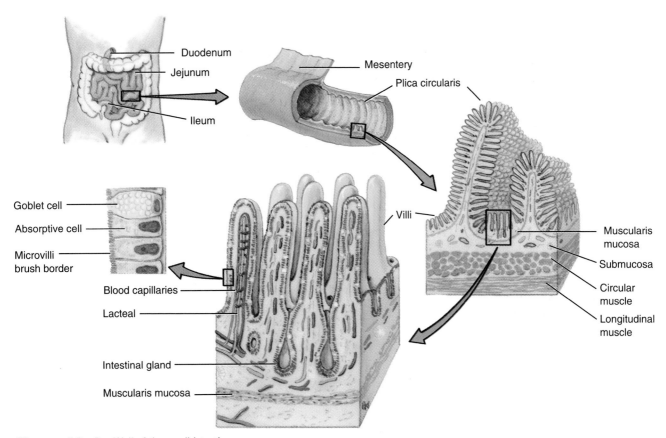

Goblet cell
Absorptive cell
Microvilli brush border
Blood capillaries
Lacteal
Intestinal gland
Muscularis mucosa

Duodenum
Jejunum
Ileum

Mesentery
Plica circularis

Villi

Muscularis mucosa
Submucosa
Circular muscle
Longitudinal muscle

Figure 16-9   Wall of the small intestine.

mucous glands in the submucosa. These are called **duodenal** (doo-oh-DEE-nal) **glands** (Brunner's glands).

The second portion of the small intestine is the **jejunum,** which is about 2.5 meters long. This is continuous with the third portion, the **ileum,** which is about 3.5 meters long. There is no distinct separation between the jejunum and ileum. They are similar in structure, are mobile, and are suspended from the dorsal abdominal wall by a fold of peritoneum, called **mesentery.** There is a gradual decrease in the number and length of the villi and an increase in the number of goblet cells in the mucosa from the beginning of the jejunum to the terminal portion of the ileum.

> The small intestine is divided into the duodenum, jejunum, and ileum.

Secretions of the Small Intestine

Intestinal glands secrete large amounts of watery fluid that is neutral or slightly alkaline in pH. It keeps the chyme in a liquid form and provides an appropriate environment for the many chemical reactions of digestion and a fluid medium for the absorption of nutrients. The fluid is readily reabsorbed by the capillaries in the microvilli.

Goblet cells in the mucosa throughout the small intestine and duodenal glands in the submucosa of the duodenum secrete mucus. The alkaline mucus protects the intestinal wall from the acid chyme and digestive enzymes.

Digestive enzymes, which have a significant role in the final stages of chemical digestion, are located in the microvilli of the mucosal epithelial cells. These enzymes, called brush border enzymes, include **peptidase,** which acts on segments of proteins called peptides; **maltase, sucrase,** and **lactase,** which act on disaccharides (double sugars); and an **intestinal lipase,** which acts on neutral fats. **Enterokinase** (en-ter-oh-KYE-nayz), although not actually a digestive enzyme, is produced by the mucosal epithelial cells. This enzyme activates a protein-splitting enzyme from the pancreas.

Lactose intolerance is caused by a deficiency of the intestinal enzyme lactase, which acts on lactose, a sugar found in milk. When people with lactose intolerance drink milk, this sugar is not digested properly. Bacterial action on the undigested sugar causes gas and a bloated feeling. The undigested lactose also prevents absorption of water from the small intestine, which leads to diarrhea. The solution to this problem is to avoid milk and milk products.

In addition to mucus and digestive enzymes, intestinal cells secrete at least two hormones, secretin and cholecystokinin. **Secretin** (see-KREE-tin) stimulates the pancreas to secrete a fluid that has a high bicarbonate ion concentration. This fluid helps to neutralize chyme so that the intestinal enzymes can function. **Cholecystokinin** (koh-lee-sis-toh-KYE-nin) stimulates the release of bile from the gallbladder and the secretion of digestive enzymes from the pancreas. It also inhibits gastric motility and secretions.

> Exocrine cells in the mucosa of the small intestine secrete mucus, peptidase, sucrase, maltase, lactase, lipase, and enterokinase. Endocrine cells secrete cholecystokinin and secretin.

The most important factor for regulating secretions in the small intestine is the presence of chyme. This is largely a local reflex action in response to chemical and mechanical irritation from the chyme and in response to distention of the intestinal wall. This is a direct reflex action; thus the greater the amount of chyme, the greater the secretion.

> The presence of chyme in the duodenum stimulates intestinal secretions.

Large Intestine

The **large intestine** is larger in diameter than the small intestine but is only about 1.5 meters long (Fig. 16–10). It begins at the **ileocecal** (ill-ee-oh-SEE-kul) **junction,** where the ileum enters the large intestine, and ends at the anus. The ileocecal junction has a circular band of smooth muscle fibers, the **ileocecal sphincter,** and a valve, the **ileocecal valve.**

Characteristic Features

The wall of the large intestine has the same types of tissue that are found in other parts of the digestive tract, but there are some distinguishing characteristics. The mucosa has large numbers of goblet cells but does not have any villi. The longitudinal muscle layer, although present, is incomplete. The longitudinal muscle is limited to three distinct bands, called **teniae coli** (TEE-nee-aye KOH-lye), that run the entire length of the colon. Contraction of the teniae coli exerts pressure on the wall and creates a series of pouches, called **haustra** (HAWS-trah), along the colon. **Epiploic** (ep-ih-PLOH-ik) **appendages,** pieces of fat-filled connective tissue, are attached to the outer surface of the colon.

> The large intestine is characterized by three bands of longitudinal muscle called teniae coli. Haustra and epiploic appendages also are features of the large intestine that are not present in other regions of the gastrointestinal tract.

Regions of the Large Intestine

The large intestine consists of the cecum, colon, rectum, and anal canal (see Fig. 16–10).

The **cecum** is the proximal portion of the large intestine. It is a blind pouch that extends inferiorly from the ileocecal junction. The **vermiform appendix** is attached to the cecum. In humans, the appendix has no function in digestion but does contain some lymphatic tissue.

The **colon** is the longest portion of the large intestine and is divided into ascending, transverse, descending, and sigmoid portions. The **ascending colon** begins at the ileocecal junction and travels upward, along the posterior abdominal wall on the right side, until it reaches the liver. Here it turns

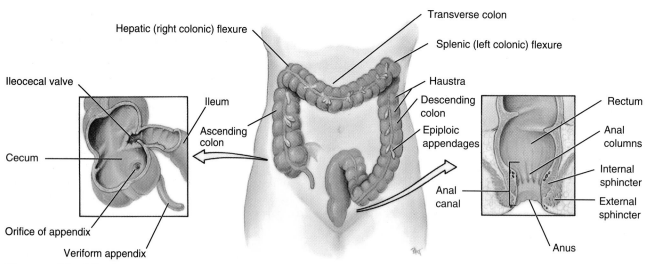

Figure 16–10 Features of the large intestine.

anteriorly and to the left, becomes the **transverse colon,** and continues across the anterior abdomen toward the spleen on the left side. Here the colon turns sharply downward and travels inferiorly along the posterior abdominal wall as the **descending colon.** At the pelvic brim, the descending colon makes a variable S-shaped curve, called the **sigmoid colon,** and then becomes the rectum. The curve between the ascending and transverse portions is the **hepatic (right colonic) flexure.** The curve between the transverse and descending portions is the **splenic (left colonic) flexure.**

> The large intestine consists of the cecum, colon, rectum, and anal canal. The colon is divided into ascending, transverse, descending, and sigmoid portions.

Appendicitis is an inflammation that sometimes occurs when infectious material becomes trapped inside the appendix. If the inflamed appendix ruptures and releases the infectious contents into the abdominal cavity, the peritoneum may become involved, resulting in a potentially life-threatening inflammation of the peritoneum, called peritonitis. Treatment for appendicitis usually is the surgical removal of the appendix.

The **rectum** continues from the sigmoid colon to the anal canal and has a thick muscular layer. It follows the curvature of the sacrum and is firmly attached to it by connective tissue. The rectum ends about 5 cm below the tip of the coccyx, at the beginning of the anal canal.

The last 2 to 3 centimeters of the digestive tract is the **anal canal,** which continues from the rectum and opens to the outside at the **anus.** The mucosa of the rectum is folded to form longitudinal **anal columns.** The smooth muscle layer is thick and forms the **internal anal sphincter** at the superior end of the anal canal. This sphincter is under involuntary control. There is an **external anal sphincter** at the inferior end of the anal canal. This sphincter is composed of skeletal muscle and is under voluntary control.

> The internal anal sphincter is under involuntary control; the external anal sphincter is controlled voluntarily.

Functions of the Large Intestine

Unlike the small intestine, the large intestine produces no digestive enzymes. Chemical digestion is completed in the small intestine before the chyme reaches the large intestine. There are no villi for the absorption of nutrients. This is also accomplished in the small intestine. The primary functions of the large intestine are the absorption of fluid and electrolytes and the elimination of waste products.

The chyme that enters the large intestine contains materials that were not digested or absorbed in the small intestine, water, electrolytes, and bacteria. Some of the water and electrolytes are absorbed in the cecum and ascending colon. Although the quantity is relatively small, this absorptive function of the large intestine is important in maintaining fluid balance in the body. The residue that remains from the chyme becomes the feces.

The large intestine has the same types of mixing and peristaltic movements as occur in other parts of the digestive tract, but they are more sluggish and occur less frequently. They are more likely to occur after a meal as a result of reflexes initiated in the small intestine. As the rectum fills with feces, the defecation reflex is triggered and the waste products are eliminated.

The only secretory product in the large intestine is mucus from the large quantity of goblet cells. The mucus protects the intestinal wall against abrasion and irritation from the chyme. It also helps hold the particles of fecal matter together. Because mucus is slightly alkaline, it helps control the pH of the material in the large intestine.

> Functions of the large intestine include the absorption of water and electrolytes and the elimination of feces.

 QuickCheck

- What muscle relaxes to permit chyme to pass from the stomach into the small intestine?

- What effect does the vagus nerve have on gastric secretions?

- How is the wall of the small intestine modified to accommodate absorption of nutrients?

- What portion of the large intestine extends inferiorly from the ileocecal junction?

Accessory Organs of the Digestive System

The salivary glands, liver, gallbladder, and pancreas are not part of the digestive tract, but they have a role in digestive activities and are considered accessory organs. Because the salivary glands are so closely associated with the mouth and their primary function is there, they are included with the oral cavity. The liver and pancreas have functions in addition to digestion, and the gallbladder is closely related to the liver; thus these three organs are described as separate accessory organs in this section.

Liver

The liver is a large reddish brown organ that is located primarily in the right hypochondriac and epigastric regions of the abdomen, just beneath the diaphragm. It is the largest gland in the body, weighs about 1.5 kg, and has numerous functions.

Structure of the Liver

On the surface, the liver is divided into two major lobes and two smaller lobes. On the anterior surface, the **falciform** (FALL-sih-form) **ligament,** a double fold of peritoneum that attaches the liver to the abdominal wall, separates the **right lobe** from the **left lobe.** Two additional small lobes are evident on the visceral surface (Fig. 16–11). The **caudate lobe** is between the **ligamentum venosum** and the **inferior vena cava.** The **quadrate lobe** is between the **ligamentum teres** and the **gallbladder.** The **porta** is also on the visceral surface. The porta is where the **hepatic artery** and **hepatic portal vein** enter the liver and where the **hepatic ducts** exit.

The substance of the liver is divided into functional units called **liver lobules** (Fig. 16–12). A liver lobule consists of **hepatocytes** (liver cells) that radiate outward from the **central vein** like spokes of a wheel. The central veins of adjacent lobules merge together to form larger vessels, until they form the **hepatic veins,** which drain into the inferior vena cava. Tiny channels, called **bile canaliculi,** are interwoven with the liver cells and carry the bile that is produced by the hepatocytes toward the periphery of the lobule. Bile canaliculi merge to form larger **right and left hepatic ducts.** These two ducts join to form the common hepatic duct, which transports bile out of the liver. The plates of hepatocytes are separated from each other by venous channels, called **sinusoids,** which carry blood from the periphery of the lobule toward the central vein. The sinusoids are lined with special phagocytic cells, called Kupffer cells, that remove foreign particles from the blood as it flows through the sinusoids. **Portal triads,** which consist of a branch of the hepatic portal vein, a branch of the hepatic artery, and a branch of a hepatic duct, are located around the periphery of the lobule.

> The functional units of the liver are lobules with sinusoids that carry blood from the periphery to the central vein of the lobule.

Cirrhosis is a chronic liver disease that may develop as a result of chronic alcoholism or severe hepatitis. The hepatic cells of the liver are destroyed and replaced with fibrous connective tissue so that the liver no longer functions properly. One effect is the buildup of bilirubin in the blood because it is not properly incorporated into the bile and excreted. The word "cirrhosis" means "orange-colored condition," which refers to the discoloration of the liver in this disease.

Blood Supply to the Liver

The liver receives blood from two sources. Freshly oxygenated blood is brought to the liver by the **common hepatic artery,** a branch of the celiac trunk from the abdominal aorta. The common hepatic artery branches into smaller and smaller vessels until it forms the small hepatic arteries in the portal triads at the periphery of the liver lobules. Blood that is rich in nutrients from the digestive tract is carried to the liver by the **hepatic portal vein.** The portal vein divides until it forms the small portal vein branches in the portal triads at the periphery of the liver lobules. Venous blood from the hepatic portal

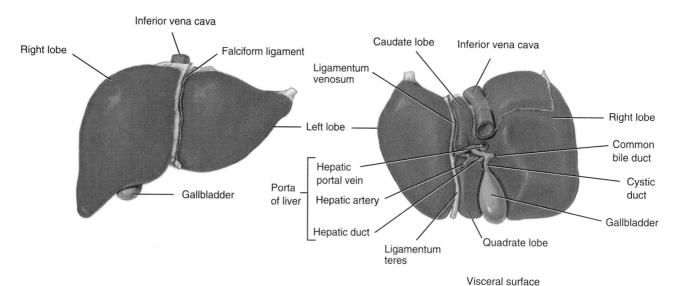

Figure 16–11   Features of the liver.

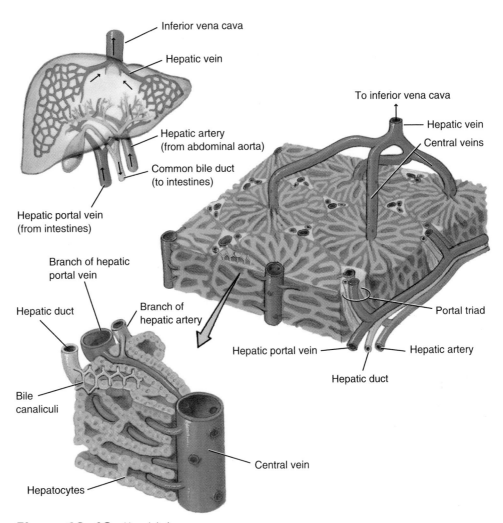

Figure 16-12   Liver lobules.

vein and the arterial blood from the hepatic arteries mix together as the blood flows through the sinusoids toward the **central vein.** The central veins of the liver lobules merge to form larger **hepatic veins** that drain into the inferior vena cava.

> The liver lobules receive nutrient-rich blood from the hepatic portal vein and oxygenated arterial blood from the hepatic artery.

Functions of the Liver

The liver has a wide variety of functions and many of these are vital to life. Hepatocytes perform most of the functions attributed to the liver, but the phagocytic Kupffer cells that line the sinusoids are responsible for cleansing the blood. Liver functions include the following:

- **Secretion**—The liver produces and secretes bile.
- **Synthesis of bile salts**—Bile salts are cholesterol derivatives that are produced in the liver and facilitate fat digestion and the absorption of fats and fat-soluble vitamins.

- **Synthesis of plasma proteins**—The liver synthesizes albumin, fibrinogen, globulins except immunoglobulins, and clotting factors.
- **Storage**—The liver stores glucose in the form of glycogen, iron, and vitamins A, B_{12}, D, E, and K.
- **Detoxification**—The liver alters the chemical composition of toxic compounds, such as ammonia, to make them less harmful. It also changes the configuration of certain drugs, such as penicillin, and excretes them in the bile to remove them from the body.
- **Excretion**—Hormones, drugs, cholesterol, and bile pigments from the breakdown of hemoglobin are excreted in the bile.
- **Carbohydrate metabolism**—The liver has a major role in maintaining blood glucose levels. It removes excess glucose from the blood and converts it to glycogen for storage; it breaks down glycogen into glucose when more is needed; it converts noncarbohydrate molecules into glucose.
- **Lipid metabolism**—The liver functions in the breakdown of fatty acids, in the synthesis of cholesterol and phospholipids, and in the conversion of excess carbohydrates and proteins into fats.

- **Protein metabolism**—The liver has the ability to convert certain amino acids into different amino acids as needed for protein synthesis in the body. It also converts ammonia, which is produced in the breakdown of proteins, into urea, which is less toxic and can be excreted in the bile.
- **Filtering**—The phagocytic **Kupffer cells** that line the sinusoids remove bacteria, damaged red blood cells, and other particles from the blood.

Bile

About 1 liter of bile, a yellowish-green fluid, is produced by liver cells each day. Bile is slightly alkaline, with a pH of 7.6 to 8.6, so it helps neutralize the acid chyme. The main components of bile are water, bile salts, bile pigments, and cholesterol. The bile salts are useful secretory products of the liver, but the bile pigments and cholesterol are waste products that are excreted in the bile and eliminated from the body.

Although they are not enzymes, bile salts have a function in the digestion of fats. Bile salts act as **emulsifying agents** that break large fat globules into tiny fat droplets. This increases the surface area of the fat for more efficient enzyme action in fat digestion. Bile salts also facilitate the absorption of fat-soluble vitamins and the end products of fat digestion.

> Bile salts act as emulsifying agents in the digestion and absorption of fats.

Bile pigments are produced in the breakdown of hemoglobin from damaged red blood cells. The hemoglobin is broken down into heme, which contains iron, and globin, a protein. The liver recycles the iron from the heme and the globin. The remainder of the heme portion is converted into bile pigments, which are normally excreted in the bile. Bile pigments are responsible for the color of the urine and feces. The principal bile pigment is **bilirubin** (bill-ih-ROO-bin).

Cholesterol is a product of lipid metabolism. Bile salts act on cholesterol to make it soluble; then it is excreted in the bile.

> Cholesterol and bile pigments from the breakdown of hemoglobin are excreted from the body in the bile.

Gallbladder

The **gallbladder** is a pear-shaped sac that is attached to the visceral surface of the liver by the **cystic duct** (see Fig. 16–11). The cystic duct joins the hepatic duct from the liver to form the **common bile duct,** which empties into the duodenum. Simple columnar epithelium lines the gallbladder, and this is surrounded by smooth muscle covered with visceral peritoneum. When the muscle layer contracts, bile is ejected from the gallbladder into the cystic duct.

Gallstones are formed in the gallbladder when cholesterol precipitates from the bile and hardens into stones because there is a lack of bile salts. Problems develop when the stones leave the gallbladder and lodge in the bile duct. This obstructs the flow of bile into the small intestine and interferes with fat absorption. Surgery may be required to remove the gallstones.

The principal functions of the gallbladder are to store and concentrate bile. Bile is continuously produced by the liver and then travels through the hepatic duct and common bile duct to the duodenum. There is a sphincter (sphincter of Oddi) where the common bile duct enters the duodenum. If the small intestine is empty, the sphincter is closed and the bile backs up through the cystic duct into the gallbladder for concentration and storage until it is needed. When chyme with fatty contents enters the duodenum, the hormone **cholecystokinin** (koh-lee-sis-toh-KYE-nin) stimulates the gallbladder to contract and the sphincter to open. This permits bile to flow from the gallbladder, through the cystic duct and common bile duct, and then into the duodenum.

> Bile is produced in the liver. The gallbladder concentrates and stores the bile until it is needed.

Pancreas

The **pancreas** is an elongated and flattened organ that is located along the posterior abdominal wall behind the parietal peritoneum (Fig. 16–13). One end of the pancreas, the **head,** is on the right side within the curve of the duodenum; the other end, the **tail,** is on the left side next to the spleen.

The pancreas has both endocrine and exocrine functions. The endocrine portion consists of the scattered **islets of Langerhans,** which secrete the hormones insulin and glucagon into the blood. These hormones and their functions are discussed in Chapter 10. The exocrine portion is the major part of the gland. It consists of **pancreatic acinar** (AS-ih-nar) **cells** that secrete digestive enzymes into tiny ducts interwoven between the cells. These tiny ducts merge to form the main **pancreatic duct,** which extends the full length of the pancreas and empties into the duodenum. The pancreatic duct usually joins the common bile duct to form a single point of entry into the duodenum. Both ducts are controlled by the hepatopancreatic sphincter (sphincter of Oddi).

> Digestive enzymes are secreted by the pancreatic acinar cells.

Pancreatic juice has a high concentration of bicarbonate ions and contains digestive enzymes that act

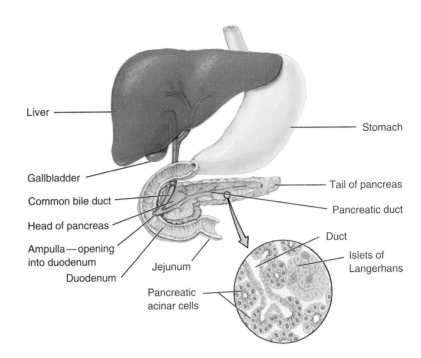

Figure 16–13 Location and features of the pancreas.

on carbohydrates, proteins, and lipids. **Pancreatic amylase** acts on starch and other complex carbohydrates to break them into simpler sugars called disaccharides. Protein-splitting enzymes from the pancreas include **trypsin,** which breaks the proteins into shorter chains of amino acids, called peptides. Like other enzymes that act on proteins, trypsin is secreted in an inactive form, **trypsinogen,** which is activated by enterokinase when it reaches the duodenum. The pancreas also secretes peptidase enzymes that break peptides into amino acids. **Pancreatic lipase** breaks fats into fatty acids and monoglycerides.

Pancreatic enzymes include amylase, trypsin, peptidase, and lipase.

Pancreatic secretion of digestive juice is regulated by the nervous system and by hormones. When parasympathetic impulses from the nervous system stimulate secretion of gastric juice, some impulses go to the pancreas and stimulate the secretion of pancreatic juice. When acid chyme enters the duodenum, the intestinal mucosa produces the hormone **secretin,** which travels in the blood to the pancreas. Secretin stimulates the pancreas to produce a fluid that has a high concentration of bicarbonate ions to neutralize the acids in the duodenum. Proteins and fats in the chyme stimulate the intestinal mucosa to secrete the hormone **cholecystokinin,** which also travels in the blood to the pancreas. This hormone stimulates the pancreas to produce a pancreatic juice that is rich in digestive enzymes. These digestive enzymes travel through the pancreatic duct to the duodenum, where they perform their actions.

Pancreatic secretions are controlled by the hormones secretin and cholecystokinin.

Chemical Digestion

Chemical digestion breaks down large complex molecules into smaller molecules that can be absorbed by the cells of the intestinal mucosa. The reactions in chemical digestion are **hydrolysis** reactions, which use water to split molecules. These reactions proceed at a slow rate. The purpose of the various digestive enzymes is to speed up the hydrolysis reactions of chemical digestion. The enzymes do not alter the reactions; they just make them occur more rapidly. Table 16–3 reviews the hormones and digestive enzymes that have been discussed in previous sections of this chapter.

Chemical digestion is the result of hydrolysis reactions.

Carbohydrate Digestion

Starches and other complex carbohydrates are first broken down into disaccharides, or double sugars, by the action of salivary amylase and pancreatic amylase. The disaccharides **sucrose, maltose,** and **lactose** are the result of this stage of digestion. Sucrase, maltase, and lactase, enzymes from the small intestine, act on the disaccharides to convert them to monosaccharides, or simple sugars, that can be absorbed. The digestion of maltose yields two molecules of glucose; sucrose produces a molecule of glucose and one of fructose; lactose yields a molecule each of glucose and galactose. The end products of complete carbohydrate digestion are the

Table 16–3 Enzymes and Hormones of the Digestive System

Secretion	Source	Action
Enzymes		
Amylase	Salivary glands Pancreas	Digestion of complex carbohydrates into disaccharides
Pepsin	Stomach	Digestion of proteins into polypeptides
Sucrase Maltase Lactase	Small intestine	Digestion of disaccharides into glucose, fructose, and galactose
Peptidase	Small intestine Pancreas	Digestion of peptides into amino acids
Lipase	Small intestine Pancreas	Digestion of fats into monoglycerides and fatty acids
Enterokinase	Small intestine	Activates trypsinogen
Hormones		
Gastrin	Stomach	Stimulates activity of the gastric glands
Secretin	Small intestine	Stimulates pancreas to secrete bicarbonate ions to neutralize acid chyme
Cholecystokinin	Small intestine	Stimulates gallbladder to contract and release bile; stimulates pancreas to secrete digestive enzymes

monosaccharides **glucose, fructose,** and **galactose.** Carbohydrate digestion is summarized by the following equation:

$$\text{Carbohydrates} \xrightarrow{\text{Salivary \& pancreatic amylase}} \text{Disaccharides}$$

Sucrose
Maltose
Lactose

$$\text{Disaccharides} \xrightarrow[\text{Lactase}]{\substack{\text{Sucrase}\\ \text{Maltase}}} \text{Monosaccharides}$$

Sucrose	Glucose + Fructose
Maltose	Glucose + Glucose
Lactose	Glucose + Galactose

Protein Digestion

The first digestive enzyme to act on proteins is pepsin in the stomach. Pepsin is secreted by the gastric glands in an inactive form, pepsinogen, which is activated by hydrochloric acid. When chyme reaches the duodenum, trypsin from the pancreas acts on the proteins. Trypsin is secreted in the inactive form, trypsinogen, which is activated by enterokinase in the small intestine. Pepsin and trypsin break down proteins into shorter chains of amino acids called

peptides. Peptidase enzymes from the small intestine and pancreas break the peptide bonds to produce **amino acids.** The amino acids are the absorbable end products of protein digestion. Protein digestion is summarized by the following equation:

$$\text{Proteins} \xrightarrow{\substack{\text{Pepsin (stomach)}\\ \text{Trypsin (pancreas)}}} \text{Peptides} \xrightarrow{\substack{\text{Peptidase}\\ \text{(small}\\ \text{intestine \&}\\ \text{pancreas)}}} \text{Amino acids}$$

Lipid Digestion

The small intestine is the only place in which lipid (fat) digestion occurs because the necessary enzymes are produced by the pancreas and enter the small intestine through the pancreatic duct. Triglycerides, glycerol molecules with three long-chain fatty acids attached, are the most abundant dietary fats. Fat molecules tend to attract each other to form large globules, which reduces the surface area for enzyme action. After the fats enter the duodenum, they are **emulsified** by bile. Emulsification does not break any chemical bonds, but it reduces the attraction between molecules so that they disperse. Pancreatic lipases act on the surfaces of the emulsified fat droplets. Lipase action breaks two fatty acid chains from the triglyceride molecules, yielding **monoglycerides** and **free fatty acids.** Lipid (fat) digestion is summarized by the following equation:

$$\text{Fats} \xrightarrow{\text{Bile}} \text{Emulsified fats} \xrightarrow{\text{Lipase}} \text{Monoglycerides and free fatty acids}$$

> The end products of digestion are glucose, fructose, galactose, amino acids, fatty acids, and monoglycerides.

Absorption

Approximately 10 liters of food, beverage, and secretions enter the digestive tract every day. Usually less than 1 liter enters the large intestine. The other 9 liters or more are absorbed in the small intestine. Absorption takes place along the entire length of the small intestine, but most of it occurs in the jejunum. By the time the chyme reaches the distal part of the ileum and large intestine, all that remains is some water, undigestible materials, and bacteria.

Water is absorbed throughout the length of the digestive tract by osmosis. Most water-soluble vitamins are easily absorbed by diffusion. Electrolytes are absorbed by diffusion and active transport. Most absorption of simple sugars and amino acids is by active transport across the cell membranes of the microvilli (Fig. 16–14). This requires cellular energy in the form of adenosine triphosphate (ATP). After transport across the cell membranes, simple sugars (monosaccharides) and amino acids passively move into the blood capillaries in the villi to be transported to the liver in the hepatic portal vein.

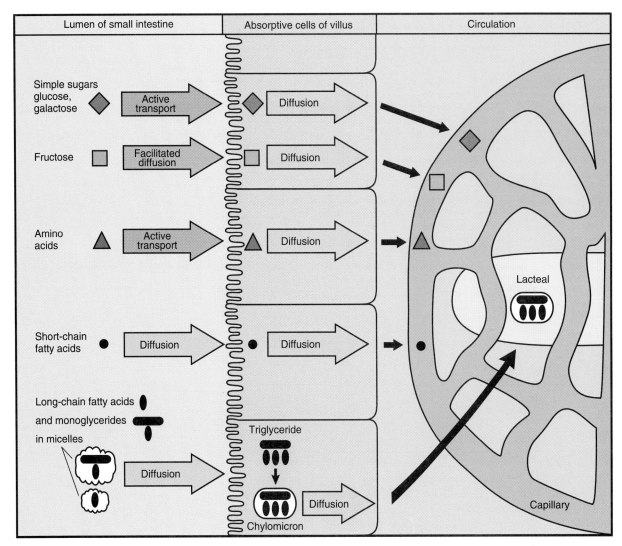

Lumen of small intestine	Absorptive cells of villus	Circulation

Simple sugars glucose, galactose — Active transport — Diffusion

Fructose — Facilitated diffusion — Diffusion

Amino acids — Active transport — Diffusion

Short-chain fatty acids — Diffusion — Diffusion

Long-chain fatty acids and monoglycerides in micelles — Diffusion — Triglyceride — Chylomicron — Diffusion

Lacteal

Capillary

Figure 16–14   Absorption of nutrients from the small intestine into blood and lymph capillaries.

Simple sugars and amino acids are absorbed into the blood capillaries in the villi of the small intestine and then are transported to the liver in the hepatic portal vein.

Monoglycerides and free fatty acids, the end products of fat digestion, are coated with bile salts to form tiny droplets, called **micelles** (mye-SELZ), in the lumen of the small intestine. The micelles come into close contact with the microvilli and because their contents, the monoglycerides and fatty acids, are lipid soluble, they diffuse across the cell membrane. The bile salts remain in the lumen to form additional micelles. Once inside the epithelial cells of the mucosa, a few short-chain fatty acids move directly into the blood capillaries of the villi. The monoglycerides and most of the fatty acids recombine to form triglycerides. These move to the Golgi apparatus where they combine with proteins to form **chylomicrons** (kye-loh-MYE-krons). The chylomicrons pass from the cells into the lacteals (lymph capillaries) in the villi. The mixture of lymph and digested fats is called **chyle.** Lymph carries the chy-

lomicrons through the lymphatic vessels into the thoracic duct, which empties into the left subclavian vein. At this point, the products of fat digestion enter the blood. Fat-soluble vitamins (A, D, E, and K) are absorbed with fats in the micelles. Table 16–4 summarizes absorption in the small intestine.

Fatty acids, monoglycerides, and fat-soluble vitamins enter the lacteals (lymph capillaries) in the villi of the small intestine.

✓ QuickCheck

● Will an obstruction of the common bile duct interfere more with the digestion of carbohydrates, digestion of proteins, or the digestion of fats? Why?

● How does the hormone cholecystokinin affect the pancreas?

● What membrane transport mechanism is responsible for the movement of nutrients from the cells of the villi into the blood and lymph capillaries?

Table 16–4 Absorption of Nutrients in the Small Intestine

Nutrient	Absorptive Mechanism	Transport Route
Water	Osmosis	Blood capillaries in villi
Glucose and galactose	Active transport into epithelial cells, then diffusion into capillaries	Blood capillaries in villi to hepatic portal circulation
Fructose	Facilitated diffusion into epithelial cells, then simple diffusion into capillaries	Blood capillaries in villi to hepatic portal circulation
Amino acids	Active transport into epithelial cells, then simple diffusion into capillaries	Blood capillaries in villi to hepatic portal circulation
Short-chain fatty acids	Simple diffusion into epithelial cells, then into capillaries	Blood capillaries of villi to hepatic portal circulation
Long-chain fatty acids, monoglycerides, and fat-soluble vitamins	Combine with bile salts to form micelles, then simple diffusion into epithelial cells; within the cell they form chylomicrons, which diffuse into lymph capillaries	Lymph capillaries (lacteals) of a villus
Electrolytes	Active transport and diffusion into epithelial cells, then into blood capillaries	Blood capillaries in villi to hepatic portal circulation
Water-soluble vitamins	Most are absorbed by diffusion into epithelial cells, then into blood capillaries; vitamin B_{12} requires intrinsic factor	Blood capillaries in villi to hepatic portal circulation

FOCUS ON AGING

Throughout life the digestive system normally functions day after day with relatively few problems. There may be an occasional episode of gastrointestinal tract inflammation, called gastroenteritis, caused by eating something that "doesn't agree," by irritation from excessively spicy foods, or from eating food that is contaminated by bacteria or toxins. Appendicitis tends to be fairly common in teenagers, but the incidence decreases with age because the opening into the appendix tends to become smaller and possibly eventually closes. Ulcers and gallbladder problems are associated with middle age, often considered to be the high stress time of life. Most of the difficulties in the digestive system before "old age" are due to external problems rather than to structural changes within the system itself.

Structural changes in the digestive system occur as part of the normal aging process. These changes affect the overall operation of the system and may influence the nutritional state of the aging individual. In the mouth, teeth may become loose, owing to periodontal disease, and have to be extracted. Because of dental problems, chewing may be uncomfortable. Salivary glands decrease their production of saliva, which reduces the salivary cleansing action and leads to a dry mouth (xerostomia). Thus, food is not adequately moistened for chewing and swallowing. Taste sensations diminish, partially because there is less saliva to dis-

solve the taste particles and partially because there are fewer taste receptors. Loneliness and the problems in the oral cavity associated with aging may make eating a chore rather than a pleasure.

The mucosa in the stomach and intestines undergoes some atrophy with advancing age. In the stomach this may lead to a deficiency in hydrochloric acid and gastric juice for digestion. Pernicious anemia may develop because there is a lack of intrinsic factor from the gastric mucosa. In the small intestine, mucosal atrophy may lead to fewer enzymes and shorter villi; however, this does not appear to impair digestion and absorption in normal healthy people. The wall of the large intestine becomes thinner and weakens. This makes older people more susceptible to diverticulosis, in which the wall bulges outward to form balloon-like pockets. Constipation is a common complaint in the elderly; statistically, however, there seems to be no basis for it. This is more likely due to lifestyle and habits than to structural changes in the digestive system.

Although structural and functional changes take place in the digestive system as part of the aging process, digestion and absorption are not altered noticeably in healthy older persons. A balanced diet, exercise, and a positive outlook on life will keep the digestive system in good working order for a long time.

Digestive System?

Eating Disorders

Food, fashion, fad, fat, and fear. What do these have in common and what do they have to do with the digestive system? The relationship of food to the digestive system is plain to see, but the connection between the others may be a little more obscure. Many Americans have an unhealthy fear of becoming fat. They are afraid that if they put on a few pounds, they will lose their friends. They feel that to be successful, they must be fashionable and to be fashionable they must be thin. Physiologic and psychological problems associated with the "fear of fat" have led to a growing concern about eating disorders. These are not new diseases. They have been mentioned in medical literature for many years, and there is evidence that the ancient Romans practiced a form of binge-purging in their orgies of feasting. The current growing interest in and concern about eating disorders arises from the dramatic increase in reported cases in recent years. Two of the most common eating disorders with a psychological basis are anorexia nervosa and bulimia.

Anorexia nervosa is self-imposed starvation with accompanying nutritional deficiencies and medical complications. It is primarily a disease of young women (90+ percent) from upwardly mobile families. Most victims are between the ages of 12 and 25. These people usually have a normal weight in the beginning but view themselves as overweight and have an intense fear of obesity. Consequently, they diet and exercise with a vengeance. Their excessive dieting and intense physical activity results in a 20 to 25 percent loss in body mass. This is accompanied by atrophy of skeletal muscle, impaired intellectual functioning, absence of menstruation in women, diminished metabolic rate, and decreased blood pressure. These individuals are likely to use laxatives and diuretics as additional methods of losing weight. This complicates their medical problems because it leads to dehydration and electrolyte imbalance.

Anorexia nervosa is fatal in approximately 10 percent of the cases. Death is often from cardiac disturbances that are the result of nutritional deficiency and electrolyte imbalance. Because anorexic individuals often have low self-esteem and are depressed, they have a higher than average suicide rate. The cause of this eating disorder is not clearly understood, but it is often brought on by anxiety and peer or family pressure. Because the cause is not well understood, treatment is varied and controversial. Both the medical and psychological problems have to be resolved for treatment to be successful.

Bulimia is characterized by binge-purge cycles. In contrast to the anorexia nervosa victims, who eat very little, bulimic individuals gorge themselves with food. The eating binge is followed by self-induced vomiting and laxatives to purge the food from the system. Because of this cycle, bulimia is sometimes referred to as the **binge-purge syndrome.** This eating disorder occurs in people who have a craving for food and an insatiable appetite but who have a fear of becoming fat. These people often have a normal weight and appear healthy. Bulimia primarily affects relatively young (mean age is 25), single women with a college education from upwardly mobile families.

Many bulimics experience low self-esteem and depression, but have a need to "succeed" at something. Their feeling of success comes from purging themselves because this is something over which they have control. Because they are depressed, these individuals frequently become chemically dependent and have a higher than normal suicide rate. Approximately 30 percent attempt suicide.

The purging half of the cycle results in a loss of stomach and intestinal contents. This leads to fluid and electrolyte imbalances that may result in convulsions, muscle spasms, and cardiac failure. Repeated vomiting increases the possibility of aspiration pneumonia. As the stomach contents flush upward, the acid damages the lining of the esophagus and mouth and causes an erosion of the tooth enamel. Bulimia may be fatal and the longer the binge-purge cycles continue, the greater the mortality from medical complications. Treatment is directed at helping the patients cope with stress and breaking the binge-purge cycles. Nutritional counseling and psychotherapy are important aspects of treatment.

Eating disorders evolve slowly over a period of time. The longer they continue, the harder it is to treat them. It is important to recognize the signs and discover the underlying stresses that prompt this behavior modification. The victims of eating disorders need support and encouragement to make the changes necessary for their own survival.

Representative Disorders of the Digestive System

Related to Malabsorption

Lactose intolerance
Crohn's disease
Pernicious anemia

Related to Motility

Dysphagia
Gastroesophageal reflux
Hiatal hernia
Obstruction

Related to Inflammation and Ulceration

Appendicitis
Peptic ulcers
Gastritis

Disorders Related to the Digestive System

Related to the Liver

Hepatitis
Cirrhosis

Related to the Pancreas

Pancreatitis
Diabetes mellitus

Related to the Gallbladder

Cholelithiasis
Cholecystitis

CHAPTER QUIZ

RECALL

Match the definitions on the left with the appropriate term on the right.

1. Fold of peritoneum that attaches small intestines to the dorsal body wall

2. Semifluid mixture that leaves the stomach

3. Movements that propel food particles through the digestive tract

4. Longitudinal folds in the stomach

5. Swallowing

6. Circular folds in the small intestine

7. Middle region of the small intestine

8. Fold of peritoneum that attaches the liver to the anterior abdominal wall

9. Phagocytic cells in the liver

10. Chemical reactions of digestion

A. Chyme

B. Deglutition

C. Falciform ligament

D. Hydrolysis

E. Jejunum

F. Kupffer cells

G. Mesentery

H. Peristalsis

I. Plicae circulares

J. Rugae

THOUGHT

1. The simple columnar epithelial cells in the stomach are a part of the
   a. serosa
   b. adventitia
   c. submucosa
   d. mucosa

2. The inactive enzyme pepsinogen is secreted by
   a. chief cells in the stomach
   b. crypts in the small intestine
   c. acinar cells in the pancreas
   d. parietal cells in the stomach

3. If the pH in the duodenum decreases to 4.0, secretion of which of the following will be increased?
   a. enterokinase
   b. bile

   c. secretin
   d. pepsinogen

4. An obstruction of the common bile duct
   a. blocks the flow of cholecystokinin into the duodenum
   b. is likely to interfere with fat digestion
   c. blocks the action of enterokinase
   d. is likely to interfere with carbohydrate digestion

5. Which one of the following does NOT increase surface area for absorption in the small intestine?
   a. plicae circulares
   b. villi
   c. taenia coli
   d. microvilli (brush border)

APPLICATION

Surgical removal of the stomach will most likely interfere with the absorption of which vitamin? Explain.

John suffers from chronic stomach ulcers. His gastroenterologist suggests a treatment that involves cutting branches of the vagus nerve that go to the stomach. Explain the rationale of this treatment.

CHAPTER 17

Metabolism and Nutrition

Outline/Objectives

Introduction 354

- Define the terms *metabolism* and *nutrition*.

Metabolism of Absorbed Nutrients 354

- Distinguish between anabolism and catabolism.
- Describe the basic steps in glycolysis, citric acid cycle, and electron transport.
- Define glycogen, glycogenesis, glycogenolysis, and gluconeogenesis.
- Describe the pathway by which fatty acids are broken down to produce adenosine triphosphate.
- Name two key molecules in the metabolism and interconversion of carbohydrates, proteins, and fats.
- State four factors that influence basal metabolism.

Basic Elements of Nutrition 361

- List the functions of carbohydrates, proteins, and fats in the body.
- State the caloric value of carbohydrates, proteins, and fats.
- Explain the importance of fiber in the diet.

- Distinguish between essential and nonessential amino acids and between complete and incomplete proteins.
- Discuss the functions of vitamins, minerals, and water in the body.

Key Terms

Acetyl-CoA

Anabolism

Basal metabolic rate

Catabolism

Citric acid cycle

Complete protein

Core temperature

Glycolysis

Thermogenesis

Building Vocabulary

WORD PART	MEANING
ana-	up
-bol-	throw, put
cata-	down
-gen-	producing
lys-	to take apart
mal-	bad, poor
neo-	new
nutri-	to nourish
pyr-	fever, fire
therm-	temperature
-tion	process of
vita-	life

Metabolism (meh-TAB-oh-lizm) is the aggregate of all the chemical reactions that take place in the body. Some of these reactions result in digestion and absorption, which are described in Chapter 16. After nutrients are absorbed by the cells, chemical reactions within the cells synthesize new materials for cellular use or secretion and produce energy for body activities. These reactions constitute **cellular metabolism,** which is described in this chapter. Each metabolic reaction, including those in cellular metabolism, requires a specific enzyme. The enzymes speed up the reactions so the rate at which they occur is consistent with life. Without the enzymes, the reaction rates are too slow to sustain life.

Nutrition (noo-TRIH-shun) is the acquisition, assimilation, and utilization of the nutrients that are contained in food. The energy for body activities ultimately comes from the food that is taken into the body. Because metabolism is the utilization of nutrients, the basic elements of nutrition are included in this chapter.

> Metabolism includes all the chemical reactions in the body, including the utilization of nutrients. Nutrition is the acquisition, assimilation, and utilization of nutrients.

Metabolism of Absorbed Nutrients

Chemical reactions either require energy or release energy. Metabolic processes are divided into two categories on this basis. **Anabolism** (ah-NAB-oh-lizm) includes the building-up, or synthesis, reactions that require energy. **Catabolism** (kah-TAB-oh-lizm) involves breaking down large molecules into smaller ones and releases energy.

> Metabolic reactions are divided into anabolism and catabolism.

Anabolism

Anabolism is the constructive portion of metabolism. These reactions use chemical energy, usually in the form of **adenosine triphosphate (ATP),** to make large molecules from smaller ones. Glucose molecules are linked together in long chains to make the larger glycogen molecules. Amino acids are connected by peptide bonds to form complex protein molecules. Glycerol and fatty acids combine to form triglycerides. In each of these examples, the smaller molecules react to produce a water molecule and a larger molecule (Fig. 17–1). Anabolic reactions such as these represent **dehydration synthesis** because a water molecule is removed and a larger molecule is synthesized. Chemical energy is required to form the new bonds in these reactions.

> The reactions of anabolism use energy to form chemical bonds and to build large molecules from smaller ones.

Catabolism

Catabolism is the part of metabolism in which large molecules are broken down into smaller ones. The **hydrolysis** reactions of digestion are examples of catabolism. Water is used to split the large molecule into two smaller parts (see Fig. 17–1). Another example of catabolism is the cellular utilization of nutrients. After the products of digestion are absorbed into the cells of the body, they are "burned," or oxidized, in the processes of **cellular respiration.** The chemical bonds break, releasing chemical energy that is used to drive the reactions of anabolism.

> The reactions of catabolism release energy when large molecules break down into smaller ones.

CLINICAL TERMS

Celiac disease (SEE-lee-ak dih-zeez) Condition in which the ingestion of gluten destroys the villi of the small intestine resulting in a malabsorption of nutrients

Heat exhaustion (HEET eks-AW-shun) Condition characterized by fluid and electrolyte loss due to profuse perspiration, but body temperature remains normal; symptoms include muscle cramps, dizziness, vomiting, low blood pressure, and fainting; also called heat prostration

Hypervitaminosis (hye-per-vye-tah-min-OH-sis) An excess of one or more vitamins, usually from the consumption of vitamin supplements; may become toxic and deadly

Hypothermia (hye-poh-THER-mee-ah) Refers to body temperature of 35° C (95° F) or below

Kwashiorkor (kwosh-ee-OR-kor) Condition in which protein intake is deficient despite normal or nearly normal calorie intake

Malnutrition (mal-noo-TRIH-shun) A state of poor nutrition

Marasmus (mar-AZ-mus) Condition in which there is deficiency in both protein and calorie intake

Pica (PYE-kah) Craving for substances not normally considered nutrients, such as dirt

Undernutrition (un-der-noo-TRIH-shun) Inadequate food intake

A Carbohydrates

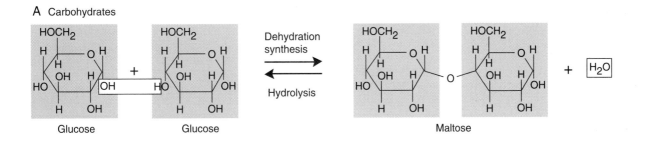

B Proteins

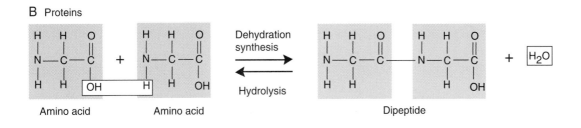

C Fats

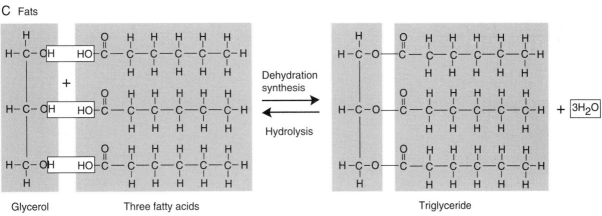

Figure 17–1   Dehydration synthesis and hydrolysis. *(A)* Carbohydrates. *(B)* Proteins. *(C)* Fats.

Energy From Foods

Within the body cells, the reactions of cellular respiration break chemical bonds and release energy. Some of this energy is captured and stored as chemical energy in molecules of ATP. The remainder is given off as heat, which is used to maintain body temperature. ATP is the energy exchange molecule in the cell (Fig. 17–2). When energy is needed for active transport, muscle contraction, or synthesis reactions, a high-energy bond in ATP breaks and gives off energy, a phosphate, and adenosine diphosphate (ADP). When energy is released from catabolic reactions, it combines with the ADP and a phosphate to form new ATP. Cellular respiration utilizes the absorbed end products of digestion and, through a series of reactions, generates ATP.

In the cell, chemical energy is stored in the high-energy bonds of ATP.

Carbohydrates

The absorbed end products of carbohydrate digestion are monosaccharides, or simple sugars. The most important of these 6-carbon molecules in cellular respiration is glucose.

The first series of reactions in the catabolism of glucose is **glycolysis** (gly-KAHL-ih-sis). These reactions take place in the cytoplasm of the cell and they are **anaerobic,** which means that they do not require oxygen. During glycolysis, a 6-carbon molecule of glucose is split into two 3-carbon molecules of **pyruvic acid** (Fig. 17–3). These reactions require two ATP molecules to get them started, but they yield four ATP molecules for a net gain of two ATP molecules.

Glycolysis takes place in the cytoplasm and does not require oxygen.

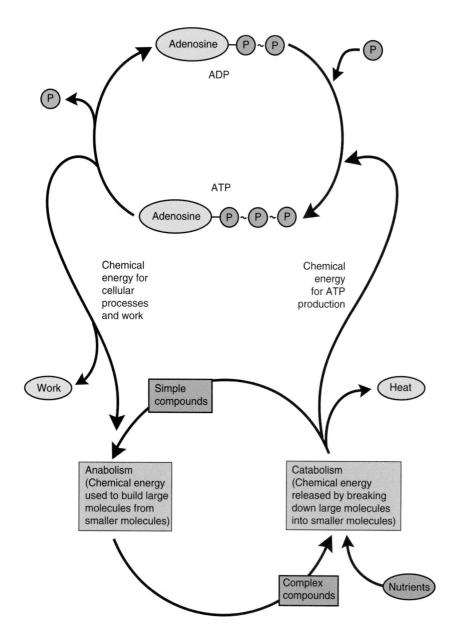

Figure 17–2 Energy exchange in ATP.

The fate of the pyruvic acid that is produced in glycolysis depends on whether oxygen is absent or present. In the absence of oxygen, the pyruvic acid is converted to **lactic acid,** which is the end product of anaerobic respiration. Most of the lactic acid diffuses out of the cells that produce it, enters the blood, and is transported to the liver. When sufficient oxygen becomes available, the liver converts lactic acid back to glucose. The oxygen necessary for this conversion is called **oxygen debt.**

If oxygen is present when pyruvic acid is produced, the pyruvic acid enters the aerobic phase of cellular respiration, which takes place in the mitochondria. Pyruvic acid enters the mitochondria and goes through a series of reactions that remove one of the carbons to form carbon dioxide and produces a 2-carbon molecule of **acetyl-CoA.** Within the mito-

chondria acetyl-CoA enters a cyclic series of reactions called the **citric acid cycle** (Krebs cycle). To start these reactions, the 2-carbon acetyl-CoA combines with a 4-carbon molecule in the cycle to form the 6-carbon molecule of citric acid. During the cycle, 2 carbons are removed to form carbon dioxide, energy is released, hydrogen ions are removed, and a 4-carbon molecule is produced. This 4-carbon molecule combines with another acetyl-CoA and the cycle is repeated. The carbon dioxide is exhaled in breathing. Carrier molecules (nicotinamide-adenine dinucleotide and flavin-adenine dinucleotide) transport the hydrogen ions to the **electron-transport chain,** a series of molecules along the inner mitochondrial membrane. Here, in reactions that require oxygen, the hydrogen ions combine with oxygen to form water; and in the process, ATP is produced.

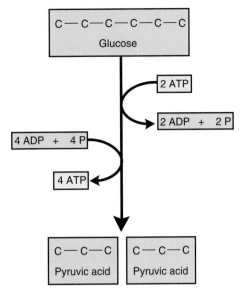

Figure 17-3   Glycolysis.

The final result of the aerobic reactions in the mitochondria is the production of carbon dioxide, water, and energy. Some of the energy forms ATP, the remainder is released as heat. The complete breakdown of a 6-carbon glucose molecule yields 36 to 38 molecules of ATP: 2 from the anaerobic glycolysis phase, and 34 to 36 from the aerobic phase within the mitochondria (Fig. 17-4).

> If oxygen is present, pyruvic acid enters the mitochondria and goes through the reactions of the citric acid cycle and electron-transport chain. The complete breakdown of glucose yields 36 to 38 molecules of ATP.

After meals, when glucose is absorbed from the digestive tract, blood glucose levels increase. The liver removes the excess glucose from the blood and stores it as **glycogen.** Some glycogen is stored in skeletal muscle and later used for skeletal muscle activity. The production of glycogen from glucose is called **glycogenesis** (gly-koh-JEN-eh-sis) (Fig. 17-5). When glycogen storage is at full capacity, glucose may be converted to fat by a process called **lipogenesis** (lip-oh-JEN-eh-sis). When blood glucose levels start to decline before the next meal, glycogen breaks down to form glucose. **Glycogenolysis** (gly-koh-jen-AHL-ih-sis) is the conversion of glycogen into glucose. Glycogenesis and glycogenolysis help keep blood glucose levels relatively constant. In addition, some noncarbohydrate nutrient sources may be converted to glucose through **gluconeogenesis** (gloo-koh-nee-oh-JEN-eh-sis).

> Blood glucose levels are maintained through the processes of glycogenesis, glycogenolysis, and gluconeogenesis.

> Many poisons function by blocking one of the steps in the metabolic pathways. This leads to a decrease in the number of ATP molecules that are produced; consequently there is not enough energy for cellular processes, which can lead to death.

Proteins

The end products of protein digestion are amino acids, which are absorbed into the capillaries in the villi of the small intestine. From the villi, the amino acids enter the hepatic portal circulation to the liver and then enter the general circulation pathways in the body so they are available to all body cells.

Amino acids are used by body cells for a wide variety of functions. Most of these involve the synthesis of proteins that are needed by the body cells. Examples of these anabolic reactions are proteins to build new tissues or to replace damaged tissues and the synthesis of hemoglobin, hormones, enzymes, and plasma proteins. The creation of proteins from amino acids involves dehydration synthesis reactions (see Fig. 17-1) in which water is removed to form peptide bonds between the amino acids.

> Amino acids are used to synthesize proteins that are needed by the body to build new tissues, to replace damaged tissues, and for the synthesis of hemoglobin, hormones, enzymes, and plasma proteins.

If there is an excess of amino acids or insufficient carbohydrates and fats, then the amino acids may be used as an energy source. This is an example of catabolism. The principal reaction that prepares an amino acid for use as an energy source is **deamination** (dee-am-ih-NAY-shun), which occurs in the liver. Deamination removes the amino group ($-NH_2$) from the amino acid to form ammonia and a deaminated portion called a keto acid. Ammonia is toxic to cells so the liver converts it to urea, which is less toxic and is excreted in the urine.

Depending on the amino acid involved, the deaminated portion is used in one of several pathways (Fig. 17-6). For some, the pathway leads directly into the citric acid cycle. Others are converted to pyruvic acid or to acetyl-CoA, which then enters the citric acid cycle. All of these pathways ultimately produce carbon dioxide, water, and energy. If energy is not needed immediately, excess amino acids may be converted into glucose by gluconeogenesis or into fat molecules by lipogenesis.

> Amino acids may be used as an energy source by removing the amino group. The resulting keto acid enters the citric acid cycle pathway to produce energy.

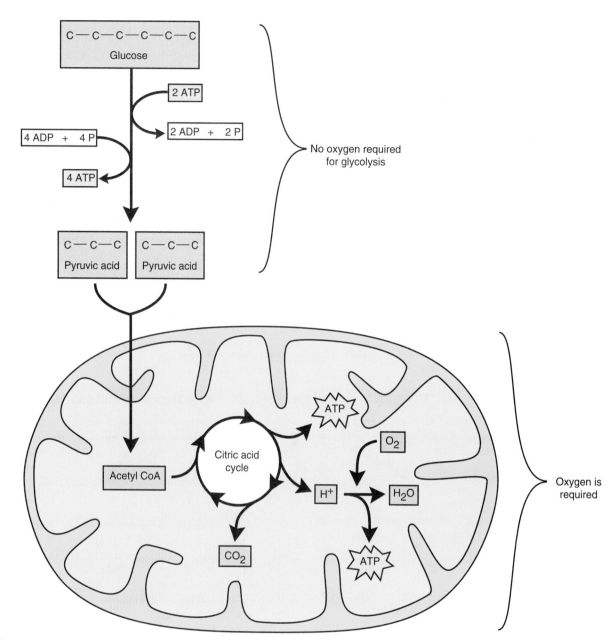

Figure 17-4 Complete breakdown of glucose.

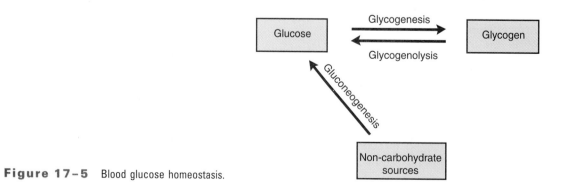

Figure 17-5 Blood glucose homeostasis.

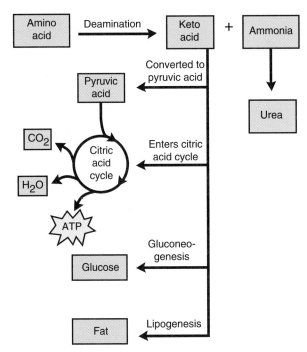

Figure 17-6 Catabolism of amino acids for energy.

Ketone bodies form when there is an excess of acetyl-CoA. In fasting and other conditions in which fats instead of carbohydrates are used as an energy source, ketone bodies form from the acetyl-CoA that is produced by beta oxidation. A buildup of ketone bodies in the blood is called ketosis. Because most of the ketone bodies are acids, the pH of the blood decreases and acidosis develops. Death results if the pH becomes too low.

Interconversion of Carbohydrates, Proteins, and Lipids

The preceding paragraphs indicate that carbohydrates, proteins, and fats can be converted to products that enter the citric acid cycle to ultimately yield energy. Pyruvic acid and acetyl-CoA are key molecules in these conversion pathways. Because the reactions are reversible, these molecules are intermediates in the pathways for the interconversion of carbohydrates, fats, and proteins. The formation of triglycerides from carbohydrates and proteins is called lipogenesis. Figure 17-8 summarizes the metabolic pathways for the nutrients that produce energy.

▎ Pyruvic acid and acetyl-CoA are key molecules in the metabolism of carbohydrates, proteins, and fats.

Lipids

Approximately 40 percent of the calories in the normal American diet are derived from fats. Furthermore, an average of 30 to 50 percent of the ingested carbohydrates are converted to triglycerides and stored. All body cells, except brain cells, can use fatty acids from triglycerides instead of glucose as an energy source. Lipids are an important factor in the body's metabolism.

▎ Lipids are an important source of energy.

Before triglycerides can be used as an energy source, they are changed into glycerol and fatty acids by hydrolysis. The glycerol enters the glycolysis pathway and continues through the citric acid cycle to yield carbon dioxide, water, and energy. Fatty acids undergo a series of reactions, called **beta oxidation** (BAY-tah oxih-DAY-shun). Beta oxidation removes 2-carbon segments from the end of a fatty acid chain and converts them into acetyl-CoA. The process keeps repeating, 2 carbon atoms at a time, until the entire fatty acid chain is converted into acetyl-CoA molecules. The acetyl-CoA molecules enter the citric acid cycle to yield carbon dioxide, water, and energy. Figure 17-7 illustrates the catabolic pathways for lipids.

▎ Fatty acids are converted to acetyl-CoA by beta oxidation. The acetyl-CoA enters the citric acid cycle to produce ATP.

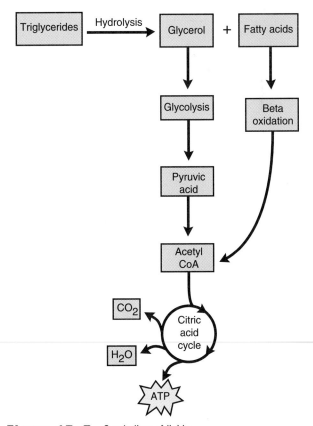

Figure 17-7 Catabolism of lipids.

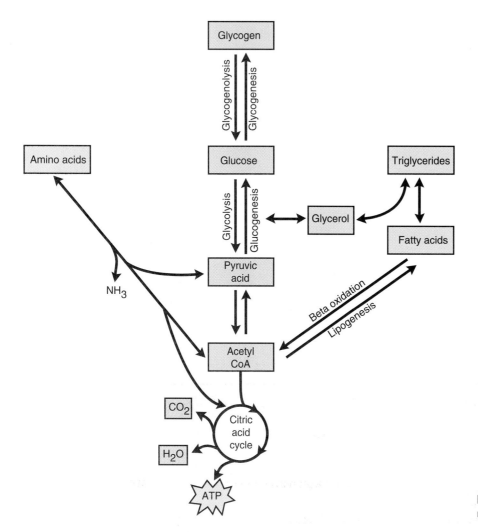

Figure 17–8 Summary of metabolic pathways.

Chronic alcoholism frequently leads to cirrhosis of the liver. Liver enzymes convert the alcohol into acetyl-CoA and in the process form reduced nicotinamide adenine dinucleotide (NADH) molecules, which enter the electron-transport chain to produce ATP. High levels of NADH in the cell from the metabolism of alcohol inhibit glycolysis and the Krebs cycle, consequently, sugars and amino acids are converted into fat instead of being used for energy. The fat is deposited in the liver cells, which die as a result of the fat accumulation. Scar tissue replaces the cells that die, resulting in cirrhosis of the liver. This condition can lead to death because the scar tissue is unable to perform the functions of viable liver cells.

☑ **Quick**Check

● Is the hydrolysis of maltose into two molecules of glucose an example of catabolism or of anabolism?

● Where in the cell does the catabolism of pyruvic acid into carbon dioxide and water and ATP occur?

● What two molecules are the keys, or central, to the interconversion of carbohydrates, proteins, and lipids?

Uses for Energy

The energy derived from food is measured in units called **kilocalories** (kcal), or "large" **Calories** (C). One Calorie is the amount of energy required to raise the temperature of 1 kg of water 1°C, for example, from 14° C to 15° C. This energy is used by the body in three different ways:

• Basal metabolism
• Physical activity
• Thermogenesis, or assimilation of food

These three factors added together make up the total metabolic rate (Fig. 17–9). If caloric intake exceeds the needs for metabolism, then there is weight gain.

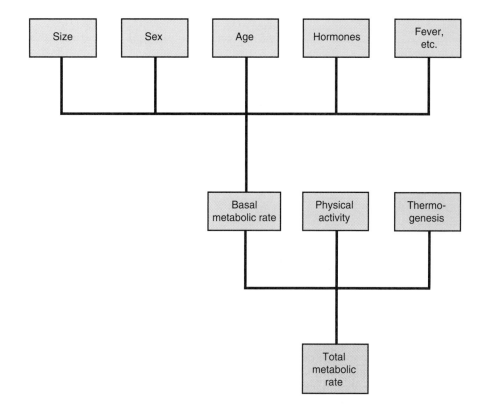

Figure 17–9 Factors that affect basal and total metabolic rates.

Basal Metabolism

The **basal metabolic rate** (BMR) is the amount of energy that is necessary to maintain life and to keep the body functioning at a minimal level. It includes the functioning of the heart, lungs, nervous system, kidney, and liver at a maintenance level in resting conditions. BMR is calculated by measuring the amount of oxygen that is used when an individual is awake but in a relaxed and resting state. The amount of oxygen used is proportional to the energy expended.

Several factors influence basal metabolism (see Fig. 17–9). Males tend to have a higher metabolic rate than females of the same age and size. Individuals with greater muscle mass usually have higher rates. Fever increases the metabolic rate, and age decreases it. Hormones such as thyroxine, growth hormone, and epinephrine increase the metabolic rate. On an average, 60 to 75 percent of the energy used each day is for basal metabolism.

> Basal metabolism is the energy that is necessary to keep the body functioning at a minimal level.

Physical Activity

Because muscle contraction requires energy, physical activity contributes to the total energy used each day. Muscular activity accounts for less than 25 percent of the total daily expenditure for an individual with a sedentary lifestyle; however, this increases with physical activity. Of the three ways in which

the body uses energy (basal metabolism, physical activity, and thermogenesis), the only one a person can reasonably control is physical activity. Assuming that calorie (energy) intake remains constant, increasing the amount of physical activity tends to encourage weight loss.

> Physical activity is the only avenue of energy expenditure that can be controlled voluntarily.

Thermogenesis

Thermogenesis (thur-moh-JEN-eh-sis) is the production of heat in response to food intake. When food is digested, transported, absorbed, and metabolized, heat is produced. In other words, it takes energy to process the food. Less than 10 percent of the caloric intake is used in the assimilation of food, or thermogenesis.

> Thermogenesis is the energy needed to utilize food. This accounts for less than 10 percent of the energy used in the body.

Basic Elements of Nutrition

Nutrition is the science that studies the relationship of food to the functioning of the living organism. The intake of food and digestive processes described in Chapter 16 are part of the broad subject of nutrition. The release of energy from metabolic processes, described in the first part of this chapter, is also a

Table 17–1 Nutrient Functions				
Carbohydrates	Proteins	Lipids	Vitamins	Minerals
Energy	Provide structure	Energy	Function with enzymes	Component of body
Bulk	Regulate body	Essential fatty acids		structures
Make other compounds	processes	Transport for fat-		Part of enzyme
	Enzymes	soluble vitamins		molecules
	Hormones	Structure components		Part of organic
	Carrier molecules	Insulation		molecules
	Fluid and elec-	Cushions organs		(hemoglobin)
	trolyte balance			Fluid and electrolyte
	Energy			balance

part of nutrition. This section primarily deals with nutrients, the substances in food that are necessary to maintain the normal functions of human organisms. Nutrients include carbohydrates, proteins, lipids, vitamins, and minerals. The functions of the nutrients are summarized in Table 17–1.

Carbohydrates

Carbohydrates have three major functions in the body. Of these, the most important is to provide energy. They are the most abundant and least expensive food sources of energy. On an average, 1 gram of pure carbohydrate yields 4 Calories of energy and 50 to 60 percent of the daily caloric intake is from this source. Carbohydrates also add bulk to the diet and are used to make other compounds, such as lipids, amino acids, and nucleic acids, in the body.

> Carbohydrates are a primary energy source, add bulk to the diet, and are used to synthesize other molecules. One gram of pure carbohydrate yields 4 Calories of energy.

Dietary carbohydrates are divided into two groups (Table 17–2):

• Simple sugars
• Complex polysaccharides

The sugars include the monosaccharides and disaccharides, which dissolve in water, form crystals, and

Table 17–2 Summary of Dietary Carbohydrates	
Simple Sugars	Complex Polysaccharides
Monosaccharides	Starch (glucose storage in
Glucose (blood sugar)	plants)
Fructose (fruit sugar, honey)	Glycogen (glucose storage in
Galactose (part of lactose)	animals)
Disaccharides	Fiber (nondigestible plant
Sucrose (table sugar)	polysaccharides)
Maltose (malt sugar)	
Lactose (milk sugar)	

taste sweet. Three monosaccharides (**glucose, fructose,** and **galactose**) are important in nutrition. Glucose is the form in which carbohydrate is carried in the blood, and it is easily broken down to provide energy. Fructose is found in honey and in many fruits. Galactose does not exist as a molecule in any food but it is a part of the disaccharide lactose molecule. Fructose and galactose are converted to glucose in the liver. When two monosaccharide molecules combine, they form a disaccharide. Three disaccharides (**sucrose, maltose,** and **lactose**) are commonly found in food. Sucrose, the familiar table sugar, is formed from glucose and fructose. It is obtained by refining sugar cane and sugar beets. It is also found in many fruits and vegetables. Maltose, which is formed from two glucose molecules, is found in sprouting grains, corn syrup, and maple syrup. It is commonly called malt sugar. Lactose, which is a combination of glucose and galactose, is found in milk and is commonly called milk sugar.

> Sugars include monosaccharides and disaccharides.

Complex polysaccharides are formed from long chains of several thousand monosaccharide units, usually glucose. In contrast to the simple sugars, these large molecules do not dissolve in water, do not form crystals, and do not taste particularly sweet. Three types of complex polysaccharides—**starch, glycogen,** and **fiber**—are important in nutrition.

Starch is the storage form of energy in plants, where it is found in the seeds and roots. Cereal grains (wheat, oats, corn, barley), starchy roots (potatoes and turnips), and legumes (peas and beans) are important sources of calories in many countries.

Glycogen is the storage form of energy in animals. Liver and muscle tissues have the ability to combine glucose molecules into highly branched long chains to form glycogen. The process of converting glucose to glycogen is called glycogenesis.

Fiber, which comes from plant sources, represents numerous polysaccharides that cannot be digested by enzymes in the human digestive system. Some of the fibers, however, are broken down by bacteria in the intestine. Fiber adds bulk to the diet, which enhances the absorption of nutrients and helps move the contents of the large intestine faster and with less effort. In unprocessed foods, starch and fiber are usually found together, but processing or refining removes the fiber. The practice of eating refined or processed carbohydrates results in too little fiber in the diet. Numerous diseases are related to decreased dietary fiber and include constipation, hemorrhoids, colon cancer, cardiovascular disease, obesity, and diabetes. Dietitians recommend diets that include 25 to 35 grams of fiber per day. Table 17–3 compares the fiber content of some common foods.

> Complex polysaccharides are starch, glycogen, and fiber. Starch is carbohydrate that is stored in plants. Glycogen is carbohydrate that is stored in animals. Fiber comes from plant sources, is not digestible, and adds bulk to the diet.

Proteins

Proteins have three major categories of functions in the body. One function is to provide structure. The matrix of bone, muscles, teeth, tendons, and other structures is composed of protein. The cell membrane and membranous organelles within the cell contain protein to provide structure. Another function of proteins is to regulate body processes. Hormones and enzymes are proteins that regulate body functions and control chemical reactions. Plasma proteins have an important role in maintaining fluid and electrolyte balance. Other proteins act as carrier molecules to transport substances across the cell membrane or to transport substances in the blood and in this way regulate body-transport processes. Proteins also supply energy for the body. If there is inadequate carbohydrate and lipid available to meet the energy needs, the amino acids in proteins are metabolized to provide the necessary calories. One

Table 17–3 Dietary Fiber in Some Common Foods

Food	Amount	Weight (grams)	Calories	Dietary Fiber (grams)
Fruit				
Apple, with peel	1 medium	138	80	3.9
Apple juice	1 cup	228	116	0.7
Banana, peeled	1 medium	110	100	2.5
Orange, peeled	1 medium	145	67	3.1
Prunes, dried	3 medium	8	60	3.5
Vegetables, Cooked				
Potato with skin, baked	1 large	200	220	3.9
Carrots, sliced	1 cup	150	60	5.0
Broccoli	1 spear	180	53	6.2
Green beans	1 cup	130	40	3.3
Corn	1 cup	164	134	7.7
Peas	1 cup	160	130	7.4
Vegetables, Raw				
Celery	1 cup	120	19	2.0
Carrots	1 medium	72	31	2.0
Tomato	1 medium	120	24	2.0
Lettuce, chopped	1 cup	56	53	0.8
Cauliflower	1 cup	100	24	2.7
Legumes and Nuts				
Navy beans, cooked	1 cup	190	225	13.0
Lima beans, cooked	1 cup	170	170	9.2
Lentils, cooked	1 cup	200	215	8.7
Pecans, dried, halves	1 cup	108	720	6.5
Walnuts, English, chopped	1 cup	120	770	8.4
Peanut butter, regular	1 tablespoon	16	95	1.0
Bread and Pasta				
White bread	1 slice	28	75	0.5
Whole wheat bread	1 slice	28	70	2.4
Spaghetti, cooked	1 cup	130	190	1.0
Brown rice, cooked	1 cup	195	232	2.8
White rice, cooked	1 cup	205	223	0.6

gram of pure protein provides 4 Calories of energy. Guidelines for protein consumption recommend that 10 to 12 percent of a normal healthy adult's daily caloric intake be in the form of proteins. Most Americans eat more than this amount.

> Proteins provide structure, regulate body-transport processes, and provide energy. One gram of protein yields 4 Calories of energy.

The purpose of proteins in the diet is to provide amino acids. The body cannot store amino acids for later use so a daily supply of protein is necessary. When there are excess amino acids, they are broken down and used to make glycogen or fat. If adequate amounts of the required amino acids are available, the body makes the various proteins that it needs. About half of the different amino acids that the body uses must be supplied because they cannot be synthesized in the body. These are called **essential amino acids.** The other amino acids are called **nonessential** because they can be made in the body and do not have to be supplied (see Table 2–4).

A **complete protein** contains all of the essential amino acids. Animal proteins such as meat, eggs, and dairy products are complete proteins. Vegetable proteins such as nuts, grains, and legumes are **incomplete proteins** because they do not contain all of the essential amino acids. Vegetable proteins, eaten in some combinations, often complement each other to provide all of the essential amino acids and are equivalent to eating a complete protein. Another point to consider is the fact that animal proteins often contain high amounts of fat and are often more expensive than vegetable proteins. Some common combinations that provide all the essential amino acids are wheat bread with peanut butter, corn and lima beans, rice with black beans, and corn bread with split pea soup.

> Incomplete proteins should be eaten in combinations that provide all the essential amino acids.

Kwashiorkor is a disease caused by protein deficiency. It occurs when the diet includes an adequate number of calories but insufficient protein. This disease results in wasting of tissues, decreased amounts of plasma proteins, abdominal bloating (ascites), and dermatitis.

Lipids

Most **lipids** in the diet are triglycerides, or neutral fats, which occur in both animal and plant food. These molecules are composed of three fatty acids attached to a glycerol molecule. Other lipids are phospholipids and steroids.

Lipids have six important functions in the body. They are stored in the body as adipose tissue, or fat, and represent a concentrated source of energy. Each gram of lipid provides 9 Calories, more than twice as much as carbohydrates or proteins. Lipids are necessary in the diet to provide essential fatty acids that cannot be synthesized in the body. Fat-soluble

Table 17–4	Common Sources of Fat and Cholesterol					
Food	Amount	Weight (grams)	Total Calories	Total Fat (grams)	Saturated Fat (grams)	Cholesterol (milligrams)
Milk, nonfat	1 cup	244	86	0.4 (4%)*	0.3 (3%)*	4
Milk, 2%	1 cup	244	121	4.8 (36%)	2.9 (2%)	22
Milk, whole	1 cup	244	151	8.2 (49%)	5.0 (30%)	33
Egg, hard boiled	1 whole	50	79	5.6 (64%)	1.7 (19%)	274
Cream cheese	1 ounce	28.3	100	10.0 (90%)	6.3 (57%)	31.4
Mayonnaise	1 tablespoon	13.8	99	10.9 (99%)	1.7 (15%)	8.1
Butter	1 tablespoon	14.2	102	11.5 (100%)	7.2 (63%)	31.1
Cheese, American	1 ounce	28.3	107	9.0 (76%)	5.7 (48%)	27.3
Cheese, Cheddar	1 ounce	28.3	115	9.2 (72%)	5.8 (45%)	27.3
Sirloin steak	3 ounces	85	240	15.0 (66%)	6.4 (24%)	74
Ground beef	3 ounces	85	230	16.0 (63%)	6.2 (24%)	74
Chicken breast (no skin)	3 ounces	86	142	3.0 (19%)	0.9 (6%)	73
Fried chicken	3 ounces	85	187	7.8 (38%)	2.1 (10%)	79.6
Frankfurter	2 ounces	57	183	16.6 (82%)	6.1 (30%)	29
Turkey, roasted	3 ounces	85	145	4.2 (26%)	1.4 (9%)	65
Cod, broiled	3 ounces	85	97	0.9 (8%)	0.8 (7%)	51
Tuna salad	½ cup	102	188	9.5 (45%)	1.6 (8%)	40
Avocado	1 medium	201	324	30.8 (86%)	4.9 (14%)	0

*Percentage of the total calories represented by the fat.

vitamins (A, D, E, K) require lipids for their absorption and transport. Numerous structural components in the body are lipid in nature. The major component of cell membranes is phospholipid, and myelin, the covering around nerve fibers, is a fatty substance. Adipose tissue under the skin helps maintain body temperature by providing insulation. Adipose also forms a cushion around body organs to protect them from bumps, jolts, and damage.

> Lipids are an important source of energy, provide essential fatty acids, transport vitamins, are components of certain structural elements, provide heat insulation, and form protective cushions. One gram of fat yields 9 Calories of energy.

The preceding paragraph indicates that fats are essential components of the diet. Less than 3 percent of the total caloric intake in the form of fats is considered to be inadequate lipid consumption to maintain health. This most often occurs in infants who are fed nonfat milk. These infants may not get sufficient amounts of the essential fatty acids that are important for growth and thus their development will be impaired.

Although fats are essential components of a healthy diet, excessive amounts are not desirable. Most Americans need to consciously strive to reduce their intake of dietary fat. The American Heart Association recommends that no more than 30 percent of the daily calorie intake should be in the form of fats. This means that a person who eats 2,200 Calories per day should eat no more than 660 Calories, or about 75 grams, of fat. In general, the American diet has 40 percent or more of its calories coming from fats. This overconsumption of fats is unhealthy and is related to cardiovascular disease, obesity, diabetes, and some cancers.

Not only does the American diet contain too much fat, it has the wrong kinds of fat. The American Heart Association recommends that less than 10 percent of the daily caloric intake, or 25 grams, be in the form of saturated fats. Currently, in the United States, 15 to 20 percent of the daily calories are from saturated fats. Most foods that contain fats have a combination of saturated and unsaturated forms. In general, if a fat is solid at room temperature it has more saturated than unsaturated fat. Animal fats also tend to have more saturated fat. Foods high in saturated fats include beef, pork, lamb, eggs, butter, and whole-milk products. Coconut oil, palm oil, and hydrogenated vegetable oils in shortening and margarine are also high in saturated fats. Many foods that are high in saturated fats are also high in cholesterol. The recommendation is that cholesterol be limited to less than 250 mg per day, which is the amount in one egg yolk. Table 17–4 compares some common sources of fats and cholesterol.

Good cholesterol. Bad cholesterol. What's the difference? Cholesterol and fats are insoluble in water and to become soluble they combine with a blood protein. This combination of cholesterol, fat, and protein is called a lipoprotein, which functions to transport cholesterol to and from the tissues. Small dense lipoproteins are called high-density lipoproteins (HDLs) and function to remove cholesterol from your arteries and carry it to the liver. This is known as "good cholesterol." Large lipoproteins are called low-density lipoproteins (LDLs) and carry cholesterol to the tissues. This "bad cholesterol" lodges in the walls or arteries; and the higher the LDL level the greater the risk of coronary artery disease. Simple ways to decrease LDL levels are through diet and exercise.

When evaluating a person's diet, the proportion of fat is a very important aspect to consider in addition to the number of calories. The conversion of dietary fat to body fat requires less energy than the conversion of carbohydrates to fat. If two people routinely eat the same number of calories but one's calories contain a higher proportion of fat, then that person is more likely to gain more weight because fewer calories are used to convert the dietary fat to body fat than are used to convert the dietary carbohydrates to body fat.

> Fats are essential in the diet, but overconsumption of fats is unhealthy.

Vitamins

Vitamins are organic compounds that are needed in minute amounts to maintain growth and good health. They do not supply energy but they are essential to release energy from the carbohydrates, lipids, and proteins. Many of the vitamins function with enzymes in the chemical reactions throughout the body. Vitamins are important in the clotting mechanism and in nucleic acid synthesis. Presently 13 vitamins have been discovered. Of these, four are **fat soluble** and nine are **water soluble.** Table 17–5 summarizes the functions, sources, and recommended daily allowances (RDA) of these vitamins.

Vitamin C is needed for the synthesis of collagen fibers in connective tissue. A vitamin C deficiency leads to **scurvy,** a condition in which the body is unable to produce and maintain healthy connective tissues, which are important in binding the body together. A condition called **rickets** is due to a deficiency of vitamin D. This vitamin is necessary for the absorption of calcium, and a lack of it causes weak bones in children. Milk is often fortified with vitamin D to enhance the absorption of the calcium in the intestines.

Table 17–5 Functions and Sources of Vitamins

Vitamin	Function	Food Source	Adult RDA
Fat Soluble			
Vitamin A	Healthy mucous membranes, skin, hair; essential for bone development and growth; component of pigments for night vision in the retina	Yellow, orange, green vegetables; milk and cheese	800–1000 μg
Vitamin D	Formation and development of bones and teeth; assists in absorption of calcium	Fortified milk, fish oils; made in the skin when exposed to sunlight	5–10 μg
Vitamin E	Conserves certain fatty acids; aids in protection against cell membrane damage	Whole grains, wheat germ, vegetable oils, nuts, green leafy vegetables	8–10 μg
Vitamin K	Needed for synthesis of factors essential in blood clotting	Green leafy vegetables, cabbage; synthesized by bacteria in intestine	65–80 μg
Water Soluble			
Thiamine (B_1)	Release of energy from carbohydrates and amino acids; growth; proper functioning of nervous system	Whole grains, legumes, nuts	1.5 mg
Riboflavin (B_2)	Helps transform nutrients into energy; involved in citric acid cycle	Whole grains, milk, green vegetables, nuts	1.7 mg
Niacin (B_3)	Helps transform nutrients in energy; involved in glycolysis and citric acid cycle	Whole grains, nuts, legumes, fish, liver	20 mg
Pyridoxine (B_6)	Involved in amino acid metabolism	Legumes, poultry, nuts, dried fruit, green vegetables	2 mg
Cyanocobalamin (B_{12})	Aids in formation of red blood cells; helps in nervous system function	Dairy products, eggs, fish, poultry	2 μg
Pantothenic acid	Part of coenzyme A; functions in steroid synthesis; helps in nutrient metabolism	Legumes, nuts, green vegetables, milk, poultry	7 mg
Folic acid	Aids in formation of hemoglobin and nucleic acids	Green vegetables, legumes, nuts, fruit juices, whole grains	200 μg
Biotin	Fatty acid synthesis; movement of pyruvic acid into citric acid cycle	Eggs; made by intestinal bacteria	0.3 mg
Ascorbic acid (C)	Important in collagen synthesis; helps maintain capillaries; aids in absorption of iron	Citrus fruits, tomatoes, green vegetables, berries	60 mg

It was originally believed that all vitamins were amines that were essential for life. Because "vita" means life, they were called "life amines," or vitamines. Later, when it was discovered than they were not all amines, the "e" was dropped from the word and the term vitamin came into usage.

Some people have the opinion that if vitamins are good for you, then more must be better. But this is not always the case. Excess fat-soluble vitamins, particularly vitamins A, D, and K, may accumulate to toxic levels in the fatty tissues of the body. Symptoms of vitamin A toxicity include anorexia, headache, irritability, enlarged liver and spleen, hair loss, scaly dermatitis, and bone thickening. Excess vitamin D is characterized by loss of weight, calcification of soft tissues, and kidney failure. Anemia, jaundice, and problems of the gastrointestinal tract may indicate vitamin K toxicity. Excessive amounts of some water-soluble vitamins also may be toxic. For example, large doses of vitamin B_6 can cause peripheral nerve damage.

Vitamins are organic molecules that are necessary for good health. Many vitamins are part of enzyme molecules.

Minerals

Minerals are inorganic substances that plants absorb from the soil and animals obtain by eating plants. They are necessary in small amounts to maintain good health in humans. Like vitamins, they do not supply energy, but they work with other nutrients to keep the body functioning properly. Some minerals, like calcium, are incorporated into body structures. Others are a part of enzymes that facilitate chemical reactions. Some help control fluid levels in the body, and others become part of organic molecules like hemoglobin. Table 17–6 summarizes the function and sources of some important minerals.

Minerals are inorganic substances that are necessary for good health. Plants absorb minerals from the soil, so fruits and vegetables are an important source of minerals in the diet.

Water

An average adult requires about 2.5 liters of water every day. A regular supply of water is more vital than food. An individual can live for several weeks without food, but only a few days without water. About two thirds of the daily intake is ingested in the form of water or other liquids. Solid food provides the remainder. Optimal health is dependent on the right balance of fluid intake and output, and abnormalities in this balance can be life threatening.

Water has numerous functions in the body. It is the principal component of the body, which is about 60 percent water by weight. It is an integral part of body cells and the fluid that surrounds the cells. Water provides an appropriate medium for the chemical reactions of the body and provides a transport medium for nutrients and waste products. It is the primary component of the lubricants for joints and muscles. The water contained in the body also helps maintain body temperature.

Water is an essential component of the diet. The average adult requires about 2.5 liters of water every day.

☑ QuickCheck

- What type of energy expenditure can be controlled voluntarily?
- Compare the amounts of energy that can be obtained from 1 gram of carbohydrate, 1 gram of protein, and 1 gram of fat.
- What is the American Heart Association recommendation regarding the amount of fat in the diet?

Body Temperature

Humans are **warm-blooded** animals, or **homeotherms** (HO-mee-oh-therms). This means that humans have the ability to maintain a constant internal body temperature even when external environmental temperatures change. Maintenance of the body's **core temperature,** the temperature of the internal organs, is essential for enzyme function. Enzymes are temperature sensitive and function only within narrow temperature ranges. Most enzymes in the

Table 17–6   Functions and Sources of Selected Minerals

Mineral	Function	Food Source	Adult RDA
Calcium	Component of bones and teeth; muscle contraction; blood clotting	Dairy products, green vegetables, legumes, nuts	800–1000 μg
Chloride	Acid–base balance of the blood; component of hydrochloric acid in the stomach	Table salt, milk, eggs, meat	750 mg
Phosphorus	Component of bones and teeth; component of adenosine triphosphate and nucleic acids; component of cell membranes	Legumes, dairy products, nuts, poultry, lean meats	800 mg
Sodium	Regulates body fluid volume; nerve impulse conduction	Table salt is the biggest source of sodium in the diet	500 mg
Potassium	Body fluid balance; muscle contraction; nerve impulse conduction	Fruits, legumes, nuts, vegetables; widely distributed	2,000 mg
Magnesium	Component of some active enzymes; releases energy from nutrients	Whole grains, legumes, green vegetables, nuts	280–350 mg
Iron	Component of hemoglobin and myoglobin; releases energy from nutrients	Whole grains, nuts, legumes, poultry, fish, lean meats	10–15 mg
Iodine	Component of thyroid hormones	Iodized table salt, dairy products, fish	150 μg
Zinc	Component of several enzymes; formation of proteins; wound healing	Legumes, poultry, nuts, whole grains, fish, lean meats	12–15 mg
Fluoride	Healthy bones and teeth	Fluoridated water is best source	1.5–4.0 mg

body function optimally at temperatures equal to the core temperature. Average normal rectal temperature is 37.6° C (99.7° F) and is considered close to the true core body temperature. Temperature at the body's surface, or skin, is the **shell temperature.** This is the heat-loss surface and has a lower value than the core temperature. Temperatures taken orally are considered close to the shell temperature. The average normal oral temperature is 37° C (98.6° F).

> Core temperature is the temperature around the internal organs. Shell temperature is the temperature near the body surface.

Heat Production

Heat is produced by the catabolism of nutrients. Approximately 40 percent of the total energy that is released by catabolism is used for biological activities in the body. The remaining 60 percent is heat energy, which is used to maintain body temperature.

When environmental temperatures are too cold and additional heat is needed to maintain core temperature, the hypothalamus initiates additional heat-conserving and heat-promoting activities. These include constriction of the cutaneous blood vessels, increase in the metabolic rate, and shivering. Constriction of the cutaneous vessels restricts the flow of blood to the skin and conserves heat by reducing heat loss through the surface. The blood maintains warmth in the core of the body. Cold stimulates the release of epinephrine and norepinephrine. These hormones increase the metabolic rate and promote heat production. Another response to cold is involuntary contraction of skeletal muscles, which results in shivering. The muscle contractions in shivering produce heat, which helps maintain core temperature.

> Heat produced by catabolism is used to maintain body temperature. When additional heat is needed to maintain core temperature, cutaneous blood vessels constrict, metabolic rate increases, and shivering develops.

Heat Loss

Heat loss mechanisms protect the body from excessive heat accumulation. Mechanisms of heat loss include **radiation, conduction, convection,** and **evaporation.** Radiation is the loss of heat as infrared energy. Any object that is warmer than its environment will transfer heat to the environment by radiation. This accounts for about 60 percent of the body's heat loss. Conduction is the transfer of heat from one object to another by direct contact between the two objects. Convection is the transfer of heat from an object (the body) to the air around it. These two processes account for 15 to 20 percent of the body's heat loss. Evaporation is the loss of heat from the body through water. This is most noticeable on a warm day when perspiration evaporates on the skin surface and has a cooling effect. Evaporation accounts for 20 to 25 percent of the body's heat loss.

> Heat is lost from the body by radiation, conduction, convection, and evaporation.

Temperature Regulation

Temperature regulation is an example of a negative feedback system that helps maintain homeostasis in the body. Review Figure 5–5 for an example of how the skin functions in this negative feedback mechanism. Temperature homeostasis requires a balance between heat production and heat loss. A small region in the hypothalamus acts as the body's thermostat with a "set point" at which it maintains body temperature. Other regions in the hypothalamus detect changes in body temperature. When the body temperature increases, the hypothalamus inhibits the mechanisms that produce heat and stimulates the mechanisms that promote heat loss. When the body temperature decreases, the hypothalamus initiates responses that produce heat and reduce heat loss. These reflex responses, along with voluntary activities such as putting on or taking off clothing, help maintain homeostasis of core body temperature.

> Body temperature is regulated by a homeostatic negative feedback mechanism.

✓ QuickCheck

- Which is greater—shell temperature or core temperature?
- By what mechanism is most heat lost from the body?
- How is internal body temperature regulated and maintained?

Heatstroke occurs when the core body temperature rises above 40.5° C (105° F). The excessive heat interferes with the temperature-regulating mechanism in the hypothalamus, and the sweat glands cease to function. A person with heatstroke has hot, dry skin. It is necessary to quickly control the rising temperature to prevent brain damage. Prolonged increases in core temperature can result in cardiovascular failure and death. The incidence of heatstroke increases in hot, humid weather.

FOCUS ON AGING

As a person grows older, there is a steady decline in energy requirements from loss of body tissue, reduced physical activity, and lowered basal metabolic rate. Although energy requirements are altered with aging, there are no major changes in nutritional needs. Older people still need a balanced diet of carbohydrates, fats, proteins, vitamins, minerals, and water. What does change is the amount of these nutrients that should be ingested.

Although the energy reduction associated with aging varies from individual to individual, it is estimated that the average decline in basal metabolic rate is 0.5 percent every year between the ages of 55 and 75. This means that a person needs 5 percent fewer calories at age 65 than at age 55, assuming other factors remain equal. Although the older person may need less carbohydrates and fats because of reduced energy requirements, the need for proteins, vitamins, and minerals continues. Nutrition in the elderly is complicated further because age-related changes in the digestive tract may affect the digestion and absorption of nutrients, production of enzymes, and kidney function.

As a person ages, the body often becomes less able to metabolize glucose efficiently and the individual is prone to fluctuations in blood sugar levels. Eating complex carbohydrates instead of refined carbohydrates helps control this problem. Reducing fat intake is a good way to reduce the calories in a diet; however, fats should not be eliminated from the diet. They are necessary for the absorption of the fat-soluble vitamins. The need for proteins does not appear to decline with aging; and this is an area of concern because the elderly tend to eliminate proteins from their diet because they often are expensive, require extra preparation time, and are sometimes difficult to chew. Because vitamins and minerals are essential in the diet, it is common practice to supplement dietary intake with over-the-counter tablets. This may help the deficiency problems but may lead to other difficulties because it is possible to produce toxic effects from excessive intake. Moderation is the key.

Because nutritional requirements do not change significantly with aging, there is no need for radical changes in dietary habits. Balanced meals provide good nutrition and contribute to a healthy lifestyle.

DO YOU KNOW THIS ABOUT

Metabolism?

Obesity

Adipose tissue, or fat, probably receives more attention than any other body tissue. Many people don't want it. They spend hard-earned money trying to get rid of it. It is sometimes the subject of ridicule, prejudice, discrimination, and jokes. It is a recurring theme in newspapers, magazines, and conversation. Yet fat is a necessary part of body composition and it performs several vital physiologic functions. Fatty tissue is incorporated into the structure of body organs such as mammary glands, nerves, and the brain. It also cushions vital organs such as the kidney. These are examples of **essential fat.** Excess fat that is stored is considered **nonessential fat,** and it is this that may lead to obesity.

The term **obesity** refers to excess body fat and is usually defined as being 20 percent or more overweight. Obesity can be classified according to the number and size of adipose cells. In **hy-**perplastic obesity, which begins in early childhood, there is a greater than normal number of adipose cells and each cell is enlarged. In all healthy children, the number of adipose cells increases between birth and 2 years of age. In nonobese children the number remains relatively stable from 2 years of age until puberty when there is another increase due to changing hormone levels, then the number stabilizes again. In children with hyperplastic obesity, the number of fat cells continues to increase during the childhood years. As teenagers and adults, these people have more fat cells than other people and once formed, the fat cells are here to stay. Losing weight does not get rid of them. They just change size as their lipid content varies. Individuals with **hypertrophic obesity** have a normal number of fat cells, but each cell enlarges as fat accumulates in it. This is the more common type of obesity and

Continued on following page

typically develops during adulthood when an individual becomes less active but eats the same amount of food. The fat cells enlarge to store the excess calories.

Obesity alone may not pose a risk of premature death, but the incidence of severe health problems increases with excess weight. Obesity increases the risk of high blood pressure, type II diabetes mellitus, and high levels of lipids in the blood. All of these contribute to a person's risk of heart disease and stroke. Gallstones, liver disease, kidney disease, and some cancers are more common in overweight individuals. Additional weight also puts stress on weight-bearing joints, which contributes to an increase in orthopedic problems. Many environmental pollutants are fat soluble, and people with excess adipose tend to retain more of these than people with "normal" weight, which may allow the pollutants to accumulate to toxic levels.

The distribution of fat in obese people can vary. Some people carry their fat in the abdomen. Others carry it in the hips and thighs. This fat distribution appears to be genetically determined, and no amount of diet or exercise changes it. When a person loses weight, it is lost from all areas and the distribution remains the same. Research has found that extra fat on the torso and abdomen is associated with a greater health risk than extra fat on the hips and thighs. Fat cells in the abdominal region have a stronger impact on fat and cholesterol metabolism because these cells release their products directly into the vein that goes to the liver, where much of the metabolism takes place. These cells are also more responsive to several hormones.

In a few cases, a specific cause of obesity can be defined. In most cases, however, the cause is multifaceted and nothing specific can be identified. Heredity may play a role because children of obese parents tend to be obese. Environment is also an issue, because adopted children tend to follow the lifestyle and habits of their adoptive parents. Psychological factors are involved when people use eating as a mechanism for coping with stress.

Whatever the cause of obesity, weight control is the interaction of energy expenditure and energy intake. When intake is greater than expenditure, the excess is stored as fat. This does not mean that obese people eat a lot more than their lean counterparts. In fact, often their calorie intake is less, but it may be that their expenditure is also less. Energy usage is through basal metabolism, physical activity, and thermogenesis, or the energy that is required to process the food. Some foods require more energy for processing than others. For example, it takes about 3 percent of the calories in dietary fat to convert it to body fat. This leaves 97 percent available for storage as adipose. In contrast, it takes about 23 percent of the calories in carbohydrates to convert them to body fat. This leaves 77 percent available for storage. This means that two people with identical caloric intake, basal-metabolism, and physical activity may have different amounts of calories for storage as fat because one eats a higher percentage of dietary fat.

Obesity is a complex issue, and there are no miracle cures. Pills, fad diets, and surgery may provide a quick fix but are not the long-term answers. The only successful way to lose weight is to eat a balanced, healthy diet that decreases energy intake and to increase physical activity over a period of time.

CHAPTER QUIZ

RECALL

Match the definitions on the left with the appropriate term on the right.

1. Anaerobic catabolism of glucose

2. Acquisition, assimilation, and utilization of nutrients

3. Smaller molecules react to produce larger molecules and water

4. Production of glycogen from glucose

5. Process in catabolism of fatty acids

6. Temperature of internal organs

7. A, D, E, K

8. Glucose, fructose, and galactose

9. Produces ammonia and a ketoacid from an amino acid

10. Production of heat in response to food intake

A. Beta oxidation

B. Core temperature

C. Deamination

D. Dehydration synthesis

E. Fat-soluble vitamins

F. Glycogenesis

G. Glycolysis

H. Monosaccharides

I. Nutrition

J. Thermogenesis

THOUGHT

1. Glycerol combines with three fatty acids to form a triglyceride and 3 molecules of water. This is an example of

   a. hydrolysis

   b. catabolism

   c. dehydration synthesis

   d. glycolysis

2. When there is oxygen deficiency (anaerobic conditions), pyruvic acid

   a. enters the citric acid cycle

   b. undergoes oxidative phosphorylation

   c. is converted to acetyl-CoA

   d. is converted to lactic acid

3. The principal reaction that prepares amino acids for use as an energy source is

   a. deamination

   b. beta oxidation

   c. glycolysis

   d. hydrolysis

4. The total body metabolic rate includes three factors. The only one of these that can be controlled voluntarily is

   a. basal metabolic rate

   b. caloric intake

   c. thermogenesis

   d. physical activity

5. The mechanism that accounts for most of the heat loss from the body is

   a. radiation

   b. conduction

   c. convection

   d. evaporation

APPLICATION

A single serving of pudding contains 4 grams of protein, 31 grams of carbohydrate, and 5 grams of fat. How many Calories (kilocalories) are in this serving?

What would happen to core body temperature if the peripheral cutaneous blood vessels constricted on a hot day?

CHAPTER 18

Urinary System and Body Fluids

Outline/Objectives

Components of the Urinary System 375

- Describe the location and structural features of the kidneys.
- Draw and label a diagrammatic representation of a nephron.
- Name the two parts of the juxtaglomerular apparatus and state where they are located.
- Trace the pathway of blood flow through the kidney from the renal artery to the renal vein.
- Describe the location, structure, and function of the ureter, urinary bladder, and urethra.

Urine Formation 381

- Describe each of the three basic steps in urine formation.
- Identify three different types of pressure that affect the rate of glomerular filtration and describe how these interact.
- Explain why some substances, such as glucose, have limited reabsorption and what happens when concentration exceeds this limit.
- Explain how kidney function has a role in maintaining blood concentration, blood volume, and blood pressure.
- Name two hormones that affect kidney function and explain the effect of each one.

- Name the enzyme that stimulates the production of angiotensin II and is produced by the kidneys.
- Describe two mechanisms by which angiotensin II increases blood pressure.

Characteristics of Urine 385

- Describe the physical characteristics and chemical composition of urine
- List five abnormal constituents of urine.

Body Fluids 386

- State the percentage of body weight that is composed of water.
- Identify the major fluid compartments in the body and state the relative amount of fluid in each compartment.
- State the sources of fluid intake and avenues of fluid output and explain how these are regulated to maintain fluid balance.
- Identify the major intracellular and extracellular ions and explain how electrolyte balance is regulated.
- State the normal pH of the blood and define the terms acidosis and alkalosis.
- Describe the three primary mechanisms by which blood pH is regulated.

Key Terms

Acidosis

Alkalosis

Glomerular capsule

Glomerulus

Interstitial fluid

Intracellular fluid

Intravascular fluid

Juxtaglomerular apparatus

Nephron

Renal tubule

Building Vocabulary

WORD PART	MEANING
-atresia	without an opening
caly-	small cup
-chrom-	color, pigment
-continence	to hold
cyst-	bladder
-ectasy	dilation
-etic	pertaining to
juxta-	near to
lith-	stone
mict-	to pass
neph-	kidney
noct-	night
peri-	around
-pexy	fixation
-phraxis	to obstruct
pyel-	renal pelvis
ren-	kidney
-rrhaphy	suture
-ur-	urine

Functional Relationships of the
Urinary System

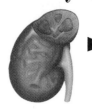

► Eliminates metabolic wastes; helps maintain pH and ion concentration of body fluids.

Integument

► Alternative excretory route for some salts and nitrogenous wastes; limits fluid loss.

► Maintains fluid and electrolyte balance which is necessary for production of sweat.

Skeletal
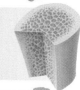

► Supports and protects organs of the urinary system.

► Conserves calcium and phosphate ions for bone growth, maintenance, and repair.

Muscular

► Supports and protects organs of the urinary system; sphincters control voluntary urination.

► Conserves calcium ions necessary for muscle contraction; eliminates wastes produced by muscle metabolism.

Nervous

► Autonomic nervous system controls renal blood pressure and blood flow, which affect rate of urine formation; regulates bladder emptying.

► Helps maintain pH and electrolyte balance necessary for neural function; eliminates metabolic wastes harmful to nerve function.

Endocrine
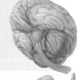

► Hormones, such as aldosterone, ADH, and atrial natriuretic hormone, regulate urine formation in the kidneys.

► Helps maintain pH and electrolyte balance necessary for hormone function; eliminates inactivated hormones and other metabolic wastes; releases renin and erythropoietin.

Cardiovascular
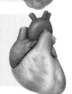

► Delivers wastes to be excreted by the kidneys; adjusts blood flow to maintain kidney function; transports hormones that regulate urine formation in the kidneys.

► Helps maintain blood pH and electrolyte composition; adjusts blood volume and pressure by altering urine composition; initiates the renin-angiotensin-aldosterone mechanism.

Lymphatic/Immune
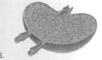

► Immune cells provide specific defense mechanisms against pathogens that enter the urinary tract.

► Helps maintain pH and electrolyte composition of body fluids for effective immune cell function; acid pH and urine flow provide a barrier against urinary tract pathogens.

Respiratory

► Assists in regulation of pH by removing carbon dioxide.

► Helps maintain pH and electrolyte composition of body fluids for effective respiratory function; eliminates metabolic waste products generated by respiratory organs.

Digestive
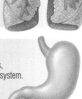

► Liver synthesizes urea, which is excreted by kidneys; liver metabolizes hormones, toxins, and drugs to forms that can be excreted in urine; absorbs nutrients for tissues of urinary system.

► Excretes toxins absorbed by the digestive system; excretes metabolic wastes produced by the liver.

Reproductive

► Prostate surrounds urethra in males and may compress it to cause urine retention; pregnant uterus pushes on bladder and causes frequent urination.

► Maintains pH and electrolyte composition for effective gonadal hormone function; maternal urinary system excretes metabolic wastes from developing fetus.

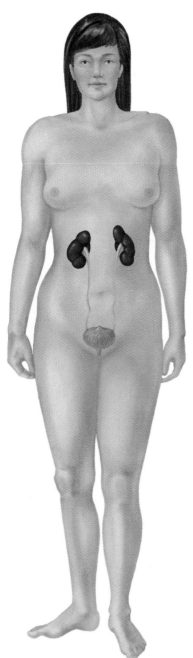

The overall function of the **urinary system** is to maintain the volume and composition of body fluids within normal limits. One aspect of this function is to rid the body of waste products that accumulate as a result of cellular metabolism, and because of this it is sometimes referred to as the excretory system. Although the urinary system has a major role in excretion, other organs contribute to the excretory function. Some waste products, such as carbon dioxide and water, are excreted by the lungs in the respiratory system. The skin is another excretory organ that rids the body of wastes through the sweat glands. The liver and intestines excrete bile pigments that result from the destruction of hemoglobin. The major task of excretion still belongs to the urinary system; and if it fails, the other organs cannot take over and compensate adequately. In addition to ridding the body of waste materials, the urinary system maintains an appropriate fluid volume by regulating the amount of water that is excreted in the urine. Other aspects of its function include regulating the concentrations of various electrolytes in the body fluids and maintaining normal pH of the blood.

In addition to maintaining fluid homeostasis in the body, the urinary system controls red blood cell production by secreting the hormone **erythropoietin** (ee-rith-roh-poy-EE-tin). The urinary system also plays a role in maintaining normal blood pressure by secreting the enzyme **renin.**

> The urinary system rids the body of waste materials, regulates fluid volume, maintains electrolyte concentrations in body fluids, controls blood pH, secretes erythropoietin, and secretes renin.

When the kidneys do not function properly and fail to remove the waste products from the blood, **uremia** may result. Uremia is a condition in which there is a toxic level of urea in the blood.

As a result of renal failure, when the kidneys fail to remove urea from the blood, the body attempts to compensate by excreting urea, through the sweat glands. After the perspiration evaporates, tiny crystals of urea remain on the skin. This is called **uremic frost.**

Components of the Urinary System

The **urinary system** consists of the kidneys, ureters, urinary bladder, and urethra. The kidneys form the urine and account for the other functions attributed to the urinary system. The ureters convey the urine away from the kidneys to the urinary bladder, which is a temporary reservoir for the urine. The urethra is a tubular structure that carries the urine from the urinary bladder to the outside. The components of the urinary system are illustrated in Figure 18–1.

> The components of the urinary system are the kidneys, ureters, urinary bladder, and urethra.

Kidneys

The **kidneys** are the primary organs of the urinary system. They are the organs that filter the blood, remove the wastes, and excrete the wastes in the urine. They are the organs that perform the functions of the urinary system. The other components

---

CLINICAL TERMS

Anuria   (an-YOU-rih-ah) Condition in which there is no formation of urine.

Azotemia   (az-oh-TEE-mee-ah) Presence of increased amounts of nitrogen waste products in the blood

Blood urea nitrogen (BUN)   (BLOOD you-REE-ah NYE-trohjen) A blood test to determine the amount of urea that is excreted by the kidneys; abnormal results indicate urinary tract disease

Dialysis   (dye-AL-ih-sis) A procedure to separate waste material from the blood and to maintain fluid, electrolyte, and acid–base balance when kidney function is impaired.

Diuresis   (dye-you-REE-sis) A condition of increased or excessive flow of urine

Diuretic   (dye-you-RET-ik) A substance that increases the production of urine

Dysuria   (dis-YOU-rih-ah) Difficult or painful urination

Enuresis   (en-you-REE-sis) Involuntary emission of urine; bedwetting

Intravenous pyelogram   (in-trah-VAYN-us PYLE-oh-gram) Radiographic procedure in which a radiopaque dye is injected into a vein and its path through the kidneys, ureters, and urinary bladder is followed to visualize abnormalities in the renal vessels and urinary tract

Lithotripsy   (lith-oh-TRIP-see) Crushing of a calculus (stone) in the bladder, urethra, ureter, or kidney

Nephrectomy   (nef-REK-toh-mee) Surgical removal of a kidney

Nephritis   (nef-RYE-tis) Inflammation of the kidney

Nocturia   (nahk-TOU-rih-ah) Excessive urination at night

Oliguria   (ahl-ig-YOU-rih-ah) Very little, or scanty, urination

Polyuria   (pahl-ee-YOU-rih-ah) Excessive urination

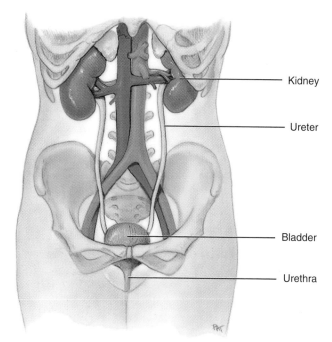

Figure 18-1 Components of the urinary system.

are accessory structures to eliminate the urine from the body.

Location

The paired kidneys are located between the 12th thoracic and 3rd lumbar vertebrae, one on each side of the vertebral column. The right kidney usually is slightly lower than the left because the liver displaces it downward. The kidneys, partially protected by the lower ribs, lie in shallow depressions against the posterior abdominal wall and behind the parietal peritoneum. This means they are retroperitoneal. Each kidney is held in place by connective tissue, called **renal fascia,** and is surrounded by a thick layer of adipose tissue, called **perirenal fat,** which helps to protect it. A tough, fibrous, connective tissue renal capsule closely envelopes each kidney and provides support for the soft tissue that is inside.

> The primary organs of the urinary system are the kidneys, which are located retroperitoneally between the levels of the 12th thoracic and 3rd lumbar vertebrae.

Nephroptosis, commonly referred to as a floating kidney, occurs when the kidney is no longer held in place by the renal fascia and it drops out of its normal position. This may make the kidney more vulnerable to injury if it is no longer protected by the ribs. Another danger is that the ureter may become twisted and block the flow of urine. Nephroptosis occurs more frequently in horseback riders, truck drivers, and people who ride motorcycles.

Macroscopic Structure

In the adult, each kidney is approximately 3 cm thick, 6 cm wide, and 12 cm long. It is roughly bean shaped with an indentation, called the **hilum,** on the medial side. The hilum leads to a large cavity, called the **renal sinus,** within the kidney. The **ureter** and **renal vein** leave the kidney, and the **renal artery** enters the kidney at the hilum.

A frontal (coronal) section through the kidney illustrates the macroscopic internal structure (Fig. 18–2). The outer, reddish region, next to the capsule, is the **renal cortex.** This surrounds a darker reddish brown region called the **renal medulla.** The renal medulla consists of a series of **renal pyramids,** which appear striated because they contain straight tubular structures and blood vessels. The wide bases of the pyramids are adjacent to the cortex and the pointed ends, called **renal papillae,** are directed toward the center of the kidney. Portions of the renal cortex extend into the spaces between adjacent pyramids to form **renal columns.** The cortex and medulla make up the parenchyma, or functional tissue, of the kidney.

The central region of the kidney contains the **renal pelvis,** which is located in the renal sinus and is continuous with the ureter. The renal pelvis is a large cavity that collects the urine as it is produced. The periphery of the renal pelvis is interrupted by cuplike projections called **calyces.** A **minor calyx** surrounds the renal papillae of each pyramid and collects urine from that pyramid. Several minor calyces converge to form a **major calyx.** From the major calyces the urine flows into the renal pelvis and from there into the ureter.

> The cortex and medulla make up the parenchyma of the kidney. The central region is the renal pelvis, which collects the urine as it is produced.

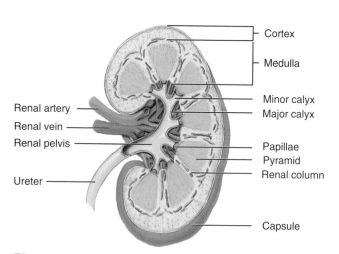

Figure 18-2 Coronal (frontal) section through the kidney.

Nephrons

Each kidney contains over a million functional units, called **nephrons,** in the parenchyma (cortex and medulla). A nephron has two parts (Fig. 18–3):

- Renal corpuscle
- Renal tubule

The number of nephrons does not increase after birth. Growth of the kidney is due to enlargement of the individual nephrons. When nephrons are damaged they are not replaced.

The renal corpuscle consists of a cluster of capillaries, called the **glomerulus** (gloh-MER-yoo-lus), surrounded by a double-layered epithelial cup, called the **glomerular capsule** (**Bowman's capsule**). Blood enters the glomerulus through an **afferent arteriole,** is filtered in the glomerulus, and leaves through an **efferent arteriole.** As the blood is filtered, the filtrate enters the glomerular capsule, which is continuous with the renal tubule. Renal corpuscles are located in the cortex of the kidney and give it a granular appearance.

The renal tubule, which carries fluid away from the glomerular capsule, consists of three regions:

- **Proximal convoluted tubule**
- **Nephron loop (Henle's loop)**
- **Distal convoluted tubule**

The first portion of the tubule, the proximal convoluted tubule, is highly coiled. Next the tubule straightens and dips into the medulla, makes a U-turn, and ascends back toward the cortex. This forms the nephron loop. The portion of the loop that descends from the proximal convoluted tubule into the medulla is the **descending limb,** and the part that ascends back toward the cortex is the **ascending limb.** The final region of the tubule, also coiled and found in the cortex, is the distal convoluted tubule.

The functional unit of the kidney is a nephron, which consists of a renal corpuscle and a renal tubule. An afferent arteriole leads into the renal corpuscle, and an efferent arteriole leaves the renal corpuscle.

Polycystic kidney disease is an inherited condition that affects the tubular portion of the nephrons. Swelling or cysts develop along the tubules; and as the cysts enlarge they crowd out and damage functional kidney tissue. This eventually leads to a total loss of kidney function. When this occurs in both kidneys, a transplant is necessary.

Collecting Ducts

Urine passes from the nephrons into **collecting ducts.** The distal convoluted tubules from several nephrons join with each collecting duct. The collecting ducts extend from the base of the pyramids to the renal papillae. These straight tubules, with the nephron loops and blood vessels, give the medulla its striated appearance. Fluid flows from the collecting ducts into the minor calyces that surround the renal papillae.

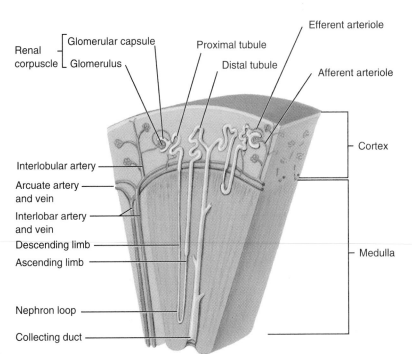

Figure 18–3   Nephron illustrating the regions in the cortex and the regions in the medulla.

Urine passes from the nephrons into collecting ducts then into the minor calyces.

Juxtaglomerular Apparatus

The ascending limb of the nephron loop, in the region where it continues into the distal convoluted tubule, comes into contact with the glomerular afferent arteriole of the same nephron (Fig. 18–4). In the region of contact, the cells of the ascending limb are modified to form the **macula densa,** and those in the afferent arteriole are modified to form the **juxtaglomerular** (juks-tah-gloh-MER-you-lar) **cells.** The macula densa monitors sodium chloride in the urine and also influences the juxtaglomerular cells. In the afferent arteriole, the juxtaglomerular cells produce the enzyme **renin,** which has a role in the regulation of blood pressure. The macula densa and juxtaglomerular cells, together, make up the **juxtaglomerular apparatus.**

The juxtaglomerular apparatus, which monitors blood pressure and secretes renin, is formed from modified cells in the afferent arteriole and the ascending limb of the nephron loop.

Blood Flow Through the Kidney

Blood flows through the kidneys at an approximate rate of 1,200 millimeters per minute. This is about one fourth of the total cardiac output. Blood is brought to the kidneys by the renal arteries, which are branches from the abdominal aorta (Fig. 18–5).

At the hilum, the renal arteries divide into **segmental arteries** that pass through the renal sinus. **Interlobar arteries** branch from the segmental arteries, pass through the renal columns, and then divide to form **arcuate arteries,** which pass over the base of the pyramids. Arcuate arteries give off branches, called **interlobular arteries,** which extend into the cortex and give rise to the **afferent arterioles.** From the afferent arteriole, the blood passes through the capillaries in the glomerulus of the renal corpuscle, and then into the efferent arteriole. Each efferent arteriole divides to form an extensive capillary network, called **peritubular capillaries,** around the tubular portion of the nephron.

The peritubular capillaries eventually reunite to form **interlobular veins.** From there, the blood flows through **arcuate veins, interlobar veins, segmental veins,** and into the **renal veins,** which return the blood to the inferior vena cava.

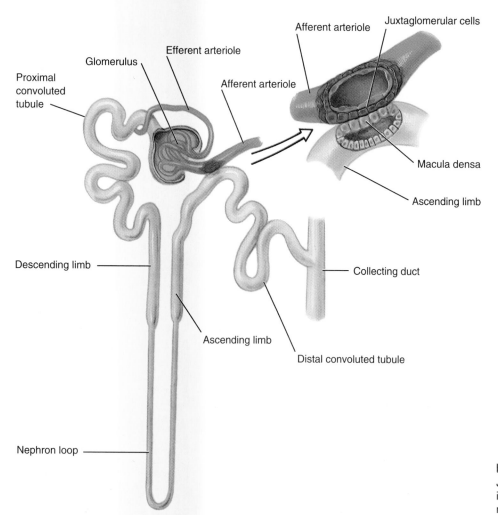

Afferent arteriole

Juxtaglomerular cells

Efferent arteriole

Glomerulus

Afferent arteriole

Proximal convoluted tubule

Macula densa

Ascending limb

Descending limb

Collecting duct

Ascending limb

Distal convoluted tubule

Nephron loop

Figure 18–4
Juxtaglomerular apparatus and its relationship to the nephron.

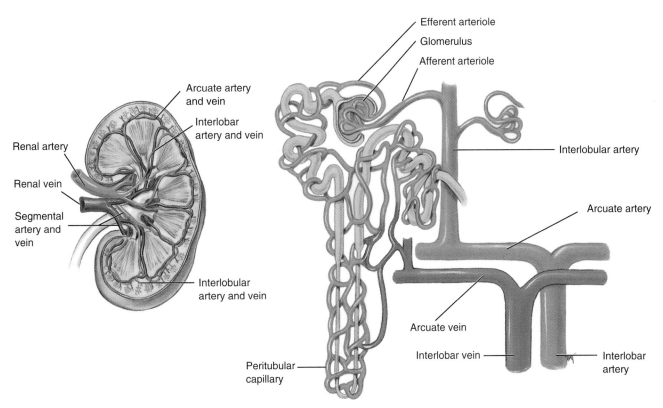

Figure 18-5   Blood flow through the kidney.

Blood flow through the kidney goes in the sequence of renal artery → segmental artery → interlobar artery → arcuate artery → interlobular artery → afferent arteriole → glomerulus → efferent arteriole → peritubular capillaries → interlobular vein → arcuate vein → interlobar vein → segmental vein → renal vein → inferior vena cava.

✓ QuickCheck

● Which portion of the kidney collects urine as it is produced?

● What are the two parts of a renal corpuscle?

● What portion of the nephron produces a substance that functions in the control of blood pressure?

Ureters

Each **ureter** is a small tube, about 25 centimeters long, that carries urine from the renal pelvis to the urinary bladder. It descends from the renal pelvis, along the posterior abdominal wall, behind the parietal peritoneum, and enters the urinary bladder on the posterior inferior surface.

The wall of the ureter consists of three layers (Fig. 18–6). The outer layer, the **fibrous coat,** is a supporting layer of fibrous connective tissue. The middle layer, the **muscular coat,** consists of inner

circular and outer longitudinal smooth muscle. The main function of this layer is peristalsis to propel the urine. The inner layer, the **mucosa,** is transitional epithelium that is continuous with the lining of the renal pelvis and the urinary bladder. This layer secretes mucus, which coats and protects the surface of the cells.

The ureter transports urine from the kidney to the urinary bladder.

Urinary Bladder

The **urinary bladder** is a temporary storage reservoir for urine (see Fig. 18–6). It is located in the pelvic cavity, posterior to the symphysis pubis, and below the parietal peritoneum. The size and shape of the urinary bladder varies with the amount of urine it contains and with pressure from surrounding organs.

The inner lining of the urinary bladder is a **mucous membrane** of transitional epithelium that is continuous with that in the ureters. When the bladder is empty, the mucosa has numerous folds called **rugae.** The rugae and transitional epithelium allow the bladder to expand as it fills. The second layer in the wall is the **submucosa** that supports the mucous membrane. It is composed of connective tissue with elastic fibers. The next layer is the **muscularis,**

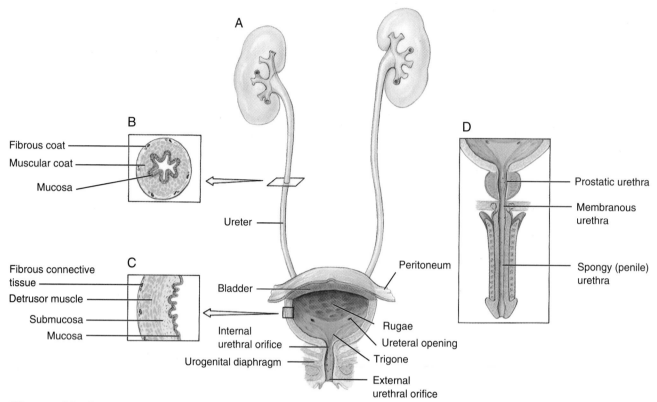

Figure 18–6 Ureter, urinary bladder, and urethra. *(A)* Urinary tract. *(B)* Cross section through the ureter. *(C)* Cross section of the bladder wall. *(D)* Regions of the male urethra.

which is composed of smooth muscle. The smooth muscle fibers are interwoven in all directions and collectively these are called the **detrusor** (dee-TROO-sor) **muscle.** Contraction of this muscle expels urine from the bladder. On the superior surface, the outer layer of the bladder wall is parietal peritoneum. In all other regions, the outer layer is fibrous connective tissue.

The lining of the urinary bladder is a mucous membrane with folds called rugae. The smooth muscle in the wall is the detrusor muscle.

There is a triangular area, called the **trigone,** formed by three openings in the floor of the urinary bladder. Two of the openings are from the ureters and form the base of the trigone. Small flaps of mucosa cover these openings and act as valves that allow urine to enter the bladder but prevent it from backing up from the bladder into the ureters. The third opening, at the apex of the trigone, is the opening into the urethra. A band of the detrusor muscle encircles this opening to form the **internal urethral sphincter.**

The trigone, in the floor of the urinary bladder, is outlined by the two ureters and the internal urethral orifice.

Infections of the urinary bladder (cystitis) tend to persist in the region of the trigone.

Urethra

The final passageway for the flow of urine is the **urethra,** a thin-walled tube that conveys urine from the floor of the urinary bladder to the outside (see Fig. 18–6). The opening to the outside is the **external urethral orifice.** The mucosal lining of the urethra is transitional epithelium. The wall also contains smooth muscle fibers and is supported by connective tissue.

The beginning of the urethra, where it leaves the urinary bladder, is surrounded by the **internal urethral sphincter.** This sphincter is smooth (involuntary) muscle. Another sphincter, the **external urethral sphincter,** is skeletal (voluntary) muscle and encircles the urethra where it goes through the pelvic floor. These two sphincters control the flow of urine through the urethra.

The flow of urine through the urethra is controlled by an involuntary internal urethral sphincter and a voluntary external urethral sphincter.

In females, the urethra is short, only 3 to 4 cm (about 1.5 inches) long. The external urethral orifice opens to the outside just anterior to the opening for the vagina.

In males, the urethra is much longer, about 20 cm (7–8 inches) in length, and transports both urine and semen. The first part, next to the urinary bladder, passes through the prostate gland and is called the **prostatic urethra.** The second part, a short region that penetrates the pelvic floor and enters the penis, is called the **membranous urethra.** The third part, the **spongy urethra,** is the longest region. This portion of the urethra extends the entire length of the penis, and the external urethral orifice opens to the outside at the tip of the penis.

> The urethra is much longer in males than in females.

QuickCheck

- Obstruction of the ureter will interfere with the flow of urine between what two structures?

- Where is the detrusor muscle located?

- What is the difference between the muscle in the internal urethral sphincter and the external urethral sphincter?

Urinary tract infections (UTIs) occur more frequently in women than in men because of differences in the urethra. In females, the urethral opening is in close proximity to the anal opening, which gives intestinal bacteria easier access to the urethra. The female urethra is short, which allows any infection to spread to the urinary bladder. An infection of the urethra is called **urethritis,** and one of the urinary bladder is called **cystitis.**

Urine Formation

The work of the kidneys, performed by the nephrons, is to maintain the volume and composition of body fluids, to regulate the pH of the blood, and to remove waste products from the blood. The result of this work is the formation of urine. As urine is excreted to the outside of the body, it carries with it the wastes, excess water, and excess electrolytes. At the same time, the kidneys conserve other electrolytes to maintain the appropriate balance. The formation of urine involves three basic steps:

- Glomerular filtration
- Tubular reabsorption
- Tubular secretion

> The work of the kidneys is accomplished through the formation of urine, which involves glomerular filtration, tubular reabsorption, and tubular secretion.

Glomerular Filtration

The first step in the formation of urine is **glomerular filtration.** During this process, blood plasma moves across the **filtration membrane** in the renal corpuscle and enters the glomerular capsule. The filtration membrane consists of the capillary endothelium of the glomerulus and the endothelium of the capsule. The force that moves the fluid across the membrane is **filtration pressure,** and the fluid that enters the capsule is the **filtrate.**

Blood flows through the kidneys at an average rate of 1,200 milliliters per minute. As the blood passes through the glomeruli, about 19 percent of the plasma enters the glomerular capsule as filtrate. This is equivalent to forming filtrate at a rate of 125 milliliters per minute or 180 liters per day. This is the total value for all the nephrons in both kidneys. The filtration membrane acts as a barrier that prevents blood cells and protein molecules from entering the capsule so they are absent from the filtrate. Normally, the filtrate in the glomerular capsule is similar in composition to blood plasma except that the filtrate lacks plasma proteins. In a diseased kidney, the filtration membrane may become too porous and allow blood cells and proteins to pass through. This alters the filtration rate, and blood cells and proteins appear in the urine.

> In glomerular filtration, plasma components cross the filtration membrane from the glomerulus into the capsule.

The filtration rate is directly related to the filtration pressure. When filtration pressure increases, filtration rate increases, more filtrate is formed, and more urine is produced. If the filtration pressure decreases, filtration rate decreases, less filtrate is formed, and less urine is produced. Filtration pressure is influenced by the blood pressure in the glomerulus, the hydrostatic pressure of the fluid in the glomerular capsule, and the osmotic pressure created by the plasma proteins. Figure 18–7 illustrates the factors that influence filtration pressure.

> The rate of glomerular filtration depends on blood pressure in the glomerulus, hydrostatic pressure in the capsule, and osmotic pressure in the blood.

Tubular Reabsorption

If the volume and composition of the filtrate in the glomerular capsule are compared with the volume and composition of urine, it is obvious that changes occur after filtration. First of all, about 180 liters (45 gallons) of filtrate are formed in a 24-hour period. This volume is reduced to 1 to 2 liters of urine. Glucose is present in the filtrate but normally absent in the urine. Urea and uric acid are present in higher concentrations in the urine than in the filtrate.

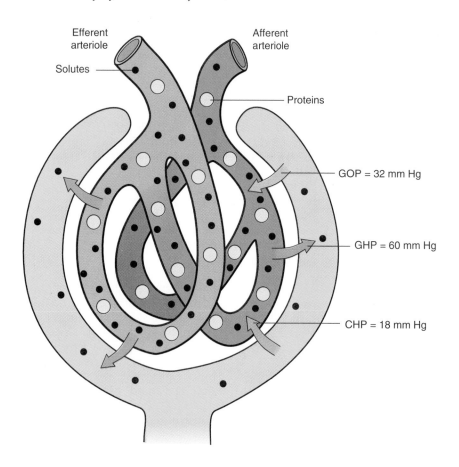

Efferent
arteriole

Afferent
arteriole

Solutes

Proteins

GOP = 32 mm Hg

GHP = 60 mm Hg

CHP = 18 mm Hg

60 mm Hg = Glomerular hydrostatic pressure (GHP)
-32 mm Hg = Glomerular osmotic pressure (GOP)
-18 mm Hg = Capsular hydrostatic pressure (CHP)
_____
10 mm Hg = Net pressure

Figure 18–7   Factors that influence
filtration pressure.

Tubular reabsorption is the first process that changes the volume and composition of the filtrate. Tubular reabsorption is the movement of substances from the filtrate in the kidney tubules into the blood in the peritubular capillaries. Only about 1 percent of the filtrate remains in the tubules and becomes urine. In general, water and other substances that are useful to the body are reabsorbed. Wastes remain in the filtrate and are excreted in the urine.

> Tubular reabsorption moves substances from the filtrate into the blood in the capillaries and reduces the volume of urine.

About 65 percent of the reabsorption takes place in the proximal convoluted tubule, 15 percent in the nephron loop (loop of Henle), and 19 percent in the distal convoluted tubule and collecting duct. This leaves about 1 percent of the filtrate to be excreted as urine. Most of the solutes (molecules and ions) are reabsorbed by active transport mechanisms. Some of the negative ions passively follow the positive ions to maintain electrical neutrality. Because active transport utilizes carrier molecules, reabsorption of some solutes is limited by the activity of the carriers. Glucose is a good example of this limitation. Under normal conditions, glucose freely passes through the filtration membrane so that the concentration in the filtrate is the same as in the blood. Glucose is then totally reabsorbed by active transport so there is no glucose present in the urine. Under certain conditions, such as with untreated diabetes mellitus, the glucose concentration in the blood and filtrate may exceed the **renal threshold,** or transport maximum. When this happens the excess glucose remains in the filtrate and appears in the urine.

Reabsorption of some solutes is limited by carrier molecules.

Renal diabetes is a condition in which there are not enough functional carrier molecules to reabsorb normal amounts of glucose. Even though blood glucose levels are normal, glucose still appears in the urine because there is inadequate reabsorption.

Water is reabsorbed by osmosis in all parts of the tubule, except in the ascending limb of the loop. Reabsorption of the molecules and ions creates concentration differences and water follows by osmosis. The exception is in the ascending limb of the nephron loop, which is impermeable to water. Here, solutes, but very little water, are removed from the filtrate.

In the cortex of the kidney, where the proximal convoluted tubules are located, the filtrate is isotonic (same concentration) to the interstitial fluid and the plasma in the peritubular capillaries. When molecules and ions are reabsorbed by active transport, water follows by osmosis and volume is reduced.

There is a concentration gradient in the interstitial fluid of the medulla in which the nephron loops are located. Near the base, next to the cortex, the concentration is nearly the same as the cortex, but in the papillae the interstitial fluid is highly concentrated. As the filtrate moves down the descending limb, water leaves the tubule by osmosis, which creates a highly concentrated filtrate. The ascending limb is impermeable to water, but solutes leave the filtrate by active transport. This creates a dilute filtrate that enters the distal convoluted tubule. Water then leaves the distal convoluted tubule and collecting duct by osmosis (Fig. 18–8).

Water is reabsorbed by osmosis.

Tubular Secretion

The final process in the formation of urine is the transport of molecules and ions into the filtrate. This is called **tubular secretion.** Most of these substances are waste products of cellular metabolism that become toxic if allowed to accumulate in the body. Tubular secretion is the method by which some drugs, such as penicillin, are removed from the body. The tubular secretion of hydrogen ions plays an important role in regulating the pH of the blood. Other molecules and ions that may enter the filtrate by tubular secretion include potassium ions, creatinine, and histamine.

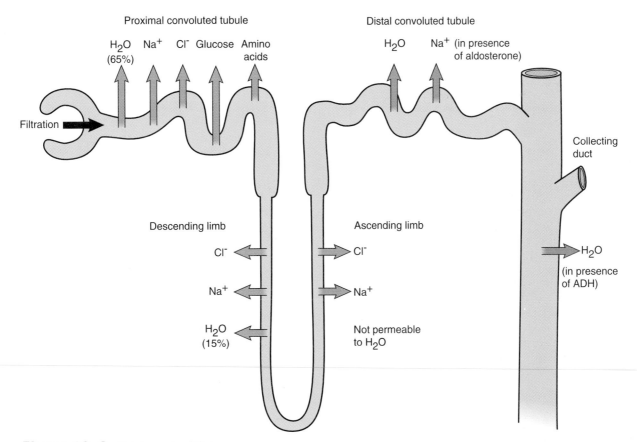

Figure 18–8   Tubular reabsorption.

The final product, urine, produced by the nephrons consists of the substances that are filtered in the renal corpuscle, minus the substances that are reabsorbed in the tubules, plus the substances that are added by tubular secretion (Fig. 18–9).

> Tubular secretion adds substances, such as drugs, hydrogen and potassium ions, creatinine, and histamine, to the urine.

Regulation of Urine Concentration and Volume

The concentration and volume of urine depends on conditions in the internal environment of the body. Cells in the hypothalamus are sensitive to changes in the composition of the blood and initiate appropriate responses that affect the kidneys. If the concentration of solutes in the blood increases above normal, the kidneys excrete a small volume of concentrated urine. This conserves water in the body and gets rid of solutes to restore the blood to normal. If the blood solute concentration decreases below normal, the kidneys conserve solutes and get rid of water by producing large quantities of dilute urine. Urine production plays an important role in maintaining homeostasis of blood concentration and volume. By regulating blood volume, the kidneys also play a role in regulating blood pressure because volume is directly related to pressure.

> By altering the concentration and volume of urine, the kidneys have a major role in maintaining blood concentration, volume, and pressure.

Three hormones, **aldosterone, antidiuretic hormone,** and **atrial natriuretic hormone,** influence urine concentration and volume. Aldosterone, secreted by cells of the adrenal cortex, acts on the kidney tubules to increase the reabsorption of sodium. When sodium is reabsorbed, water follows by osmosis. This reduces urine output.

Antidiuretic hormone (ADH) is produced by cells in the hypothalamus and is released from the posterior lobe of the pituitary gland. ADH makes the distal convoluted tubule and collecting duct more permeable to water. When ADH is present, more water is reabsorbed, which reduces the volume of urine and makes it more concentrated. Water is conserved in the body. In the absence of ADH, the tubules are less permeable to water and there is less reabsorption. This results in large quantities of dilute urine and water is lost from the body.

Special cells in the heart produce a hormone called atrial natriuretic hormone, or atriopeptin, which is secreted when the atrial cells are stretched. This hormone promotes the excretion of sodium and water by acting directly on the kidney tubules and by inhibiting the secretion of ADH, renin, and aldosterone. The result of atrial natriuretic hormone is a decrease in blood volume and blood pressure.

> Aldosterone increases sodium reabsorption, and ADH increases water reabsorption in the kidney tubules. Atrial natriuretic hormone inhibits both ADH and aldosterone.

> Alcohol inhibits the secretion of ADH so when people drink alcohol, they experience diuresis, or excessive urination. It is believed that the dehydration caused by diuresis contributes to "hangover" symptoms.

Renin is an enzyme that is produced by the juxtaglomerular cells in the kidney in response to low blood pressure or decreased blood sodium concentration. Renin promotes the production of **angiotensin II** in the blood. Angiotensin II is a powerful vasoconstrictor, which increases the blood pressure. Angiotensin II also stimulates the adrenal gland to secrete aldosterone, which acts on the kidney tubules to conserve sodium and water. This increases blood volume and, consequently, increases blood pressure.

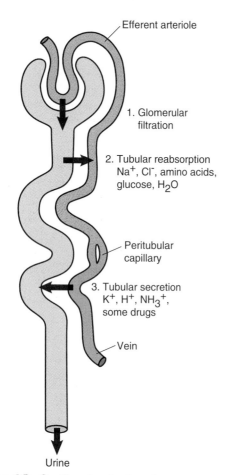

1. Glomerular filtration

2. Tubular reabsorption Na^+, Cl^-, amino acids, glucose, H_2O

Efferent arteriole

Peritubular capillary

3. Tubular secretion K^+, H^+, NH_3^+, some drugs

Vein

Urine

Figure 18–9 Steps in urine formation.

Renin from the kidneys increases the production of angiotensin II, which increases blood pressure and volume.

✓ QuickCheck

- How does the glomerular filtrate differ from blood plasma?
- Where does most tubular reabsorption occur?
- Why does glucose appear in the urine of persons with diabetes mellitus?
- Name three hormones that regulate urine concentration and volume.

Micturition

Micturition (mik-tou-RISH-un), commonly called urination or voiding, is the act of expelling urine from the bladder. The bladder can hold up to a liter of urine, but normally when it contains 200 to 400 milliliters, stretch receptors in the bladder wall trigger impulses that initiate the **micturition reflex.** This is an automatic and involuntary response that is coordinated in the spinal cord. Then, impulses are transmitted along parasympathetic nerves to the detrusor muscle. Even though the micturition reflex is involuntary, it can be inhibited or stimulated by higher brain centers.

Urinary incontinence is the inability to control urination and to retain urine in the bladder. Temporary incontinence may result when the muscles around the bladder and urethra become weakened and lose muscle tone. This sometimes is caused by stretching of the muscles during childbirth. Because these muscles help restrict the outlet of the bladder, their weakness contributes to a leakage of urine. A cough or sneeze may increase pressure within the bladder sufficiently to force urine to escape. Permanent incontinence usually is due to damage of the central nervous system or extensive damage to the bladder or urethra.

Characteristics of Urine

The volume, physical characteristics, and chemical composition of urine changes with diet, physical activity, and state of health. A chemical and microscopic examination of urine, called **urinalysis** (you-rin-AL-ih-sis), reveals a lot about the physiologic condition of a person.

Physical Characteristics

A normal, healthy individual excretes 1 to 2 liters of urine per day; however, the volume varies considerably. Even under conditions of water deprivation, the body needs to excrete a certain volume of urine

to get rid of toxic metabolic wastes. Freshly voided urine is normally clear and has a yellowish color. The color is due to the presence of **urochrome** (YOO-roh-krohm), a substance produced by the breakdown of bile pigments. The pH ranges between 4.6 and 8.0 with an average of about 6.0. High-protein diets increase the acidity and lower the pH. Vegetarian diets generally make the urine more alkaline and increase the pH. The specific gravity of urine varies from 1.001 to 1.035, which means that it is slightly heavier than water. This is due to the presence of solutes in the urine. The higher the concentration of solutes, the higher the specific gravity. These characteristics are summarized in Table 18–1.

Urine is clear, yellow, and heavier than water and has a normal pH range from 4.6 to 8.0.

Chemical Composition

Urine is about 95 percent water by volume. The remaining 5 percent consists of various solutes that are present. Most of the solutes are metabolic waste products that need to be eliminated from the body. Others, such as drugs, come from outside sources.

Kidney stones develop when uric acid or calcium salts precipitate instead of remaining dissolved in the urine. The stones usually form in the renal pelvis, but they may also develop in the urinary bladder. If small enough, they may pass naturally with urine flow but usually cause a lot of discomfort. If kidney stones cause a serious obstruction, they may need to be surgically removed. A newer method of treatment called lithotripsy uses high-frequency sound waves to break the stone into small pieces so that it may pass naturally. The formation of stones in the urine is called **urolithiasis.**

Abnormal Constituents

Certain substances, although normally not present in the urine, may appear from time to time. Their pres-

Table 18–1   Physical Characteristics of Urine
Characteristic	**Description**
Volume	1–2 liters per 24-hour period; average 1500 milliliters
pH	Varies between 4.6 and 8; average about 6; more acid with high-protein diets and more alkaline with vegetarian diets
Specific gravity	Varies between 1.001 and 1.035; slightly heavier than water
Color	Yellow due to presence of urochrome
Composition	95% water and 5% solutes; predominate solute is urea

ence in the urine may suggest some pathologic condition. Examples of abnormal constituents include albumin, glucose, blood cells, ketone bodies, and microbes (Table 18–2).

Body Fluids

Fluids make up 60 percent of the adult body weight. This fluid is not evenly distributed throughout the body but is separated into compartments. Even though separated by cell membranes, fluids can move back and forth between compartments. Fluid balance suggests that there is equilibrium or homeostasis between fluid intake and fluid output and in the movement of fluid between the compartments. The urinary system has an important role in maintaining homeostasis of body fluids by adjusting total fluid volume, by modifying electrolyte concentration, and by secreting varying quantities of hydrogen ions to regulate the pH of the blood.

Fluid Compartments

About two thirds of the total body fluid is found inside the cells of the body and is called **intracellular** (intrah-SELL-yoo-lar) **fluid** (ICF). The remaining

one third is outside the cells and includes all other body fluids. It is called **extracellular** (eks-trah-SELL-yoo-lar) **fluid** (ECF). About one fourth of the extracellular fluid is **intravascular** (in-trah-VAS-kyoo-lar) **fluid** (**blood plasma**), and the remaining three fourths is the **interstitial** (in-ter-STISH-al) **fluid** in the tissue spaces. Figure 18–10 illustrates the fluid compartments. A small amount of the extracellular fluid is localized as cerebrospinal fluid, aqueous and vitreous humors of the eyes, endolymph and perilymph in the ears, the serous fluid between the layers of serous membranes, and the synovial fluid in joints.

> Fluid makes up 60 percent of the adult's body weight. This is two thirds intracellular fluid and one third extracellular fluid. The extracellular fluid is further divided into intravascular and interstitial fluid.

Table 18–2	Abnormal Constituents of Urine	
Constituent	Clinical Term	Comment
Albumin	Albuminuria	Presence indicates increased permeability of filtration membrane due to disease, injury, or high blood pressure
Glucose	Glucosuria	Usually indicates diabetes mellitus
Erythrocytes (red blood cells)	Hematuria	Usually indicates kidney inflammation, trauma, or disease
Leukocytes (white blood cells)	Pyuria	Indicates infection in the kidney or urinary tract
Ketone bodies	Ketosis	Usually indicates diabetes mellitus, but occurs in any condition in which large quantities of fatty acids are metabolized
Bilirubin	Bilirubinuria	Usually indicates excessive destruction of red blood cells
Microbes		Indicates infection in the urinary tract

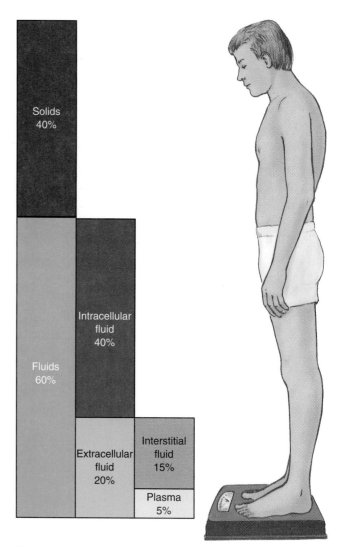

Figure 18–10 Fluid compartments.

Edema is a condition in which fluid accumulates in the interstitial compartment. This is sometimes due to a blockage of lymphatic vessels, which reduces the return of the fluid to the blood it may also be caused by a lack of plasma proteins or sodium retention.

Intake and Output of Fluid

Normally fluid intake equals fluid output so that the total amount of fluid in the body remains constant. Average fluid intake is 2,500 milliliters per day and comes from three sources (Fig. 18–11). Beverages account for about 1,600 milliliters and ingested foods provide another 700 milliliters. Water is produced as a by product of metabolism, and this metabolic water accounts for another 200 milliliters. The greatest regulator of fluid intake is the thirst mechanism. When body fluids become too concentrated, the increased osmotic pressure stimulates the thirst center in the hypothalamus. This results in a desire to drink fluids.

Sources of fluid intake are beverages, food, and metabolic water.

Under normal conditions, fluid output equals fluid intake to maintain fluid balance. There are four avenues of fluid loss (see Fig. 18–11). On an average, the kidneys excrete about 1,500 milliliters of water per day. The skin loses about 400 milliliters per day through evaporation and 150 milliliters per day through perspiration for a total of 550 milliliters per day. Water vapor is exhaled with each breath, and this loss through the lungs accounts for 300 milliliters per day. Finally, about 150 milliliters is lost through the gastrointestinal tract each day. Added together, these four avenues account for 2,500 milliliters of fluid output per day. The kidneys, under the influence of ADH, are the main regulators of fluid loss. If fluid intake remains constant and excess fluid is lost through diarrhea, vomiting, or perspiration, the kidneys excrete less urine to maintain fluid balance.

Avenues of fluid loss are through the kidneys, skin, lungs, and gastrointestinal tract.

Electrolyte Balance

Electrolytes are in balance when the concentration of individual electrolytes in the body fluid compartments is normal and remains relatively constant. This implies that the total electrolyte concentration is also normal and constant. Because electrolytes are dissolved in the body fluids, electrolyte balance and fluid balance are interrelated. When fluid volume changes, the concentration of the electrolytes also changes.

Sodium is the predominant cation (positive ion), and chloride is the predominant anion (negative ion) in the extracellular fluid. Bicarbonate ions are also extracellular ions. These three ions account for over 90 percent of the extracellular electrolytes. In the intracellular fluid compartment, potassium is the most abundant cation and phosphates are the major anions.

Sodium, chloride, and bicarbonate are the major ions in the extracellular fluid. Potassium and phosphates are intracellular ions.

The primary regulation of electrolyte balance is through active reabsorption of positive ions. The negative ions follow by electrochemical attraction. Because sodium and potassium are the predominant cations, they are the most important ones to be reg-

TOTAL INTAKE—2500 mL

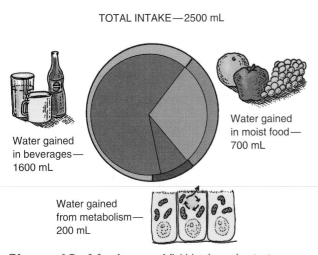

Water gained in beverages— 1600 mL

Water gained in moist food— 700 mL

Water gained from metabolism— 200 mL

TOTAL OUTPUT—2500 mL

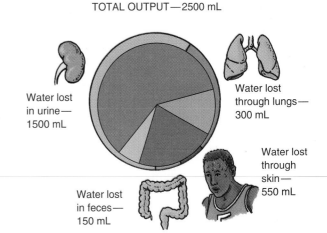

Water lost in urine— 1500 mL

Water lost through lungs— 300 mL

Water lost through skin— 550 mL

Water lost in feces— 150 mL

Figure 18-11 Avenues of fluid intake and output.

ulated. Aldosterone, acting on the kidney tubules, regulates sodium and potassium levels by stimulating the reabsorption of sodium ions from the filtrate into the blood and the excretion of potassium ions in the urine. This adds sodium to the extracellular fluid and deceases the potassium.

> Aldosterone from the adrenal cortex is the primary hormone that regulates sodium and potassium concentrations.

Because sodium (Na+) is the predominate cation in the interstitial fluid and potassium (K+) is the predominate cation in the intracellular fluid, changes in either of their concentrations within their respective compartments will cause a movement of fluid between the two compartments. For example, if a person has a high Na+ concentration in the extracellular fluid (plasma and interstitial fluid), the increased osmotic pressure causes water to move from the intracellular compartment into the extracellular compartment. This movement results in edema and a reduction of fluid volume inside the cells. This illustrates that fluid balance depends on electrolyte balance. However, the opposite is also true. If the amount of water in a compartment increases, the concentration of the electrolyte will decrease. This shows that electrolyte balance depends on fluid balance. Fluid balance and electrolyte balance are interdependent.

> Fluid moves from one compartment to another when there is a change in electrolyte concentration in the compartments.

Acid–Base Balance

Blood, the intravascular fluid, has a normal pH range of 7.35 to 7.45. Deviations below this range are called **acidosis** (AS-id-oh-sis), and an increase in pH above the normal is called **alkalosis** (AL-kah-loh-sis). Cellular metabolism produces substances that tend to upset the pH balance. Lactic acid is produced in the anaerobic breakdown of glucose. When carbon dioxide from aerobic metabolism combines with water, it produces carbonic acid. The metabolism of fatty acids produces acidic ketone bodies. All of these products tend to make the blood more acidic and to lower the pH. The body has three mechanisms by which it attempts to maintain a normal blood pH:

- Buffers
- Removal of carbon dioxide by the lungs
- Removal of hydrogen ions by the kidneys

> Blood has a normal pH range of 7.35 to 7.45. Acidosis occurs when pH of the blood decreases below normal, and alkalosis occurs when there is an increase above normal.

Buffers (see Chapter 2) are substances that prevent significant changes in pH. If the hydrogen ion concentration is too high (acid), the buffer combines with some of the hydrogen ions to bring the pH back to normal. If the hydrogen ion concentration is too low (alkaline), the buffer releases hydrogen ions to lower the pH. Buffers are important for adjusting small changes in hydrogen ion concentration.

Carbon dioxide is a byproduct of cellular metabolism. When carbon dioxide combines with water, it produces carbonic acid, which releases hydrogen ions and lowers the pH of the blood. As the blood flows through the lungs, carbon dioxide is removed and exhaled. This reduces the amount of carbonic acid that is present. The lungs are important in regulating pH because they remove one of the sources (CO_2) of acids. Without the work of the lungs in removing carbon dioxide, the buffers are quickly overloaded and the pH decreases below normal.

The kidneys function in acid–base balance by the tubular secretion of hydrogen ions and excreting them in the urine. If the blood is too acid (excess hydrogen ions), the kidney tubules actively secrete hydrogen ions from the peritubular capillaries into the filtrate, and they are removed from the body. If the blood is too alkaline, the kidney tubules conserve hydrogen ions.

> Buffer systems in the blood, the lungs, and the kidneys are the primary regulators of blood pH.

✓ QuickCheck

- Approximately what percentage of the adult body weight is due to fluids?
- Where is most of the body fluid located?
- What is the predominant cation in extracellular fluid?
- What is the normal pH for blood?

FOCUS ON AGING

Some of the more obvious and familiar aging changes occur in the urinary bladder and urethra. Muscles in the wall of these structures tend to weaken and become less elastic with age. As a person ages, the bladder is unable to expand or contract as much as in younger people. This reduces the capacity of the bladder and makes it more difficult to completely empty it during urination. Awareness of the need to urinate, which usually occurs when the bladder is half full in younger people, may be delayed in the elderly until the bladder is nearly full. Thus, urgency accompanies awareness. The external urethral sphincter also weakens, which adds to the problems.

Several anatomical changes occur in the kidneys as a person ages, and these changes are reflected in their related functions. There is a general atrophy of nephrons so that by the age of 80, the kidney is about 80 percent of its young, but mature, size. Some of the remaining glomeruli are modified, and this, along with the decrease in number, results in decreased glomerular filtration rate so that the blood is not filtered as quickly as before.

The tubules also undergo changes as a person ages. In general, the tubule walls thicken, which makes them less able to reabsorb water to form a concentrated urine. The collecting ducts are less responsive to ADH and this, along with a diminished thirst mechanism, may result in dehydration. The ability to reabsorb glucose and sodium is also diminished. The tubules become less efficient in the secretion of ions and drugs. They have diminished ability to compensate for drastic changes in acid–base balance. Drugs that are normally eliminated from the body by tubular secretion may accumulate to toxic levels because they are not cleared from the blood as quickly as they are in younger people.

Amazingly, even with the changes due to aging, the kidneys of elderly persons are capable of maintaining relatively stable balances in the blood and body fluids under normal conditions. However, their ability to compensate for drastic changes and abnormal conditions is diminished.

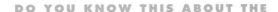

DO YOU KNOW THIS ABOUT THE

Urinary System?

Acid–Base Imbalances

The normal pH range of the blood and interstitial fluid is 7.35 to 7.45. A person can live for only a few hours if the pH falls to 7.0 or increases to 8.0, which means that deviations of only a few tenths of a unit can be disastrous. Chemical buffers, the respiratory system, and the kidneys work together to keep the body fluids within the specified normal range. If any one of these mechanisms fails, then acid–base imbalances occur. **Acidosis** occurs if the blood pH falls below 7.35. The physiologic effect of acidosis is depression of synaptic transmission in the central nervous system. If the pH falls below 7.0, the depression is so severe that the person becomes disoriented and lapses into a coma, and death soon follows. In **alkalosis,** the pH of the blood is above 7.45 and the principal effect is hyperexcitability in both the central nervous system and the peripheral nerves. This leads to extreme nervousness and muscle spasms. If untreated, alkalosis may lead to convulsions and death.

Acidosis and alkalosis can be classified according to cause as either **respiratory** or **metabolic.** Respiratory acidosis or alkalosis represents a problem with respiratory mechanisms, and the most important indicator of these conditions is the partial pressure of carbon dioxide (P_{CO_2}). Normal arterial P_{CO_2} ranges between 35 mm Hg and 45 mm Hg. Values above 45 mm Hg represent respiratory acidosis, and values below 35 mm Hg represent respiratory alkalosis. **Metabolic** acidosis or alkalosis includes all acid–base imbalances that are not caused by deviations in carbon dioxide. In other words, if it is not a respiratory problem, then it is considered metabolic. The most important indicator of imbalances that are caused by metabolic problems is the concentration of bicarbonate (HCO^-_3) ions. The normal range of bicarbonate ion concentration is 22 to 26 mEq per liter. A bicarbonate ion concentration below 22 mEq per liter is an indication of metabolic acidosis, and a concentration

Continued on following page

above 26 mEq per liter represents metabolic alkalosis.

Changes in blood pH that lead to acidosis or alkalosis can be returned to normal by physiologic responses called **compensation.** If a person has metabolic acidosis or alkalosis, the respiratory system attempts to bring the pH back to normal by changing the rate and depth of breathing. Respiratory compensation for metabolic pH imbalances occurs within minutes, and maximum compensation is achieved within hours. If the pH imbalance is caused by some problem in the respiratory system, the kidneys attempt to compensate for the imbalance by changing the amount of hydrogen and bicarbonate ions that are excreted. Metabolic compensation for respiratory pH imbalances begins within minutes, but it takes several days to achieve maximum compensation. Respiratory and metabolic mechanisms for compensation may be successful in restoring the blood pH to normal range, but evidence of the original pH imbalance still exists in the altered CO_2 and bicarbonate ion concentrations.

Respiratory acidosis is indicated when the arterial P_{CO_2} is above 45 mm Hg and the pH is below 7.35. When CO_2 accumulates in the blood, the amount of carbonic acid and hydrogen ions increases and the pH decreases. Any condition that hinders the movement of CO_2 from the blood to the alveoli and into the atmosphere may result in respiratory acidosis. Such conditions include emphysema, airway obstruction, depression of the medullary respiratory center, weakness of the muscles used in breathing, and pulmonary edema. The kidneys compensate by excreting hydrogen ions in the urine and by reabsorbing bicarbonate ions. Renal compensation for respiratory acidosis is indicated by an increased bicarbonate ion concentration in the blood.

Respiratory alkalosis is caused by a loss of CO_2 from the lungs through hyperventilation. The low levels of CO_2 in the lungs lead to an excessive loss of CO_2 from the blood, which causes alkalosis and an increase in pH. The primary indicators of respiratory alkalosis are P_{CO_2} below 35 mm Hg and pH above 7.45. Conditions that may lead to respiratory alkalosis are those that stimulate the respiratory center in the medulla. Such conditions include severe anxiety, hysterical hyperventilation, oxygen deficiency due to high altitude, and the early stages of aspirin overdose. The kidneys attempt to compensate for the alkalosis by decreasing the excretion of hydrogen ions and by increasing bicarbonate ion excretion. Renal compensation for respiratory alkalosis is indicated by a decreased bicarbonate ion concentration in the blood.

Metabolic acidosis is indicated by a decrease in bicarbonate ion concentration below 22 mEq per liter, which causes the pH to fall below 7.35. This may be due to a loss of bicarbonate ions or to an accumulation of metabolic acids. Severe diarrhea or renal dysfunction leads to a loss of bicarbonate ions. Metabolic acids accumulate when the kidneys fail to excrete hydrogen ions or when fats instead of carbohydrates are used for energy. Diabetes mellitus is a good example of a condition that leads to metabolic acidosis because acidic ketone bodies are produced as a byproduct of fat utilization. The respiratory system attempts to compensate for metabolic acidosis by hyperventilation, which removes CO_2 from the body. Respiratory compensation for metabolic acidosis is indicated by a decreased P_{CO_2} value in the blood.

In **metabolic alkalosis** there is an increase in bicarbonate ion concentration above 26 mEq per liter and a pH above 7.45. The increase in pH may be caused by a nonrespiratory loss of acid or by an excessive intake of alkaline substances. Repeated vomiting of gastric contents causes a loss of hydrochloric acid, and this probably is the most frequent cause of metabolic alkalosis. Excessive ingestion of sodium bicarbonate and other antacids also contributes to the problem. The respiratory system compensates by hypoventilation, which retains carbon dioxide in the body and lowers the pH. Respiratory compensation for metabolic alkalosis is indicated by an increased P_{CO_2} value in the blood.

Table 18–3 is a summary of the blood indicators for the different types of acid–base imbalances.

Table 18–3 Acid–Base Indicators

	pH	PCO$_2$	HCO$_3^-$
Normal	7.35–7.45	35–45 mm Hg	22–26 mEq/liter
Respiratory acidosis	↓	↑	Normal or ↑ if compensating
Respiratory alkalosis	↑	↓	Normal or ↓ if compensating
Metabolic acidosis	↓	Normal ↓ if compensating	↓
Metabolic alkalosis	↑	Normal ↑ if compensating	↑

REPRESENTATIVE DISORDERS OF THE URINARY SYSTEM

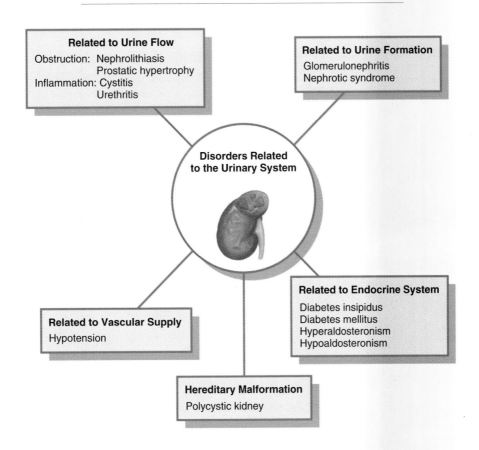

Related to Urine Flow
Obstruction: Nephrolithiasis
                      Prostatic hypertrophy
Inflammation: Cystitis
                      Urethritis

Related to Urine Formation
Glomerulonephritis
Nephrotic syndrome

**Disorders Related
to the Urinary System**

Related to Vascular Supply
Hypotension

Related to Endocrine System
Diabetes insipidus
Diabetes mellitus
Hyperaldosteronism
Hypoaldosteronism

Hereditary Malformation
Polycystic kidney

CHAPTER QUIZ

RECALL

Match the definitions on the left with the appropriate term on the right.

1. Functional unit in kidney

2. Cluster of capillaries in the renal corpuscle

3. Cortical substance between adjacent renal pyramids

4. Modified cells in the ascending limb of the nephron loop

5. Enzyme produced by juxtaglomerular cells

6. Folds in the mucosa of the urinary bladder

7. Urination or voiding

8. Responsible for yellow color of urine

9. Accounts for about two thirds of the body fluid

10. Increase in pH above normal

   A. Alkalosis

   B. Glomerulus

   C. Intracellular fluid

   D. Macula densa

   E. Micturition

   F. Nephron

   G. Renal columns

   H. Renin

   I. Rugae

   J. Urochrome

THOUGHT

1. When blood is filtered in the kidney, the filtrate passes from the
   a. efferent arteriole into the glomerulus
   b. glomerulus into the glomerular capsule
   c. afferent arteriole into the glomerulus
   d. glomerulus into the proximal convoluted tubule

2. Which of the following is NOT true about the juxtaglomerular apparatus?
   a. it produces an enzyme called renin
   b. it secretes a substance that functions in the regulation of blood pressure
   c. it occurs where the efferent arteriole contacts the afferent arteriole
   d. it contains a region called the macula densa

3. The greatest amount of fluid is reabsorbed from the filtrate in the
   a. proximal convoluted tubule
   b. nephron loop
   c. distal convoluted tubule
   d. collecting duct

4. Which of the following statements about body fluids is NOT true?
   a. the volume of plasma is greater than the volume of interstitial fluid
   b. the volume of intracellular fluid is greater than the volume of extracellular fluid
   c. the interstitial fluid is a part of extracellular fluid
   d. fluids account for about 60% of the total body weight

5. Which of the following blood pH values represents alkalosis?
   a. 7.3 and 7.6
   b. 6.7 and 6.9
   c. 7.1 and 7.3
   d. 7.5 and 7.6

APPLICATION

Name three hormones that influence urine volume, state the source of each hormone, and describe how it affects the volume.

When a child learns to control micturition, he or she controls what muscle?

CHAPTER 19

Reproductive System

Outline/Objectives

Male Reproductive System 395

- Distinguish between primary and secondary reproductive organs.
- Describe the location and structure of each component of the male reproductive system.
- Draw and label a diagram or flow chart that illustrates spermatogenesis and describe the process by which spermatids become mature sperm.
- Trace the pathway of sperm from the testes to the outside of the body.
- Outline the physiologic events in the male sexual response.
- Describe the role of GnRH, FSH, LH, and testosterone in male reproductive functions.

Female Reproductive System 402

- Describe the location and structure of each component of the female reproductive system, including the mammary glands.
- Draw and label a diagram or flow chart that illustrates oogenesis.
- Describe the development of ovarian follicles as they progress from primordial follicles to primary follicles, secondary follicles, vesicular follicles, corpus luteum, and, finally, the corpus albicans.
- Outline the physiologic events in the female sexual response.
- Describe the roles of GnRH, FSH, LH, estrogen, and progesterone in female reproductive functions.
- Describe what happens in each phase of the ovarian and uterine cycles, when each phase occurs, and how the cycles interact.

Key Terms

Gametes

Gonads

Oogenesis

Ovarian cycle

Ovarian follicle

Spermatogenesis

Spermiogenesis

Uterine cycle

Building Vocabulary

WORD PART	MEANING
andr-	male
balan-	glans
colpo-	vagina
crypt-	hidden
ejacul-	to shoot forth
fimb-	fringe
follic-	small bag
gynec-	female
hyster-	womb or uterus
labi-	lip
mamm-	breast
meno-	month
metr-	uterus
oo-	egg, ovum
oophor-	ovary
orch-	testicle
prostat-	prostate
-rrhagia	to burst forth
salping-	tube
spadias	an opening

Functional Relationships of the
Reproductive System

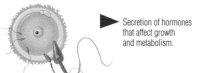

Secretion of hormones that affect growth and metabolism.

Integument
Skin forms scrotum that protects testes; tactile receptors in skin provide sensations associated with sexual behaviors.

Gonads provide hormones that promote growth, and maintenance of skin; gonadal hormones affect growth and distribution of body hair and activity of sebaceous glands.

Skeletal
Provides protection for reproductive organs in pelvis; pelvis may hinder vaginal delivery of fetus.

Gonads produce hormones that influence bone growth, maintenance, and closure of epiphyseal plates.

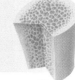

Muscular
Provides support for reproductive organs in the pelvis; muscle contractions contribute to orgasm in both sexes; aid in childbirth.

Gonads produce hormones that influence muscle development and size.

Nervous
Regulates sex drive, arousal, and orgasm; stimulates the release of numerous hormones involved in sperm production, menstrual cycle, pregnancy, and parturition.

Gonads produce hormones that affect CNS development and sexual behavior; menstrual hormones affect the activity of the hypothalamus.

Endocrine
Hormones have a major role in differentiation and development of reproductive organs, sexual development, sex drive, gamete production, menstrual cycle, pregnancy, parturition, and lactation.

Gonads produce hormones that feedback to influence pituitary function.

Cardiovascular
Transports reproductive hormones to target tissues; provides nutrients and oxygen to developing fetus, and removes wastes; vasodilation responsible for erection.

Gonads produce hormones that help maintain healthy blood vessels; testosterone stimulates erythropoiesis; some evidence that estrogens may decrease cholesterol levels.

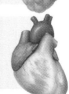

Lymphatic/Immune
Provides specific defense against pathogens that enter the body through the reproductive tract; surveillance against cancer cells.

Acids and enzymes along the reproductive tract provide nonspecific defense against pathogens; blood-testis barrier prevents immune destruction of sperm.

Respiratory
Supplies oxygen and removes carbon dioxide to maintain metabolism in tissues of reproductive system; helps maintain pH for gonadal hormone function.

Sexual arousal stimulates changes in rate and depth of breathing; during pregnancy, the expanding uterus reduces depth of breathing, but rate of breathing increases.

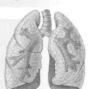

Urinary
Maintains pH and electrolyte composition for effective gonadal hormone function; maternal urinary system excretes metabolic wastes from developing fetus.

Prostate surrounds urethra and may compress it to cause urine retention; pregnant uterus pushes on urinary bladder to cause frequent urination.

Digestive
Provides nutrients for growth, maintenance, and repair of reproductive tissues; provides nutrients for repair of endometrium following menstruation and for developing fetus during pregnancy.

During pregnancy, expanding uterus may crowd intestines causing constipation and heartburn; gonadal steroids have an effect on metabolic rate.

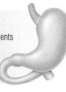

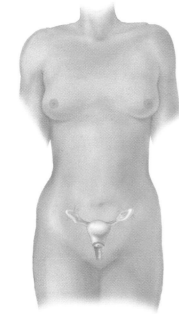

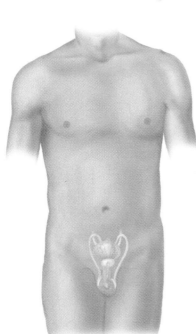

he major function of the reproductive system is to produce offspring. Other systems in the body, such as the endocrine and urinary systems, work continuously to maintain homeostasis for survival of the individual. The reproductive system, on the other hand, functions for the survival of the species. An individual may live a long, healthy, and happy life without producing offspring, but if the species is to continue, at least some individuals must produce offspring.

Within the context of producing offspring, the reproductive system has four functions:

- To produce egg and sperm cells
- To transport and sustain these cells
- To nurture the developing offspring
- To produce hormones

These functions are divided between the **primary reproductive organs** and the **secondary,** or **accessory, reproductive organs.** The primary reproductive organs, also called **gonads,** are the ovaries and testes. These organs are responsible for producing the egg and sperm cells, also called **gametes,** and for producing hormones. These hormones function in the maturation of the reproductive system and the development of sexual characteristics and have important roles in regulating the normal physiology of the reproductive system. All other organs, ducts, and glands in the reproductive system are considered secondary, or accessory, reproductive organs. These structures transport and sustain the gametes and nurture the developing offspring.

> The primary reproductive organs are the gonads, which produce the gametes and hormones. The secondary, or accessory, structures transport and sustain the gametes and nurture the developing offspring.

Male Reproductive System

The male reproductive system produces, sustains, and transports sperm; introduces the sperm into the female vagina; and produces hormones. Figure 19–1 shows the organs of the male reproductive system.

Testes

The **testes,** or **testicles,** the male gonads, begin their development high in the abdominal cavity, near the kidneys. During the last 2 months before birth, or shortly after birth, they descend through the inguinal canal into the **scrotum,** a pouch that extends below the abdomen, posterior to the penis. Although this location of the testes, outside the abdominal cavity, may seem to make them vulnerable to injury, it provides a temperature about 3° C below normal body temperature. This lower temperature is necessary for the production of viable sperm. The scrotum consists of skin and subcutaneous tissue. A vertical septum, or partition, of subcutaneous tissue in the center divides it into two parts, each containing one testis. Smooth muscle fibers, called the **dartos muscle,** in the subcutaneous tissue contract to give the scrotum its wrinkled appearance. When these fibers are relaxed, the scrotum is smooth. Another muscle, the **cremaster muscle** in the spermatic cord, consists of skeletal muscle fibers and controls the position of the scrotum and testes. When it is cold or a man is sexually aroused, this muscle contracts to pull the testes closer to the body for warmth.

> The male gonads are the testes. They develop within the abdominal cavity, but usually descend into the scrotum before birth. Their location within the scrotum is necessary for the production of viable sperm.

CLINICAL TERMS

Amenorrhea (ah-men-oh-REE-ah) A lack of the monthly flow or menstruation

Coitus (KOH-ih-tus) Sexual intercourse between a man and a woman

Dysmenorrhea (dis-men-oh-REE-ah) Difficult or painful menstruation

Endometriosis (en-doh-mee-trih-OH-sis) A condition in which endometrial tissue occurs in various abnormal sites in the abdominal or pelvic cavity; it may be caused when pieces of menstrual endometrium pass backward through the uterine tube into the peritoneal cavity

Episiotomy (eh-peez-ee-AHT-oh-mee) Incision of the perineum to prevent tearing of the perineum and to facilitate delivery during childbirth

Hysterectomy (his-ter-ECK-toh-mee) Surgical removal of the uterus

Mittelschmerz (MIT-el-shmairts) Abdominal pain that occurs midway between the menstrual periods, at the time of ovulation

Oligospermia (ahl-ih-goh-SPER-mee-ah) A condition in which there are few sperm in the semen; low sperm count

Oophorectomy (oh-ahf-oh-RECK-toh-mee) Surgical removal of an ovary

Orchidectomy (or-kih-DECK-toh-mee) Surgical excision of a testis

Phimosis (fye-MOH-sis) A condition in which the opening of the prepuce is narrow and cannot be drawn back over the glans penis

Prostatitis (prahs-tah-TYE-tis) Inflammation of the prostate

Salpingectomy (sall-pin-JECK-toh-mee) Surgical removal of a uterine tube

Spermicide (SPER-mih-syde) An agent that kills sperm

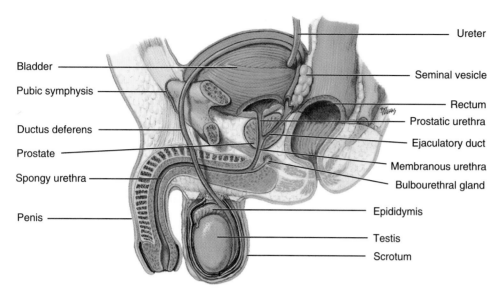

Figure 19–1 Structures in the male reproductive system.

The inguinal canal represents a weakened area in the abdominal wall which may open, resulting in an inguinal hernia. A portion of the intestine may pass through the opening into the scrotum. This is painful and potentially dangerous if the blood supply to the intestine is constricted. This condition is more common in men than in women. Inguinal hernias are frequently repaired by surgery.

The condition in which the testes do not descend into the scrotum is called **cryptorchidism**. Crypt means hidden and orchid refers to the testis, so the term means hidden testis. Cryptochidism results in sterility if it is not corrected before puberty because the cooler temperature of the scrotum is necessary for sperm productiion.

Structure

Each testis is an oval structure about 5 cm long and 3 cm in diameter (Fig. 19–2). A tough, white fibrous connective tissue capsule, the **tunica albuginea** (TOO-nik-ah al-byoo-JIN-ee-ah), surrounds each testis and extends inward to form **septa** that partition the organ into **lobules**. There are about 250 lobules in each testis. Each lobule contains one to four highly coiled **seminiferous** (seh-mye-NIFF-er-us) **tubules** that converge to form a single **straight tubule**, which leads into the **rete testis** (REE-tee TEST-is), a tubular network on one side of the testis. Short efferent ducts exit the testes. **Interstitial cells** (cells of Leydig), which produce male sex hormones, are located between the seminiferous tubules within a lobule.

The testes are divided into lobules. Each lobule contains seminiferous tubules and interstitial cells.

Spermatogenesis

Sperm are produced by **spermatogenesis** (spur-mat-oh-JEN-eh-sis) within the seminiferous tubules. A transverse section of a seminiferous tubule shows that it is packed with cells in various stages of spermatogenesis (Fig. 19–3). Interspersed with these cells, there are large cells that extend from the periphery of the tubule to the lumen. These large cells are the **supporting,** or **sustentacular, cells** (Sertoli's cells), which support and nourish the other cells.

Early in embryonic development, **primordial germ cells** enter the testes and differentiate into **spermatogonia** (spur-mat-oh-GOH-nee-ah), imma-

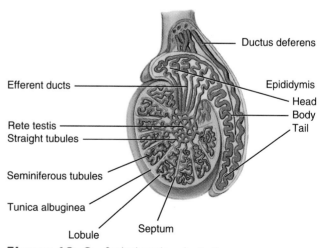

Figure 19–2 Sagittal section of a testis.

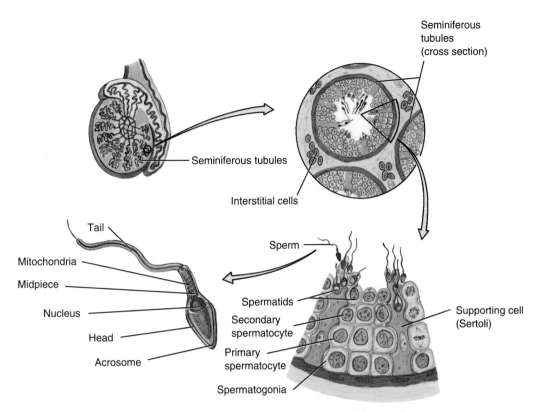

Figure 19-3   Cross section of a seminiferous tubule showing the different cell types.

ture cells that remain dormant until puberty. Spermatogonia are diploid cells, each with 46 chromosomes (23 pairs), that are located around the periphery of the seminiferous tubules. At puberty, hormones stimulate these cells to begin dividing by mitosis. Some of the daughter cells produced by mitosis remain at the periphery as spermatogonia. Others are pushed toward the lumen, undergo some changes, and become **primary spermatocytes.** Because they are produced by mitosis, primary spermatocytes, like spermatogonia, are diploid and have 46 chromosomes.

Each primary spermatocyte goes through the first meiotic division, meiosis I, to produce two **secondary spermatocytes,** each with 23 chromosomes (haploid). Just before this division, the genetic material is replicated so that each chromosome consists of two strands, called **chromatids,** that are joined by a centromere. During meiosis I, one chromosome, consisting of two chromatids, goes to each secondary spermatocyte. In the second meiotic division, meiosis II, each secondary spermatocyte divides to produce two **spermatids.** There is no replication of genetic material in this division, but the centromere divides so that a single-stranded chromatid goes to each cell. As a result of the two meiotic divisions, each primary spermatocyte produces four spermatids (Fig. 19–4). During spermatogenesis there are two cellular divisions, but only one replication of DNA so that each spermatid has 23 chromosomes (hap-

loid), one from each pair in the original primary spermatocyte. Each successive stage in spermatogenesis is pushed toward the center of the tubule so that the more immature cells are at the periphery and the more differentiated cells are nearer the center (see Fig. 19–3).

Spermatogenesis (and oogenesis in the female) differs from mitosis (review Chapter 3) because the resulting cells have only half the number of chromosomes as the original cell. When the sperm cell nucleus unites with an egg cell nucleus, the full number of chromosomes is restored. If sperm and egg cells were produced by mitosis, then each successive generation would have twice the number of chromosomes as the preceding one.

Spermatogenesis takes place inside the seminiferous tubules. Each primary spermatocyte produces four spermatids, each with 23 chromosomes.

The final step in the development of sperm is called **spermiogenesis** (spur-mee-oh-JEN-eh-sis). In this process, the spermatids formed from spermatogenesis become mature spermatozoa, or sperm. The mature sperm cell has a **head, midpiece,** and **tail** (see Fig. 19–3). The head, also called the nuclear region, contains the 23 chromosomes surrounded by a nuclear membrane. The tip of the head is covered by an **acrosome** (Ak-roh-sohm), which contains enzymes that help the sperm penetrate the female

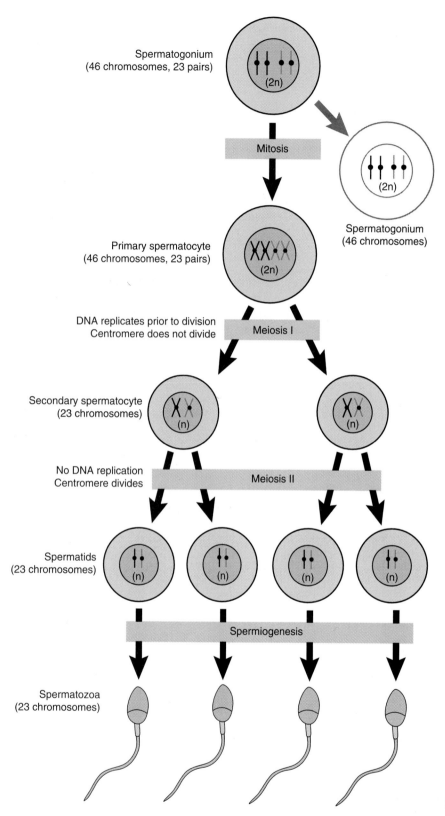

Spermatogonium
(46 chromosomes, 23 pairs)

(2n)

Mitosis

Spermatogonium
(46 chromosomes)

(2n)

Primary spermatocyte
(46 chromosomes, 23 pairs)

(2n)

DNA replicates prior to division
Centromere does not divide

Meiosis I

Secondary spermatocyte
(23 chromosomes)

(n)

(n)

No DNA replication
Centromere divides

Meiosis II

Spermatids
(23 chromosomes)

(n)

(n)

(n)

(n)

Spermiogenesis

Spermatozoa
(23 chromosomes)

Figure 19–4 Spermatogenesis.

gamete. The midpiece, also called the metabolic region, contains mitochondria that provide adenosine triphosphate (ATP). The tail, also called the locomotor region, is a typical flagellum for locomotion. The sperm are released into the lumen of the seminiferous tubule, leave the testes, and enter the epididymis, where they undergo their final maturation and become capable of fertilizing a female gamete.

| Spermiogenesis changes a spermatid into a mature sperm cell with a head, midpiece, and tail.

Sperm production begins at puberty and continues throughout the life of a male. The entire process, beginning with a primary spermatocyte, takes about 74 days. After ejaculation, the sperm can live for about 48 hours in the female reproductive tract.

Duct System

Sperm cells pass through a series of ducts to reach the outside of the body. After they leave the testes, the sperm pass through the epididymis, ductus deferens, ejaculatory duct, and urethra.

Epididymis

Sperm leave the testes through a series of efferent ducts that enter the **epididymis** (ep-ih-DID-ih-mis) (see Fig. 19–2). The epididymis is a long (about 6 meters) tube that is tightly coiled to form a comma-shaped organ located along the superior and posterior margins of the testes. When the sperm leave the testes, they are immature and incapable of fertilizing ova. They complete their maturation process and become fertile as they move through the epididymis. Mature sperm are stored in the lower portion, or tail, of the epididymis.

| Sperm move from the testis into the epididymis, where they mature and become fertile.

Ductus Deferens

The **ductus deferens,** also called **vas deferens,** is a fibromuscular tube that is continuous with the epididymis. It begins at the bottom (tail) of the epididymis then turns sharply upward along the posterior margin of the testes (see Fig. 19–2). The ductus deferens enters the abdominopelvic cavity through the inguinal canal and passes along the lateral pelvic wall. It crosses over the ureter and posterior portion of the urinary bladder, then descends along the posterior wall of the bladder toward the prostate gland (see Fig. 19–1). Just before it reaches the prostate gland, each ductus deferens enlarges to form an **ampulla.** Sperm are stored in the proximal portion of the ductus deferens, near the epididymis, and peristaltic movements propel the sperm through the tube.

The proximal portion of the ductus deferens is a component of the **spermatic cord,** which contains vascular and neural structures that supply the testes. The spermatic cord contains the ductus deferens, testicular artery and veins, lymph vessels, testicular nerve, cremaster muscle (which elevates the testes for warmth and at times of sexual stimulation), and a connective tissue covering.

A **vasectomy** is a surgical procedure, usually accomplished through a tiny incision in the scrotum, that severs the vas deferens. This results in sterility because it interrupts the pathway of the sperm to the outside of the body.

Ejaculatory Duct

Each ductus deferens, at the ampulla, joins the duct from the adjacent seminal vesicle (one of the accessory glands) to form a short **ejaculatory** (ee-JAK-yoo-lah-to-ree) **duct** (see Fig. 19–1). Each ejaculatory duct passes through the prostate gland and empties into the urethra.

| The ductus deferens conveys sperm from the epididymis to the ejaculatory duct. The ejaculatory duct penetrates the prostate gland and empties into the urethra.

Urethra

The **urethra** (yoo-REE-thrah) extends from the urinary bladder to the external urethral orifice at the tip of the penis. It is a passageway for sperm and fluids from the reproductive system and urine from the urinary system. While reproductive fluids are passing through the urethra, sphincters contract tightly to keep urine from entering the urethra.

The male urethra is divided into three regions (see Fig. 19–1). The **prostatic urethra** is the proximal portion that passes through the prostate gland. It receives the ejaculatory duct, which contains spermatozoa and secretions from the seminal vesicles, and numerous ducts from the prostate gland. The next portion, the **membranous urethra,** is a short region that passes through the pelvic floor. The longest portion is the **penile urethra** (also called spongy urethra or cavernous urethra), which extends the length of the penis and opens to the outside at the external urethral orifice. The ducts from the bulbourethral glands open into the penile urethra.

| The male urethra is a passageway for sperm, fluids from the reproductive system, and urine. It is divided into the prostatic urethra, membranous urethra, and penile urethra.

Benign prostatic hyperplasia is a common condition in older men. The prostate enlarges and compresses the urethra making urination difficult. This tends to retain urine in the bladder, which makes the individual more susceptible to urinary tract infections.

Accessory Glands

The accessory glands of the male reproductive system are the seminal vesicles, prostate gland, and the bulbourethral glands. These glands secrete fluids that enter the urethra.

Seminal Vesicles

The paired **seminal vesicles** are saccular glands posterior to the urinary bladder (see Fig. 19–1). Each gland has a short duct that joins with the ductus deferens at the ampulla to form an ejaculatory duct that empties into the urethra. The fluid from the seminal vesicles is viscous and contains fructose, which provides an energy source for the spermatozoa; prostaglandins, which contribute to the motility and viability of the sperm; and proteins, which cause slight coagulation reactions in the semen after ejaculation.

> Cancer of the prostate is the second most common cancer in men. It usually starts in one of the secretory glands, and as it continues, it produces a lump on the surface of the prostate. In many cases by the time the lump can be palpated through the wall of the rectum, the cancer has metastasized to other areas of the body. It is hoped that using some new blood screening techniques in addition to rectal palpation will result in earlier detection of the tumor and treatment can begin before metastasis occurs.

Prostate

The **prostate gland** is a firm, dense structure that is located just inferior to the urinary bladder (see Fig. 19–1). It is about the size of a walnut and encircles the urethra as it leaves the urinary bladder. Numerous short ducts from the substance of the prostate gland empty into the prostatic urethra. The secretions of the prostate are thin, milky colored, and alkaline. They function to enhance the motility of the sperm.

Bulbourethral Glands

The paired **bulbourethral (Cowper's) glands** (see Fig. 19–1) are small, about the size of a pea, and are located near the base of the penis. A short duct from each gland enters the proximal end of the penile urethra. In response to sexual stimulation, the bulbourethral glands secrete an alkaline mucuslike fluid. This fluid neutralizes the acidity of the urine residue in the urethra, helps to neutralize the acidity of the vagina, and provides some lubrication for the tip of the penis during intercourse.

> The seminal vesicles, prostate, and bulbourethral glands secrete fluids that nourish the spermatozoa, enhance the motility and viability of the spermatozoa, neutralize the acidity of the urethra and vagina, and provide some lubrication during intercourse.

Seminal Fluid

Seminal fluid, or **semen,** is the slightly alkaline (pH 7.5) mixture of sperm cells and secretions from the accessory glands. Secretions from the seminal vesicles make up about 60 percent of the volume of the **semen,** with most of the remainder coming from the prostate gland. The spermatozoa and secretions from the bulbourethral gland contribute only a small volume.

The volume of semen in a single ejaculation may vary from 1.5 to 6.0 milliliters. There are usually between 50 and 150 million sperm per milliliter of semen. Sperm counts below 10 to 20 million per milliliter usually present fertility problems. Although only one spermatozoon actually penetrates and fertilizes the ovum, it takes several million spermatozoa in an ejaculation to ensure that fertilization will take place.

> Seminal fluid, or semen, is slightly alkaline. Approximately 60 percent of the volume comes from the seminal vesicles.

✓ QuickCheck

- Why is it necessary for the testes to descend into the scrotum?
- Specifically, where in the testes does spermatogenesis occur?
- What duct is ligated or severed in a vasectomy?
- Which of the male accessory glands contributes the greatest volume to seminal fluid?

Penis

The **penis,** the male copulatory organ, is a cylindrical pendant organ located anterior to the scrotum and functions to transfer sperm to the vagina. Figure 19–5 illustrates that the penis consists of three columns of erectile tissue that are wrapped in connective tissue and covered with skin. The two dorsal columns are the **corpora cavernosa** (KOR-por-ah kav-er-NOH-sah). The single, midline ventral column surrounds the urethra and is called the **corpus spongiosum** (KOR-pus spun-jee-OH-sum).

> The penis consists of three columns of erectile tissue. The two dorsal columns are the corpora cavernosa, and the ventral column is the corpus spongiosum.

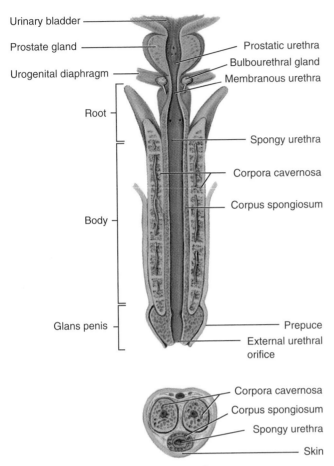

Urinary bladder

Prostate gland

Urogenital diaphragm

Root

Body

Glans penis

Prostatic urethra

Bulbourethral gland

Membranous urethra

Spongy urethra

Corpora cavernosa

Corpus spongiosum

Prepuce

External urethral orifice

Corpora cavernosa

Corpus spongiosum

Spongy urethra

Skin

Figure 19–5   Structure of the penis.

The penis has a **root, body** (or **shaft**), and **glans penis.** The root of the penis attaches it to the pubic arch and the body is the visible, pendant portion. The corpus spongiosum expands at the distal end to form the glans penis. The urethra, which extends throughout the length of the corpus spongiosum, opens through the external urethral orifice at the tip of the glans penis. A loose fold of skin, called the **prepuce** (PREE-pyoos), or **foreskin,** covers the glans penis.

Circumcision is the surgical removal of the prepuce of the penis. Sometimes this is done to correct **phimosis,** a condition in which the prepuce is too tight and obstructs urine flow. In certain cultures circumcision is performed as a religious rite or an ethnic custom. For others, it is a matter of family preference. The medical benefits of circumcision are the subject of debate in the medical community. Some believe it is practical for hygienic reasons. There also is evidence that circumcision may reduce the risk of penile cancer.

Male Sexual Response

In the absence of sexual arousal the vascular sinusoids in the erectile tissue of the penis contain only a small volume of blood and the penis is flaccid. During sexual excitement, parasympathetic impulses dilate the arterioles that supply blood to the erectile tissue and constrict the veins that remove the blood. As a result, the spaces in the erectile tissue become engorged with blood, causing the penis to enlarge and become rigid. This is called **erection** and is necessary to allow the penis to enter the female vagina. The erection reflex may be initiated by stimuli such as anticipation, memory, and visual sensations, or it may be the result of stimulation of touch receptors on the glans penis and skin of the genital area. Emotions and thoughts can inhibit erection.

Impotence is the inability to achieve an erection. Psychological stresses are often blamed for impotence, but other causes can lead to the difficulty. Impotence may result from an abnormality of the erectile tissue or failure of the parasympathetic reflexes that produce an erection. Drugs and alcohol may cause temporary impotence because they can interfere with the nerve and blood vessel actions that are necessary.

Continued sexual stimulation causes the parasympathetic reflexes that promote an erection to become more and more intense until they reach a level that prompts a surge of sympathetic impulses to the genital organs. These sympathetic impulses stimulate rhythmic contractions of the epididymides, vasa deferentia, and ejaculatory ducts, along with contractions of the accessory glands. This results in **emission,** the forceful discharge of semen into the urethra. **Ejaculation,** which immediately follows emission, is the forceful expulsion of semen from the urethra to the exterior. Contraction of smooth muscle in the wall of the urethra and skeletal muscle at the base of the penis forcefully eject the semen from the urethra. Concurrently with emission and ejaculation, the sphincters of the urinary bladder constrict to prevent semen from entering the bladder and the flow of urine from the bladder.

The rhythmic muscle contractions of ejaculation are accompanied by feelings of intense pleasure, increased heart rate, elevated blood pressure, and increased respiration. Together, these physiologic activities are referred to as **climax,** or **orgasm.** This is quickly followed by relaxation, and blood leaves the penis so it becomes flaccid. After orgasm, there is a latent period, lasting from several minutes to several hours, during which another erection is impossible.

The male sexual response includes erection and orgasm accompanied by ejaculation of semen. Orgasm is followed by a variable time period during which it is not possible to achieve another erection.

Hormonal Control

The hypothalamus, anterior pituitary, and testes have significant roles in the hormonal control of male reproductive functions. The relationship between these areas is sometimes referred to as the **brain testicular axis.**

Puberty in males usually begins between the ages of 10 and 12 and continues until ages 16 to 18. During this period the male reproductive organs become sexually mature. The sequence of events that triggers the onset of puberty is unknown. It begins when certain unknown stimuli cause the hypothalamus to start secreting **gonadotropin-releasing hormone** (GnRH), which enters the blood and goes to the anterior pituitary gland.

In response to GnRH, the anterior pituitary secretes **luteinizing hormone** (LH) and **follicle-stimulating hormone** (FSH). Luteinizing hormone is often referred to as **interstitial cell–stimulating hormone** (ICSH) because it promotes the growth of the interstitial cells (cells of Leydig) in the testes and stimulates the cells to secrete **testosterone.** FSH binds with receptor sites on the sustentacular cells (Sertoli's cells) in the seminiferous tubules. This action makes the spermatogenic cells respond to stimulation by testosterone. Testosterone and FSH, acting together, stimulate spermatogenesis in the seminiferous tubules. Figure 19–6 summarizes the hormonal control of testicular functions.

Male sex hormones are collectively called **androgens.** The most abundant androgen is testosterone. Before birth and for a brief period after, testosterone from the adrenal cortex stimulates the development of the male reproductive organs. Between birth and puberty testosterone levels are low. Then at puberty, under the influence of LH, the interstitial cells begin secreting high levels of testosterone. The adrenal cortex continues to secrete small amounts of androgens. The increase in testosterone at puberty promotes the maturation of the male reproductive organs, stimulates spermatogenesis, and promotes the development of the male secondary sex characteristics. After puberty, testosterone production is controlled by a negative feedback mechanism that involves the hypothalamus (see Fig. 19–6). High blood testosterone levels inhibit GnRH, which removes the stimulus for LH, which reduces the testosterone level back to normal. Testosterone production continues from puberty throughout the rest of a man's life, although there is some decline in quantity in old age.

Three hormones are the principal regulators of the male reproductive system. FSH stimulates spermatogenesis; LH stimulates the production of testosterone; and testosterone stimulates the development of male secondary sex characteristics and spermatogenesis.

✓ **Quick**Check

- What will occur if the arteries to the penis dilate due to parasympathetic impulses?
- At puberty, what is the effect of luteinizing hormone in the male?
- What will occur if there is a deficiency of testosterone before birth?

Female Reproductive System

The organs of the female reproductive system produce and sustain the female sex cells (egg cells, or ova), transport these cells to a site where they may be fertilized by sperm, provide a favorable environment for the developing offspring, move the offspring to the outside at the end of the development period, and produce the female sex hormones. The system includes the ovaries, uterine tubes, uterus, vagina, accessory glands, and external genital organs (Fig. 19–7).

Ovaries

The primary reproductive organs, or gonads, in the female are the paired **ovaries.** Each ovary is a solid, ovoid structure about the size and shape of an almond, about 3.5 cm in length, 2 cm wide, and 1 cm thick. The ovaries are located in shallow depressions, called **ovarian fossae,** one on each side of the uterus, in the lateral wall of the pelvic cavity. They are held loosely in place by peritoneal ligaments.

The female gonads are the ovaries, which are located on each side of the uterus in the pelvic cavity.

Carcinomas of the ovary account for more deaths than those of cervical and uterine cancers together. Because there are no screening tests and few symptoms in the early stages, ovarian carcinomas are usually in an advanced stage when they are discovered. Surgery, radiation therapy, and chemotherapy are used as therapeutic measures.

Structure

The ovaries are covered on the outside by a layer of simple cuboidal epithelium called **germinal (ovar-**

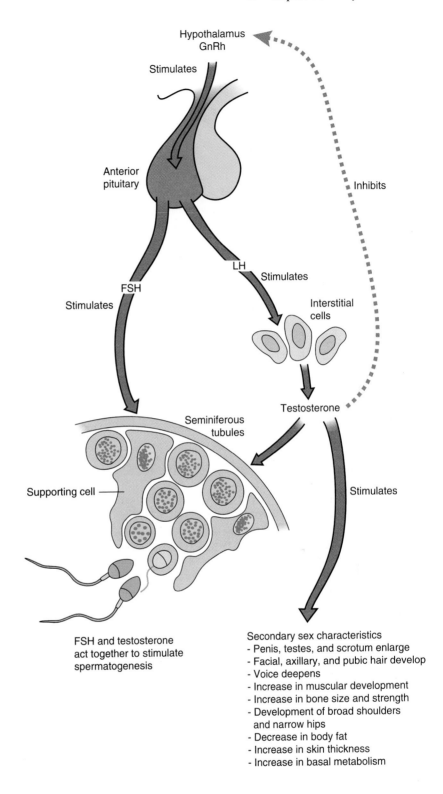

Hypothalamus
GnRh

Stimulates

Anterior
pituitary

Inhibits

LH   Stimulates

FSH

Stimulates

Interstitial
cells

Testosterone

Seminiferous
tubules

Supporting cell

Stimulates

FSH and testosterone
act together to stimulate
spermatogenesis

Secondary sex characteristics
- Penis, testes, and scrotum enlarge
- Facial, axillary, and pubic hair develop
- Voice deepens
- Increase in muscular development
- Increase in bone size and strength
- Development of broad shoulders
  and narrow hips
- Decrease in body fat
- Increase in skin thickness
- Increase in basal metabolism

Figure 19–6   Hormonal regulation of
testicular function.

ian) epithelium (Fig. 19–8). This is actually the visceral peritoneum that envelops the ovaries. Underneath this layer there is a dense connective tissue capsule, the **tunica albuginea.** The substance of the ovaries is indistinctly divided into an outer **cortex** and an inner **medulla.** The cortex appears more dense and granular due to the presence of numerous **ovarian follicles** in various stages of development. Each of the follicles contains an **oocyte,** a female germ cell. The medulla is loose connective tissue with abundant blood vessels, lymphatic vessels, and nerve fibers.

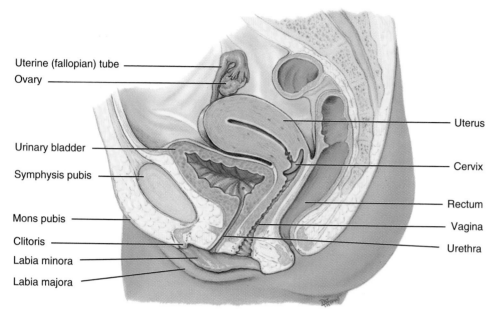

Figure 19–7 Organs of the female reproductive system.

Ovaries contain numerous follicles, each with an oocyte, around a central region of connective tissue and vessels.

Oogenesis

Female sex cells, or gametes, develop in the ovaries by a form of meiosis called **oogenesis** (oh-oh-JEN-eh-sis). The sequence of events in oogenesis is similar to the sequence in spermatogenesis, but the timing and final result are different (Fig. 19–9). Early in fetal development, primitive germ cells in the ovaries differentiate into **oogonia** (oh-oh-GO-nee-ah). These divide rapidly to form thousands of cells, still called oogonia, which have a full complement of 46

(23 pairs) chromosomes. Oogonia then enter a growth phase, enlarge, and become **primary oocytes.** The diploid (46 chromosomes) primary oocytes replicate their DNA and begin the first meiotic division, but the process stops in prophase and the cells remain in this suspended state until puberty. Many of the primary oocytes degenerate before birth, but even with this decline, the two ovaries together contain approximately 700,000 oocytes at birth. This is the lifetime supply, and no more will develop. This is quite different than the male in whom spermatogonia and primary spermatocytes continue to be produced throughout the reproductive lifetime. By puberty the number of primary oocytes has further declined to about 400,000.

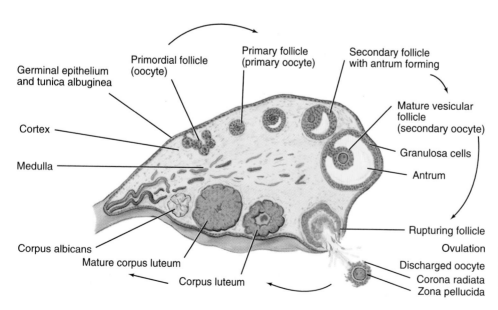

Figure 19–8 Structure of an ovary illustrating the stages in follicle development and corpus luteum formation.

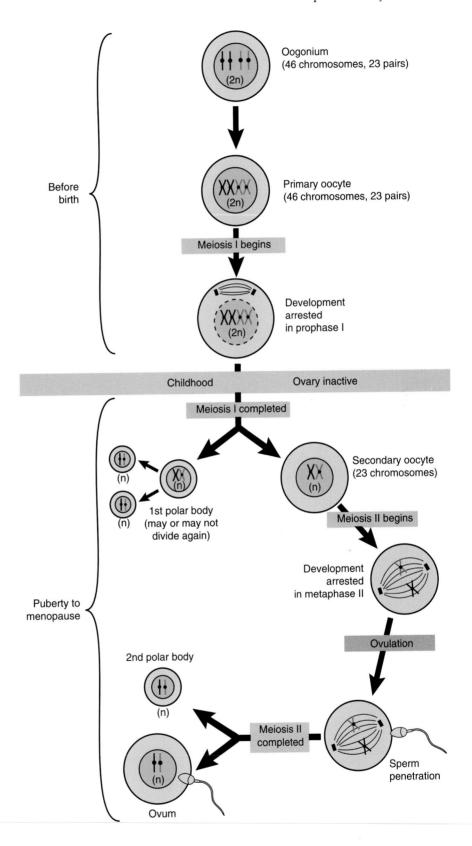

Figure 19-9   Oogenesis.

Beginning at puberty, under the influence of FSH, several primary oocytes start to grow again each month. One of the primary oocytes seems to outgrow the others and it resumes meiosis I. The other cells degenerate. The large cell undergoes an unequal division so that nearly all the cytoplasm, organelles, and half the chromosomes go to one cell, which becomes a **secondary oocyte.** The remaining half of the chromosomes go to a smaller cell called the **first polar body.** The secondary oocyte begins the second meiotic division, but the process stops in metaphase. At this point ovulation occurs. If fertilization occurs, meiosis II continues. Again this is an unequal division with all of the cytoplasm going to the ovum, which has 23 single-stranded chromosomes. The smaller cell from this division is a **second polar body.** The first polar body also usually divides in meiosis II to produce two even smaller polar bodies. If fertilization does not occur, the second meiotic division is never completed and the secondary oocyte degenerates. Here again there are obvious differences between the male and female. In spermatogenesis, four functional spermatozoa develop from each primary spermatocyte. In oogenesis, only one functional fertilizable cell develops from a primary oocyte. The other three cells are polar bodies and they degenerate.

> All primary oocytes develop before birth and remain dormant until puberty. After puberty a primary oocyte resumes division each month to form a secondary oocyte and a polar body. If a spermatozoon penetrates the oocyte, meiosis continues. If not, the oocyte degenerates.

Ovarian Follicle Development

An ovarian follicle consists of a developing oocyte surrounded by one or more layers of cells called **follicular cells.** At the same time the oocyte is progressing through meiosis, corresponding changes are taking place in the follicular cells (see Fig. 19–8). **Primordial follicles,** which consist of a primary oocyte surrounded by a single layer of flattened cells, develop in the fetus and are the stage that is present in the ovaries at birth and throughout childhood.

Beginning at puberty FSH stimulates changes in the primordial follicles. The follicular cells become cuboidal, the primary oocyte enlarges, and it is now a **primary follicle.** The follicles continue to grow under the influence of FSH, and the follicular cells proliferate to form several layers of **granulosa cells** around the primary oocyte. Most of these primary follicles degenerate along with the primary oocytes within them, but usually one continues to develop each month. The granulosa cells start secreting estrogen, and a cavity, or antrum, forms within the follicle. When the antrum starts to develop, the follicle becomes a **secondary follicle.** The granulosa cells also secrete a glycoprotein substance that forms a clear membrane, the **zona pellucida** (ZOH-nah peh-LOO-sih-dah), around the oocyte. After about 10 days of growth the follicle is a mature vesicular (graafian) follicle, which forms a "blister" on the surface of the ovary and contains a secondary oocyte ready for ovulation.

> A mature vesicular follicle contains a secondary oocyte surrounded by the zona pellucida and granulosa cells.

Ovulation

Ovulation, prompted by LH from the anterior pituitary, occurs when the mature follicle at the surface of the ovary ruptures and releases the secondary oocyte into the peritoneal cavity. The ovulated secondary oocyte, ready for fertilization, is still surrounded by the zona pellucida and a few layers of cells called the **corona radiata** (koh-ROH-nah ray-dee-AH-tah). If it is not fertilized, the secondary oocyte degenerates in a couple of days. If a spermatozoon passes through the corona radiata and zona pellucida and enters the cytoplasm of the secondary oocyte, the second meiotic division resumes to form a polar body and a mature ovum.

> At ovulation, a secondary oocyte, surrounded by the zona pellucida and corona radiata, is released from the ovary.

After ovulation and in response to LH, the portion of the follicle that remains in the ovary enlarges and is transformed into a **corpus luteum** (see Fig. 19–8). The corpus luteum is a glandular structure that secretes progesterone and some estrogens. Its fate depends on whether fertilization occurs. If fertilization does not take place, the corpus luteum remains functional for about 10 days and then begins to degenerate into a **corpus albicans,** which is primarily scar tissue, and its hormone output ceases. If fertilization occurs, the corpus luteum persists and continues its hormone functions until the placenta develops sufficiently to secrete the necessary hormones. Again, the corpus luteum ultimately degenerates into a corpus albicans; it just remains functional for a longer period of time.

> After ovulation, the portion of the mature follicle that remains in the ovary develops into a corpus luteum. The corpus luteum secretes progesterone and estrogen.

Genital Tract

Uterine Tubes

There are two **uterine tubes,** also called **fallopian** (fah-LOH-pee-an) **tubes** or **oviducts.** Each tube is about 4 cm long and about 1 cm in diameter and extends laterally from the upper portion of the uterus to the region of the ovary on that side (Fig. 19–10). There is one tube associated with each ovary. The end of the tube near the ovary expands to form a funnel-shaped **infundibulum,** which is surrounded by fingerlike extensions called **fimbriae.** Because there is no direct connection between the infundibulum and the ovary, the oocyte enters the peritoneal cavity before it enters the uterine tube. At the time of ovulation, the fimbriae increase their activity and create currents in the peritoneal fluid that help propel the oocyte into the uterine tube. Once inside the uterine tube, the oocyte is moved along by the rhythmic beating of cilia on the epithelial

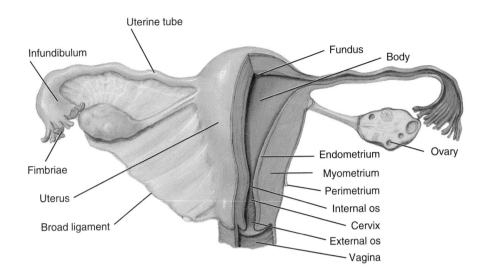

Figure 19–10 Uterus and uterine tubes.

lining and by peristaltic action of the smooth muscle in the wall of the tube. The journey through the uterine tube takes about 7 days. Because the oocyte is fertile for only 24 to 48 hours, fertilization usually occurs in the uterine tube.

> The uterine tubes, also called fallopian tubes or oviducts, transport the oocyte to the uterus. Fertilization normally occurs within the uterine tubes.

Tubal ligation is a surgical procedure in which the uterine tubes are burned or severed and tied off. This is a permanent method of birth control because sperm are unable to reach the egg for fertilization. The technique involves making a small incision in the abdomen and inserting a small tube through which the ligation instruments can be introduced.

Uterus

The **uterus** is a muscular organ that receives the fertilized oocyte and provides an appropriate environment for the developing offspring. It is located in the pelvic cavity, between the rectum and urinary bladder (see Fig. 19–10). Before the first pregnancy, the uterus is about the size and shape of a pear, with the narrow portion directed inferiorly. After childbirth, the uterus is usually larger, then regresses after menopause.

The upper, bulging surface of the uterus, above the entrance of the uterine tubes, is the **fundus.** The large main portion is the **body,** and the narrow region that is directed inferiorly into the vagina is the **cervix.** The opening between the body and cervix is the **internal os,** and the opening from the cervix into the vagina is the **external os.** Normally the uterus is bent forward between the body and cervix so that the body projects anteriorly over the superior surface of the urinary bladder. In this position the

uterus is said to be **anteflexed** (see Fig. 19–7). Several ligaments hold the uterus in place. The largest of these is the **broad ligament,** which drapes over the uterus like a sheet and extends laterally to the lateral pelvic wall. The broad ligament also encloses the uterine tubes.

> The uterus receives the fertilized egg from the uterine tubes and provides an appropriate environment for its development.

An **ectopic pregnancy** occurs when a fertilized egg implants in some place other than the uterus. Frequently, ectopic pregnancies occur in the uterine tubes. Because the tubes are not equipped to sustain and nourish the developing embryo miscarriages often occur. The uterine tubes are unable to expand like the uterus and may rupture with subsequent hemorrhage. Surgery may be indicated to remove the implant and to preserve the uterine tube before rupture occurs.

The wall of the uterus consists of perimetrium, myometrium, and endometrium. The outer serous layer, the **perimetrium,** is visceral peritoneum. The thick middle layer, the **myometrium,** is smooth muscle and makes up the bulk of the uterine wall. The inner layer, the **endometrium,** is a mucous membrane and is subdivided into two regions. The **stratum functionale** of the endometrium is the portion that is sloughed off during menstruation. The deeper, thinner **stratum basale** is more constant and provides the materials to rebuild the stratum functionale after menstruation.

> The lining of the uterus is the endometrium. The stratum functionale of the endometrium sloughs off during menstruation. The deeper stratum basale provides the foundation for rebuilding the stratum functionale.

The **Papanicolaou smear (Pap test)** is a frequently used screening method for cervical and vaginal cancer. In this technique, the physician uses a swab or spatula to remove cells from the cervix. These cells are microscopically examined for abnormalities. This is an important tool in the early detection of cervical cancer, and every woman should take advantage of its availability.

Vagina

The **vagina** is a fibromuscular tube, about 10 cm long, that extends from the cervix of the uterus to the outside. It is located between the rectum and the urinary bladder. Because the vagina is tilted posteriorly as it ascends and the cervix is tilted anteriorly, the cervix projects into the vagina at nearly a right angle. The vagina provides a passageway for menstrual flow to reach the outside, receives the penis and semen during sexual intercourse (coitus), and serves as the birth canal during the birth of a baby. The smooth muscle and mucosal lining of the vaginal wall are capable of stretching to accommodate the erect penis and to permit passage of a baby. The opening of the vagina to the outside, the **vaginal orifice,** may be incompletely covered by a thin fold of mucous membrane called the **hymen.**

> The vagina serves as a passageway for menstrual flow, receives the erect penis during intercourse, and is the birth canal during the birth of a baby.

External Genitalia

The external genitalia are accessory structures of the female reproductive system that are outside the vagina. They are also referred to as the **vulva** or **pudendum** (pyoo-DEN-dum). The external genitalia include the labia majora, mons pubis, labia minora, clitoris, and glands within the vestibule (Fig. 19–11).

> Collectively, the female external genitalia are referred to as the vulva or pudendum.

The **labia majora** (*labium majus*) are two large fat-filled folds of skin that enclose the other external genitalia. Anteriorly the labia majora merge to form the **mons pubis,** a rounded elevation of fat that overlies the pubic symphysis. After puberty the mons pubis and lateral surfaces of the labia majora are covered with coarse pubic hair. The skin on the medial surfaces of the labia majora is thinner than that on the lateral surfaces and contains numerous sebaceous and sweat glands. The **labia minora** (*labium minus*) are two smaller folds of skin medial to the labia majora. The skin on the labia minora contains sebaceous glands but does not have hair, sweat glands, or adipose tissue.

The area between the two labia minora is called the **vestibule.** At the anterior end of the vestibule, where the two labia minora meet, there is a small mass of erectile tissue called the **clitoris** (KLY-toh-ris). The clitoris is homologous to the male penis and becomes erect in response to sexual stimulation. The labia minora merge and form a hood, or **prepuce,** over the clitoris. Posterior to the clitoris, the urethra and vagina open into the vestibule. **Paraurethral glands** (Skene's glands) open into the vestibule on each side of the urethral orifice. These glands secrete mucus. Adjacent to the vaginal orifice, between the vagina and labia minora, the **greater vestibular glands** (Bartholin's glands) open into the vestibule. These glands produce a mucus-like secretion for lubrication during sexual intercourse.

> The clitoris is an erectile organ, similar to the male penis, that responds to sexual stimulation. Posterior to the clitoris, the urethra, vagina, paraurethral glands, and greater vestibular glands open into the vestibule.

Female Sexual Response

The female sexual response is similar to that of the male and consists of erection and orgasm. Parasympathetic responses to sexual stimuli produce increased blood flow to the erectile tissue in the clitoris, the vaginal mucosa, breasts, and nipples. The

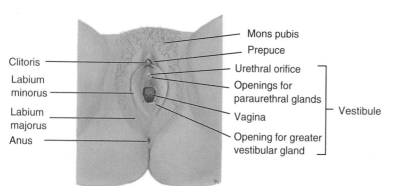

Clitoris
Labium minorus
Labium majorus
Anus

Mons pubis
Prepuce
Urethral orifice
Openings for paraurethral glands
Vagina
Opening for greater vestibular gland

Vestibule

Figure 19–11 Female external genitalia.

clitoris and nipples become rigid and erect. The breasts and vaginal mucosa enlarge. Glands in the cervix and the vestibular glands secrete fluids that lubricate the vaginal mucosa and aid the entry of the penis. These responses correspond to the erection phase of the male response.

With continued stimulation the female response culminates in orgasm, but this is not accompanied by ejaculation. Sympathetic responses produce rhythmic contractions of the uterus and muscles of the pelvic floor. This helps the movement of sperm through the uterus toward the uterine tubes. The rhythmic muscle contractions are accompanied by feelings of intense pleasure, increased heart rate, elevated blood pressure, and increased respiration rate. This is followed by a general relaxation and feeling of warmth throughout the body. It is not necessary for a woman to experience orgasm to become pregnant.

> The female sexual response includes erection and orgasm, but there is no ejaculation. A woman may become pregnant without having an orgasm.

✓ QuickCheck

- What happens to the follicle cells after ovulation?
- Where does fertilization usually occur?
- Which layer of the uterus is sloughed off during menstruation?
- Which component of the vulva is homologous to the male penis and becomes erect during sexual arousal?

Hormonal Control

As in the male, the hypothalamus, anterior pituitary, and gonads secrete hormones that have significant roles in the control of reproductive functions (Fig. 19–12). The hypothalamus secretes **gonadotropin-releasing hormone** (GnRH); the anterior pituitary secretes **follicle-stimulating hormone** (FSH) and **luteinizing hormone** (LH); and the ovaries secrete the sex hormones **estrogen** and **progesterone.** Unlike the male, the secretion of these hormones follows monthly cyclic patterns that affect the ovaries and the uterus. These cycles, referred to as the **ovarian cycle** and the **menstrual** (uterine) **cycle,** begin at puberty and continue for about 40 years.

> FSH, LH, estrogen, and progesterone have major roles in regulating the functions of the female reproductive system.

At puberty, when the ovaries and uterus are mature enough to respond to hormonal stimulation, certain stimuli cause the hypothalamus to start secreting (GnRH). This hormone enters the blood and goes to the anterior pituitary gland where it stimulates the secretion of FSH and LH. These hormones, in turn, affect the ovaries and uterus and the monthly cycles begin. In females, the beginning of

puberty is marked by the first period of menstrual bleeding, called **menarche** (meh-NAHR-kee). After this the cycles continue, more or less regularly, until the late 40s or early 50s. At this time, the cycles become increasingly irregular until they finally stop. **Menopause** is the cessation of the reproductive cycles.

> A woman's reproductive cycles last from menarche to menopause.

Ovarian Cycle

The ovarian cycle reflects the changes that occur within the ovaries as the follicles develop (follicular phase), ovulation occurs (ovulatory phase), and the corpus luteum develops (luteal phase) (Fig. 19–13).

The **follicular phase** of the cycle begins when GnRH from the hypothalamus stimulates increased secretion of FSH (and small amounts of LH) from the anterior pituitary. FSH stimulates growth of the ovarian follicles. As the follicles enlarge, estrogen secretion increases. Low levels of estrogens exert a negative feedback effect on the hypothalamus and anterior pituitary, but also increase the effect of FSH on the follicle. The follicle continues to grow and mature until the middle of the cycle.

The **ovulatory phase** is the result of high levels of estrogen from the mature follicles. Low levels of estrogen have a negative feedback effect on the pituitary, but high levels have a positive feedback effect. This results in a surge of LH and a smaller increase in FSH. The surge of LH stimulates resumption of meiosis in the oocyte and causes the rupture of the follicle, and estrogen levels decline.

The **luteal phase** results when the surge of LH stimulates the development of the corpus luteum from the ruptured follicle. LH also stimulates the corpus luteum to secrete progesterone and some estrogen. These have a negative feedback on the hypothalamus and anterior pituitary so that FSH and LH levels decline. As LH declines, corpus luteum activity declines and the inhibitory effect is removed. The cycle starts over.

> The monthly ovarian cycle begins with the follicle development during the follicular phase, continues with ovulation during the ovulatory phase, and concludes with the development and regression of the corpus luteum during the luteal phase.

Mittelschmerz is a distress that some women experience during ovulation. Typical symptoms include one-sided lower abdominal pain, which may switch sides from one month to another, at or around the time of ovulation. The pain is usually described as sharp or cramping and lasts from 24 to 48 hours. There is no known prevention, and treatment consists of analgesics.

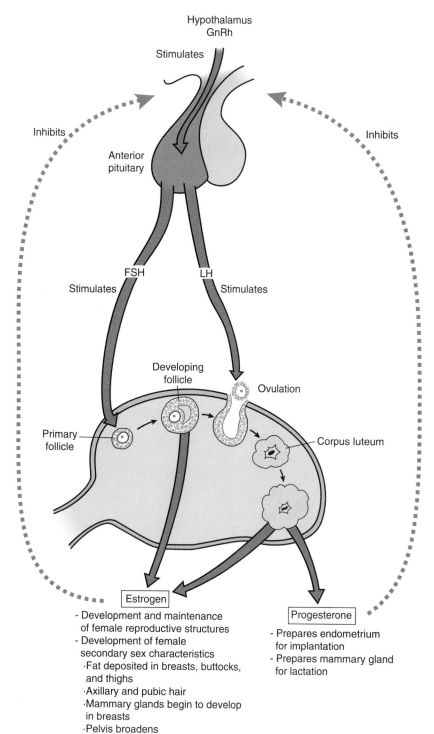

Hypothalamus
GnRh

Stimulates

Inhibits

Inhibits

Anterior
pituitary

FSH   LH
Stimulates   Stimulates

Developing
follicle
Ovulation

Primary
follicle

Corpus luteum

Estrogen
- Development and maintenance
  of female reproductive structures
- Development of female
  secondary sex characteristics
  ·Fat deposited in breasts, buttocks,
   and thighs
  ·Axillary and pubic hair
  ·Mammary glands begin to develop
   in breasts
  ·Pelvis broadens

Progesterone
- Prepares endometrium
  for implantation
- Prepares mammary gland
  for lactation

Figure 19–12 Hormonal regulation of ovarian functions.

Uterine (Menstrual) Cycle

The uterine (menstrual) cycle reflects changes in the stratum functionale of the endometrium of the uterus. Changes in estrogen and progesterone levels during the ovarian cycle are responsible for the changes in the uterus. The uterine cycle is divided into the menstrual phase, proliferative phase, and secretory phase (see Fig. 19–13).

The **menstrual phase** begins on the first day of the cycle and continues for 3 to 5 days. The thick stratum functionale detaches from the uterine wall and, accompanied by bleeding, passes through the vagina as the menstrual flow. Follicles are growing in the ovary during this time.

The **proliferative phase** begins with the end of the menstrual phase and lasts for about 8 days. In-

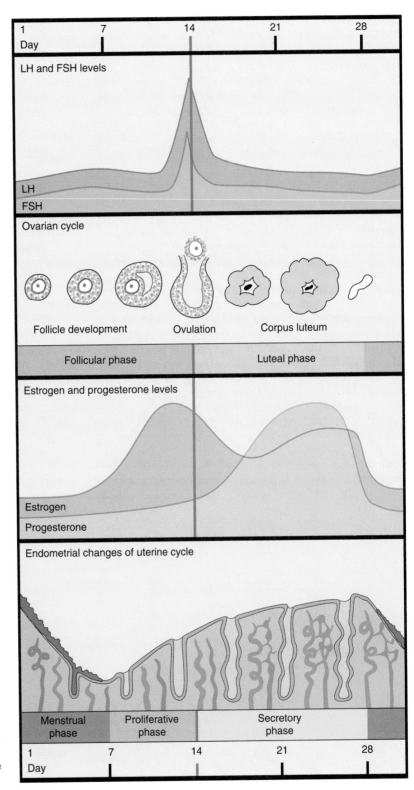

Figure 19–13   Correlation of events in the ovarian and uterine cycles.

creasing levels of estrogen from the growing follicles in the ovary stimulate repair of the endometrium in the uterus. The endometrium thickens, glands develop, and blood vessels grow in the new tissue. Ovulation in the ovarian cycle occurs at the end of this uterine phase.

The **secretory phase** corresponds to the luteal phase of the ovarian cycle. Progesterone from the corpus luteum stimulates continued growth and thickening of the endometrium. Arteries and glands proliferate and enlarge. The glands secrete glycogen, which will nourish a developing embryo if fertilization occurs. If fertilization does not occur, the corpus luteum in the ovary begins to degenerate. This leads to menstruation, and the cycle starts over.

> The uterine cycle takes place simultaneously with the ovarian cycle. The uterine cycle begins with menstruation during the menstrual phase, continues with repair of the endometrium during the proliferative phase, and ends with the growth of glands and blood vessels during the secretory phase.

Menopause

Menopause is the cessation of the female reproductive cycles. Even though menopause is marked by the lack of menstrual cycles, the first changes are in the ovary. By the age of 45 or 50, ovarian follicles cease responding to FSH and LH from the pituitary gland. As a result, the follicle cells do not produce estrogen and there is no ovulation, no corpus luteum, and no progesterone. Without estrogen and progesterone, the cyclic changes in the uterus stop and menstruation ceases. This is the visible evidence of menopause. As estrogen and progesterone levels decline, FSH and LH increase because of the lack of ovarian hormone feedback. These high levels of pituitary hormones with the low levels of ovarian hormones are believed to be responsible for a variety of symptoms associated with the onset of menopause. Some women experience hot flashes, sweating, depression, headaches, irritability, and insomnia. However, many women experience few, if any, of these symptoms.

> Menopause occurs when a woman's reproductive cycles stop. This period is marked by decreased levels of ovarian hormones and increased levels of pituitary FSH and LH. The changing hormone levels are responsible for the symptoms associated with menopause.

Mammary Glands

Functionally, the mammary glands are the organs of milk production; structurally, they are modified sweat glands. Mammary glands, which are located in the breast overlying the pectoralis major muscles, are present in both sexes, but usually are functional only in the female.

Externally, each breast has a raised **nipple**, which is surrounded by a circular pigmented area called the **areola** (ah-REE-oh-lah). The nipples are sensitive to touch, and they contain smooth muscle that contracts and causes them to become erect in response to stimulation.

Internally, the adult female breast contains 15 to 20 lobes of glandular tissue that radiate around the nipple (Fig. 19–14). The **lobes** are separated by connective tissue and adipose. The connective tissue helps support the breast. Some bands of connective tissue, called **suspensory** (Cooper's) **ligaments** extend through the breast from the skin to the underlying muscles. The amount and distribution of the adipose determines the size and shape of the breast. Each lobe consists of **lobules** that contain the glandular units. A **lactiferous** (lak-TIFF-er-us) **duct** collects the milk from the lobules within each lobe and carries it to the nipple. Just before the nipple the

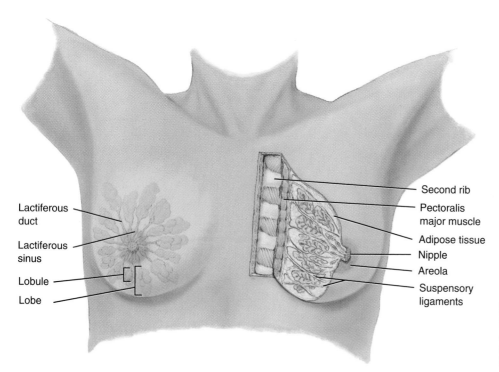

Figure 19–14 Breast and mammary glands. (From Jarvis C: Physical Examination and Health Assessment. Philadelphia, WB Saunders, 1992.)

lactiferous duct enlarges to form a **lactiferous sinus (ampulla),** which serves as a reservoir for milk. After the sinus, the duct again narrows and each duct opens independently on the surface of the nipple.

> The mammary glands, located within the breast, consist of lobules of glandular units that produce milk. Lactiferous ducts transport the milk to the nipple.

Mammary gland function is regulated by hormones. At puberty, increasing levels of estrogen stimulate the development of glandular tissue in the female breast. Estrogen also causes the breasts to increase in size through the accumulation of adipose tissue. Progesterone stimulates the development of the duct system. During pregnancy these hormones enhance further development of the mammary glands. Prolactin from the anterior pituitary stimulates the production of milk within the glandular tissue, and oxytocin causes the ejection of milk from the glands.

> Estrogen and progesterone stimulate the development of glandular tissue and ducts in the breast. Prolactin stimulates the production of milk, and oxytocin causes the ejection of the milk.

 Quick Check

- What are two effects of luteinizing hormone in the ovarian cycle?
- What is the primary source of progesterone in the nonpregnant female?
- What happens in the uterus in response to increased estrogen levels during the second week of the menstrual cycle?

Fibrocystic disease is a common benign condition of the breast. Small sacs of tissue and fluid develop in the breast tissue and the patient notices lumps in the breast often associated with premenstrual tenderness. Mammography and surgical biopsy may be indicated to differentiate between fibrocystic disease and carcinoma of the breast.

 ## FOCUS ON AGING

Men normally do not experience a sudden decline in reproductive function comparable to menopause in women. Instead, they experience a gradual and subtle decline over many years. After age 50, men have some testicular atrophy, partially due to a decrease in the size of the seminiferous tubules and partially due to a reduction in the number of interstitial cells. These changes are accompanied by a decline in sperm and testosterone production. Both the seminal vesicles and the prostate show a decrease in secretory activity, which results in a reduction in the volume of semen. The portion of the prostate gland that surrounds the urethra often enlarges and may constrict the urethra, making urination difficult. The penis may undergo some atrophy and become smaller with age. The blood vessels and erectile tissue in the penis become less elastic, which hinders the ability to attain an erection. Although there is a general decline in the aging male reproductive system, many men are capable of achieving erection and ejaculation into old age.

After menopause, there is a gradual decline in the female reproductive system. Most of the changes are believed to be due to the reduction in estrogen. The ovaries undergo progressive atrophy. The uterus becomes smaller, and fibrous connective tissue replaces much of the myometrium. The vagina becomes narrower and shorter, and its walls become thin and less elastic. Glands that lubricate the vagina reduce their secretory activity, and the vagina becomes dry. The vaginal secretions that remain are less acid, which makes older women more susceptible to vaginal infections. The external genitalia and mammary glands undergo atrophic changes. The lack of estrogen also affects nonreproductive organs. This is particularly true in the case of bone metabolism, which is indicated by the increased incidence of osteoporosis in postmenopausal women. There is also increased cardiovascular disease.

Estrogen replacement therapy is prescribed for many women to combat osteoporosis and other symptoms of menopause. However, there is controversy about the risks involved with this treatment, particularly the risks of uterine and breast cancer. Consideration should be given to the risks and benefits before beginning estrogen replacement therapy. Current practice often prescribes progesterone in conjunction with estrogen, which seems to reduce some of the risks.

There is a growing awareness that elderly people have sexual needs and enjoy sexual relations. Although age-related physical and hormonal changes that take place in the reproductive system may alter these needs and sexual functioning, studies demonstrate that sexuality remains important to many older people.

Reproductive System?

Birth Control

Birth control is the voluntary regulation of the number of offspring produced and the time at which they are conceived. There are numerous methods of birth control, some more effective than others; and for maximum effectiveness, each method must be used correctly. Most of the generally accepted methods prevent fertilization of the oocyte after intercourse. These are called contraceptives because they prevent conception and include behavioral, barrier, surgical, and chemical methods. Intrauterine devices do not interfere with fertilization; therefore they are not contraceptives, but they prevent implantation in the uterus after fertilization has occurred. Abortion is the removal of an embryo after it has become implanted in the uterus.

Behavioral methods do not utilize drugs, surgery, or any type of apparatus, but they require action by the participants. The surest way to prevent pregnancy is to abstain from sexual intercourse. The **rhythm method** is a modification of this practice in which couples abstain from intercourse for a few days before and a few days after ovulation. A major factor in the failure of this method is the inability to predict the exact time of ovulation. Theoretically, ovulation occurs on the fourteenth day of a 28 day cycle. However, relatively few women have absolutely regular menstrual cycles and the part of the cycle that varies occurs before ovulation, which makes it more difficult to predict the time of ovulation. Some women, but not all, show a temperature increase of about 0.35° C (0.6° F) immediately after ovulation. Morning temperatures measured over a period of months may help predict the time of ovulation. The rhythm method has about a 30 percent failure rate, which is the result of both the inability to accurately predict the time of ovulation and the failure to abstain from intercourse during the fertile period. **Coitus interruptus** is a behavioral method that involves withdrawing the penis from the vagina before ejaculation. This is an unreliable method of preventing pregnancy because some males find it emotionally difficult to withdraw. Also, small quantities of semen may be expelled from the penis before ejaculation.

Barriers prevent sperm cells from reaching the oocyte. **Mechanical barriers** prevent sperm cells from entering the reproductive tract during sexual intercourse. The **condom** is a thin rubber or plastic sheath that is placed over the erect penis prior to intercourse. The condom collects the semen and prevents it from entering the female reproductive tract. This method is about 90 percent effective when used correctly. It has the added advantage of providing protection against sexually transmitted diseases. The **diaphragm** is a rubber or plastic dome-shaped barrier that is inserted into the vagina so that it covers the cervix and prevents sperm cells from entering the uterus. To be effective the diaphragm must be fitted for the right size by a physician, and it must be inserted properly before each sexual contact. **Chemical barriers** include creams, foams, and jellies with spermicidal properties that create an unfavorable environment for sperm within the vagina. Used alone, chemical barriers result in a relatively high pregnancy rate. They are most effective when used with the mechanical barriers. A diaphragm used with a spermicide is about 90 percent effective.

Surgical methods of contraception include **vasectomy** in males and **tubal ligation** in females. Vasectomy is a surgical procedure in which the ductus deferentia, within the scrotum, are cut and tied. This prevents sperm cells from becoming part of the semen. In the female, the uterine tubes are tied and cut in a procedure called tubal ligation. This prevents sperm cells from coming in contact with the oocyte. Neither procedure alters the concentrations of hormones or sexual drives of the individuals involved. Both procedures are usually considered permanent and are nearly 100 percent effective.

Chemical methods of birth control use hormones to suppress fertility. These are the oral contraceptives, commonly called "the pill." Oral contraceptives contain synthetic hormones similar to estrogen and progesterone that disrupt the normal pattern of reproductive hormone secretion and prevent ovulation. These must be prescribed by a physician. When instructions for their use are explicitly followed, oral contraceptives are nearly 100 percent effective and are considered the most reliable method of temporary birth control. They may cause side effects such as nausea and fluid retention in some women.

An **intrauterine device** (IUD) is a small object, usually metallic, that is placed in the uterus by a physician to prevent implantation of the developing embryo. The presence of an IUD in the uterus apparently causes inflammatory reactions that interfere with implantation. They are an effective method of preventing pregnancy; however, some have caused serious side effects and have been withdrawn from the market. An IUD should be checked regularly by a physician.

The behavioral, barrier, and chemical methods of temporary birth control depend on some action by the user. Often the effectiveness of these methods is reduced because the user "forgets" or doesn't follow the correct procedure.

Reproductive System?

Sexually Transmitted Diseases

Sexually transmitted diseases (STDs), also called venereal diseases, are infectious diseases caused by microorganisms that are spread from person to person through sexual contact. They are rarely contracted by casual dry contact with objects or people. As a group, they are the most important cause of reproductive system disorders. The most common sexually transmitted diseases are gonorrhea, syphilis, nongonococcal urethritis, and genital herpes.

Gonorrhea primarily affects the moist mucous membranes of the reproductive and urinary tracts. It may also affect the eyes. Gonorrhea, called the "clap" in common usage, is caused by the bacterium *Neisseria gonorrhoeae*. In males, it causes a painful inflammation of the urethra and a discharge of pus from the penis. If it spreads throughout the male reproductive tract, it may result in inflammation of the epididymis and swelling of the testes. In females, gonorrhea affects the vagina and causes a greenish yellow discharge from the cervix. Untreated, it may spread to the uterus, uterine tubes, and into the pelvic cavity where it causes **pelvic inflammatory disease.** Unfortunately, it often is unnoticed in females until it spreads into the pelvic cavity. By this time, the disease has caused sterility by blocking the uterine tube with scar tissue. One complication of gonorrhea affects newborns of infected mothers. The gonococcal organism infects the eyes of newborns as they pass through the birth canal of infected mothers. Before treatment of the eyes of newborns with 1 percent silver nitrate solution became routine, gonorrhea contracted during birth caused blindness in thousands of infants. If left untreated, gonorrhea becomes difficult to cure, but it can usually be cured by antibiotics if it is diagnosed and treated early. The disease is becoming more difficult to cure, however, because antibiotic-resistant strains of the causative organism are more prevalent.

Syphilis is potentially more dangerous than gonorrhea, especially when untreated, because it can irreversibly damage the central nervous system. This sexually transmitted disease is caused by a corkscrew-shaped bacterium called *Treponema pallidum*. The first sign of infection is a red open sore, called a **chancre.** This usually appears 2 to 3 weeks after contact and is located where the organism penetrated the mucous membrane. In the male, the chancre is typically on the penis, but in females, it is frequently hidden in the vagina and goes undetected. The chancre persists for about a week then spontaneously heals. After a latent period ranging from 1 to 6 months, the symptoms of **secondary syphilis** appear. These include muscle and joint pain, fever, and rash. The symptoms last about a month then spontaneously disappear, and the disease enters a variable **latent** period, during which the disease is detectable only by a diagnostic blood test. During the latent period, the organism invades and destroys body organs, often the central nervous system and liver. The latent period may last a lifetime, but frequently after weeks, months, or years, the disease reappears as **tertiary syphilis,** characterized by destructive lesions of the nervous system, blood vessels, and skin. Paralysis, insanity, and death follow. Antibiotics are effective treatment during the first two stages. Prognosis is poor after the symptoms of tertiary syphilis appear. One of the most unfortunate aspects of syphilis is that it can pass through the placenta during pregnancy. Thus the developing fetus can contract syphilis from the mother and show symptoms of the disease at birth.

Continued on following page

Nongonococcal urethritis, the most common sexually transmitted disease in the United States, is caused by the bacterium *Chlamydia trachomatis*. It is responsible for nearly half of all diagnosed cases of pelvic inflammatory disease and has symptoms similar to gonorrhea. In men, it produces infection in the urethra, prostate gland, and epididymis. In women, it affects the cervix and uterine tubes. If left untreated, it may result in sterility in both sexes. If a woman has a chlamydial infection during pregnancy, she may transmit it to her newborn as it passes through the birth canal, and the affected infant may develop conjunctivitis or pneumonia. Antibiotics are an effective treatment for nongonococcal urethritis.

Genital herpes is caused by the type II herpes simplex virus. There are two familiar types of herpes simplex viruses, both of which cause painful blisterlike lesions. The type I herpes simplex virus causes lesions above the waist and is the one responsible for cold sores on the lips and in the mouth. The type II virus causes similar lesions below the waist, often in the genital area.

In men, they are likely to appear on the penis; and in women, they are likely to be on the vulva or in the vagina. The lesions usually heal after 1 or 2 weeks, but the viruses retreat to nerves near the lower part of the spinal cord where they remain dormant for a variable period of time until the next episode of lesions. Usually there are no serious consequences to genital herpes. It is a painful nuisance more than a threat to life. An infant may become infected as it passes through the birth canal, and genital herpes infections have been implicated as a cause of cervical cancer. Unlike the other three sexually transmitted diseases discussed here, which are caused by bacteria and are curable, genital herpes is caused by a virus and is incurable. The virus may be dormant for a period but may reactivate at any time.

It is true that the current array of antibiotics makes treating most sexually transmitted diseases easier than ever before if they are treated in the early stages. The most effective treatment, however, is prevention.

REPRESENTATIVE DISORDERS OF THE REPRODUCTIVE SYSTEM

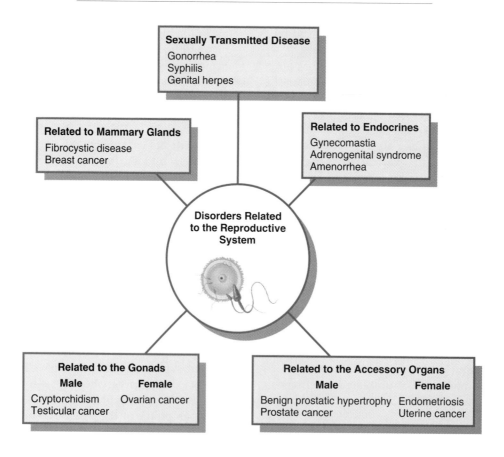

CHAPTER QUIZ

RECALL

Match the definitions on the left with the appropriate term on the right.

1. Ovaries and testes

2. Egg and sperm cells

3. Smooth muscle in the subcutaneous tissue of the scrotum

4. Skeletal muscle in the spermatic cord

5. Produce testosterone

6. Occurs within seminiferous tubules

7. Clear membrane around the oocyte

8. Produces progesterone

9. Normal site of fertilization

10. Smooth muscle in the uterus

A. Corpus luteum

B. Cremaster

C. Dartos

D. Gametes

E. Gonads

F. Interstitial cells

G. Myometrium

H. Spermatogenesis

I. Uterine tube

J. Zona pellucida

THOUGHT

1. The correct pathway for passage of sperm is

   a. seminiferous tubules, ductus deferens, epididymis, rete testis, urethra

   b. rete testis, seminiferous tubules, ductus deferens, epididymis, urethra

   c. ductus deferens, seminiferous tubules, rete testis, epididymis, urethra

   d. seminiferous tubules, rete testis, epididymis, ductus deferens, urethra

2. Spermiogenesis is

   a. a part of meiosis

   b. the formation of mature spermatozoa from spermatids

   c. the formation of spermatids

   d. the formation of testosterone by spermatozoa

3. More than half of the volume of seminal fluid comes from the

   a. prostate gland

   b. seminal vesicles

   c. bulbourethral gland

   d. sperm

4. The term *vulva* refers to the

   a. ovary, uterus, and vagina

   b. cervix, vagina, and clitoris

   c. labia majora and minora, mons pubis, and clitoris

   d. penis, scrotum, and testes

5. The luteal phase of the ovarian cycle

   a. is characterized by high levels of progesterone

   b. occurs at the same time as the proliferative phase of the uterine cycle

   c. occurs just before ovulation

   d. is characterized by high levels of luteinizing hormone

APPLICATION

A 36-year-old mother of four is considering tubal ligation (constricting the uterine tubes) as a means of ensuring that her family gets no larger. She asks her gynecologist if she will become "menopausal" after the surgery. Answer her question and explain.

Sexually transmitted diseases such as gonorrhea sometimes cause peritonitis (inflammation of the peritoneum) in females. However, peritonitis from this cause does not develop in males. Explain.

CHAPTER 20

Development

Outline/Objectives

Fertilization 420

- Describe the events in the process of fertilization, state where it normally occurs, and name the cell that is formed as a result of fertilization.
- Name the three divisions of prenatal development and state the period of time for each.

Preembryonic Period (Two weeks) 422

- Describe three significant developments that take place during the preembryonic period.

Embryonic Development (Six weeks) 424

- Describe three significant developments that take place during the embryonic period.
- List five derivatives from each of the primary germ layers.

Fetal Development (Thirty weeks) 427

- State the two fundamental processes that take place during fetal development.
- Name, describe the location, and state the function of five structures that are unique in the circulatory pattern of the fetus.

Parturition and Lactation 428

- Describe the roles of the hypothalamus, estrogen, progesterone, oxytocin, and prostaglandins in promoting labor.
- Describe the three stages of labor.
- Describe the changes that take place in the infant's respiratory system and circulatory pathway at birth or soon after birth.

Postnatal Development 430

- Name and define six periods in postnatal development.

Key Terms

Amnion

Chorion

Cleavage

Embryo

Fetus

Implantation

Parturition

Zygote

Building Vocabulary

WORD PART	MEANING
amnio-	a fetal membrane, a lamb
-cente	to puncture surgically
cleav-	to divide
cyesi-	pregnancy
cyst-	bag, hollow
galacto-	referring to milk
gravid-	filled, pregnant
morpho-	shape, form
morul-	mulberry
nat-	birth
oxy-	sharp, quick, rapid
para-	to bear
partur-	bring forth, give birth
sen-	old
-toc-	birth
umbil-	navel
zyg-	paired together, union

he previous chapter focused on the male and female reproductive systems and the formation of the spermatozoa and oocytes. This chapter continues with the events that result in the union of the gametes and the subsequent development of a new individual. Development is a continuous process that starts with fertilization (conception) and ends with death. Birth is an awesome event that divides the total span of development into two portions. It is the culmination of 38 weeks of **prenatal development** within the uterus. Prenatal development is divided into preembryonic, embryonic, and fetal periods. The period of **postnatal development** begins with birth and lasts until death.

Embryologists describe the timing of events in development by using the term **developmental age,** which begins at fertilization. The medical community uses **clinical age,** which begins at the last menstrual period (LMP). Developmental age is 2 weeks less than clinical age. Pregnancy is also divided into three equal periods called trimesters. Three calendar months constitute a trimester.

Fertilization

Fertilization, or conception, is the union of the sperm cell nucleus with an egg cell nucleus. The product of fertilization, a single cell, is called a **zygote.**

During ovulation, a secondary oocyte, surrounded by the zona pellucida and corona radiata, is released from an ovary and enters the uterine tube. Sperm cells, deposited in the vagina during sexual intercourse, travel through the cervix and body of the uterus to the uterine tube where they encounter the secondary oocyte. The upward movement through the female reproductive tract is accomplished by the movements of the sperm tail (flagellum) and contractions of the uterus. Sperm have a high mortality rate, and many never reach the uterine tube. While moving through the female reproductive tract, which takes about an hour, the sperm undergo a process called **capacitation** (kah-pass-ih-TAY-shun). This weakens the membrane around the acrosome so that the enzymes can be released. When the sperm reach the egg (secondary oocyte) in the uterine tube, the acrosomal enzymes from thousands of sperm break down the corona radiata and zona pellucida to create a tiny opening. As soon as one sperm enters the cell membrane of the oocyte, changes occur in the membrane that prevent other sperm from entering.

Enzymes in the acrosome break down the corona radiata and zona pellucida around the oocyte so that a single sperm can enter the oocyte for fertilization.

CLINICAL TERMS

Abruptio placentae (ab-RUP-tee-oh plah-SEN-tay) Complete separation of the placenta from the uterine wall after 20 weeks but before labor; results in immediate death of the fetus and severe hemorrhage in the mother

Apgar score (APP-gar score) System of scoring an infant's physical condition 1 minute after birth; heart rate, respiration, color, muscle tone, and response to stimuli are rated as 0, 1, 2, with a maximum total score of 10; infants with low Apgar scores require prompt medical attention

Cesarean section (seh-SAIR-ee-an SECK-shun) Removal of the fetus by abdominal incision into the uterus

Dystocia (dihs-TOH-see-ah) Difficult and painful childbirth

Eclampsia (ee-KLAMP-see-ah) A critical condition during pregnancy or shortly after, marked by high blood pressure, proteinuria, edema, uremia, convulsions, and coma

Eutocia (yoo-TOH-see-ah) Good, normal childbirth

Miscarriage (miss-KAIR-ayj) Loss of an embryo or fetus before the 20th week; most common cause is a structural or functional defect in the developing offspring; technically known as spontaneous abortion

Multipara (mull-TIP-ah-rah) A woman who has borne more than one child

Nullipara (null-IP-ah-rah) A woman who has borne no offspring

Pelvimetry (pel-VIM-eh-tree) Measurement of the dimensions of the mother's pelvis to determine its capacity to allow passage of the fetus through the birth canal

Preeclampsia (pree-ee-KLAMP-see-ah) A condition during pregnancy or shortly after, marked by acute hypertension, proteinuria, and edema; may progress to the more severe form, eclampsia; also called toxemia of pregnancy

Stillbirth (STILL-berth) Delivery of a lifeless infant after the 20th week

Sperm penetration of the oocyte membrane is the stimulus for the second meiotic division to resume. This division produces a small polar body, which is pushed to the side, and a large ovum with all the cytoplasm and 23 single-stranded chromosomes. When this division is completed, the sperm nucleus moves toward the center of the egg cell, the membranes of the two nuclei (sperm and egg) disintegrate, and their chromosomes combine. This completes the process of fertilization. The resulting cell, a **zygote,** has a full complement, or diploid number (46), of chromosomes; 23 came from the sperm and 23 from the egg. The zygote is the first cell of the future offspring. Figure 20–1 depicts the events in fertilization.

> Fertilization is completed when the chromosomes from the ovum and sperm nuclei combine to form a new cell nucleus with a full complement of 46 chromosomes. This new cell, the fertilized egg, is called a zygote.

The zygote occasionally divides resulting in **monozygotic twins.** Because these twins have the same genetic make-up, they are called "identical" twins. Sometimes a woman may ovulate two or more oocytes at the same time and both oocytes are subsequently fertilized. This results in **dizygotic twins** because more than one zygote is formed. These are also called "fraternal" twins.

Ovulated secondary oocytes are viable and fertile for only about 24 hours. Most sperm are fertile in the female reproductive tract for only about 48 hours, but some may retain fertility for 3 days. This means that for conception to occur, sexual intercourse must take place between 3 days before to 1 day after ovulation. Again, because the eggs are fertile for only 24 hours, fertilization usually occurs in the uterine tube near the infundibulum.

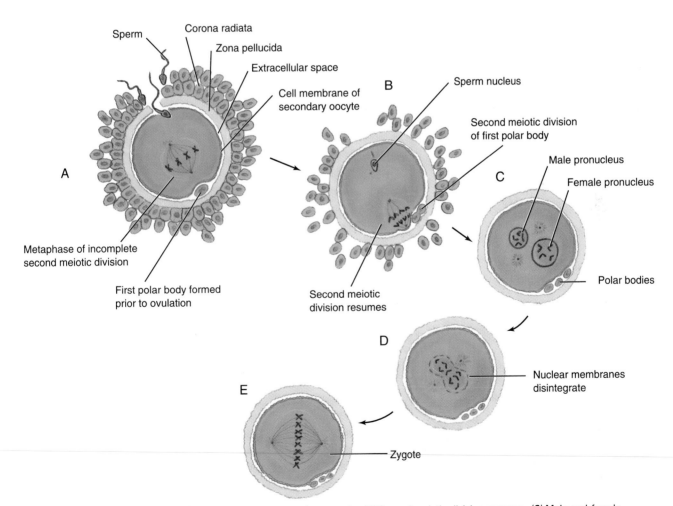

Figure 20–1   Fertilization. (A) Sperm penetrates secondary oocyte. (B) Second meiotic division resumes. (C) Male and female pronuclei come together. (D) Nuclear membranes disintegrate. (E) Fertilization completed with formation of zygote.

For fertilization to take place, sexual intercourse must occur approximately between 3 days before and 1 day after ovulation.

Multiple ovulations may occur naturally, or they may be the result of drugs that are used to treat infertility.

Preembryonic Period

The **preembryonic period** lasts for about 2 weeks after fertilization. During this time the zygote and subsequent stages move through the uterine tube into the cavity of the uterus. Significant developments in this period are **cleavage** (KLEE-vayj), **implantation** in the uterine wall, and formation of the **primary germ layers.**

The preembryonic period, which lasts for 2 weeks, includes cleavage, implantation, and the formation of the primary germ layers.

Cleavage

After fertilization, the zygote undergoes a series of mitotic cell divisions that produce increasing numbers of cells. These early cell divisions are called **cleavage** (Fig. 20–2). The first cleavage division is completed about 36 hours after fertilization and results in two cells, called **blastomeres** (BLAS-tohmeerz). Subsequent divisions of the blastomeres occur at approximately 12-hour intervals. By the end of the third day after fertilization, there are 16 cells in a solid ball, called a **morula** (MOR-yoo-lah). Still enclosed within the zona pellucida, each division produces cells that are smaller and smaller so that the total volume stays about the same.

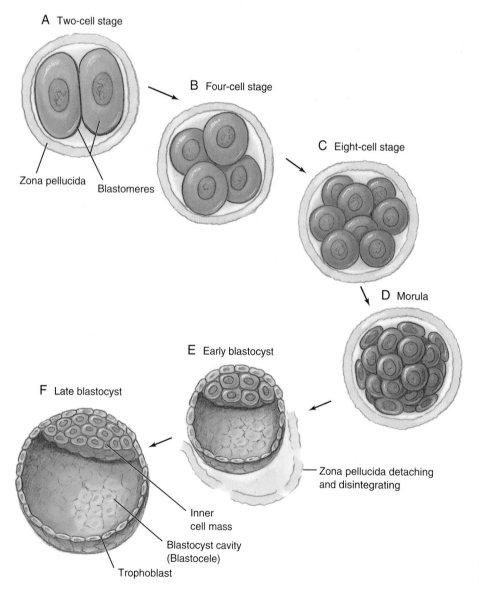

Figure 20–2 Cleavage and formation of blastocyst.

The root morul means mulberry. The solid ball of cells produced by cleavage is called a **morula** because it looks like a tiny mulberry.

The morula moves into the uterine cavity, floats freely in the cavity, and continues cell division. By the fifth day, the zona pellucida breaks down and a cavity forms in the ball of cells. The resulting hollow sphere of cells is called a **blastocyst** (BLAS-toh-syst). It receives nourishment from glycogen that is secreted by the endometrial glands in response to high levels of progesterone. The blastocyst consists of a single layer of flattened cells around a cavity and a cluster of cells at one side. The cavity is the **blastocele** (BLAS-toh-seel), the cells around the cavity make up the **trophoblast** (TROH-foh-blast), and the cluster of cells is the **inner cell mass.** The trophoblast functions in the formation of the chorion, which forms the fetal portion of the placenta, and the inner cell mass becomes the embryo. The blastocyst is now ready for implantation to begin. Figure 20–3 summarizes the events that occur during the first week of prenatal development.

Cleavage is a rapid series of cell divisions that results in a hollow ball of cells called a blastocyst. The blastocyst consists of the trophoblast, which develops into the chorion, and the inner cell mass, which becomes the embryo.

By the eighth day after fertilization, the trophoblast cells of the blastocyst secrete the hormone **human chorionic gonadotropin** (hCG). This hormone normally is not produced in a woman unless she is pregnant. Pregnancy tests are based on the presence of this hormone in the blood or urine.

Implantation

By the seventh day after ovulation (21st day of the menstrual cycle), the endometrium of the uterus is ready to receive the blastocyst. The blastocyst approaches the endometrium, usually high in the uterus, and if the endometrium is ready, the blastocyst attaches to it. This begins the process of **implantation** (Fig. 20–4).

The blastocyst is oriented so that the inner cell mass is toward the endometrium. The trophoblast cells in this region secrete enzymes that erode the endometrium to form a hole. The blastocyst "burrows" into the thick endometrial tissue. Cells of the endometrium grow over the blastocyst until it is fully implanted. Implantation is usually completed by the 14th day after ovulation. If fertilization had not taken place, the corpus luteum would regress and the endometrium would slough off as menstrual flow at this time. The blastocyst saves itself from being aborted by secreting **human chorionic gonadotropin** (hCG), a hormone that acts like luteinizing hormone (LH). hCG travels in the blood to the ovary where it causes the corpus luteum to remain functional and secrete progesterone to maintain the endometrium. The secretion of hCG reaches a peak about 8 weeks after fertilization, then declines as the placenta develops and is able to secrete sufficient quantities of progesterone to maintain pregnancy.

Implantation occurs as endometrial tissue grows around the blastocyst. The entire process takes about 7 days.

☑ **Quick**Check

● Why is capacitation of sperm necessary? Where does it occur?

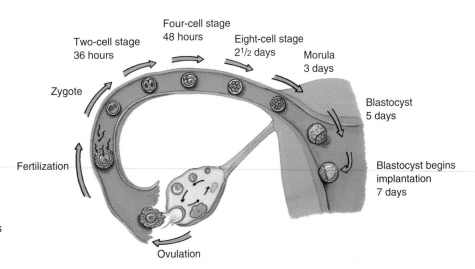

Figure 20–3 Summary of events during the first week of prenatal development.

Two-cell stage
36 hours

Four-cell stage
48 hours

Eight-cell stage
2½ days

Morula
3 days

Zygote

Blastocyst
5 days

Fertilization

Blastocyst begins implantation
7 days

Ovulation

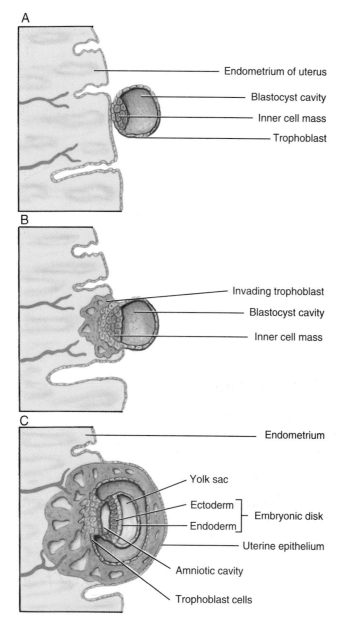

Figure 20–4 Implantation. *(A)* Blastocyst approaches endometrium. *(B)* Trophoblast invades endometrium. *(C)* Endometrial tissue grows over blastocyst to complete implantation.

● What develops from the inner cell mass?

● About how many days after ovulation does implantation begin?

In a small number of women, a normal pregnancy is impossible because of an obstruction or other defect in the uterine tubes. In such cases, pregnancy may be possible by **in vitro fertilization.** The root vitr- means "glass," so this is literally fertilization in a glass. Prescribed drugs induce the woman to ovulate multiple oocytes, which are then harvested and placed with sperm in a glass container. After the zygotes begin cleavage, several are introduced into the uterus for implantation.

Formation of Primary Germ Layers

While the blastocyst is implanting itself in the endometrium, changes are taking place in the inner cell mass that result in the formation of the primary germ layers. A cavity, called the **amniotic** (am-nee-AH-tik) **cavity,** develops in the inner cell mass. The portion of the inner cell mass that is adjacent to the blastocele flattens into a two-layered **embryonic disk** (see Fig. 20–4). The upper layer, next to the amniotic cavity, becomes **ectoderm,** and the lower layer becomes **endoderm.** A short time later a third layer, the **mesoderm,** appears between the ectoderm and endoderm. All of the tissues and organs in the body come from these three primary germ layers.

> The three primary germ layers, which develop while implantation is taking place, are the ectoderm, mesoderm, and endoderm.

Embryonic Development

Implantation and the formation of the three primary germ layers mark the end of the preembryonic period and the beginning of the embryonic period. The period of embryonic development lasts from the beginning of the third week to the end of the eighth week. The developing offspring is called an **embryo** during this time. Significant changes during this 6-week period include the formation of the **extraembryonic membranes, placenta,** and all of the **organ systems** in the body.

> The period of embryonic development lasts for 6 weeks, from the beginning of the third week to the end of the eighth week.

> The most critical time of development is during the embryonic period because this is when there is a lot of tissue differentiation and the organs are forming. Often a woman is not yet aware that she is pregnant. For this reason, a woman should always be concerned about good nutrition and a healthy lifestyle—if not for herself, then just in case she might be pregnant!

Formation of Extraembryonic Membranes

The **extraembryonic membranes** form outside the developing embryo and are responsible for its protection, nutrition, and excretion (Fig. 20–5). At birth these membranes are expelled, along with the placenta, as the **afterbirth.** The extraembryonic membranes are the amnion, chorion, yolk sac, and allantois.

The **amnion** (AM-nee-on) is a thin membrane that forms as the embryonic disk separates from the outer layer of the inner cell mass. The membrane and enclosed space enlarge to form a sac that com-

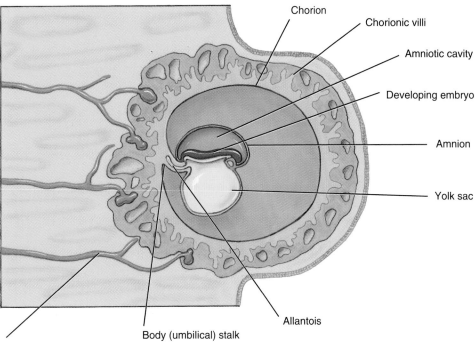

Figure 20-5
Extraembryonic membranes.

Labels: Chorion, Chorionic villi, Amniotic cavity, Developing embryo, Amnion, Yolk sac, Allantois, Body (umbilical) stalk, Blood vessel in endometrium

pletely surrounds the developing embryo. The **amniotic sac** is filled with **amniotic fluid,** which is formed initially by absorption from the maternal blood. The amniotic fluid cushions and protects the developing offspring from bumps and jolts, helps maintain a constant temperature and pressure around it, provides a medium for symmetrical development, and allows freedom of movement, which is necessary for development of muscles and skeleton and for blood flow. Before delivery, the amnion ruptures, either naturally or surgically, and the fluid is released.

Amniocentesis is a procedure in which a sample of aminiotic fluid is aspirated from the amniotic sac. The fluid contains cells from the fetus, which are removed and cultured in the laboratory. The cells and fluid are analyzed to detect chromosomal and biochemical abnormalities in the fetus. This procedure is usually performed during the fourth month of development.

The **chorion** (KOR-ee-on), which develops from the trophoblast, is the outermost extraembryonic membrane. It develops numerous finger like projections called chorionic villi. The villi on the side of the uterine wall enlarge, penetrate the maternal tissue, and become highly vascular. This region contributes to the formation of the placenta. The villi on the side next to the uterine cavity degenerate, and the surface becomes smooth. As the fetus enlarges, the chorion fuses with the amnion.

The **yolk sac** develops from the endoderm side of the embryonic disk. The yolk sac produces the pri-

mordial germ cells, which then migrate to the developing gonads during the fourth week. It also produces blood until the sixth week when the liver is developed sufficiently to take over the task. During the sixth week, the yolk sac detaches, shrinks, and has no further purpose.

The allantois (ah-LAN-toys) develops as a small outgrowth of the yolk sac. It contributes to the development of the urinary bladder and the umbilical arteries and vein. During the second month, it degenerates and becomes part of the umbilical cord.

The amnion, chorion, yolk sac, and allantois are membranes that form outside the embryo and function in protection, nutrition, and excretion.

Formation of the Placenta

The **placenta** is a highly vascular disk, 15 to 20 centimeters in diameter and 2.5 centimeters thick, that develops from both embryonic and maternal tissue. It is usually formed and fully functioning by the end of the embryonic period. After the infant is born, the placenta is expelled from the uterus as the afterbirth.

The placenta develops as chorionic villi from the embryo penetrate the endometrium of the uterus (Fig. 20-6). As this occurs, the villi become highly vascular and these vessels extend to the umbilical arteries and veins. The spaces in the endometrium surrounding the villi are filled with maternal blood. Oxygen and nutrients diffuse from the mother's blood into the fetal blood, and metabolic wastes, including carbon dioxide, diffuse from the fetal

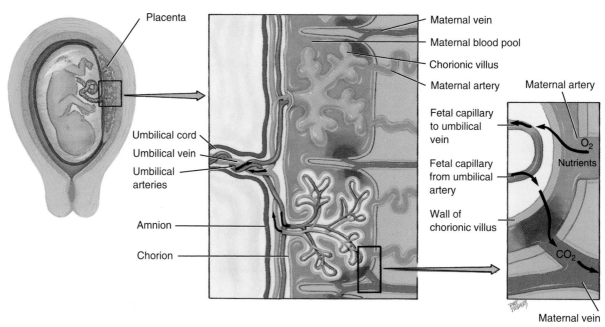

Figure 20–6 Structural features of the placenta and exchange of nutrients and wastes between maternal and fetal blood.

blood into the maternal blood. The membranes of the fetal capillaries and chorionic villi normally keep the fetal and maternal blood from actually mixing.

By the diffusion of substances across the membranes, the placenta functions as a nutritive, respiratory, and excretory organ. It also secretes hormones and thus functions as a temporary endocrine gland. Table 20–1 lists some of the hormones secreted by the placenta and their effects.

> The placenta develops from the endometrium of the uterus and the chorion of the embryo. It functions in nutrition, respiration, and excretion for the embryo/fetus and as an endocrine gland for the mother.

Normally, implantation occurs and the placenta develops in the upper portion of the uterus. In **placenta previa,** the placenta forms in the lower portion of the uterus and grows over the internal os of the cervix. This condition may result in reduced oxygen supply to the fetus and increases the risk of hemorrhage and infection for the mother. Cesarean delivery usually is recommended when placenta previa is diagnosed.

Organogenesis

Organogenesis (or-gan-oh-JEN-eh-sis) is the formation of body organs and organ systems. The formation of the primary germ layers sets the stage for this process because all body organs develop from them. Table 20–2 lists some examples of the derivatives of the primary germ layers. The skin, one of the earliest organs to develop, forms during the third week. By the end of the fourth week, the heart is pumping blood to all parts of the embryo. By the end of the eighth week, all the main internal body organs are established and the embryo has a human-like appearance even though it is only about 25 millimeters (1 inch) long and weighs about 1 gram.

> All body organs develop from the ectoderm, mesoderm, and endoderm that are formed during the preembryonic period. All organ systems are formed by the end of the embryonic period.

Table 20–1	Hormones Secreted by the Placenta
Hormone	**Effects**
Human chorionic gonadotropin	Similar to luteinizing hormone from the anterior pituitary; maintains mother's corpus luteum for the first 2 months of pregnancy
Estrogen	Helps maintain the endometrium; stimulates mammary gland development; inhibits follicle-stimulating hormone; increases uterine sensitivity to oxytocin
Progesterone	Helps maintain endometrium; stimulates mammary gland development; inhibits prolactin; inhibits follicle-stimulating hormone

Table 20–2 Derivatives of the Three Primary Germ Layers

Ectoderm	Mesoderm	Endoderm
Epidermis of the skin	Dermis of the skin	Epithelial lining of digestive tract
Hair, nails, skin glands	Skeletal, smooth, cardiac muscle	Epithelium of the liver and pancreas
Lens of the eye	Connective tissue including cartilage and bone	Epithelium of urinary bladder and urethra
Enamel of the teeth	Epithelium of serous membranes	Epithelium of the respiratory tract
All nervous tissue	Epithelium of joint cavities	Thyroid, parathyroid, and thymus glands
Adrenal medulla	Epithelium of blood vessels	
Sense organ receptor cells	Kidneys and ureters	
Linings of the oral and nasal cavities, vagina, and anal canal	Adrenal cortex	
	Epithelium of gonads and reproductive ducts	

Fetal Development

The **fetal stage** of development starts at the beginning of the ninth week and lasts until birth. The developing offspring is called a **fetus** at this time. Because all the organ systems are formed during the embryonic period, the fetus is less vulnerable than the embryo to malformations due to radiation, viruses, and drugs. The fetal stage is a period of growth and maturation. Table 20–3 describes some developments in each month of development.

By the end of the 20th week, the mother commonly feels the fetus moving within the uterus. This is called **quickening.** At this time in development, the fetal skin is coated with **vernix caseosa,** a cheesy mixture of sebum and dead epidermal cells, which protects the skin from the amniotic fluid that surrounds it. Fine **lanugo hair** covers the body and helps keep the vernix caseosa intact. By the end of

28 weeks, the fetus may survive outside the uterus with medical support. Mortality rate is high with infants born at this time because their temperature control mechanisms are not mature enough to maintain constant body temperature, and their respiratory system is not ready to maintain regular respiration. By 38 weeks, the fetus is considered full term and ready for life outside the uterus.

The fetus is dependent on its mother for oxygen and nutrients, which are supplied by diffusion through membranes in the placenta. Carbon dioxide and other wastes diffuse from the fetus into the maternal blood in the lacunae of the placenta. Gases, nutrients, and wastes are carried to and from the fetus in the umbilical vessels. This arrangement necessitates that the pattern of blood flow in the fetus be different from the pattern after birth. These differences, which are discussed in Chapter 13, are reviewed in Table 20–4.

Table 20–3 Monthly Changes During Prenatal Development

End of Month*	Size	Developments During the Month
1	6 mm	Arm and leg buds form; heart forms and starts beating; body systems begin to form
2	25–30 mm, 1 g	Head nearly as large as body; major brain regions present; ossification begins; arms and legs distinct; blood vessels form and cardiovascular system fully functional; liver large
3	75 mm, 10–45 g	Facial features present; nails develop on fingers and toes; can swallow and digest amniotic fluid; urine starts to form; fetus starts to move; heartbeat detected; external genitalia develop
4	140 mm, 60–200 g	Facial features well formed; hair appears on head; joints begin to form
5	190 mm, 250–450 g	Mother feels fetal movement; fetus covered with fine hair called lanugo hair; eyebrows visible; skin coated with vernix caseosa, a cheesy mixture of sebum and dead epidermal cells
6	220 mm, 500–800 g	Skin reddish because blood in the capillaries is visible; skin wrinkled because it lacks adipose in the subcutaneous tissue
7	260 mm, 900–1300 g	Eyes open; capable of survival but the mortality rate is high; scrotum develops; testes begin their descent
8	280–300 mm, 1400–2100 g	Testes descend into the scrotum; sense of taste is present
9	310–340 mm, 2200–2900 g	Reddish skin fades to pink; nails reach tips of fingers and toes or beyond
10	350–360 mm, 3000–3400 g	Skin smooth and plump because of adipose in subcutaneous tissue; lanugo hair shed; fetus usually turns to a head-down position; full term

*These are 4-week (28-day) months.

Table 20–4 Summary of Special Features in Fetal Circulation

Feature	Location	Before Birth	After Birth
Umbilical arteries (2)	Umbilical cord	Transport blood from fetus to the placenta	Degenerate to become lateral umbilical ligaments
Umbilical vein (1)	Umbilical cord	Transports blood from placenta to the fetus	Becomes the ligamentum teres (round ligament) of the liver
Ductus venosus	Between the umbilical vein and the inferior vena cava	Carries blood directly from umbilical vein to inferior vena cava; bypasses the liver	Becomes ligamentum venosum of the liver
Foramen ovale	Interatrial septum	Allows blood to go directly from right atrium into the left atrium to bypass pulmonary circulation	Closes after birth to become the fossa ovalis
Ductus arteriosus	Between the pulmonary trunk and aorta	Permits blood in the pulmonary trunk to go directly into the descending aorta and bypass pulmonary circulation	Becomes a fibrous cord, the ligamentum arteriosum

The fetal period is one of growth and maturation of the organ systems.

 QuickCheck

● What is the purpose of the amniotic fluid? List four functions.

● What are the two primary functions of the placenta?

● What is the basic process that occurs during fetal development?

Parturition and Lactation

The time of prenatal development, or pregnancy, is referred to as the **gestation** (jes-TAY-shun) period. In humans, the normal gestation period is 266 days from fertilization. Because it is difficult to determine the actual time of fertilization, "due dates" are calculated as 280 days after the beginning of the last menstrual period. **Parturition** (par-too-RIH-shun) refers to the birth of an infant, and **labor** is the process by which forceful contractions expel the fetus from the uterus.

The normal human gestation period is 266 days from fertilization or 280 days from the beginning of the last menstrual period.

Labor and Delivery

The onset of **true labor** is marked by rhythmic contractions, dilation of the cervix, and "show," which is a discharge of bloody mucus from the cervix and vagina. In **false labor** the contractions are weak and irregular and there is no cervical dilation and no "show."

Although the physiologic mechanisms are unclear, labor appears to be the result of hormone interactions. Near the end of pregnancy, progesterone levels decline and estrogen levels increase. This removes progesterone's inhibitory effects on uterine contractions and at the same time estrogen sensitizes the uterus to the effects of oxytocin. Pressure of the fetal head on the cervix signals the hypothalamus to secrete oxytocin from the posterior pituitary. Oxytocin stimulates the production of prostaglandins, and together oxytocin and prostaglandins cause contractions of the myometrium. As soon as the hypothalamus becomes involved, a positive feedback cycle is set up in which the uterine contractions stimulate more oxytocin and the oxytocin stimulates uterine contractions.

Oxytocin and prostaglandins stimulate uterine contractions during labor.

Labor is divided into three stages (Fig. 20–7):

• The **dilation stage** begins with the onset of true labor and lasts until the cervix is fully dilated. This is the longest part of labor and lasts from 6 to 24 hours, or even longer. It is characterized by rhythmic and forceful uterine contractions. The amniotic sac ruptures, and the cervix dilates to a diameter of 10 centimeters.

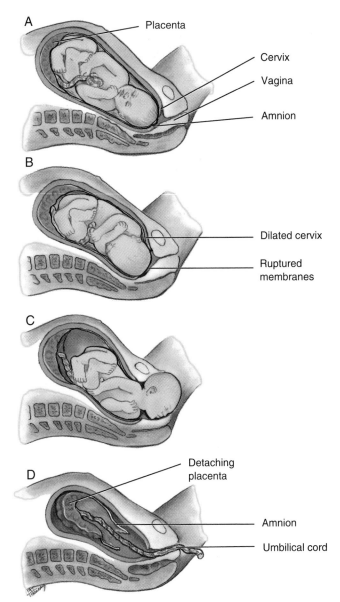

Figure 20–7 Three stages of labor. *(A)* Before labor begins. *(B)* Dilation stage. *(C)* Expulsion stage. *(D)* Placental stage.

Labels: Placenta, Cervix, Vagina, Amnion, Dilated cervix, Ruptured membranes, Detaching placenta, Amnion, Umbilical cord

• The **expulsion stage** lasts from full cervical dilation until delivery of the fetus. This stage usually lasts less than an hour. In normal position, the head appears first (cephalic presentation) and helps dilate the cervix. This makes it easier for the rest of the body to pass through the birth canal. The head-first position also allows mucus to be suctioned from the respiratory passages so that the newborn can breathe before the rest of the body is completely through the birth canal. At the end of this stage, the umbilical cord is clamped and cut.
• The final phase is the **placental stage.** Within 10 to 15 minutes after parturition, the placenta separates from the uterine wall. Forceful uterine contractions expel the placenta and the attached membranes as the afterbirth. The forceful contractions constrict torn blood vessels to prevent hemorrhage. Nor-

mally less than half a liter of blood is lost during delivery.

> Labor is divided into dilation, expulsion, and placental stages.

> Breech presentation occurs in about 5 percent of all deliveries. In a breech presentation, the buttocks appear first rather than the head. The major concern is the time and difficulty of the expulsion stage of parturition. A cesarean section must be performed if the infant cannot be delivered breech.

Adjustments of the Infant at Birth

The fetal lungs are collapsed or partially filled with amniotic fluid and are nonfunctional. As soon as the umbilical cord is cut, the oxygen supply from the mother ceases. Blood continues to circulate through the fetus, however, and the increasing carbon dioxide levels, decreasing pH (acidosis), and decreasing oxygen stimulate the respiratory center in the medulla. The respiratory muscles contract and the infant draws its first breath. This first breath is normally strong and deep as the infant inflates the collapsed alveoli.

Numerous changes take place in the circulatory pathway at birth or soon after (Fig. 20–8 and Table 20–4). The foramen ovale, between the right and left atria, functionally closes at the moment of birth so that the blood will flow through the pulmonary arteries to pick up oxygen in the lungs. Eventually two flaps of tissue fuse across the opening to permanently seal it off, and it becomes the fossa ovalis. As soon as the lungs begin to function, smooth muscle in the ductus arteriosus contracts to close that vessel, again to encourage blood flow to the lungs. The remnant of the ductus arteriosus is the ligamentum arteriosum. The ductus venosus takes blood from the umbilical vein to the inferior vena cava in the fetus. As soon as the umbilical cord is severed, this shunt is no longer needed and the ductus venosus degenerates into the ligamentum venosum.

> An infant's first breath is normally strong and deep to inflate the lungs. When the lungs begin to function with the first breath and the umbilical cord is cut, the circulatory pattern changes so that the blood goes to the lungs for oxygenation.

Physiology of Lactation

Lactation (lak-TAY-shun) refers to the production of milk by the mammary glands and the ejection of milk from the breasts. The most important hormone that stimulates milk production is **prolactin.** During pregnancy, the increasing levels of estrogen and progesterone from the placenta stimulate the enlargement of the mammary glands. Prolactin levels

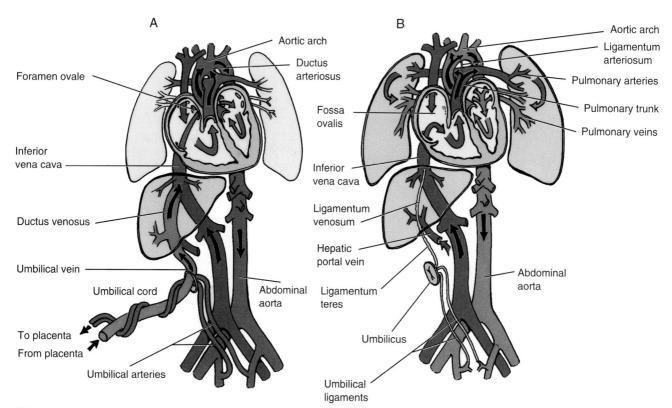

Figure 20-8 Circulation patterns before and after birth. *(A)* Fetal circulation. *(B)* Circulation after birth.

also increase during this time, but the prolactin stimulus for milk production is inhibited by the estrogen and progesterone. During parturition, when the placenta is expelled from the uterus, estrogen and progesterone dramatically decrease and remove the inhibition for milk production. The infant's sucking action triggers impulses to the posterior pituitary by means of the hypothalamus. These impulses stimulate the release of **oxytocin,** which causes the ejection (let-down) of milk from the breasts (Fig. 20-9).

Normally, there is a 2- to 3-day delay in the start of milk production after birth. During this time a cloudy yellowish fluid, called colostrum (koh-LAHS-trum), is secreted by the mammary glands. Colostrum has less lactose than milk, has almost no fat, but has more protein, vitamin A, and minerals than milk. Colostrum and maternal milk contain antibodies that help provide immunity for the infant.

Prolactin levels soon return to normal after birth, and milk is not produced unless prolactin is stimulated by the infant's suckling. Each time a mother nurses her infant, impulses from the nipple to the hypothalamus stimulate the release of **prolactin-releasing hormone** (PRH). This causes a temporary surge in prolactin, which stimulates milk production for the next nursing period. If a mother stops nursing her infant, milk production ceases within a few days.

Prolactin stimulates production of milk in the mammary glands. Oxytocin causes contractions that eject the milk from the breasts.

✓ **Quick**Check

- What is the longest stage of labor?

- Describe three changes that occur in the circulatory pattern of the infant after birth.

- What are the functions of prolactin and oxytocin in lactation?

The oxytocin that stimulates the ejection of milk also causes uterine contractions, so it is believed that breast feeding hastens the return of the uterus to its normal prepregnant size.

Postnatal Development

Development after birth is termed **postnatal development.** It lasts from parturition until death and is divided into the following stages:

- Neonatal period
- Infancy

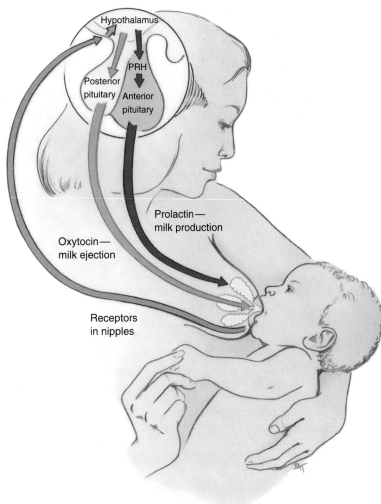

Figure 20–9   Stimulus for lactation.

PRH = Prolactin releasing hormone

- Childhood
- Adolescence
- Adulthood
- Senescence

Neonatal Period

The **neonatal** (nee-oh-NAY-tal) **period** begins at the moment of birth and lasts until the end of the first 4 weeks. During this time, the infant is called a newborn or **neonate** (NEE-oh-nayt). These 4 weeks are characterized by dramatic changes, which occur at a rapid rate. In addition to the respiratory and circulatory changes mentioned earlier, the neonate faces other adjustments to life outside the uterus. The neonate needs vitamins C and D to help harden the skeleton and iron to aid the liver in the production of red blood cells. This period is critical also because the temperature-regulating mechanism and immune system are not fully developed, which means that the neonate is vulnerable to environmental temperature changes and infections.

Infancy

The period of **infancy** lasts from the end of the first month to the end of the first year. During this time body weight generally triples and many developmental changes take place. There is a myelinization of the nervous system, which is manifest in more coordination of motor activities. The infant learns to sit, crawl, stand, and perhaps walk by the end of the first year. The deciduous incisor teeth erupt during this time, and the infant learns to communicate by smiling, laughing, and making sounds.

Childhood

The period of **childhood** lasts from the end of the first year until puberty. Bone ossification is rapid. Bone growth slows in late childhood then accelerates again just before puberty. Bladder and bowel controls are established. The deciduous teeth erupt, then are shed, and are replaced by permanent teeth. Motor coordination develops more fully. Language, reading, writing, reasoning, and other intellectual skills become more refined. The child is maturing emotionally.

Adolescence

The period of **adolescence** lasts from puberty until adulthood. Puberty is the period when an individual becomes physiologically capable of reproduction. In females, the first sign of puberty is usually development of the breasts. In males, the first sign is enlargement of the testes. The changes that occur during this period are largely controlled by hormones. The secondary sex characteristics appear, and there is a rapid growth in the muscular and skeletal systems. The adolescent shows increasing levels of motor skills, intellectual ability, and emotional maturity.

Adulthood

Adulthood is the period from adolescence to old age. The progression from adolescence to adulthood is vague and has physical, emotional, and behavioral implications. Generally, adulthood is characterized by a maintenance of existing body tissues so that the body remains unchanged anatomically and physiologically for many years. Sometime after the age of 30, degenerative changes start to occur. These changes may not be noticeable at first, but later become more significant as the individual progresses into old age.

Senescence

Senescence (seh-NESS-ens) is the period of old age and ends in death. As the degenerative changes that begin in adulthood continue throughout old age, the body becomes less and less capable of coping with the demands placed on it. Changes related to aging take place in all body systems; however, the rate at which they occur varies from individual to individual and from system to system. The central nervous system may become less efficient so that memory fails and motor skills are impaired. Homeostatic mechanisms may fail so the individual is more vulnerable to fluid and electrolyte changes, acid–base imbalances, and temperature variations. Sensory functions often decline and are manifest in a hearing loss, poor vision, and reduced senses of taste, smell, and touch. The aging section that is presented with each body system in this book describes some of the changes in more detail. Even though there are degenerative changes in all body systems, death usually results from cardiovascular disturbances, failure of the immune system, or disease processes that affect vital organs.

> Postnatal development is a continuum that is divided into several periods based on physical and psychological development. These periods are neonatal, infancy, childhood, adolescence, adulthood, and senescence.

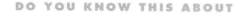

DO YOU KNOW THIS ABOUT

Development?

Teratogens

A **teratogen** is any agent or factor that causes the production of physical defects in the developing embryo. The word is derived from the Greek word *teras*, which means "monster." These factors interfere with development and cause deformities without changing the DNA in the embryo. Examples of teratogens include alcohol, cigarette smoke, cocaine and other drugs, ionizing radiation, rubella virus (German measles), pesticides, and industrial chemicals. One of the best known and saddest examples of a teratogenic drug is thalidomide. This drug was commonly used to diminish the nausea of "morning sickness" and as a sedative in sleeping pills during the early 1960s, primarily in Europe. Later, it was discovered that thalidomide, when taken by a woman during early pregnancy, caused serious physical

deformities in the fetus. In thalidomide cases, the infant was often born without arms and/or legs.

In general, the effect of the teratogen is greater if the exposure is early in pregnancy. For example, exposure to teratogens during the first 2 weeks after conception, before a woman knows she is pregnant, usually causes death of the embryo and spontaneous abortion because this is a period of rapid cell division and primary germ layer formation. Exposure during the period of organogenesis, from days 15 to 60, frequently causes physical deformities in the developing embryo. Later exposure, during the period of growth and maturation of the organ systems, usually results in relatively minor abnormalities.

Alcohol is the number one fetal teratogen. Like most other drugs, alcohol easily diffuses through the placenta and enters the fetal circulation. No one knows if there is a "safe" level of alcohol consumption during pregnancy. Even small amounts of alcohol are associated with increased miscarriages and decreased birth weight. In the crucial early period of an infant's development, often before pregnancy is recognized, maternal consumption of alcohol increases the risk of fetal abnormalities. Women who regularly drink alcoholic beverages during pregnancy may give birth to infants with **fetal alcohol syndrome (FAS).** Infants affected with FAS have severe mental and physical problems, including lifelong mental retardation, slow growth and development, a defective heart, malformed arms and legs, a small head, and abnormal eye features. They also have behavioral problems such as hyperactivity and a short attention span. Maternal alcohol consumption may result in intoxication of the fetus and subsequent withdrawal symptoms in the newborn. The United States Surgeon General recommends that pregnant women and those who are considering pregnancy do not drink any alcoholic beverages.

Maternal smoking during pregnancy appears to be a significant factor in the development of cardiac abnormalities, cleft lip, and cleft palate in the fetus. Women who smoke have a much higher risk of ectopic pregnancy. Cigarette smoking also is directly associated with premature birth, low infant birth weight, miscarriage, increased fetal and infant mortality rate, and physical abnormalities. Infants born to mothers who smoked while pregnant and after delivery have a higher incidence of **sudden infant death syndrome (SIDS)** and are more susceptible to respiratory problems in early childhood. Even exposure to cigarette smoke in the air they breathe predisposes infants to increased incidence of bronchitis and pneumonia. Not smoking is one of the best gifts parents can give their children.

Drugs of all kinds may be detrimental to the fetus when they are used by the mother during pregnancy. Even supposedly "safe" drugs such as aspirin, antibiotics, antihistamines, and tranquilizers may cause problems ranging from bleeding and miscarriage to physical abnormalities. A pregnant woman should always check with her physician before taking any medication. Illegal drugs such as heroine, cocaine, and morphine may cause the fetus to be addicted to those drugs at birth. In addition to infant addiction, these drugs are associated with a higher incidence of premature infants, low birth weight, slow growth of the infant after birth, mental retardation, and physical deformities. Of the illegal drugs, cocaine and crack are considered to be the worst and cause the most damage to the fetus. It takes only a single use of cocaine during pregnancy to damage the developing fetal brain. Part of its detrimental effect is because cocaine crosses the placenta readily and has a longer half-life in the fetus than other drugs. The enzymes involved in cocaine metabolism are not fully developed and immature renal function delays its excretion so that the drug tends to accumulate and stay in the fetal circulation for a long time. This gives the drug more time in which to damage body cells and organs.

There is no safe amount of alcohol, cigarettes, or illegal drugs. Even small quantities increase risks for the developing fetus. Whatever a mother eats or drinks crosses the placenta and gets to her fetus.

CHAPTER QUIZ

RECALL

Match the definitions on the left with the appropriate term on the right.

1. The single cell produced by fertilization

2. Early cell divisions after fertilization

3. Develops from the trophoblast and contributes to the formation of the placenta

4. Hollow sphere of cells during the preembryonic period

5. Develops into three primary germ layers

6. Develops into muscle

7. Develops into epidermis and its derivatives

8. Develops into the lining of the digestive and respiratory tracts

9. Longest stage of labor

10. Stimulates uterine contractions and the ejection of milk

A. Blastocyst

B. Chorion

C. Cleavage

D. Dilation

E. Ectoderm

F. Endoderm

G. Inner cell mass

H. Mesoderm

I. Oxytocin

J. Zygote

THOUGHT

1. Capacitation

    a. dissolves the corona radiata so a sperm can fertilize the egg

    b. occurs in the female reproductive tract and weakens the acrosomal membrane

    c. occurs in the epididymis and energizes the mitochondria for locomotion

    d. occurs in the vagina and weakens the zona pellucida

2. Which of the following statements about human chorionic gonadotropin is NOT true?

    a. it is secreted by the blastocyst

    b. it causes the corpus luteum to continue secreting progesterone

    c. levels reach a peak about 8 weeks after fertilization

    d. it has the same effect as follicle-stimulating hormone

3. Implantation begins

    a. about 3 days after ovulation

    b. about 7 days after ovulation

    c. about 14 days after ovulation

    d. about 21 days after ovulation

4. Which of the following is NOT true about the placenta?

    a. it develops from both embryonic and maternal tissue

    b. it secretes progesterone, estrogen, and human chorionic gonadotropin

    c. it develops before the fetal period begins

    d. it develops from the amnion and chorion

5. Fetal blood is carried to the placenta by the

    a. umbilical artery

    b. umbilical vein

    c. ductus venosus

    d. ductus arteriosus

APPLICATION

Mary Smith recently gave birth to her first baby, a daughter she named Sarah. One day while nursing Sarah, she felt "cramps" in her uterus. Concerned, she called her obstetrician. Explain what was happening to cause the cramps.

How do the amnion and chorion differ in function?

Answers for QuickCheck Questions

CHAPTER 1

Page 4: 1) physiologist, because immunology is a part of the study of functions in the human body; 2) structure, because anatomy is the study of structure and structural relationships; 3) organs are more complex than tissues. **Page 9:** 1) respiratory system; 2) cardiovascular; 3) water, oxygen, nutrients, heat, and pressure. **Page 14:** 1) negative feedback; 2) sagittal; 3) in the area behind the knee.

CHAPTER 2

Page 19: 1) oxygen; 2) there are 17 protons, 17 electrons, and 18 neutrons; 3) three energy levels with 2 electrons in the first level, 8 in the second level, and 7 in the third level. **Page 23:** 1) covalent bonds; 2) intermolecular bonds. **Page 24:** 1) sodium, hydrogen, carbon, and oxygen; 2) a molecule. **Page 27:** 1) decomposition reaction; 2) the coal dust has a much greater surface area than the briquet; therefore it has a much faster reaction rate. **Page 30:** 1) the pH is less than 7.0 because all acids have a pH less than 7.0; 2) the acids are neutralized by buffers in the body. **Page 35:** 1) RNA because DNA does not contain uracil but RNA does; 2) a lipid because carbohydrates have a higher oxygen content, proteins contain nitrogen, and nucleic acids contain phosphates and nitrogenous bases.

CHAPTER 3

Page 45: 1) Golgi apparatus; 2) cilia. **Page 56:** 1) they shrink or crenate; 2) lysosomes to digest the material they engulf; 3) telophase.

CHAPTER 4

Page 70: 1) epithelium; 2) connective tissue; 3) heart. **Page 71:** 1) serous membranes; 2) synovial membranes.

CHAPTER 5

Page 80: 1) stratum basale; 2) dermis; 3) stratum basale of the epidermis. **Page 82:** 1) stratum ba-

sale; 2) merocrine sweat glands; **Page 84:** 1) because the epidermis, which protects against fluid loss and acts as a barrier against pathogen entry, has been destroyed; 2) evaporation of perspiration cools the body, and cutaneous blood vessels dilate to bring warm blood to the surface where heat is lost to the surrounding air.

CHAPTER 6

Page 97: 1) compact bone; 2) appositional growth produces an increase in the diameter of bone and is accomplished by osteoblasts depositing bone tissue on the outside of the bone and osteoclasts absorbing bone tissue on the inside of the bone; growth at the epiphyseal plate increases the length of the bone. **Page 106:** 1) frontal, maxilla, ethmoid, and sphenoid; 2) vomer and perpendicular plate of the ethmoid; 3) thoracic vertebrae. **Page 113:** 1) radius; 2) forms a deep socket for the head of the femur; 3) calcaneus. **Page 115:** 1) the knee, which is a synovial joint, is affected; 2) diarthrosis or synovial joint.

CHAPTER 7

Page 126: 1) epimysium; 2) I band. **Page 133:** 1) prolonged contraction or spastic paralysis because there would be no acetylcholinesterase to inactivate the acetylcholine, which would remain bound with receptors to provide stimulus for contraction; 2) calcium ions, because the presence of calcium changes the configuration of troponin and exposes the myosin binding sites on actin myofilaments; 3) multiple motor unit summation where additional motor units are recruited to counteract the increased load; 4) aerobic pathway yields nearly 20 times more ATP than the anaerobic pathway. **Page 145:** 1) masseter muscle; 2) triceps brachii; 3) the hamstring muscle group on the posterior surface of the thigh flexes the knee; the antagonist is the quadriceps femoris group on the anterior surface of the thigh.

CHAPTER 8

Page 157: 1) association neurons; 2) myelin; 3) sensory functions because afferent neurons are sensory neurons that conduct impulses to the CNS. **Page 163:** 1) action potential; 2) nodes of Ranvier, which are the gaps between myelin segments; 3) divergence circuit. **Page 171:** 1) parietal lobe; 2) myelinated fibers; 3) third ventricle; 4) sensory impulses of touch, pain, pressure, and temperature. **Page 177:** 1) facial nerve, cranial nerve VII; 2) sympathetic or thoracolumbar division; 3) localization is because one preganglionic fiber synapses with only a few postganglionic fibers; and the short-term effect is because the neurotransmitter is acetylcholine, which is quickly inactivated.

CHAPTER 9

Page 186: 1) because taste receptors are localized on the tongue but temperature receptors are widely distributed; 2) free nerve endings interspersed between epithelial cells of the skin. **Page 188:** 1) taste; 2) taste and smell. **Page 194:** 1) the fovea centralis is the area of sharpest vision because it has the highest concentration of cones; 2) there are no photoreceptors in the region of the optic disk; 3) the lens. **Page 199:** 1) because the ossicles transmit the sound vibrations from the tympanic membrane, through the middle ear, to the inner ear where the receptors are located; 2) base of the cochlea near the oval window; 3) within the membranous labyrinth of the vestibule and semicircular canals.

CHAPTER 10

Page 207: 1) receptor sites for protein hormones are located on the surface of the plasma membrane; receptor sites for steroids are located in the cytoplasm; 2) tropic hormones cause secretion of other hormones. **Page 212:** 1) anterior region is controlled by factors from the hypothalamus, posterior region is controlled by neural stimulation; 2) the posterior pituitary gland will secrete increased amounts of antidiuretic hormone to reduce urine output and conserve water to restore homeostasis. **Page 217:** 1) an iodine deficiency decreases the amount of active thyroxine, which increases the amount of thyroid-stimulating hormone released from the anterior pituitary gland; 2) calcitonin from the thyroid gland reduces calcium levels, and parathyroid hormone from the parathyroid gland increases blood calcium levels; 3) aldosterone stimulates the reabsorption, or conservation, of sodium in the kidney and water follows the sodium so this increases water retention and decreases urine output. **Page 220:** 1) insulin is secreted to reduce the glucose levels; 2) injections of testosterone will inhibit the release of luteinizing hormone from the anterior pituitary; 3) melatonin is secreted by the pineal gland.

CHAPTER 11

Page 233: 1) decrease in albumins produced by the liver would reduce osmotic pressure of the blood and affect fluid/electrolyte balance, decrease in fibrinogen would impair blood clotting process, decrease in globulins would interfere with transport of fats and fat-soluble vitamins; 2) an increase in oxygen delivery to the kidneys decreases the amount of renal erythropoietic factor, which decreases the amount of active erythropoietin in the blood; 3) diapedesis. **Page 238:** 1) blood clotting will be impaired because the megakaryocytes form platelets that function in blood clotting; 2) because there is a decrease in fibrinogen and prothrombin that are produced by the liver and function in blood clotting; 3) yes, because the AB+ recipient has no agglutinins to attack the antigens from the A+ blood.

CHAPTER 12

Page 249: 1) ascending aorta; 2) papillary muscles and chordae tendineae; 3) left atrium and left ventricle. **Page 253:** 1) heart rate will decrease because the AV node, which has a slower rate, will take over as pacemaker; 2) the atria are in diastole and receiving blood from the IVC and SVC; 3) sympathetic stimulation and increased end-diastolic volume.

CHAPTER 13

Page 263: 1) veins contain almost 70% of total blood volume at any given time; 2) prevent backflow of blood due to gravity and keep the blood moving toward the heart; 3) when the precapillary sphincters relax there is increased blood flow through a given capillary bed. **Page 269:** 1) fluid leaves the blood vessel and enters tissue spaces; 2) capillaries; 3) there is increased heart rate and increased venous return, both of which increase cardiac output; 4) decreased pressure in the carotid sinus increases heart rate and causes vasoconstriction to return blood pressure to normal levels. **Page 280:** 1) liver, stomach, pancreas, spleen; 2) hepatic portal vein; 3) pulmonary capillaries.

CHAPTER 14

Page 291: 1) respiratory movements, skeletal muscle contraction; and contraction of smooth muscle within the vessel walls; 2) as the infectious agents and cellular debris are filtered/trapped by the lymph nodes, they accumulate and cause an enlargement; 3) there is massive hemorrhage because the spleen is a reservoir for blood. **Page 293:** 1) inflammation, phagocytosis, and the chemical action of complement and interferon; 2) virus infections. **Page 301:** 1) helper T cells stimulate B-cell activity; 2) IgG; 3) passive natural immunity.

CHAPTER 15

Page 312: 1) three; 2) pleura. **Page 315:** 1) it increases the intrapleural pressure so that intrapulmonary pressure is no longer greater than intrapleural pressure; 2) reduces the surface tension of the fluid within the alveoli so they expand more readily; 3) it will reduce her vital capacity because the fluid displaces the air. **Page 323:** 1) it decreases the effectiveness of external respiration because the surface area for gas exchange is reduced; 2) attached to hemoglobin is the primary way by which oxygen is transported in the blood and if there is reduced hemoglobin, there is reduced oxygen transport and reduced delivery; 3) this will lower the pH; 4) stimulate the medullary respiratory centers to increase the rate and depth of breathing; 5) phrenic nerve.

CHAPTER 16

Page 335: 1) crown; 2) the esophagus has to expand into the soft part of the trachea to permit the bolus to pass through; 3) the lower esophageal, or cardiac, sphincter. **Page 341:** 1) pyloric sphincter; 2) vagus nerve stimulation increases gastric secretions; 3) surface area is increased by the plicae circulares, villi, and microvilli; 4) cecum. **Page 347:** 1) digestion of fats because the bile transported in the common bile duct emulsifies the fats so they can be hydrolyzed by the lipases; 2) increases the production of pancreatic enzymes; 3) diffusion.

CHAPTER 17

Page 360: 1) catabolism; 2) inside mitochondria; 3) pyruvic acid acetyl Co-A. **Page 367:** 1) physical activity; 2) carbohydrates and proteins yield 4 C per gram and fats yield 9 C per gram; 3) no more than 30% of caloric intake should be in the form of fats and less than 10% of caloric intake should be in the form of saturated fats. **Page 368:** 1) core temperature is slightly greater than shell temperature; 2) radiation; 3) by homeostatic negative feedback mechanisms.

CHAPTER 18

Page 379: 1) renal pelvis; 2) glomerulus and glomerular (Bowman's) capsule; 3) juxtaglomerular apparatus, specifically the juxtaglomerular cells in the afferent arteriole. **Page 381:** 1) renal pelvis of the kidney and the urinary bladder; 2) in the wall of the urinary bladder; 3) the internal urethral sphincter is involuntary smooth muscle and the external urethral sphincter is voluntary skeletal muscle. **Page 385:** 1) glomerular filtrate lacks plasma proteins; 2) proximal convoluted tubule (about 65%); 3) glucose content of the blood exceeds renal threshold so it is not all reabsorbed and the excess appears in the urine; 4) aldosterone, antidiuretic hormone, and atrial natriuretic hormone. **Page 388:** 1) 60%; 2) inside the cells as intracellular fluid; 3) sodium; 4) 7.4, normal range is 7.35–7.45.

CHAPTER 19

Page 400: 1) abdominal temperature is too high for production of viable sperm; 2) seminiferous tubules; 3) ductus (vas) deferens; 4) seminal vesicles (about 60%). **Page 402:** 1) penis will become filled with blood—erection; 2) stimulates the interstitial cells to produce testosterone; 3) male reproductive organs will fail to develop properly. **Page 409:** 1) converted into the corpus luteum; 2) uterine tube; 3) stratum functionale of the endometrium; 4) clitoris. **Page 413:** 1) ovulation and development of the corpus luteum; 2) corpus luteum; 3) the cells of the endometrium proliferate to restore the uterine lining.

CHAPTER 20

Page 423: 1) capacitation of sperm, which occurs in the female reproductive tract, weakens the membrane around the acrosome so the enzymes necessary for fertilization can be released; 2) embryo; 3) 7 days. **Page 428:** 1) cushions and protects developing embryo/fetus, maintains constant temperature and pressure, provides medium for symmetrical development, permits freedom of movement for musculoskeletal development; 2) placenta functions as an endocrine organ for the mother and in the nutrition, excretion, and respiration of the fetus; 3) growth and maturation. **Page 430:** 1) dilation stage; 2) foramen ovale functionally closes so blood doesn't bypass the lungs, ductus arteriosus closes so blood flows to the lungs, ductus venosus closes so blood doesn't bypass the liver; 3) prolactin stimulates the production of milk and oxytocin causes contractions that eject the milk.

Glossary of Disorders

Acne vulgaris (AK-nee vul-GAIR-is) Inflammatory condition of sebaceous glands frequently occurring during puberty and adolescence; characterized by increased production of sebum and formation of blackheads that plug the pores. **(Ch 5)**

Acromegaly (ack-roh-MEG-ah-lee) Abnormal enlargement of the extremities caused by hypersecretion of growth hormone in the adult. **(Ch 10)**

Addison's disease (ADD-ih-sunz dih-ZEEZ) A syndrome resulting from insufficient secretion of glucocorticoids and mineralocorticoids from the adrenal cortex; potentially life-threatening hypoglycemia and fluid and electrolyte disturbances may develop. **(Ch 10)**

Adrenogenital syndrome (ah-DREE-noh-jen-ih-tal SIN-drohm) Group of symptoms associated with alterations in secondary sex characteristics as a result of increased sex hormones from the adrenal cortex; increased amounts of androgens in the female lead to masculinization and increased amounts of estrogens in the male lead to breast enlargement (gynecomastia). **(Ch 10, 19)**

Alopecia (al-oh-PEE-shee-ah) Absence of hair from skin areas where it normally grows; baldness; may be hereditary or due to disease, injury, or chemotherapy or may occur as part of aging. **(Ch 5)**

Alzheimer's disease (ALTZ-hye-merz dih-ZEEZ) Irreversible senile dementia characterized by increasing loss of mental abilities, including memory, recognition, reasoning, and judgment, and by mood changes, including irritability, agitation, and restlessness. **(Ch 8)**

Amenorrhea (a-men-oh-REE-ah) Absence of menstruation; may be due to abnormal development or malformation of the reproductive organs, endocrine disturbances, excessive weight loss, emotional shock, or pregnancy. **(Ch 19)**

Anaphylaxis (an-ah-fill-AKS-is) An exaggerated or unusual hypersensitivity to foreign protein or other substances, characterized by a systemic vasodilation with a dramatic decrease in blood pressure that can be life threatening. **(Ch 14)**

Anemia (ah-NEE-mee-ah) Condition in which there is decreased oxygen delivery to the tissues; may be from decreased erythrocyte production, blood loss, or increased erythrocyte destruction. **(Ch 11, 12, 13)**

Anencephaly (an-en-SEF-ah-lee) Congenital disorder with cranial vault and cerebral hemispheres missing. **(Ch 8)**

Aneurysm (AN-yoo-rizm) A saclike protrusion formed by a localized dilatation in the wall of a weakened blood vessel, usually an artery. **(Ch 11, 12, 13)**

Angina pectoris (an-JYE-nah PECK-tohr-is) Acute chest pain caused by decreased blood supply to the heart muscle. **(Ch 11, 12, 13)**

Anosmia (an-OZ-mee-ah) Lack of sense of smell. **(Ch 9)**

Appendicitis (ah-pen-dih-SYE-tis) Inflammation of the vermiform appendix; usually requires surgical removal of the organ. **(Ch 16)**

Arrhythmia (ah-RITH-mee-ah) Variations from the normal rhythm of the heartbeat; often described as palpitations. **(Ch 11, 12, 13)**

Arthritis (ahr-THRYE-tis) Inflammation of a joint. **(Ch 6)**

Asthma (AZ-mah) A condition characterized by recurrent attacks of difficult breathing with wheezing due to spasmodic constriction of the bronchi; often caused by an allergy to antigens. **(Ch 15)**

Atherosclerosis (ath-er-oh-skleh-ROH-sis) A form of arteriosclerosis in which deposits of cholesterol and other fatty material form within the tunica intima of large and medium-sized arteries. **(Ch 11, 12, 13)**

Bacterial endocarditis (back-TEER-ee-al en-doh-kar-DYE-tis) Inflammation of the endocardium, particularly the heart valves and chordae tendineae, caused by any of a number of bacteria; characterized by the presence of vegetations on the surface of the endocardium. **(Ch 11, 12, 13)**

Basal cell carcinoma (BAY-sal SELL kar-sih-NOH-mah) Malignant tumor of the basal cell layer of the epidermis; most common form of skin cancer and usually grows slowly. **(Ch 5)**

Boil (BOYL) A localized and painful bacterial infection originating in a hair follicle or skin gland; furuncle. **(Ch 5)**

Botulism (BOTCH-yoo-lizm) A severe form of food poisoning due to a neurotoxin produced by *Clostridium botulinum*; toxin inhibits transmission of nerve impulse at neuromuscular junctions. **(Ch 7, 8)**

Breast cancer (BREST KAN-ser) Malignancy of the breast. **(Ch 19)**

Bronchitis (brong-KYE-tis) Inflammation of one or more bronchi; may be acute or chronic; characterized by restricted air movements. **(Ch 15)**

Bursitis (burr-SYE-tis) Inflammation of a bursa, most commonly in the shoulder, often caused by excessive use of the joint and accompanied by severe pain and limitation of motion. **(Ch 6)**

Cataract (KAT-ah-rakt) The lens of the eye or its capsule becomes opaque, resulting in blurry or dim vision. **(Ch 9)**

Cellulitis (sell-yoo-LYE-tis) Infection of connective tissue with severe inflammation of the dermis and subcutaneous layer of the skin. **(Ch 5)**

Cholecystitis (kohl-ee-sis-TYE-tis) Inflammation of the gallbladder; sometimes caused by obstruction of the cystic duct with gallstones. **(Ch 16)**

Cholelithiasis (kohl-ee-lith-EYE-ah-sis) Presence or formation of gallstones. **(Ch 16)**

Cirrhosis (sih-ROH-sis) Liver disease characterized by the loss of normal liver tissue that is replaced by fibrous bands of connective tissue. **(Ch 16)**

Concussion (kon-KUSH-un) Loss of consciousness as the result of a blow to the head; usually clears within 24 hours; no evidence of permanent structural damage to the brain tissue. **(Ch 8)**

Conductive hearing loss (konn-DUCK-tiv HEER-ing LOSS) Defective hearing caused by conditions that interfere with the transmission of sound from the outer ear to the inner ear. **(Ch 9)**

Congestive heart failure (kahn-JES-tiv HART FAIL-yer) Condition in which the heart's pumping ability is impaired and results in fluid accumulation in vessels and tissue spaces; various stages of difficult breathing occur as fluid accumulates in pulmonary vessels and lung tissue. **(Ch 15)**

Contact dermatitis (KAHN-takt der-mah-TYE-tis) A rash caused by direct contact between the skin and a substance to which the individual is sensitive; characterized by itching, swelling, blistering, oozing, and scaling; most common form is poison ivy. **(Ch 5, 14)**

Contusion (kon-TOO-shun) Bruising of brain tissue as a result of direct trauma to the head; neurologic problems persist longer than 24 hours. **(Ch 8)**

Coronary artery disease (KOR-oh-nair-ee ART-er-ee dih-ZEEZ) Degenerative changes in the coronary circulation, usually caused by the formation of fatty deposits in the walls of the coronary vessels; also called CAD. **(Ch 11, 12, 13)**

Cretinism (KREE-tin-izm) Arrested physical development and mental retardation caused by congenital hyposecretion of the thyroid gland in the child; if untreated, the child is permanently dwarfed, mentally retarded, and sterile. **(Ch 10)**

Crohn's disease (KRONZ dih-ZEEZ) Chronic, relapsing inflammation of the intestinal tract, usually the terminal ileum; genetic disorder that produces abdominal cramps and diarrhea with malabsorption of nutrients. **(Ch 16)**

Cryptorchidism (krip-TOR-kid-izm) Failure of one or both of the testes to descend into the scrotum; if both testes are involved and untreated, sterility results. **(Ch 19)**

Cushing's disease (KOOSH-ingz dih-ZEEZ) A group of symptoms produced by excess production of cortisol from the adrenal cortex; characterized by excessive deposition of fat in the scapular area and in the face, high blood pressure, and generalized weakness and loss of muscle mass due to excessive protein catabolism. **(Ch 10)**

Cystic fibrosis (SIS-tick fye-BROH-sis) Hereditary disorder associated with the accumulation of excessively thick and adhesive mucus, which obstructs bronchioles and restricts air movement. **(Ch 15)**

Cystitis (sis-TYE-tis) Inflammation of the urinary bladder; may be caused by an infection descending from the kidney or one ascending from the urethra. **(Ch 18)**

Diabetes insipidus (di-ah-BEE-teez in-SIP-ih-dus) A metabolic disorder due to a deficient quantity of antidiuretic hormone (ADH) resulting in a large quantity of dilute urine and accompanied by great thirst. **(Ch 10, 18)**

Diabetes mellitus (di-ah-BEE-teez mell-EYE-tus) Disorder caused by a deficiency of insulin from the beta cells of the pancreatic islets; characterized by a disturbance in the utilization of blood glucose and manifested by polyuria, polyphagia, and polydipsia. **(Ch 10, 16, 18)**

Dislocation (dis-loh-KAY-shun) Displacement of a bone from its joint with tearing of ligaments, tendons, and articular capsule; also called luxation. **(Ch 6)**

Disuse atrophy (dis-YOOS AT-troh-fee) Skeletal muscle deterioration with reduction in size and weakness due to bed rest, immobility (casting), or local nerve damage. **(Ch 7)**

Dwarfism (DWAR-fizm) Underdevelopment of the body, usually refers to the small body stature that occurs when there is insufficient growth hormone from the anterior pituitary gland during childhood; in this case the size of the limbs is proportional to body size and mental development may be normal. **(Ch 10)**

Dysphagia (dis-FAY-jee-ah) Difficulty in swallowing; condition ranges from mild discomfort to inability to control muscles needed for chewing and swallowing. **(Ch 16)**

Eczema (ECK-zeh-mah) An inflammatory skin disease with red, itching, vesicular lesions that may crust over; common allergic reaction, but may occur without any obvious cause. **(Ch 5)**

Emphysema (em-fih-SEE-mah) A lung disorder in which the terminal bronchioles become plugged with mucus; eventually there is a loss of elasticity in the lung tissue, which makes breathing, especially expiration, difficult. **(Ch 15)**

Encephalitis (en-sef-ah-LYE-tis) Inflammation of the brain; frequently caused by viruses. **(Ch 8)**

Endometriosis (en-doh-mee-tree-OH-sis) Condition in which an area of endometrial tissue grows outside the uterus; cause is unknown but thought to be due to retrograde menstruation or hormonal disturbances; symptoms vary. **(Ch 19)**

Fibrocystic disease (figh-broh-SIS-tick dih-ZEEZ) Condition characterized by the development of benign cysts in the breast; cysts may be fluid-filled sacs or solid growths containing connective tissue. **(Ch 19)**

Gastritis (gas-TRY-tis) Inflammation of the stomach lining; may be acute or chronic. **(Ch 16)**

Gastroesophageal reflux (gas-troh-ee-sahf-ah-JEE-al REE-fluks) Reflux of chyme from the stomach into the esophagus; irritation from the acid in the chyme may cause an inflammation of the esophagus. **(Ch 16)**

Genital herpes (JEN-ih-tal HER-peez) Highly contagious disease of the reproductive organs caused by the herpes simplex virus and transmitted by direct person-to-person contact; characterized by periods of dormancy and recurrent outbreaks; second most prevalent sexually transmitted disease in the United States. **(Ch 19)**

Gigantism (jye-GAN-tizm) Excessive size and stature; usually refers to the abnormal growth that occurs if there is hypersecretion of growth hormone in the child; body proportions are generally normal. **(Ch 10)**

Glaucoma (glaw-KOH-mah) Disease of the eye characterized by increased pressure within the eye, which causes pathologic changes in the optic disk. **(Ch 9)**

Glomerulonephritis (glo-mair-yoo-low-neh-FRY-tis) Inflammation of the capillary loops in the glomeruli of the kidney; usually secondary to an infection. **(Ch 18)**

Gonorrhea (gahn-oh-REE-ah) Highly contagious bacterial (*Neisseria gonorrhoeae*) infection of the genitourinary system; most prevalent sexually transmitted disease in the United States. **(Ch 19)**

Gout (GOWT) A form of acute arthritis in which uric acid crystals develop within a joint and irritate the cartilage, causing acute inflammation, swelling, and pain; most commonly occurs in middle-aged and older men. **(Ch 6)**

Guillain-Barré syndrome (gee-YAN bah-RAY SIN-drohm) A relatively rare disorder that affects the peripheral nervous system, particularly the spinal nerves; characterized by muscular weakness or flaccid paralysis, usually beginning in the lower extremities and progressing upward; respiratory manifestations are the result of respiratory muscle involvement. **(Ch 15)**

Gynecomastia (jin-eh-koh-MAS-tee-ah or gy-neh-koh-MAS-tee-ah) Excessive development of the mammary glands in the male as a result of hormonal disorders, especially the estrogen/testosterone ratio. **(Ch 19)**

Heart block (HART BLAHK) Condition resulting from damage to the conduction pathways in the heart and alters the normal rhythm; may be caused by mechanical distortion, ischemia, infection, or inflammation; also called conduction deficit. **(Ch 11, 12, 13)**

Heavy metal poisoning (HEH-vee MET-ahl POY-sun-ing) Irreversible demyelination of axons and damage to glial cells due to chronic exposure to heavy metal ions, such as arsenic, lead, or mercury. **(Ch 8)**

Hemophilia (hee-moh-FILL-ee-ah) A hereditary disorder characterized by a tendency to bleed and caused by a deficiency of certain clotting factors. **(Ch 11, 12, 13)**

Hemorrhage (HEM-ohr-ij) Escape of blood from a ruptured blood vessel; if severe, it may lead to hypovolemia and circulatory shock; in the brain, it may be epidural, subdural, or into the brain tissue; cerebral hemorrhage is one of the three main causes of strokes (cerebrovascular accidents). **(Ch 8, 11, 12, 13)**

Hepatitis (hep-ah-TYE-tis) Inflammation of the liver; may be caused by alcoholism, parasites, and viruses. **(Ch 16)**

Herniated intervertebral disk (HER-nee-ayt-ed in-ter-VER-tee-bruhl DISK) Protrusion of the inner region of an intervertebral disk through the outer fibrous ring of the disk; distorts the sensory nerves and may compress nerve roots, with resulting pain from the affected area; frequently occurs in the lumbar region. **(Ch 8)**

Herpes simplex (HER-peez SIM-plecks) Acute viral skin condition characterized by groups of vesicles on the skin, often around the margins of the lips and/or nose; cold sores or fever blisters. **(Ch 5)**

Herpes zoster (HER-peez ZAH-stir) Acute viral skin condition caused by the virus of chickenpox and characterized by vesicular eruptions along the pathway of a sensory nerve; also called shingles. **(Ch 5)**

Hiatal hernia (hi-A-tal HER-nee-ah) Protrusion of a structure, usually a portion of the stomach, through the opening in the diaphragm for the esophagus. **(Ch 16)**

Hirsutism (HER-soo-tizm) Abnormal hairiness, especially in women. **(Ch 5)**

Human immunodeficiency virus (HIV) disease (HYOO-man im-yoo-noh-dee-FISH-ehn-see VYE-rus dih-ZEEZ) An impairment of the immune system caused by a virus that destroys helper T cells; in time, the number of circulating antibodies declines and cellular immunity is reduced, leaving the body defenseless against numerous microbial invaders; the acquired immunodeficiency syndrome (AIDS) is late-stage HIV disease. **(Ch 14)**

Hydrocephalus (high-droh-SEF-ah-lus) Abnormal accumulation of cerebrospinal fluid within the ventricles of the cerebrum; in the child, this results in enlargement of the cranium. **(Ch 8)**

Hyperaldosteronism (high-per-al-DOS-ter-ohn-izm) Condition in which there is excessive secretion of aldosterone from the adrenal cortex causing sodium and fluid retention by the kidneys, accompanied by a loss of potassium. **(Ch 18)**

Hyperopia (high-per-OH-pee-ah) A visual defect in which light rays focus beyond the retina; farsightedness. **(Ch 9)**

Hyperparathyroidism (high-purr-pair-ah-THIGH-royd-izm) Abnormally increased activity of the parathyroid gland, which causes a generalized decalcification of bone (osteomalacia), increased blood calcium levels, and kidney stones. **(Ch 6)**

Hypoaldosteronism (high-poh-al-DOS-ter-ohn-izm) Condition in which there is reduced secretion of aldosterone from the adrenal cortex causing excessive sodium and fluid loss by the kidneys, accompanied by a retention of potassium. **(Ch 18)**

Hypogeusia (high-poh-GOO-zee-ah) Diminished sense of taste. **(Ch 9)**

Hypogonadism (high-poh-GO-nad-izm) Sterility and lack of secondary sexual characteristics due to lack of estrogens in the female and androgens in the male. **(Ch 10)**

Hypoparathyroidism (high-poh-pair-ah-THIGH-royd-izm) Abnormally decreased activity of the parathyroid gland, which leads to increased bone density, decreased blood calcium levels, neuromuscular excitability, and tetany. **(Ch 6)**

Hyposmia (high-PAHZ-mee-ah) Diminished sense of smell. **(Ch 9)**

Hypotension (high-poh-TEN-shun) Reduced blood pressure; consistent low blood pressure is usually no cause for concern, but sudden and/or extremely low pressures may be symptomatic and, along with other problems, interfere with blood flow to the kidneys resulting in impaired renal function. **(Ch 18)**

Hypovolemia (high-poh-voh-LEE-mee-ah) Abnormally decreased amount of circulating plasma in the body. **(Ch 11, 12, 13)**

Immunosuppression (im-yoo-noh-soo-PRESH-un) Inhibition of the formation of antibodies to antigens that may be present; suppression of the immune system. **(Ch 14)**

Impetigo (im-peh-TYE-go) Superficial skin infection caused by staphylococcal or streptococcal bacteria and characterized by vesicles, pustules, and crusted-over lesions; most common in children. **(Ch 5)**

Infarction (in-FARK-shun) A localized area of damage caused by interrupted blood supply, usually as the result of an occluded artery. **(Ch 11, 12, 13)**

Lactose intolerance (LACK-tose in-TAHL-er-ans) Inability to digest the sugar lactose, because of a deficiency of the intestinal enzyme lactase; symptoms include abdominal pain and diarrhea after drinking milk. **(Ch 16)**

Leukemia (loo-KEE-mee-ah) A chronic or acute progressive cancer of blood-forming tissues. **(Ch 11, 12, 13)**

Lymphadenopathy (lim-fad-eh-NAH-pah-thee) Disease of the lymph nodes. **(Ch 14)**

Lymphedema (lim-feh-DEE-mah) Swelling of tissues due to fluid accumulation resulting from obstruction of lymph vessels or disorders of the lymph nodes. **(Ch 14)**

Lymphoma (lim-FOH-mah) Malignant tumor of lymph nodes and lymph tissue. **(Ch 14)**

Malignant melanoma (mah-LIG-nant mel-ah-NOH-mah) Cancerous growth composed of melanocytes; often arises in preexisting mole; an alarming increase in the incidence of malignant melanoma is attributed to excessive exposure to sunlight. **(Ch 5)**

Meningitis (men-in-JYE-tis) Inflammation of the meninges; may be caused by anything that activates the inflammatory process, including bacteria, viruses, fungi, and chemical toxins. **(Ch 8)**

Multiple sclerosis (MULL-tih-pull sclair-OH-sis) Chronic, progressive demyelination of axons that produces muscular paralysis and sensory loss; may affect respiratory centers in the brain stem; recent evidence suggests the disease may be due to a defect in the immune system. **(Ch 7, 8, 14, 15)**

Muscular bruises (MUSS-kyoo-lar BROOZ-ehz) Muscle strain in which the muscle remains intact but there is mild bleeding into the surrounding tissue. **(Ch 7)**

Muscular dystrophy (MUSS-kyoo-lar DIS-troh-fee) An inherited, chronic, progressive wasting and weakening of muscles without involvement of the nervous system. **(Ch 7)**

Muscular tears (MUSS-kyoo-lar TAIRS) Severe muscle strain in which there is tearing of the fascia and bleeding; may require surgery and/or immobility to promote healing. **(Ch 7)**

Myasthenia gravis (mye-as-THEE-nee-ah GRAY-vis) An autoimmune disease characterized by skeletal muscle weakness due to a defect in nerve impulse conduction at the neuromuscular junction; severe forms may involve respiratory muscles, resulting in respiratory insufficiency. **(Ch 7, 15)**

Myopia (mye-OH-pee-ah) A visual defect in which light rays focus in front of the retina; nearsightedness. **(Ch 9)**

Myositis (mye-oh-SYE-tis) Inflammation of muscle tissue. **(Ch 7)**

Nephrolithiasis (nef-roh-lith-EYE-ah-sis) Condition marked by presence of renal calculi, or kidney stones; common cause of urinary tract obstruction in adults. **(Ch 18)**

Nephrotic syndrome (nef-RAH-tick SIN-drohm) Condition marked by excessive protein in the urine (3.5 g/day or more); characteristic of glomerular injury; accompanied by massive edema and reduced albumin in the blood. **(Ch 18)**

Nerve gas (NURV GAS) A toxic gas that interferes with normal nerve impulse conduction by blocking cholinesterase activity at the synapse, resulting in sustained skeletal muscle contraction; also affects smooth and cardiac muscle; used in warfare. **(Ch 8)**

Neurotoxins (new-row-TAHK-sins) Substances that are poisonous or destructive to nerve tissue; many affect acetylcholine activity at synapses and neuromuscular junctions resulting in paralysis. **(Ch 15)**

Nevus (NEE-vus) An elevated, pigmented lesion on the skin; commonly called a mole; a dysplastic nevus is a mole that does not form properly and may progress to a type of skin cancer; plural, nevi. **(Ch 5)**

Nystagmus (nihs-TAG-muss) Involuntary, rapid, rhythmic movements of the eyeball. **(Ch 9)**

Obstruction (ob-STRUCK-shun) Any blockage or clogging of the digestive tract; pyloric obstruction is a narrowing of the opening between the stomach and duodenum; intestinal obstruction interferes with the flow of chyme through the tract; causes include hernia, telescoping of one part of the intestine into another; twisting of the intestine, diverticulosis, tumors, and loss of peristaltic motor activity. **(Ch 16)**

Osteomalacia (ahs-tee-oh-mah-LAY-shee-ah) Softening of bone, occurring in the adult, because of inadequate amounts of calcium and phosphorus; bones bend easily and become deformed; in childhood this is called rickets. **(Ch 6)**

Osteomyelitis (ahs-tee-oh-my-eh-LYE-tis) Inflammation of the bone marrow caused by bacteria. **(Ch 6)**

Osteoporosis (ahs-tee-oh-por-OH-sis) Decrease in bone density and mass; commonly occurs in postmenopausal women as a result of increased osteoclast activity due to diminished estrogen; bones fracture easily. **(Ch 6)**

Osteosarcoma (ahs-tee-oh-sahr-KOH-mah) Malignant tumor derived from bone; also called osteogenic sarcoma; osteoblasts multiply without control and form large tumors in bone. **(Ch 6)**

Ovarian cancer (oh-VAIR-ee-an KAN-ser) Malignant tumor of the ovary, usually arising from epithelial cells; most dangerous reproductive cancer among women because it is seldom detected early. **(Ch 19)**

Pancreatitis (pan-kree-ah-TYE-tis) Inflammation of the pancreas due to autodigestion of pancreatic tissue by its own enzymes; associated with other conditions such as alcoholism, biliary tract obstruction, peptic ulcers, trauma, and certain drugs. **(Ch 16)**

Parageusia (par-ah-GOO-zee-ah) An abnormal or perverted sense of taste; also a bad taste in the mouth. **(Ch 9)**

Parkinson's disease (PAR-kin-sunz dih-ZEEZ) A slowly progressive disease, usually appearing after the age of 60, characterized by increased motor activity and caused by a lack of dopamine; symptoms include muscle tremors, rigidity, and difficulty in initiating movements and speech. **(Ch 8)**

Paronychia (pair-oh-NICK-ee-ah) Bacterial infection of the cuticle involving either fingers or toes. **(Ch 5)**

Parosmia (par-AHZ-mee-ah) An abnormal or perverted sense of smell. **(Ch 9)**

Patent foramen ovale (PAY-tent foh-RAY-men oh-VAL-ee) Congenital heart defect occurring when the opening between the right and left atria fails to close after birth, permitting mixing of blood between the right and left sides of the heart. **(Ch 11, 12, 13)**

Peptic ulcer (PEP-tick UL-ser) A deterioration of the mucous membrane lining of the esophagus, stomach, or duodenum caused by the action of the acid in gastric juice. **(Ch 16)**

Pernicious anemia (per-NISH-us ah-NEE-me-ah) A type of anemia caused by a lack of intrinsic factor from the gastric mucosa, which is necessary for the absorption of vitamin B$_{12}$; results in a deficiency of normal blood cells. **(Ch 16)**

Pleural effusion (PLOO-rahl eh-FEW-shun) Accumulation of fluid in the space between the parietal and visceral layers of the pleura, which threatens collapse of the lung; may be due to trauma, inflammatory processes, or cardiac dysfunction. **(Ch 15)**

Pneumoconiosis (new-moh-koh-nee-OH-sis) General term for lung disease that occurs after long-term inhalation of pollutants; characterized by chronic inflammation, infection, and bronchitis; includes coal miners' disease and asbestosis. **(Ch 15)**

Pneumonia (new-MOW-nee-ah) Inflammation of the lung usually caused by bacteria or viruses; inflammation and edema from the immune response cause the alveoli and terminal bronchioles to fill with exudate, which restricts ventilation and perfusion. **(Ch 15)**

Pneumothorax (new-mow-THOH-racks) Accumulation of air or gas in the space between the parietal and visceral layers of the pleura, resulting in collapse of the lung on the affected side; may be due to trauma or may occur spontaneously as a result of pulmonary disease. **(Ch 15)**

Polio (POH-lee-oh) Abbreviated term for poliomyelitis; an acute, contagious, viral disease that attacks the central nervous system where it damages or destroys nerve cells that control muscles and causes paralysis. **(Ch 7)**

Polycystic kidney (pah-lee-SIS-tick KID-nee) Hereditary disease in which there is massive enlargement of the kidney and accompanied by the formation of cysts, which interfere with kidney function; results in renal failure; renal dialysis and kidney transplant during end-stage renal failure may prolong life. **(Ch 18)**

Polycythemia (pahl-ee-sye-THEE-mee-ah) An increase in the mass of red blood cells (hematocrit) in the blood. **(Ch 11, 12, 13)**

Precocious puberty (pre-KOH-she-us PEW-burr-tee) Unusually early sexual maturation due to overproduction of estrogens in the female and androgens in the male. **(Ch 10)**

Presbyopia (prez-bih-OH-pee-ah) Impairment of vision due to aging characterized by decreased ability to accommodate for close vision due to diminished elasticity of the lens. **(Ch 9)**

Prostate cancer (PRAH-state KAN-ser) Malignant tumor of the prostate, usually originating in a secretory portion; early detection is important because metastasis soon involves the lymphatic system, bones, and lungs. **(Ch 19)**

Prostatic hypertrophy (prah-STAT-ick high-PER-troh-fee) Enlargement of the prostate gland, common in men older than age 50; because the prostate surrounds the urethra it may obstruct the flow of urine from the bladder. **(Ch 18, 19)**

Pulmonary embolism (PULL-moh-nair-ee EM-boh-lizm) Obstruction of a pulmonary artery or one of its branches by an embolus, usually a blood clot, which interrupts blood supply and interferes with gas exchange. **(Ch 15)**

Pulmonary hypertension (PULL-moh-nair-ee high-per-TEN-shun) excessive pressure in the pulmonary arteries resulting in respiratory and cardiac dysfunction. **(Ch 15)**

Respiratory distress syndrome (reh-SPY-rah-toh-ree dis-TRESS SIN-drohm) Condition resulting from abnormalities in the surfactant and causing the alveoli to collapse; often occurs in premature infants when surfactant production fails to reach normal levels. **(Ch 15)**

Rheumatic fever (roo-MAT-ik FEE-ver) A childhood (usually) disease associated with the presence of hemolytic streptococci bacteria in the body and characterized by fever and joint pain. **(Ch 6)**

Rheumatic heart disease (roo-MAT-ik HART dih-ZEEZ) A consistent clinical effect of rheumatic fever in which, over a period of time, the heart valves become thickened and often calcified, seriously affecting cardiac function. **(Ch 11, 12, 13)**

Rheumatoid arthritis (ROO-mah-toyd ahr-THRYE-tis) A chronic systemic disease with changes occurring in the connective tissues of the body; also known as collagen disease; evidence indicates it may be an autoimmune disease in which the body abnormally produces antibodies against its own cells and proteins. **(Ch 14)**

Rickets (RICK-ehts) Softening of bone, occurring in childhood, because of inadequate amounts of calcium and phosphorus; bones bend easily and become deformed. **(Ch 6)**

Ringworm (RING-wurm) Superficial fungal infection of the skin; also called tinea infections; tinea capitis is ringworm of the scalp; tinea pedis is athlete's foot; tinea cruris is jock itch. **(Ch 5)**

Sensorineural hearing loss (sen-soh-ree-NEW-rahl HEER-ing LOSS) Defective hearing caused by impairment of the organ of Corti or in its nerve connections. **(Ch 9)**

Septal defects (SEP-tull DEE-fekts) Openings in the atrial, ventricular, and/or atrioventricular septa of the heart, causing disturbances in blood flow patterns through the heart and pulmonary circulation. **(Ch 11, 12, 13)**

Spina bifida (SPY-nah BIFF-ih-dah) A developmental anomaly in which the vertebral laminae do not close around the spinal cord, leaving an opening through which the cord and meninges may or may not protrude. **(Ch 8)**

Spinal cord injuries (SPY-nuhl KORD IN-juhr-ees) Depending on severity, trauma to the spinal cord results in temporary or permanent disruption of cord-mediated functions, including motor impulses to skeletal muscles, with subsequent loss of muscle function; extent of muscle paralysis depends on location of trauma. **(Ch 7)**

Splenomegaly (spleh-noh-MEG-ah-lee) Enlargement of the spleen. **(Ch 14)**

Sprain (SPRAYN) Twisting of a joint with pain, swelling, and injury to ligaments, tendons, muscles, blood vessels, and nerves; most often occurs in the ankle; more serious than a strain, which is the overstretching of the muscles associated with a joint. **(Ch 6)**

Squamous cell carcinoma (SKWAY-mus SELL kar-sih-NOH-mah) Tumor of the epidermis in regions of the skin exposed to the sun; may become invasive and malignant. **(Ch 5)**

Strabismus (strah-BIHZ-muss) Deviation of one eye from the other when looking at an object; caused by weakened or hypertonic muscle in one of the eyes. **(Ch 9)**

Strain (STRAYN) Overstretching or overexertion of a muscle; less serious than a sprain. **(Ch 6)**

Stroke syndrome (STROHK SIN-drohm) A complex of symptoms caused by disrupted blood supply to the brain due to thrombosis, embolism, or hemorrhage; symptoms depend on region of the brain affected, but frequently involve disturbed muscular function including paralysis; also called cerebrovascular accident (CVA). **(Ch 7, 8)**

Subluxation (sub-luck-SAY-shun) Incomplete or partial dislocation. **(Ch 6)**

Syphilis (SIFF-ih-lis) Contagious sexually transmitted disease caused by the spirochete *Treponema pallidum*; it leads to many structural and cutaneous lesions; if untreated, it may lead to serious cardiovascular and neurologic disturbances years after infection and may be spread to the fetus during pregnancy. **(Ch 19)**

Systemic lupus erythematosus (SLE) (sih-STEM-ik LOO-pus air-ith-eh-mah-TOE-sis) An autoimmune connective tissue disease in which the body attacks its own cells and proteins; characterized by injury to the skin, joints, kidneys, and mucous membranes. **(Ch 14)**

Tendinitis (ten-dih-NYE-tis) Inflammation of tendons and tendon-muscle attachments, frequently associated with calcium deposits; common cause of acute shoulder pain. **(Ch 6)**

Testicular cancer (tess-TICK-yoo-lar KAN-ser) Malignant tumor of the testes, usually arising from the germ cells; relatively rare and usually curable if treated early in tumor development. **(Ch 19)**

Tetanus (TET-ah-nus) A highly fatal disease caused by the toxin from *Clostridium tetani* bacteria; the toxin attacks the central nervous system and is characterized by muscle spasms and convulsions. **(Ch 8)**

Tetralogy of Fallot (the-TRAL-oh-jee of fah-LOH) A complex group of congenital heart defects that combines four structural anomalies: the pulmonary trunk is abnormally narrow, obstructing blood flow to the lungs; the interventricular septum is incomplete; the aortic opening overrides the interventricular septum and receives blood from both ventricles; enlargement of the right ventricle. **(Ch 11, 12, 13)**

Thrombus (THROM-buss) An abnormal clot within blood vessels that is stationary or adheres to the vessel wall; a floating clot is an embolus. **(Ch 11, 12, 13)**

Tonsillitis (tahn-sih-LYE-tis) Inflammation and enlargement of the tonsils, especially the palatine tonsils. **(Ch 14)**

Tuberculosis (too-ber-kyoo-LOH-sis) An infectious, inflammatory disease, usually in the lungs, that results in the formation of an exudate that restricts diffusion; original lesion may become dormant, then reactivate at a later time; may spread to other parts of the body and may become chronic. **(Ch 15)**

Urethritis (yoo-reth-RYE-tis) Inflammation of the urethra, usually caused by infectious organisms; urethra may swell and impede the flow of urine. **(Ch 18)**

Urticaria (er-tih-KAY-ree-ah) Vascular skin eruption characterized by redness and severe itching; most commonly associated with hypersensitivity reactions to drugs, certain foods, or physical agents; also called hives. **(Ch 5)**

Uterine cancer (YOO-ter-in KAN-ser) Malignant tumor of the uterus, usually a carcinoma that arises from the basal cells of the epithelial lining; may be detected by dysplasia of the epithelial cells in a Papanicolaou (Pap) smear; progresses to carcinoma in situ and finally to an invasive malignant carcinoma. **(Ch 19)**

Varicose veins (VAIR-ih-kohs VAINS) Swollen, distended, and knotted veins, usually in the subcutaneous tissues of the leg resulting from sluggish flow of blood; varicosities in the veins of the anus are called hemorrhoids. **(Ch 11, 12, 13)**

Glossary of Word Parts

WORD PART	MEANING
-a	lack of
a-	without, lacking
acetabul-	little cup
act-	motion
ad-	toward
aden-	gland
adip-	fat
af-	toward
agglutin-	sticking together
-agon	gather together
al-	pertaining to
albin-	white
-algia	pain
alkal-	basic
alveol-	tiny cavity
amnio-	a fetal membrane
amyl-	starch
ana-	up
ana-	apart
andr-	male, maleness
angi-	vessel
anthrac-	coal
anti-	against
aort-	lift up
appendicul-	little attachment
arter-	artery
arthr-	joint
artic-	joint
-ary	pertaining to
-ase	enzyme
astro-	star
ather-	yellow fatty plaque
-atresia	without an opening
atri-	entrance room
audi-	to hear
balan-	glans
bi-	two
bili-	bile, gall

WORD PART	MEANING
-blast	to form, sprout
-bol-	throw, put
brachi-	arm
brady-	slow
bronchi-	bronchi
burs-	pouch
caly-	small cup
carb/o-	charcoal, coal, carbon
cardi-	heart
carotid-	put to sleep
cata-	down
-cente	to puncture surgically
cephal-	head
cer-	wax
chole-	gall, bile
-chrom-	color, pigment
chrondr-	cartilage
-clast-	to break
cleav-	to divide
coagul-	clotting
conch-	snail
colpo-	vagina
-coni-	dust
-continence	to hold
corac-	beak
corpor-	body
cortic-	outer region, cortex
cribr-	sieve
cric-	ring
crin-	to secrete
crist-	crest, ridge
crypt-	hidden
cusp-	point
cutane-	skin
cyesi-	pregnancy
cyst-	bladder
cyt-	cell

WORD PART	MEANING
delt-	triangle
dendr-	tree
dent-	tooth
derm-	skin
di-	two
dia-	through
diastol-	expand, separate
dips-	thirst
dors-	back
duct-	movement
dys-	difficult
-ectasis	dilation
-ectomy	surgical removal
edem-	to swell
ef-	away from
ejacul-	to shoot forth
-elle	little, small
embol-	stopper, wedge
-emesis	vomit
-emia	blood condition
encephal-	within the head, brain
end-	within, inner
enter-	intestine
epi-	upon, above
erg-	work, energy
erythr-	red
esthes-	feeling
ethm-	sieve
-etic	pertaining to
eu-	good
ex-	out of, away from
extra-	outside, beyond
-fer-	to carry
fibr-	fiber
-fic-	make
fimb-	fringe
flex-	bend
follic-	small bag

445

WORD PART	MEANING
fove-	pit
galacto-	referring to milk
gangli-	knot
gastr-	stomach
-gen-	to produce
-genesis	to form, produce
-gest-	to carry, pregnancy
gingiv-	gums
glia-	glue
glob-	globe
gloss-	tongue
gravid-	filled, pregnant
gust-	taste
gynec-	female
hem-	blood
hepat-	liver
hex-	six
hidr-	sweat
hist-	tissue
homeo-	alike, same
hydro-	water
hyper-	excessive, above
hypo-	beneath, below
hyster-	womb or uterus
-ic-	pertaining to
ichthy-	scaly, dry
-ide	pertaining to
immun-	protection
-in	neutral substance
integ-	a covering
intra-	within, inside
irid-	iris
isch-	deficiency
-ism	process of
iso-	equal, same, alike
-itis	inflammation
juxta-	near to
kary-	nucleus
kerat-	hard, horny tissue
kerat-	cornea
kyph-	hump
labi-	lip
lacr-	tears
lact-	milk

WORD PART	MEANING
lemm-	peel, rind
leuk-	white
lingu-	tongue
lip/o-	fat
lith-	stone
-logy	study of, science of
-lucid-	clear, light
lun-	moon shaped
lute-	yellow
lymph-	lymph
-lys	to take apart, destroy
macro-	large
macul-	spot
mal-	bad, poor
mamm-	breast
masset-	chew
meat-	passage
meg-	large
melan-	black
mening-	membrane
meno-	month
metabol-	change
metr-	uterus
metr-	measure
mict-	to pass
mono-	one
morpho-	shape, form
morul-	mulberry
multi-	many
myo-, mys-	muscle
nat-	birth
neo-	new
neph-	kidney
neur-	nerve
noct-	night
nutri-	to nourish
ocul-	eye
odont-	tooth
-oid	like, resembling
olfact-	smell
-oma	tumor, swelling, mass
onychi-	nail
oo-	egg, ovum
oophor-	ovary

WORD PART	MEANING
op-	eye
ophthalm-	eye
orch-	testicle
-orexia	appetite
-ose	sugar
-osis	condition of
oste-, oss-	bone
ot-	ear
oxy-	oxygen
oxy-	rapid, sharp, sour
pachy-	thick
para-	to bear
para-	beside
partur-	bring forth, give birth
path-	disease
pelv-	basin
-penia	deficiency, lack of
pent-	five
peri-	all around
-pexy	fixation
-phag-	to eat, devour
pharyng-	throat
phas-	speech
-phil	love, affinity for
phleb-	vein
-phob-	hate, dislike
phon-	voice
phragm-	fence, partition
-phraxis	to obstruct
physi-	nature, function
pin-	pine cone
pino-	to drink
-plasm-	matter
-plasty	surgical repair
pleg-	paralysis
plex-	interweave, network
-pnea	breathing
pneum-	lung, air
-poie-	making, forming
poly-	many
prandi-	meal
presby-	old
proct-	rectum, anus

WORD PART	MEANING	WORD PART	MEANING	WORD PART	MEANING
prostat-	prostate	-spadias	an opening	-tom-	to cut
proxim-	nearest	sphen-	wedge	ton-	tone, tension
pseudo-	false	sphygm-	pulse	tox-	poison
-ptysis	spitting	spir-	breath	tri-	three
pulmon-	lung	splen-	spleen	-tripsy	crushing
pyel-	renal pelvis	squam-	flattened, scale	trop-	to change, influence
pyr-	fever, fire	-sta-	to control, staying	troph-	nourish, develop
ren-	kidney			tympan-	drum
-reti-	network, lattice	-stasis	control	-ul-, -ule	small, tiny
rhin-	nose	sten-	narrowing	-um	presence of
rhytido-	wrinkles	ster-	steroid	umbil-	navel
-rrhage	burst forth, flow	strat-	layer	-ur-	urine
-rrhaphy	suture	sud-	sweat	-uria	urine condition
-rrhea	flow or discharge	sulc-	furrow, ditch	valvu-	valve
		syn-	together	vas-	vessel
sacchar-	sugar, sweet	systol-	contraction	ventilat-	to fan or blow
salping-	tube	tachy-	fast, rapid	verm-	worm
sarco-	flesh, muscle	test-	eggshells, eggs	viscer-	internal organs
scler-	hard	tetan-	stiff	vita-	life
seb-	oil	therm-	temperature	vitre-	glass
sen-	old	thromb-	clot	-y	process, condition
sial-	saliva	thym-	thymus		
skelet-	a dried, hard body	thyr-	shield	zyg-	paired together, union
		-tion	act or process of		
-som-	body	-toc-	birth		

General Glossary

Abdomen (ab-DOH-men or AB-doh-men) Portion of the trunk below the diaphragm; between the thorax and pelvis

Abdominal cavity (ab-DAHM-ih-nal KAV-ih-tee) Superior portion of the abdominopelvic cavity; contains the stomach, spleen, liver, pancreas, gallbladder, small intestine, and most of the large intestine

Abdominopelvic cavity (ab-dahm-ih-no-PEL-vik KAV-ih-tee) Inferior part of the ventral body cavity; subdivided into the abdominal cavity and pelvic cavity

Abducens nerve (ab-DOO-sens NERV) Cranial nerve VI; motor nerve; responsible for eye movements

Abduction (ab-DUCK-shun) Movement away from the midline or axis of the body; opposite of adduction

Absolute refractory period (AB-soh-loot ree-FRACK-toar-ee PEE-ree-od) Time during which an excitable cell cannot respond to a second stimulus regardless of the strength of the second stimulus

Absorption (ab-SOARP-shun) The passage of digestive end products from the gastrointestinal tract into the blood or lymph

Accessory nerve (ak-SES-oar-ee NERV) Cranial nerve XI; motor nerve; responsible for contraction of the trapezius and sternocleidomastoid muscles

Accommodation (ah-kahm-o-DAY-shun) Mechanism that allows the eye to focus at various distances, primarily achieved through changing the curvature of the lens

Acetabulum (as-sah-TAB-yoo-lum) Large depression in the hip bone for articulation with the femur

Acetyl CoA (as-SEE-til CO-A) A molecule formed from pyruvic acid in the mitochondria when oxygen is present

Acetylcholine (ah-see-till-KOH-leen) A chemical substance that is released at the axon terminals of many neurons to carry the impulse across a synaptic cleft; one of the neurotransmitters

Acetylcholinesterase (ah-see-till-koh-lin-ES-ter-ase) An enzyme that causes the decomposition of acetylcholine; also called cholinesterase

Acid (AS-id) A substance that ionizes in water to release hydrogen ions; a proton donor; a substance with a pH less than 7.0

Acidosis (AS-id-oh-sis) Condition in which the blood has a lower pH than normal

Acinar (AS-ih-nur) Shaped like a small sac

Acinar cells (AS-ih-nar SELZ) Cells in the pancreas that secrete digestive enzymes

Acromion (ah-KRO-mee-on) A process on the scapula that forms the tip of the shoulder

Acrosome (AK-roh-sohm) Structure on the head of a sperm that contains enzymes neccessary to break down the coverings around an ovum to facilitate fertilization

Actin (AK-tin) Contractile protein in the thin filaments of skeletal muscle cells

Action potential (AK-shun po-TEN-shall) A nerve impulse; a rapid change in membrane potential that involves depolarization and repolarization

Active immunity (AK-tiv ih-MYOO-nih-tee) Immunity that is produced as the result of an encounter with an antigen, with subsequent production of memory cells

Active transport (AK-tive TRANS-port) Membrane transport process that requires cellular energy (ATP)

Addison's disease (ADD-ih-sons dys-EEZ) Condition caused by hyposecretion of glucocorticoids from the adrenal cortex

Adduction (ad-DUCK-shun) Movement toward the midline or axis of the body; opposite of abduction

Adenohypophysis (add-eh-noe-hye-PAH-fih-sis) Anterior portion of the pituitary gland

Adenoids (AD-eh-noyds) Paired masses of lymphoid tissue in the nasopharynx; pharyngeal tonsils

Adenosine diphosphate (ADP) (ah-DEN-oh-sin di-FOS-fate) A molecule that is formed when the terminal phosphate group is removed from adenosine triphosphate

Adenosine triphosphate (ATP) (ah-DEN-oh-sin try-FOS-fate) Compound that stores chemical energy within the cell and provides energy for use by body cells

Adipose (ADD-ih-pose) Fat tissue

Adolescence (add-oh-LESS-ens) Period from puberty until adulthood

Adrenal cortex (ah-DREE-null KOR-teks) Outer portion of the adrenal gland that secretes hormones called corticoids

Adrenal gland (ah-DREE-null GLAND) Endocrine gland that is located on the superior pole of each kidney; divided into cortex and medulla regions; also called suprarenal gland

Adrenal medulla (ah-DREE-null meh-DOO-lah) Inner portion of the adrenal gland; secretes epinephrine and norepinephrine

Adrenaline (ah-DREN-ah-lihn) Neurotransmitter released by some neurons in the sympathetic nervous system; also called epinephrine

Adrenergic fiber (add-rih-NER-jik FYE-ber) A nerve fiber that releases epinephrine (adrenaline) or norepinephrine (noradrenaline) at a synapse

Adrenocorticotropic hormone (ACTH) (ah-dree-noh-kor-tih-koh-TROH-pik HOAR-moan) A hormone secreted by the anterior pituitary gland that stimulates the cortex of the adrenal gland

Adulthood (ah-DULT-hood) Period from the end of adolescence to old age

Aerobic (air-OH-bik) Requiring molecular oxygen

Aerobic respiration (air-ROE-bik res-pih-RAY-shun) Catabolic process in cells that requires oxygen

Afferent nervous system (AF-fur-ent NER-vus SIS-tem) The portion of the peripheral nervous system that consists of all the incoming sensory nerves

Afferent neuron (AF-fur-ent NOO-ron) Nerve cell that carries impulses toward the central nervous system from the periphery; sensory neuron

Agglutination (ah-GLOO-tih-nay-shun) Clumping of red blood cells or microorganisms; typically an antigen–antibody reaction

Agglutinin (ah-GLOO-tih-nin) A specific substance in plasma that is capable of causing a clumping of red blood cells; an antibody

Agglutinogen (ah-gloo-TIN-oh-jen) A genetically determined antigen on the cell membrane of a red blood cell that determines blood types

Agranulocyte (a-GRAN-yoo-loh-syte) A white blood cell that lacks granules in the cytoplasm

Albinism (AL-bih-nizm) Lack of pigment in the skin, hair, and eyes

Albumin (al-BYOO-min) The most abundant plasma protein, which is primarily responsible for regulating the osmotic pressure of the blood

Aldosterone (al-DAHS-ter-own) Primary mineralocorticoid secreted by the adrenal cortex; helps maintain sodium homeostasis by promoting the reabsorption of sodium in the renal tubules

Alimentary canal (al-ih-MEN-tah-ree kah-NAL) Long, continuous tube that extends from the mouth to the anus; the digestive tract or gastrointestinal tract

Alkaline (AL-kuh-lihn) Pertaining to a base; having a pH greater than 7.0

Alkalosis (AL-kah-lo-sis) Condition in which the blood has a higher pH than normal

Allantois (ah-LAN-toys) Small extraembryonic membrane that develops between the amnion and chorion and contributes to the formation of the urinary bladder; degenerates and becomes part of the umbilical cord during the second month

Alpha cell (AL-fah sell) Type of cell that produces glucagon in the pancreatic islets

Alveolar processes (al-VEE-oh-lar PRAH-sess-es) Bony sockets for the teeth

Alveolus (al-VEE-oh-lus) Small sac-shaped structure; most often used to denote the microscopic dilations of terminal bronchioles in the lungs where diffusion of gases occurs; air sacs in the lungs

Amino acid (ah-MEEN-oh AS-id) The structural unit of a protein molecule; an organic compound that contains an amino group ($-NH_2$) and a carboxyl group ($-COOH$)

Amnion (AM-nee-on) The innermost fetal membrane; transparent sac that holds the developing fetus suspended in fluid

Amniotic cavity (am-nee-AH-tik KAV-ih-tee) Fluid-filled cavity within the amnion

Amniotic fluid (am-nee-AH-tik FLOO-id) Fluid surrounding the fetus within the amnion

Amphiarthrosis (am-fee-ahr-THROH-sis) A slightly movable joint; plural, amphiarthroses

Amylase (AM-ih-lays) An enzyme that breaks down starches into disaccharides

Anabolism (ah-NAB-oh-lizm) Building up, or synthesis, reactions that require energy and make complex molecules out of two or more smaller ones; opposite of catabolism

Anaerobic (an-air-OH-bik) Not requiring molecular oxygen

Anaerobic respiration (an-air-ROE-bik res-pih-RAY-shun) Catabolic process in cells that does not require oxygen

Anaphase (AN-ah-faze) Third stage of mitosis; stage in which spindle fibers shorten and duplicate chromosomes move to opposite ends of the cell

Anatomical position (an-ah-TOM-ih-kull poh-ZIH-shun) Standard reference position for the body; body is erect, facing the observer, upper extremities are at the sides; palms and toes are directed forward

Anatomy (ah-NAT-o-mee) Study of body structure and the relationships of its parts

Androgens (AN-droh-jenz) Male sex hormones; primary androgen is testosterone; produced by the interstitial cells of the testes and a small amount by the adrenal cortex

Anemia (ah-NEE-mee-ah) Condition of the blood in which the number of red blood cells or their hemoglobin content is below normal

Angiotensin (an-jee-oh-TEN-sin) A substance formed in the blood that helps regulate blood pressure; a vasoconstrictor

Anion (AN-eye-on) A negatively charged ion

Anisotropic (an-eye-soh-TROH-pik) Dark bands in skeletal and cardiac muscle fibers, do not allow light to pass through

Antagonist (an-TAG-oh-nist) A muscle that has an action opposite to the prime mover

Antebrachial region (an-te-BRAY-kee-al REE-jun) Region between the elbow and the wrist; forearm; cubital region

Antecubital (an-te-KYOO-bih-tal) Space in front of the elbow

Anterior (an-TEER-ee-or) Toward the front or ventral; opposite of posterior or dorsal

Antibody (AN-tih-bahd-ee) Substance produced by the body that inactivates or destroys another substance that is introduced into the body; immunoglobulin

Antibody-mediated immunity (AN-tih-bahd-ee MEE-dee-ate-ed ih-MYOO-nih-tee) Immunity that is the result of B-cell action and the production of antibodies; also called humoral immunity

Anticoagulant (an-tih-koh-AG-yoo-lant) A substance that delays, suppresses, or prevents the clotting of blood

Anticodon (an-tih-KO-don) A sequence of three nucleotide bases on transfer RNA that is complementary to a codon on messenger RNA; represents a single amino acid

Antidiuretic hormone (ADH) (an-tih-dye-yoo-RET-ik HOAR-moan) Hormone produced by the hypothalamus and secreted from the posterior pituitary gland that promotes water reabsorption from the kidney tubules

Antigen (AN-tih-jen) A substance that triggers an immune response when it is introduced into the body

Antiserum (AN-tih-see-rum) A preparation that contains antibodies from a source other than the recipient and that provides short-term protection against a specific antigen

Aorta (ay-OR-ta) The main systemic vessel that emerges from the left ventricle and carries blood to systemic arteries

Aortic semilunar valve (ay-OR-tik seh-mee-LOO-nar VALVE) The valve between the left ventricle and the aorta that keeps blood from flowing back into the ventricle

Apical foramen (A-pik-al foh-RAY-men) Opening in the root of a tooth where nerves and blood vessels enter the root canal

Apneustic center (ap-NOO-stick SEN-ter) A group of neurons in the pons that affects the rate of respiration by stimulating inspiration

Apocrine gland (AP-oh-krin GLAND) Gland in which the secretory product accumulates in the apex of the cells; then that portion pinches off and is discharged with the secretion

Aponeurosis (ah-pah-noo-ROE-sis) Broad, flat sheet of connective tissue that connects one muscle to another or a muscle to bone

Appendicular (ap-pen-DIK-yoo-lar) Pertaining to the upper and lower extremities, or arms and legs

Appendicular skeleton (ap-pen-DIK-yoo-lar SKEL-eh-ton) Bones of the upper and lower extremities of the body

Appositional growth (ap-poh-ZISH-un-al GROWTH) Growth due to material deposited on the surface, such as the growth in diameter of long bones

Aqueous humor (AY-kwee-us HYOO-mer) Fluid that fills the anterior cavity of the eye, in front of the lens

Arachnoid (ah-RAK-noyd) The middle layer of the coverings around the brain and spinal cord

Arachnoid granulations (ah-RACK-noyd gran-yoo-LAY-shuns) Small projections of arachnoid that protrude into the superior sagittal sinus and function in returning cerebrospinal fluid into the blood; also called arachnoid villi

Arachnoid villi (ah-RACK-noyd VILL-eye) Small projections of arachnoid that protrude into the superior sagittal sinus and function in returning cerebrospinal fluid into the blood; also called arachnoid granulations

Arbor vitae (AR-bor VYE-tay) Arrangement of the internal white matter of the cerebellum

Areola (ah-REE-oh-lah) Circular pigmented area that surrounds the nipple

Areolar (ah-REE-oh-lar) Type of connective tissue that contains fibers and a variety of cells in a soft, loose, matrix; loose connective tissue

Arteriole (ar-TEER-ee-ohl) A small branch of an artery that delivers blood to a capillary

Arteriovenous anastomosis (ar-teer-ee-oh-VAY-nus ah-NAS-toh-moh-sis) Direct connection between a small arteriole and a small venule without the intervening capillary

Artery (AR-ter-ee) A blood vessel that carries blood away from the heart

Articular cartilage (ahr-TIK-yoo-lar KAR-tih-layj) Thin layer of hyaline cartilage that covers the ends of long bones

Articulation (are-TIK-yoo-lay-shun) A joint; a point of contact between bones

Artificial immunity (art-ih-FISH-al ih-MYOO-nih-tee) Immunity that requires some deliberate action, such as a vaccination, to achieve exposure to the potentially harmful antigen

Ascending tract (ah-SEND-ing TRACT) Spinal cord nerve tract that conducts sensory impulses up to the brain

Association neuron (ah-soh-see-AY-shun NOO-ron) Nerve cell, totally within the central nervous system, that carries impulses from a sensory neuron to a motor neuron; also called an interneuron

Astrocyte (AS-troh-syte) A star-shaped neuroglial cell that supports neurons in the brain and spinal cord

Atom (AT-tum) The smallest unit of a chemical element that retains the properties of that element

Atomic number (ah-TOM-ik NUM-ber) The number of protons in the nucleus of an atom

Atrioventricular bundle (ay-tree-oh-ven-TRIK-yoo-lar BUN-dul) Portion of the conduction system of the heart that begins at the atrioventricular node and continues for a short way down the interventricular septum, then divides into the right and left bundle branches; involved in coordination of heart muscle contraction; also called the bundle of His

Atrioventricular node (ay-tree-oh-ven-TRIK-yoo-lar NODE) Mass of specialized cardiac muscle cells that form a part of the conduction system of the heart and that are located in the right atrium near the opening for the coronary sinus

Atrioventricular valve (ay-tree-oh-ven-TRIK-yoo-lar VALVE) Valve between an atrium and a ventricle in the heart

Atrium (A-tree-um) Thin-walled chamber of the heart that receives blood from veins

Auditory tube (AW-dih-toar-ee TOOB) Passageway between the throat and middle ear that functions to equalize pressure between the middle ear and the exterior; also called the eustachian tube

Auditory ossicles (AW-dih-toar-ee OS-sih-kulls) Three tiny bones in the middle ear that function to amplify sound waves: malleus, incus, stapes

Auerbach's plexus (OUR-bahks PLEK-sus) A network of autonomic nerves between the circular and longitudinal muscle layers of the gastrointestinal tract; also called myenteric plexus

Auricle (AW-rih-kull) Visible portion of the external ear; also called the pinna; also used to denote earlike projections of the atria of the heart

Autoimmune disease (aw-toh-im-YOON dih-ZEEZ) Tissue destruction that results when an individual produces antibodies that attack his or her own tissues

Autonomic ganglion (aw-toe-NOM-ic GANG-lee-on) A cluster of cell bodies of neurons from the autonomic nervous system that are outside the central nervous system; the region of synapse between the two neurons in an autonomic pathway

Autonomic nervous system (aw-toe-NOM-ic NER-vus SIS-tem) The portion of the peripheral efferent nervous system consisting of motor neurons that control involuntary actions

Avascular (ay-VAS-kyoo-lar) Without blood vessels

Axial (AK-see-al) Pertaining to the head, neck, and trunk

Axial skeleton (ACK-see-al SKEL-eh-ton) Bones of the head, neck, and torso

Axillary (AK-sih-lair-ee) Pertaining to the armpit region

Axon (AKS-on) The single efferent process of a neuron that carries impulses away from the cell body

Axon collateral (AKS-on koh-LAT-er-al) One or more side branches of an axon

B lymphocytes (B LIM-foh-sytes) A cell of the immune system that develops into a plasma cell and produces antibodies; B cell

Basal ganglia (BAY-sal GANG-lee-ah) Paired regions of gray matter located within the white matter of the cerebrum

Basal metabolic rate (BAY-sal met-ah-BAHL-ik RAYT) Amount of energy that is necessary to maintain life and keep the body functioning at a minimal level

Base (BASE) A substance that ionizes in water to release hydroxyl (OH^-) ions or other ions that combine with hydrogen ions; a proton acceptor; a substance with a pH greater than 7.0; alkaline

Basilar membrane (BAYS-ih-lar MEM-brayn) Floor of the cochlear duct; separates cochlear duct from scala tympani

Basophil (BAY-soh-fill) A white blood cell with granules in the cytoplasm that stain readily with basic dyes

Beta cell (BAY-tah SELL) Type of cell that produces insulin in the pancreatic islets

Beta oxidation (BAY-tah ox-ih-DAY-shun) Catabolic reaction in which a 2-carbon segment is removed from a fatty acid and is converted to acetyl-CoA

Bicuspid valve (bye-KUS-pid VALVE) Valve between the left atrium and left ventricle; also called the mitral valve

Bile (BYLE) Yellowish green fluid that is produced by the liver, stored in the gallbladder, and functions to emulsify fats

Bilirubin (bill-ih-ROO-bin) A pigment that is produced in the breakdown of hemoglobin and excreted in bile

Blastocele (BLAS-toh-seel) Cavity within a blastocyst

Blastocyst (BLAS-toh-syst) Hollow sphere of cells that forms when a cavity develops in a morula; usually present by the fifth day after conception

Blastomeres (BLAS-toh-meerz) Cells formed by early mitotic divisions of a zygote

Blood pressure (BLUHD PRESH-ur) Pressure exerted by the blood against the vessel walls; usually refers to arterial blood pressure

Bony labyrinth (BOH-nee LAB-ih-rinth) A series of interconnecting chambers in the petrous portion of the temporal bone that includes the cochlea, vestibule, and semicircular canals of the inner ear

Bowman's capsule (BOE-mans KAP-sool) Double-layered epithelial cup that surrounds the glomerulus in a nephron; also called glomerular capsule

Brachial (BRAY-kee-al) Pertaining to the arm; proximal portion of the upper limb

Brain stem (BRAYN STEM) The portion of the brain, between the diencephalon and spinal cord, that contains the midbrain, pons, and medulla oblongata

Broad ligament (BRAWD LIG-ah-ment) Largest peritoneal ligament that supports the uterus; double fold of peritoneum that extends laterally from the uterus to the pelvic wall

Bronchial tree (BRONG-kee-al TREE) The bronchi and all their branches that function as passageways between the trachea and the alveoli

Bronchopulmonary segment (brong-koh-PUL-moh-nair-ee SEG-ment) Portion of a lung surrounding a tertiary, or segmental, bronchus; lobule of the lung

Brunner's glands (BROO-nerz GLANDS) Mucous glands in the submucosa of the duodenum; also called duodenal glands

Buccal (BUK-al) Pertaining to the region of the mouth and cheek

Buffer (BUFF-fur) A substance that prevents, or reduces, changes in pH when either an acid or a base is added

Bulbourethral glands (bul-boh-yoo-REE-thral GLANDS) Small accessory glands near the base of the penis in the male; also called Cowper's glands

Bundle branches (BUN-dul BRAN-chez) Specialized cardiac muscle cells that form a part of the conduction system of the heart, are located on either side of the interventricular septum, and carry impulses from the atrioventricular node to the conduction myofibers

Bursae (BUR-see) Fluid-filled sacs that act as cushions at friction points in certain freely movable joints; singular, bursa (BUR-sah)

Calcaneus (kal-KAY-nee-us) Heel bone, one of the tarsal bones

Calcitonin (kal-sih-TOH-nin) A hormone produced by the thyroid gland that reduces calcium levels in the blood

Calorie (c) (KAL-or-ee) Unit of heat energy; amount of energy required to raise the temperature of 1 gram of water 1° C from 14° C to 15° C

Calorie (C) (KAL-or-ee) Unit of heat energy used in metabolic and nutritional studies; equivalent to 1,000 calories or a kilocalorie; amount of energy required to raise the temperature of 1 kilogram of water 1° C from 14° C to 15° C

Calyx (KAY-liks) Cup-like extensions of the renal pelvis that collect the urine

Canaliculi (kan-ah-LIK-yoo-lye) Small tubular channels or passages that connect lacunae with other lacunae or the haversian canal in compact bone; singular, canaliculus

Capacitation (kah-pass-ih-TAY-shun) Process that enables sperm to penetrate an egg; membrane around the acrosome weakens so the enzymes can be released

Capillary (KAP-ih-lair-ee) Microscopic blood vessel between an arteriole and a venule, where gaseous exchange takes place

Carbaminohemoglobin (kar-bah-meen-oh-HEE-moh-gloh-bin) Compound that is formed when carbon dioxide combines with the protein portion of a hemoglobin molecule; accounts for approximately 23% of carbon dioxide transport in the blood

Carbohydrate (kar-boh-HYE-drayt) An organic compound that contains carbon, hydrogen, and oxygen with the hydrogen and oxygen present in a 2:1 ratio; sugar, starch, cellulose

Cardiac cycle (KAR-dee-ak SYE-kul) A complete heartbeat consisting of contraction and relaxation of both atria and both ventricles

Cardiac muscle (KAR-dee-ak MUS-el) Muscle tissue that is found only in the heart; involuntary striated muscle

Cardiac output (KAR-dee-ak OUT-put) The volume pumped from one ventricle in one minute; usually measured from the left ventricle

Cardiovascular (car-dee-oh-VAS-kyoo-lar) Relating to the heart and blood vessels

Carina (kah-RYE-nah) Ridge of hyaline cartilage in the region where the trachea divides into the right and left bronchi

Carotene (KAIR-oh-teen) Yellowish pigment that contributes to skin color

Carpal (KAR-pul) Pertaining to the wrist

Carpals (KAR-puls) Small bones in the wrist

Carpus (KAR-pus) Wrist, which consists of eight small carpal bones

Cartilage (KAR-tih-layj) A type of connective tissue in which cells and fibers are embedded in a semisolid gel matrix

Catabolism (kah-TAB-oh-lizm) Reactions that break down complex molecules into two or more smaller ones with the release of energy; opposite of anabolism

Catalyst (KAT-ah-list) A substance that speeds up chemical reactions without being changed itself

Cation (KAT-eye-on) A positively charged ion

Cauda equina (KAW-dah ee-KWYNE-ah) Collection of spinal nerve roots at the distal end of the spinal cord; literally means "horse's tail"

Cecum (SEE-kum) Proximal portion of the large intestine, below the ileocecal valve

Celiac (SEE-lee-ak) Pertaining to the abdomen

Cell (SEL) Basic unit of life; structural and functional unit of the body

Cell-mediated immunity (SEL MEE-dee-ate-ed ih-MYOO-nih-tee) Immunity that is the result of T-cell action; also called cellular immunity

Cell membrane (SEL MEM-brane)

Phospholipid membrane that separates the contents of the cell from the material outside the cell

Cellular metabolism (SEL-yoo-lar meh-TAB-oh-lizm) Chemical reactions that take place inside cells

Cellular respiration (SEL-yoo-lar res-per-RAY-shun) Utilization of oxygen by the tissue cells

Central nervous system (CNS) (SEN-tral NER-vus SIS-tem) The portion of the nervous system that consists of the brain and spinal cord

Central sulcus (SEN-tral SULL-kus) The groove between the frontal and parietal lobes of the cerebrum; also called the fissure of Rolando

Central venous pressure (SEN-tral VAYN-us PRESH-ur) Blood pressure in the right atrium

Centrioles (SEN-tree-ohlz) Collection of microtubules that function in cell division

Centromere (SEN-tro-meer) Portion of the chromosome where the two chromatids are joined; serves as point of attachment for spindle fibers

Centrosome (SEN-tro-sohm) Dense area near the nucleus that contains the centrioles

Cephalic (seh-FAL-ik) Pertaining to the head

Cerebellar hemisphere (sair-eh-BELL-ar HEM-ih-sfeer) Either of the two halves of the cerebellum

Cerebellar peduncles (sair-eh-BELL-ar pee-DUNK-als) Bundles of nerve fibers that connect the cerebellum with other parts of the central nervous system

Cerebellum (sair-eh-BELL-um) Second largest part of the human brain, located posterior to the pons and medulla oblongata, and involved in the coordination of muscular movements

Cerebral aqueduct (seh-REE-brull AH-kweh-dukt) A narrow channel through the midbrain, between the third and fourth ventricles, that contains cerebrospinal fluid

Cerebral cortex (seh-REE-brull KOR-teks) Thin layer of gray matter, composed of neuron cell bodies and dendrites, on the surface of the brain

Cerebral hemisphere (seh-REE-brull HEM-ih-sfeer) Either of the two halves of the cerebrum

Cerebral peduncles (seh-REE-brull pee-DUNK-als) Two bands of connecting fibers on the ventral aspect of the midbrain that contain voluntary motor tracts descending from the cerebral cortex

Cerebrospinal fluid (seh-ree-broh-SPY-null FLOO-id) A fluid, similar to plasma, that fills the subarachnoid space around the brain and spinal cord and is in the ventricles of the brain

Cerebrum (seh-REE-brum) The largest and uppermost part of the human brain, which is concerned with consciousness, learning, memory, sensations, and voluntary movements

Cerumen (see-ROOM-men) Ear wax

Ceruminous gland (see-ROOM-in-us GLAND) A gland in the ear canal that produces cerumen or ear wax

Cervical (SER-vih-kal) Pertaining to the neck region

Cervix (SIR-viks) The lower, narrow portion of the uterus that projects into the vagina

Chemical bond (KEM-ih-kal BOND) Force that holds atoms together; involved in the sharing or exchange of electrons

Chemoreceptor (kee-moh-ree-SEP-tor) A sensory receptor that detects the presence of chemicals; responsible for taste, smell, and monitoring the concentration of certain chemicals in body fluids

Chief cells (CHEEF SELZ) Cells in the gastric mucosa that secrete pepsinogen

Childhood (CHYLD-hood) Period from the second year until puberty

Cholecystokinin (koh-lee-sis-toe-KYE-nin) A hormone that is produced in the small intestine and stimulates the release of bile from the gallbladder

Cholinergic fiber (koh-lih-NER-jik FYE-ber) A nerve fiber that releases acetylcholine at a synapse

Cholinesterase (koe-lin-ES-ter-ase) An enzyme that causes the decomposition of acetylcholine; also acetylcholinesterase

Chondrocyte (KON-droh-syte) Cartilage cell

Chordae tendineae (KOR-dee ten-DIN-ee) Fibrous, stringlike structures that attach the atrioventricular valves to the papillary muscles of the heart wall

Chorion (KOR-ee-on) Outermost extraembryonic, or fetal, membrane; contributes to the formation of the placenta

Chorionic villi (kor-ee-ON-ik VILL-eye) Fingerlike projections of the chorion that grow into the endometrium of the uterus and contain fetal blood vessels

Choroid (KOR-oyd) Dark pigmented portion of the vascular tunic of the eye; prevents scattering of light rays

Choroid plexus (KOR-oyd PLEKS-us) Specialized capillary network within the ventricles of the brain that secretes cerebrospinal fluid

Chromatid (KRO-mah-tid) One member of a duplicate pair of chromosomes

Chromatin (KRO-ma-tin) Long, slender threads of DNA in the nucleus of a cell; gives rise to chromosomes during mitosis

Chromosomes (KRO-mo-sohmz) Dark staining structures that appear in the nucleus when chromatin condenses during mitosis

Chylomicrons (kye-loh-MY-krons) Small fat droplets that are covered with a protein coat in the epithelial cells of the mucosa of the small intestine

Chyme (KYME) The semifluid mixture of food and gastric juice that leaves the stomach through the pyloric sphincter

Cilia (SIL-ee-ah) Hairlike processes that project outward from the cell membrane and move substances across the surface of the cell

Ciliary body (SILL-ee-air-ee BAH-dee) Part of the vascular tunic of the eye; includes the ciliary muscle and ciliary processes

Ciliary muscle (SILL-ee-air-ee MUSS-el) Smooth muscle in the ciliary body that functions in accommodation for near vision

Ciliary processes (SILL-ee-air-ee PRAH-sess-es) Fingerlike structures in the ciliary body that secrete the aqueous humor

Circumcision (SIR-kum-sih-shun) Surgical removal of the prepuce

Circumduction (sir-kum-DUCK-shun) A conelike movement of a body part; the distal end of the part outlines a circle but the proximal end remains relatively stationary

Cisterna chyli (sis-TER-nah KY-lee) A dilation that forms the beginning of the thoracic duct

Citric acid cycle (SIT-rik AS-id SYE-kul) Aerobic series of reactions that follows glycolysis in glucose metabolism to release energy and carbon dioxide; also called Krebs cycle

Clavicle (KLAV-ih-kul) Collarbone

Cleavage (KLEE-vayj) Series of mitotic cell divisions after fertilization; resulting cells are called blastomeres

Clitoris (KLY-toe-ris) Small mass of erectile tissue at the anterior end of the vestibule in females; homologous to the penis in males

Coagulant (koh-AG-yoo-lant) A substance that promotes the clotting of blood

Coagulation (koh-ag-yoo-LAY-shun) The process of blood clotting

Coccyx (KOK-siks) Lowest part of the vertebral column, composed of four vertebrae fused together

Cochlea (KOK-lee-ah) The spiral, or coiled, portion of the bony labyrinth

Cochlear duct (KOK-lee-ar DUKT) Portion of the membranous labyrinth that is inside the cochlea; contains endolymph and the organ of hearing

Codon (KO-don) A set of three nucleotides on a messenger RNA molecule; contains the code for a single amino acid

Collateral ganglion (koh-LAT-er-al GANG-lee-on) An autonomic ganglion outside the sympathetic chain and located near selected abdominal blood vessels; part of the sympathetic pathway; also called prevertebral ganglion

Colostrum (koh-LAHS-trum) Fluid secreted by the mammary glands before the beginning of true milk production

Columnar (ko-LUM-nar) Shaped like a column; vertical dimension is greater than horizontal dimension

Columns (KOLL-ums) Regions of white matter in the spinal cord; also called funiculi

Complement (KOM-pleh-ment) A group of proteins normally found in serum that provides nonspecific resistance by promoting phagocytosis and inflammation

Complete protein (kum-PLEET PRO-teen) A protein that contains all of the essential amino acids

Compound (KAHM-pownd) A substance formed from two or more elements joined by chemical bonds in a definite, or fixed, ratio; smallest unit of a compound is a molecule

Concentration gradient (kon-sen-TRAY-shun GRAY-dee-ent) Difference in concentration of substances between two different areas

Conception (kon-SEP-shun) Union of a sperm cell nucleus with an egg cell nucleus; fertilization

Conchae (KONG-kee) Scroll-like bones or projections of bones; also called turbinates; singular, concha (KONG-kah)

Conduction myofibers (kon-DUK-shun my-o-FYE-bers) Cardiac muscle cells specialized for conducting action potentials to the myocardium; part of the conduction system of the heart; also called Purkinje fibers

Conductivity (kon-duck-TIV-ih-tee) The ability of neurons to transmit an impulse from one point in the body to another

Condyle (KON-dial) Smooth, rounded articular surface on a bone

Cone (KONE) A photoreceptor in the retina that is specialized for color vision

Connective tissue (ko-NEK-tiv TISH-yoo) Most abundant and widespread tissue in the body; includes bone, cartilage, adipose, blood, and various fibrous tissues

Contractility (kon-track-TILL-ih-tee) The ability of muscle cells to shorten to produce movement

Conus medullaris (KOE-nus med-yoo-LAIR-is) Tapered distal portion of the spinal cord below the lumbar enlargement

Convergence circuit (kon-VER-jens SIR-cut) A conduction pathway in which several presynaptic neurons synapse with a single postsynaptic neuron within a neuronal pool

Coracoid (KOR-ah-koyd) A process on the scapula that projects forward and downward below the clavicle and provides attachments for arm and chest muscles

Core temperature (KOR TEM-per-ah-chur) The temperature deep in the body; temperature of the internal organs

Cornea (KOR-nee-ah) Transparent anterior portion of the outer layer of the eyeball; anterior portion of the fibrous tunic

Corona radiata (koh-ROH-nah ray-dee-AH-tah) Several layers of cells that surround a secondary oocyte when it is released from the ovary

Coronal plane (ko-ROH-nal PLANE) A vertical plane that extends from side to side and divides the body or part into anterior and posterior portions; also called a frontal plane

Coronary artery (KOR-oh-nair-ee AHR-tur-ee) Vessel that carries oxygenated blood to the myocardium

Coronary sinus (KOR-oh-nair-ee SYE-nus) A large venous channel on the posterior surface of the heart that collects deoxygenated blood from coronary circulation and returns it to the right atrium

Corpora cavernosa (KOR-por-ah kav-er-NOH-sah) Two dorsal columns of erectile tissue found in the penis

Corpora quadrigemina (KOR-por-ah kwad-rih-JEM-ih-nah) Four rounded structures composed of the superior and inferior colliculi on the dorsal surface of the midbrain

Corpus albicans (KOR-pus AL-bih-kans) Scar tissue in the ovary that forms when the corpus luteum degenerates

Corpus callosum (KOR-pus kah-LOH-sum) Large band of myelinated nerve fibers that connects the two halves of the cerebrum

Corpus luteum (KOR-pus LOO-tee-um) Under the influence of luteinizing hormone, the structure that develops from the mature follicle after ovulation

Corpus spongiosum (KOR-pus spun-jee-OH-sum) Ventral column of erectile tissue found in the penis

Cortex (KOR-tex) The outer portion of an organ

Corticospinal tract (kor-tih-koh-SPY-null TRACT) Descending, or motor, tract that begins in the cerebral cortex and ends in the spinal cord; also called pyramidal tract

Cortisol (KOR-tih-sahl) Primary glucocorticoid secreted by the adrenal cortex; functions in the regulation of carbohydrate metabolism and also has anti-inflammatory effects

Costal (KAHS-tal) Pertaining to the ribs

Covalent bond (koe-VAY-lent BOND) Chemical bond formed by two atoms sharing one or more pairs of electrons

Cowper's glands (KOW-pers GLANDS) Small accessory glands near the base of the penis in the male; also called bulbourethral glands

Cranial (KRAY-nee-al) Pertaining to the skull

Cranial cavity (KRAY-nee-al KAV-ih-tee) Part of the dorsal body cavity that contains the brain

Craniosacral division (kray-nee-oh-SAY-kral dih-VIH-shun) One of two divisions of the autonomic nervous system; primarily concerned with processes that involve the conservation and restoration of energy; sometimes referred to as the "rest and repose" division; also called the parasympathetic division

Cranium (KRAY-nee-um) Bones of the skull that surround the brain; includes the frontal, parietal, occipital, temporal, ethmoid, and sphenoid bones

Creatine phosphate (KREE-ah-tin FOS-fate) High-energy molecule in muscle cells that is used to rapidly regenerate ATP

Crenation (kree-NAY-shun) Shrinkage of red blood cells when they are placed in a hypertonic solution

Crest (KREST) Narrow ridge of bone

Cretinism (KREE-tin-izm) Dwarfism caused by insufficient thyroid hormone in children

Cribriform plate (KRIB-rih-form PLATE) Portion of the ethmoid bone that contains olfactory foramina

Cricoid cartilage (KRY-koyd KAR-tih-layj) Most inferior cartilage of the larynx

Crista ampullaris (KRIS-tah amp-yoo-LAIR-is) Receptor organ located within the ampulla of the semicircular canals; functions in dynamic equilibrium

Crista galli (KRIS-tah GAL-lee) Upward projecting process on the ethmoid bone

Cristae (KRIS-tee) Shelflike ridges formed by folds of the inner membrane of the mitochondria

Cubital (KYOO-bih-tal) Pertaining to the forearm; region between the elbow and wrist; antebrachial

Cuboidal (kyoo-BOYD-al) Shaped like a cube; horizontal and vertical dimensions approximately equal

Cupula (KEW-pew-lah) A gelatinous mass over the crista ampullaris in the ampulla of the semicircular canals; functions in dynamic equilibrium

Cushing's syndrome (KOOSH-ings SIN-drohm) Condition caused by hypersecretion of glucocorticoids from the adrenal cortex

Cutaneous (kyoo-TAY-nee-us) Pertaining to the skin

Cutaneous membrane (kyoo-TAY-nee-us MEM-brayn) One of the types of epithelial membranes; primary organ of the integumentary system; the skin

Cuticle (KEW-tih-kuhl) A fold of stratum corneum at the proximal border of the visible portion of a nail; also called eponychium

Cystic duct (SIS-tik DUKT) Duct from the gallbladder

Cytokinesis (sye-toe-kih-NEE-sis) Division of the cytoplasm at the end of mitosis to form two separate daughter cells

Cytoplasm (SYE-toe-plazm) Gel-like fluid inside the cell, exclusive of the organelles

Cytoskeleton (sye-toe-SKEL-eh-ton) Complex network of filaments and tubules that function in support and movement of the cell and organelles

Deamination (dee-am-ih-NAY-shun) Catabolic reaction in which an amino group is removed from an amino acid to form ammonia and a keto acid; occurs in the liver as part of protein catabolism

Deciduous teeth (dee-SID-yoo-us TEETH) The teeth that appear first and then are shed and replaced by permanent teeth; also called primary teeth or baby teeth

Decussation (dee-kuh-SAY-shun) A crossing over; usually refers to motor fibers that cross over to the opposite side in the medulla oblongata

Deep (DEEP) Away from the surface; opposite of superficial

Defecation (def-eh-KAY-shun) The removal of indigestible wastes, or feces, through the anus

Deglutition (dee-gloo-TISH-un) The process of swallowing

Dehydration synthesis (dee-hye-DRAY-shun SIN-the-sis) A reaction in which a larger molecule is made from two or more smaller molecules by removing a water molecule

Dendrite (DEN-dryte) The branching afferent process of a neuron that receives impulses from other neurons and transmits them toward the cell body

Deoxyhemoglobin (dee-ok-see-hee-moh-GLOH-bin) The reduced form of hemoglobin; hemoglobin that is not combined with a full load of oxygen

Deoxyribonucleic acid (DNA) (dee-ahk-see-rye-boh-noo-KLEE-ik AS-id) A nucleic acid that contains deoxyribose sugar; genetic material of the cell

Depolarization (dee-poh-lar-ih-ZAY-shun) A reduction in membrane potential; the interior side of the cell membrane becomes less negative (more positive) relative to the exterior

Dermis (DER-mis) Inner layer of the skin, which contains the blood vessels, nerves, glands, and hair follicles; also called stratum corium

Descending tract (dee-SEND-ing TRACT) Spinal cord nerve tract that conducts motor impulses down the cord from the brain

Detrusor muscle (dee-TROO-sor MUSS-el) The smooth muscle in the wall of the urinary bladder

Diabetes mellitus (dye-ah-BEE-teez MEL-ih-tus) Condition caused by insufficient insulin and characterized by high blood glucose levels

Diapedesis (dye-ah-peh-DEE-sis) The process by which white blood cells squeeze between the cells in a vessel wall to enter the tissue spaces outside the blood vessel

Diaphysis (dye-AF-ih-sis) The long straight shaft of a long bone

Diarthrosis (dye-ahr-THROW-sis) Freely movable joint characterized by a joint cavity; also called a synovial joint; plural diarthroses (dye-ahr-THROW-sees)

Diastole (dye-AS-toh-lee) Relaxation phase of the cardiac cycle; opposite of systole

Diastolic pressure (dye-ah-STAHL-ik PRESH-ur) Blood pressure in the arteries during relaxation of the ventricles

Diencephalon (dye-en-SEF-ah-lon) Part of the brain between the cerebral hemispheres and the midbrain; includes the thalamus, hypothalamus, and epithalamus

Differentiation (dif-er-en-she-AY-shun) Process by which cells become structurally and functionally specialized

Diffusion (dif-YOO-zhun) Movement of atoms, ions, or molecules from a region of high concentration to a region of low concentration

Digestive (dye-JES-tiv) Relating to digestion

Diploë (DIP-loh-ee) Layer of spongy bone between the inner and outer tables of compact bone in the flat bones of the skull

Disaccharide (die-SAK-ah-ride) A sugar formed from two monosaccharide molecules; double sugar such as sucrose, maltose, and lactose

Distal (DIS-tal) Farther from a point of attachment or origin; opposite of proximal

Divergence circuit (dye-VER-jens SIR-cut) A conduction pathway in which a single neuron synapses with multiple neurons within a neuronal pool

Dopamine (DOH-pah-meen) One of several neurotransmitters

Dorsal (DOR-sal) Toward the back or posterior; opposite of ventral or anterior

Dorsal root (DOR-sal ROOT) Sensory branch of a spinal nerve by which the nerve is attached to the spinal cord

Dorsal root ganglion (DOR-sal ROOT GANG-lee-on) Collection of sensory neuron cell bodies in the dorsal root of a spinal nerve

Dorsiflexion (dor-sih-FLEK-shun) A movement in which the top of the foot is lifted upward to decrease the angle between the foot and leg; opposite of plantar flexion

Ductus arteriosus (DUCK-tus ar-teer-ee-OH-sus) A small vessel between the pulmonary trunk and the aorta in the fetus, which permits blood to bypass the lungs in the fetal circulatory pathway

Ductus deferens (DUCK-tus DEFF-er-enz) Tubular structure that is continuous with the epididymis, ascends through the inguinal canal, and transports sperm to the ejaculatory duct

Ductus venosus (DUCK-tus veh-NOH-sus) A small vessel that connects the umbilical vein to the inferior vena cava in the fetus and permits blood to bypass the liver in the fetal circulatory pathway

Duodenal glands (doo-oh-DEE-nal GLANDS) Mucous glands in the submucosa of the duodenum; also called Brunner's glands

Duodenum (doo-oh-DEE-num) The first part of the small intestine, about 25 cm long

Dura mater (DOO-rah MAY-ter) Tough, outermost layer of the coverings around the brain and spinal cord; one of the meninges; literally means "tough mother"

Dural sinus (DOO-ral SYE-nus) A channel, or large vein, within the dura mater of the cranial cavity

Dynamic equilibrium (dye-NAM-ik ee-kwi-LIB-ree-um) Equilibrium of motion; maintaining balance when the head or body is moving

Ectoderm (EK-toh-derm) The outermost of the three primary germ layers, which gives rise to the nervous system and the epidermis of the skin

Efferent ducts (EF-fur-ent DUCTS) Tubules that convey sperm from the rete testis to the epididymis

Efferent nervous system (EF-fur-ent NER-vus SIS-tem) The portion of the peripheral nervous system that consists of all the outgoing motor nerves

Efferent neuron (EF-fur-ent NOO-ron) Nerve cell that carries impulses away from the central nervous system toward the periphery; motor neuron

Ejaculation (ee-jak-yoo-LAY-shun) Forceful expulsion of seminal fluid from the urethra

Ejaculatory duct (ee-JAK-yoo-lah-tor-ee DUKT) Short duct that penetrates the prostate gland and empties sperm and fluid from the seminal vesicles into the prostatic urethra

Elasticity (ee-lass-TIS-ih-tee) The ability of tissue to return to its original shape after contraction or extension

Electrocardiogram (ECG) (ee-lek-troh-KAR-dee-oh-gram) A graphic recording of the electrical changes that occur during a cardiac cycle

Electroencephalogram (EEG) (ee-lek-troh-en-SEF-ah-loh-gram) A graphic recording of the electrical activity associated with the function of neural tissue

Electrolyte (ee-LEK-troh-lite) A substance that forms positive and negative ions in a solution, which makes it capable of conducting an electric current

Electron (ee-LEK-tron) A negatively charged particle found in the nucleus of an atom

Embryo (EM-bree-oh) Stage of development that lasts from the beginning of the third week to the end of the eighth week after fertilization; period during which the organ systems develop in the body

Embryonic disk (em-bree-ON-ik DISK) Cells of the early embryo that give rise to the three primary germ layers

Emission (ee-MISH-un) Discharge of seminal fluid into the urethra

Endergonic reaction (en-der-GAHN-ik ree-AK-shun) A chemical reaction that uses energy

Endocardium (en-doh-KAR-dee-um) The thin, smooth inner lining of each chamber of the heart

Endochondral ossification (en-doh-KON-dral ah-sih-fih-KAY-shun) Method of bone formation in which cartilage is replaced by bone

Endocrine (EN-doh-krin) Relating to glands that secrete their product directly into the blood; opposite of exocrine

Endocytosis (en-doh-sye-TOH-sis) Formation of vesicles to transfer substances from outside the cell to the inside of the cell

Endoderm (EN-doh-derm) The innermost of the three primary germ layers, which gives rise to the digestive tract, urinary organs, respiratory structures, and other organs and glands

Endolymph (EN-doh-lymf) Fluid that fills the membranous labyrinth of the inner ear

Endometrium (end-oh-MEE-tree-um) Innermost layer of the uterus, which is a mucous membrane

Endomysium (end-oh-MY-see-um) Connective tissue that surrounds individual muscle fibers (cells)

Endoneurium (end-oh-NOO-ree-um) Connective tissue that surrounds individual nerve fibers

Endoplasmic reticulum (end-oh-PLAZ-mik ree-TIK-yoo-lum) Membrane-enclosed channels within the cytoplasm

Endorphin (en-DOR-fin) A chemical in the central nervous system that influences pain perception and acts as a natural painkiller

Endosteum (end-AH-stee-um) The membrane that lines the medullary cavity of bones

Enkephalin (en-KEF-ah-lin) A chemical in the central nervous system that influences pain perception and acts as a natural painkiller

Enterokinase (en-ter-oh-KYE-nays) An enzyme in the small intestine that activates trypsinogen from the pancreas

Enzyme (EN-zime) An organic catalyst; a substance that affects the rates of biochemical reactions; usually a protein

Eosinophil (ee-oh-SIN-oh-fill) A white blood cell with granules in the cytoplasm that stain readily with acid (eosin) dyes

Ependymal cell (ee-PEN-dih-mal CELL) Neuroglial cell that lines the ventricles of the brain and the central canal of the spinal cord

Epicardium (eh-pih-KAR-dee-um) The outer layer of the heart wall; the visceral pericardium

Epicondyle (ep-ih-KON-dial) Bony bulge adjacent to, or above, a condyle on a bone

Epidermis (ep-ih-DER-mis) Outermost layer of the skin

Epididymis (ep-ih-DID-ih-mis) Tightly coiled tubule along the posterior margin of each testis; functions in the maturation and storage of sperm

Epidural space (ep-ih-DOO-ral SPACE) The space between the dura mater and surrounding bone, especially between the spinal dura mater and the vertebrae

Epigastric region (ep-ih-GAS-trik REE-jun) The upper middle portion of the abdomen

Epiglottis (eh-pih-GLAHT-is) Long, leaf-shaped, movable cartilage of the larynx that covers the opening of the larynx and prevents food from entering during swallowing

Epimysium (ep-ih-MY-see-um) Fibrous connective tissue that surrounds a whole muscle

Epinephrine (ep-ih-NEFF-rihn) Hormone secreted by the adrenal medulla that produces effects similar to the sympathetic nervous system; neurotransmitter released by some neurons in the sympathetic nervous system; also called adrenaline

Epineurium (ep-ih-NOO-ree-um) Fibrous connective tissue that surrounds a whole nerve

Epiphyseal plate (ep-ih-FIZ-ee-al PLATE) The cartilaginous plate between the epiphysis and diaphysis of a bone; responsible for the lengthwise growth of a long bone

Epiphyseal line (ep-ih-FIZ-ee-al

LINE) The remnant of the epiphyseal plate after the cartilage calcifies and growth ceases

Epiphysis (ee-PIF-ih-sis) The end of a long bone

Epiploic appendages (ep-ih-PLOH-ik ah-PEN-day-jez) Pieces of fat-filled connective tissue attached to the outer surface of the colon

Epithalamus (ep-ih-THAL-ah-mus) A tiny region, located superior to the thalamus and hypothalamus in the diencephalon, that includes the pineal body

Epithelial tissue (ep-ih-THEE-lee-al TISH-yoo) Tissue that covers the body and its parts; lines parts of the body; classified according to shape and arrangement

Eponychium (eh-poh-NICK-ee-um) A fold of stratum corneum at the proximal border of the visible portion of a nail; also called cuticle

Equilibrium (ee-kwi-LIB-ree-um) A state of balance between opposing forces

Erection (ee-REK-shun) Condition when the erectile tissue of the penis is filled with blood

Erythrocyte (ee-RITH-roh-syte) Red blood cell

Erythropoiesis (ee-rith-roh-poy-EE-sis) The process of red blood cell formation

Erythropoietin (ee-rith-roh-POY-ee-tin) A hormone released by the kidneys that stimulates red blood cell production

Esophagus (ee-SAHF-ah-gus) Collapsible muscular tube that serves as a passageway for food between the pharynx and stomach

Essential amino acids (ee-SEN-chul ah-MEEN-oh AS-ids) Amino acids that cannot be synthesized in the human body and must be supplied in the diet

Estrogen (ESS-troh-jen) Hormone secreted by the ovarian follicles that stimulates the development and maintenance of female secondary sex characteristics and the cyclic changes in the uterine lining

Ethmoid bone (ETH-moyd BONE) Cranial bone that occupies most of the space between the nasal cavity and the orbits of the eyes

Eustachian tube (yoo-STAY-shee-an TOOB) Tubular passageway that connects the middle ear cavity and the nasopharynx and functions to equalize pressure between the middle ear cavity and the exterior; also called auditory tube

Eversion (ee-VER-zhun) Movement of the sole of the foot outward or laterally; opposite of inversion

Excitability (eks-eye-tah-BILL-ih-tee) The ability of muscle and nerve tissue to receive and respond to stimuli; also called irritability

Excitatory transmission (eks-EYE-tah-toar-ee trans-MIH-shun) Nerve impulse conduction in which the neurotransmitter causes a depolarization (excitation) of the postsynaptic membrane

Exergonic reaction (eks-er-GAHN-ik ree-AK-shun) A chemical reaction that releases energy

Exhalation (eks-hah-LAY-shun) Process of letting air out of the lungs during the breathing cycle; also called expiration

Exocrine gland (EKS-oh-krihn GLAND) A gland that secretes its product to a surface or cavity through ducts

Exocytosis (eks-oh-sye-TOE-sis) Formation of vesicles to transfer substances from inside the cell to the outside of the cell

Exophthalmos (eks-off-THAL-mus) An abnormal bulging or protruding eyeball

Expiration (eks-per-RAY-shun) Process of letting air out of the lungs during the breathing cycle; also called exhalation

Expiratory reserve volume (ERV) (eks-PYE-rah-tor-ee ree-ZERV VOL-yoom) Maximum amount of air that can be forcefully exhaled after a tidal expiration

Extensibility (eks-ten-sih-BILL-ih-tee) The ability of muscle tissue to stretch when pulled

Extension (ek-STEN-shun) A movement that increases the angle between two parts; opposite of flexion

External auditory meatus (eks-TER-nal AW-dih-toar-ee mee-AY-tus) The curved tube that extends from the auricle of the ear into the temporal bone, and ends at the tympanic membrane; also called the ear canal or external auditory canal

External ear (eks-TER-nal EER) The outer portion of the ear; includes the pinna and external auditory canal, and terminates at the tympanic membrane

External nares (eks-TER-nal NAY-reez) Openings through which air enters the nasal cavity; nostrils

External respiration (eks-TER-nal res-per-RAY-shun) Exchange of gases between the lungs and the blood

Extracellular (eks-trah-SELL-yoo-lar) Outside the cell

Extracellular fluid (ECF) (eks-trah-SELL-yoo-lar FLOO-id) Fluid in the body that is not inside cells; includes plasma and interstitial fluid

Extrapyramidal tract (eks-trah-pih-RAM-ih-dal TRACT) Any descending, or motor, tract in the spinal cord that is not a pyramidal tract

Extrinsic eye muscles (eks-TRIN-sik eye MUSS-els) Six skeletal muscles external to the eyeball that control movements of the eye

Facet (FASS-et) Smooth, nearly flat articular surface on a bone

Facial nerve (FAY-shall NERV) Cranial nerve VII; mixed nerve; responsible for taste sensations and for stimulating the muscles of facial expression

Facilitated diffusion (fuh-SIL-ih-tay-ted dif-YOO-zhun) A type of passive membrane transport that requires a carrier molecule

Falciform ligament (FALL-sih-form LIG-ah-ment) Fold of peritoneum that attaches the anterior surface of the liver to the anterior abdominal wall

Fallopian tubes (fah-LOH-pee-an TOOBS) The tubes that extend laterally from the upper portion of the uterus to the region of the ovaries; also called uterine tubes or oviducts

Falx cerebelli (FALKS sair-ee-BELL-eye) Small extension of dura mater between the cerebellar hemispheres

Falx cerebri (FALKS SAYR-ee-brye) A fold of dura mater that extends into the longitudinal fissure between cerebral hemispheres

Fasciculus (fah-SICK-yoo-lus) A small bundle or cluster of muscle or nerve fibers (cells); also called fascicle (FAS-ih-kull); plural, fasciculi (fah-SICK-yoo-lye)

Fatty acid (FAT-tee AS-id) Building blocks of fat molecules; consists of a long chain of carbon and hydrogen atoms

Fauces (FAW-seez) Opening from the oral cavity into the oropharynx

Feces (FEE-seez) Material discharged from the rectum consisting of bacteria, indigestible food residue, and secretions

Femoral (FEM-or-al) Pertaining to the thigh; the part of the lower extremity between the hip and the knee

Femur (FEE-mer) Large, long bone in the thigh

Fertilization (fir-tih-lih-ZAY-shun) Union of a sperm cell nucleus with an egg cell nucleus; conception

Fetal period (FEE-tal PEER-ee-od) Stage of development that starts at the beginning of the ninth week after fertilization and lasts until birth

Fetus (FEE-tus) Term used for the developing offspring from the beginning of the ninth week after fertilization until birth

Fiber (FYE-bur) Complex polysaccharides that cannot be digested by enzymes in the human digestive system but add bulk to the diet

Fibrin (FYE-brin) An insoluble, fibrous protein that is formed by the action of thrombin on fibrinogen during the process of blood clotting

Fibrinogen (fye-BRIN-oh-jen) A soluble plasma protein that is converted to insoluble fibrin by the action of thrombin during the process of blood clotting

Fibrinolysis (fye-brin-AHL-ih-sis) Mechanism by which a blood clot dissolves

Fibroblast (FYE-broh-blast) Connective tissue cell that produces fibers

Fibrosis (fye-BROH-sis) Replacement of damaged tissue with fibrous connective tissue

Fibrous pericardium (FYE-brus pair-ih-KAR-dee-um) The outer, tough, white fibrous connective tissue layer of the pericardial sac

Fibrous tunic (FYE-bruss TOO-nik) Outermost layer of the eyeball

Fibula (FIB-yoo-lah) Small bone on the lateral side of the leg

Filtrate (FILL-trayt) The fluid that enters the glomerular capsule when blood is filtered by the glomerulus in a nephron of the kidney

Filtration (fil-TRAY-shun) The movement of a fluid through a membrane in response to hydrostatic pressure

Filum terminale (FYE-lum term-ih-NAL-ee) Slender thread of pia mater that extends inferiorly from the conus medullaris of the spinal cord to the coccyx

Fissure (FISH-ur) Narrow cleft or slit between bones or separating body parts

Fissure of Rolando (FISH-ur of roh-LAN-doh) The groove between the frontal and parietal lobes of the cerebrum; also called the central sulcus

Fissure of Sylvius (FISH-ur of SYL-vee-us) The deep groove between the temporal lobe below and the frontal and parietal lobes above; also called the lateral fissure or lateral sulcus

Flagellum (fluh-JELL-um) Long projection of the cell membrane that functions in the motility of the cell; plural, flagella

Flexion (FLEK-shun) A movement that decreases the angle between two parts; opposite of extension

Follicle-stimulating hormone (FSH) (FAHL-ik-yool STIM-yoo-lay-ting HOAR-moan) Hormone secreted by the anterior pituitary gland in both males and females; one of the gonadotropins

Foramen (foh-RAY-men) A hole or opening

Foramen of Monro (foh-RAY-men of mun-ROH) A small opening between each lateral ventricle and the third ventricle of the brain for the passage of cerebrospinal fluid; also called the interventricular foramen

Foramen ovale (foh-RAY-men oh-VAL-ee) An opening in the interatrial septum of the fetal heart that permits blood to flow directly from the right atrium into the left atrium and to bypass the lungs in the fetal circulatory pathway; also an opening in the sphenoid bone that transmits the mandibular branch of the trigeminal nerve

Formed elements (formed EL-eh-ments) Red blood cells, white blood cells, and platelets in the blood

Fossa (FAW-sah) A smooth, shallow depression

Fossa ovalis (FAW-sah oh-VAL-is) A region in the interatrial septum of the heart that represents the region of the foramen ovale in the fetus

Fovea (FOE-vee-ah) A small pit or depression

Fovea centralis (FOE-vee-ah sen-TRAL-is) Depression in the center of the macula lutea where vision is sharpest because the cones are most numerous there

Free nerve ending (FREE NERV END-ing) A nerve ending that has no connective tissue covering; responds to pain

Frenulum (FREN-yoo-lum) Membranous fold of tissue that loosely attaches the tongue to the floor of the mouth

Frontal (FRUN-tal) Pertaining to the forehead region

Frontal bone (FRUN-tal BONE) Bone of the cranium that forms the forehead

Frontal plane (FRUN-tal PLANE) A vertical plane that extends from side to side and divides the body or part into anterior and posterior portions; also called a coronal plane

Functional residual capacity (FRC) (FUNK-shun-al ree-ZID-yoo-al kah-PASS-ih-tee) Amount of air remaining in the lungs after a tidal expiration; equals residual volume plus expiratory reserve volume

Funiculi (fuh-NIK-yoo-lee) Regions of white matter in the spinal cord; also called columns

Gametes (GAM-eets) Sex cells; sperm and ova

Gamma-aminobutyric acid (GABA) (gam-mah-ah-meen-oh-byoo-TEER-ik AS-id) One of several neurotransmitters

Ganglion (GANG-lee-on) A group of nerve cell bodies that lie outside the central nervous system; plural, ganglia

Gaster (GAS-ter) The fleshy part of a muscle; also called the belly

Gastrointestinal tract (gas-troh-in-TEST-ih-nal TRACT) Long, continuous tube that extends from the mouth to the anus; the digestive tract or alimentary canal

Gene (JEEN) Portion of a DNA molecule that contains the genetic information for making one particular protein molecule

Gestation (jes-TAY-shun) Time of prenatal development or pregnancy

Gingiva (JIN-jih-vah) The soft tissue that covers the alveolar processes of the mandible and maxillae; also called gums

Glans penis (glanz PEE-nis) Distal end of the penis through which the urethra opens to the exterior

Glenoid cavity (GLEN-oyd KAV-ih-tee) A large depression on the lateral side of the scapula that articulates with the head of the humerus to form the shoulder joint

Globulin (GLOB-yoo-lin) One type of protein in the blood plasma

Glomerular capsule (gloh-MER-yoo-lar KAP-sool) Double-layered epithelial cup that surrounds the glomerulus in a nephron; also called Bowman's capsule

Glomerulus (gloh-MER-yoo-lus) Cluster of capillaries in the nephron through which blood is filtered

Glossopharyngeal nerve (glos-so-fah-RIN-jee-al NERV) Cranial nerve IX; mixed nerve; responsible for taste sensations and for stimulating the muscles used in swallowing

Glucagon (GLOO-kah-gahn) A hormone secreted by the alpha cells of the pancreatic islets; increases the glucose level in the blood

Glucocorticoids (gloo-koh-KOR-tih-koyds) A group of hormones secreted by the adrenal cortex that regulate carbohydrate and fat metabolism; primary glucocorticoid is cortisol

Gluconeogenesis (gloo-koh-nee-oh-JEN-eh-sis) Process of forming glucose from noncarbohydrate nutrient sources such as proteins and lipids

Gluteal (GLOO-tee-al) Pertaining to the buttock region

Glycogen (GLY-koh-jen) Complex

polysaccharide that is the storage form of energy in animals

Glycogenesis (gly-koh-JEN-eh-sis) Series of reactions that convert glucose or other monosaccharides into glycogen for storage

Glycogenolysis (gly-koh-jen-AHL-ih-sis) Series of reactions that convert glycogen into glucose

Glycolysis (gly-KAHL-ih-sis) Anaerobic series of reactions that produces two molecules of pyruvic acid from one molecule of glucose; first series of reactions in the catabolism of glucose

Goiter (GOY-ter) An enlargement of the thyroid gland

Golgi apparatus (GOAL-jee ap-ah-RA-tus) Membranous sacs within the cytoplasm that process and package cellular products

Golgi tendon organ (GOAL-jee TEN-don OAR-gan) A receptor, usually found near the junction of a muscle and tendon, that is stimulated by changes in muscle length or tension; a type of proprioceptor

Gonadocorticoids (go-nad-oh-KOR-tih-koyds) Sex hormones secreted by the adrenal cortex

Gonadotropic hormones (go-nad-oh-TROH-pik HOAR-moans) Hormones secreted by the anterior pituitary gland that stimulate the ovaries or testes; also called gonadotropins

Gonads (GO-nads) Primary reproductive organs; organs that produce the gametes; testes in the male and ovaries in the female

Granulocyte (GRAN-yoo-loh-syte) White blood cell that has granules in the cytoplasm

Granulosa cells (gran-yoo-LOH-sah SELZ) Cells that surround an oocyte during the development of ovarian follicles

Gray commissure (GRAY KOM-ih-shur) Narrow strip of gray matter that connects the two larger regions of gray matter in the spinal cord

Greater vestibular glands (GRAY-ter ves-TIB-yoo-lar GLANDS) Female accessory glands located adjacent to the vaginal orifice; also called Bartholin's glands

Growth hormone (GH) (GROWTH HOAR-moan) A hormone secreted by the anterior pituitary gland that influences the rate of skeletal growth; also called somatotropic hormone

Gustatory (GUS-tah-toar-ee) Refers to taste

Gustatory cell (GUS-tah-toar-ee SELL) Specialized chemoreceptor in the tongue for the sense of taste

Gyrus (JYE-rus) One of the raised folds on the surface of the cerebrum; also called convolution; plural, gyri (JYE-rye)

Hair follicle (HAIR FAH-lih-kal) Cells that surround the root of the hair

Hair root (HAIR ROOT) The part of the hair that is below the surface of the skin

Hair shaft (HAIR SHAFT) The visible part of hair

Hard palate (HARD PAL-at) Anterior portion of the floor of the nasal cavity and roof of the mouth, which is supported by bone

Haustra (HAWS-trah) A series of pouches along the length of the colon

Haversian canal (hah-VER-shun kah-NAL) Central canal in a haversian system, contains blood vessels and nerves; also called osteonic canal

Haversian system (hah-VER-shun SIS-tem) Structural unit of bone consisting of concentric rings of cells and matrix around a central canal; also called osteon

Head (HED) Enlarged, often rounded, end of a bone

Hematocrit (hee-MAT-oh-krit) The percentage of red blood cells in a given volume of blood

Hematopoiesis (hee-mat-oh-poy-EE-sis) Blood cell production, which occurs in the red bone marrow; also called hemopoiesis

Hemocytoblast (hee-moh-SYTE-oh-blast) A stem cell in the bone marrow from which the blood cells arise

Hemoglobin (hee-moh-GLOH-bin) The iron-containing protein in red blood cells that is responsible for the transport of oxygen

Hemolysis (hee-MAHL-ih-sis) The escape of hemoglobin from a red blood cell into the surrounding medium, usually caused by rupture of the cell

Hemopoiesis (hee-moh-poy-EE-sis) Blood cell production, which occurs in the red bone marrow; also called hematopoiesis

Hemostasis (hee-moh-STAY-sis) The stoppage of bleeding

Heparin (HEP-ah-rihn) A substance that inhibits blood clotting

Hepatic flexure (heh-PAT-ik FLEK-shur) Curve between the ascending colon and transverse colon; also called the right colonic flexure

Hepatocytes (heh-PAT-oh-sytes) Liver cells

Hering-Breuer reflex (HER-ing BREW-er REE-fleks) Stretch reflex in the lungs that prevents overinflation of the lungs

Histamine (HISS-tah-meen) A substance that promotes inflammation

Histology (hiss-TAHL-oh-jee) Branch of microscopic anatomy that studies tissues

Holocrine gland (HOH-loh-krin GLAND) Gland in which the cells are discharged with the secretory product

Homeostasis (hoh-mee-oh-STAY-sis) A normal stable condition in which the body's internal environment remains the same; constant internal environment

Homeotherms (HOH-mee-oh-therms) Warm-blooded animals; have the ability to maintain a constant internal temperature

Homunculus (hoh-MUNK-yoo-lus) An imaginary figure that represents the distribution of body regions in the primary sensory and motor areas of the cerebral cortex

Hormone (HOAR-moan) A substance secreted by an endocrine gland

Horn (HORN) Regions of gray matter in the spinal cord

Human chorionic gonadotropin (HCG) (HYOO-man kor-ee-ON-ik goh-nad-oh-TROH-pin) Hormone secreted by the trophoblast, which has an effect similar to luteinizing hormone and causes the corpus luteum to remain functional to maintain pregnancy

Humerus (HYOO-mur-us) Bone in the arm, or brachium

Humoral immunity (HYOO-mur-al ih-MYOO-nih-tee) Immunity that is the result of B-cell action and the production of antibodies; also called antibody-mediated immunity

Hyaline cartilage (HYE-ah-lihn KAR-tih-layj) Most abundant type of cartilage; appears glossy

Hydrogen bond (HYE-droh-jen BOND) Weak chemical bond that is formed between the partial positive charge on a covalently bound hydrogen atom and the partial negative charge on another covalent molecule

Hydrolysis (hye-DRAHL-ih-sis) Chemical breakdown of complex molecules by the addition of water

Hydrophilic (hye-droh-FILL-ik) "Water loving"; attracts water

Hydrophobic (hye-droh-FOE-bik) "Water fearing"; will not mix with water

Hydrostatic pressure (hye-droh-STAT-ik PRESH-ur) Pressure or force due to a fluid

Hymen (HYE-men) Thin fold of mucous membrane that may cover the vaginal orifice

Hyoid (HYE-oyd) Bone in the neck, between the mandible and the larynx, which supports the tongue

Hyperextension (hye-per-eks-TEN-shun) A movement in which a part of the body is extended beyond the anatomical position

Hyperpolarization (hye-per-poh-lar-ih-ZAY-shun) An increase in the difference of electrical charges between the inside and outside of the cell membrane, which makes it more difficult to generate an action potential

Hypertonic (hye-per-TAHN-ik) A solution that has a greater concentration of solutes than another solution

Hypochondriac region (hye-poh-KAHN-dree-ak REE-jun) The upper lateral portions of the abdomen, on either side of the epigastric region

Hypodermis (hye-poh-DER-miss) Below the skin; a sheet of areolar connective tissue and adipose beneath the dermis of the skin; also called the subcutaneous layer or superficial fascia

Hypogastric region (hye-poh-GAS-trik REE-jun) The central portion of the abdomen inferior to the umbilical region

Hypoglossal nerve (hye-poh-GLAHS-al NERV) Cranial nerve XII; motor nerve; responsible for tongue movements

Hypophysis (hye-PAH-fih-sis) See pituitary gland

Hypothalamus (HYE-poh-thal-ah-mus) A small region, located just below the thalamus in the diencephalon, which is important in autonomic and neuroendocrine functions

Hypotonic (hye-poh-TAHN-ik) A solution that has a lesser concentration of solutes than another solution

Ileocecal junction (ill-ee-oh-SEE-kul JUNK-shun) Connection between the small intestine and large intestine

Ileum (ILL-ee-um) Terminal portion of the small intestine

Iliac region (ILL-ee-ak REE-jun) The lateral inferior portions of the abdomen, on either side of the hypogastric region; also called the inguinal region

Iliosacral (ill-ee-oh-SAY-kral) Pertaining to the ilium and sacrum

Ilium (ILL-ee-um) One of the parts of the os coxa or hip bone

Immunity (ih-MYOO-nih-tee) Specific defense mechanisms that provide resistance to invading pathogens

Immunoglobulins (ih-myoo-noh-GLAHB-yoo-lins) Substances produced by the body that inactivate or destroy another substance that is introduced into the body; antibodies

Implantation (im-plan-TAY-shun) Process by which the developing embryo becomes embedded in the uterine wall; usually takes about a week and is completed by the 14th day after fertilization

Incomplete protein (IN-kum-pleet PRO-teen) A protein that does not contain all of the essential amino acids

Incus (INK-us) One of the tiny bones in the middle ear, between the malleus and the stapes

Infancy (IN-fan-see) Period from the end of the first month to the end of the first year after birth

Inferior (in-FEER-ee-or) Lower; one part is below another; opposite of superior

Inferior colliculi (in-FEER-ee-or koh-LIK-yoo-lye) Two lower bodies of the corpora quadrigemina on the dorsal surface of the midbrain, which function in auditory reflexes

Inferior vena cava (in-FEER-ee-or VEE-nah KAY-vah) Large vein that collects blood from all parts of the body inferior to the heart and returns it to the right atrium

Inflammation (in-flah-MAY-shun) Nonspecific defense mechanism that involves a group of responses to tissue irritants and is characterized by redness, heat, swelling, and pain

Ingestion (in-JEST-chun) The process of taking in food

Inguinal (IN-gwih-nal) Pertaining to the depressed region between the abdomen and the thigh; groin

Inguinal canal (IN-gwih-nal kah-NAL) A passageway in the abdominal wall that transmits the spermatic cord in the male and the round ligament of the uterus in the female

Inguinal region (IN-gwih-nal REE-jun) The lateral inferior portions of the abdomen, on either side of the hypogastric region; also called the iliac region

Inhalation (in-hah-LAY-shun) Process of taking air into the lungs; also called inspiration

Inhibitory transmission (in-HIB-ih-toar-ee trans-MIH-shun) Nerve impulse conduction in which the neurotransmitter causes hyperpolarization of the postsynaptic membrane and reduces the chances of generating an action potential

Inner cell mass (IN-ner SELL MASS) Cluster of cells at one side of a blastocyst; cells that develop into the embryo

Inner ear (IN-er EER) The internal ear or labyrinth, located in the temporal bone, and containing the organs of hearing and balance

Insertion (in-SIR-shun) The end of a muscle that is attached to a relatively movable part; the end opposite the origin

Inspiration (in-spur-RAY-shun) Process of taking air into the lungs; also called inhalation

Inspiratory capacity (IC) (in-SPY-rah-tor-ee kah-PASS-ih-tee) Maximum amount of air that can be inhaled; equals tidal volume plus inspiratory reserve volume

Inspiratory reserve volume (IRV) (in-SPY-rah-tor-ee ree-ZERV VOL-yoom) Maximum amount of air that can be forcefully inhaled after a tidal inspiration

Insula (IN-sull-ah) A triangular area of cerebral cortex that lies deep within the lateral sulcus, beneath the frontal, parietal, and temporal lobes and hidden from view; also called the island of Reil (RY-al)

Insulin (IN-suh-lin) A hormone secreted by the beta cells of the pancreatic islets; decreases the glucose level in the blood

Integumentary (in-teg-yoo-MEN-tar-ee) Pertaining to the skin and related structures

Interatrial septum (in-ter-AY-tree-al SEP-tum) The partition between the right atrium and left atrium

Intercalated disk (in-TER-kuh-lay-ted DISK) Specialized intercellular connection that appears as a dark band in cardiac muscle

Intercellular matrix (in-ter-SEL-yoo-lar MAY-triks) Nonliving material that fills the spaces between cells in a tissue

Interferon (in-ter-FEER-on) A substance that is produced by the body in response to the presence of a virus, which in turn, offers some protection against that virus by inhibiting its multiplication

Internal nares (in-TER-nal NAY-reez) Openings from the nasal cavity into the pharynx

Internal respiration (in-TER-nal res-per-RAY-shun) Exchange of gases between the blood and tissue cells

Interneuron (in-ter-NOO-ron) Nerve cell, totally within the central nervous system, that carries impulses from a sensory neuron to a motor neuron; also called association neuron

Interphase (IN-ter-faze) The period of the cell cycle between active cell divisions

Interstitial cells (in-ter-STISH-al SELZ) Cells between the seminiferous tubules in the testes; produce testosterone; also called cells of Leydig

Interstitial cell–stimulating hormone (ICSH) (in-ter-STISH-al SELL STIM-yoo-lay-ting HOAR-moan) Hormone secreted by the anterior pituitary gland in males, which is the same as luteinizing hormone in females; one of the gonadotropins

Interstitial fluid (in-ter-STISH-al FLOO-id) Portion of the extracellular fluid that is found in the microscopic spaces between cells

Interventricular foramen (in-ter-ven-TRICK-yoo-lar for-RAY-men) Opening between the lateral and third ventricles in the brain; also called the foramen of Monro

Interventricular septum (in-ter-ven-TRIK-yoo-lar SEP-tum) The partition between the right ventricle and left ventricle

Intra-alveolar pressure (in-trah-al-VEE-oh-lar PRESH-ur) Pressure inside the alveoli of the lungs; also called intrapulmonary pressure

Intracellular (in-trah-SEL-yoo-lar) Inside the cell

Intracellular fluid (ICF) (in-trah-SELL-yoo-lar FLOO-id) The fluid inside body cells

Intramembranous ossification (in-trah-MEM-bran-us ah-sih-fih-KAY-shun) Method of bone formation in which the bone is formed directly in a membrane

Intrapleural pressure (in-trah-PLOO-ral PRESH-ur) Pressure within the pleural cavity, between the visceral and parietal layers of the pleura

Intrapulmonary pressure (in-trah-PUL-mon-air-ee PRESH-ur) Pressure inside the alveoli of the lungs; also called intra-alveolar pressure

Intravascular fluid (in-trah-VAS-kyoo-lar FLOO-id) Portion of extracellular fluid that is in the blood; plasma

Intrinsic factor (in-TRIN-sik FAK-tor) A substance produced by cells in the stomach lining that facilitates the absorption of vitamin B_{12}

Inversion (in-VER-zhun) Movement of the sole of the foot inward or medially; opposite of eversion

Ion (EYE-on) Electrically charged atom or group of atoms; an atom that has gained or lost one or more electrons

Ionic bond (eye-ON-ik BOND) Chemical bond that is formed when one or more electrons are transferred from one atom to another

Ionic compound (eye-ON-ik KAHM-pownd) Chemical compounds that are formed by the force of attraction between cations and anions

Iris (EYE-rihs) The colored portion of the eye that is seen through the cornea; contains smooth muscle that regulates the size of the pupil; part of the middle layer of the eye

Ischium (IS-kee-um) One of the parts of the os coxa or hip bone

Island of Reil (EYE-land of RY-al) A triangular area of cerebral cortex that lies deep within the lateral sulcus, beneath the frontal, parietal, and temporal lobes and hidden from view; also called the insula

Islets of Langerhans (EYE-lets of LAHNG-er-hanz) See pancreatic islets

Isometric contraction (eye-so-MET-rik kon-TRACK-shun) Type of muscle contraction in which the muscle tension increases but no movement is produced

Isotonic (eye-soh-TAHN-ik) A solution that has the same concentration of solutes as another solution

Isotonic contraction (eye-soh-TAHN-ik kon-TRACK-shun) Type of muscle contraction in which the muscle maintains the same tension and there is movement between two parts

Isotropic (eye-soh-TROH-pik) Bands in skeletal and cardiac muscle fibers that appear light; light passes through

Jejunum (jeh-JOO-num) Middle portion of the small intestine

Jugular notch (JUG-yoo-lar NOTCH) Depression on the superior margin of the manubrium of the sternum

Juxtaglomerular apparatus (juks-tah-gloh-MER-yoo-lar ap-pah-RAT-us) Complex of modified cells in the afferent arteriole and the ascending limb/distal tubule in the kidney, which helps regulate blood pressure by secreting renin; consists of the macula densa and juxtaglomerular cells

Keratin (KER-ah-tin) Hard, fibrous protein found in the epidermis, hair, and nails

Keratinization (ker-ah-tin-ih-ZAY-shun) Process by which the cells of the epidermis become filled with keratin and move to the surface where they are sloughed off

Kidney (KID-nee) Organ of the urinary system that filters the blood and functions to maintain the homeostasis of body fluids

Kilocalorie (KILL-oh-kal-or-ee) Unit of heat energy used in metabolic and nutritional studies; equivalent to 1,000 standard calories; Calorie

Korotkoff sounds (koh-ROT-kof SOUNDS) The sounds heard in the stethoscope while taking blood pressure

Krebs cycle (KREBZ SYE-kul) Aerobic series of reactions that follows glycolysis in glucose metabolism to release energy and carbon dioxide; also called citric acid cycle

Labia majora (LAY-bee-ah mah-JOR-ah) Two large fat-filled folds of skin that enclose the other female external genitalia; homologous to the scrotum in the male

Labia minora (LAY-bee-ah mye-NOR-ah) Two small folds of skin medial to the labia majora

Labor (LAY-bor) Process by which forceful contractions expel the fetus from the uterus

Lacrimal (LAK-rih-mal) Small bone anterior to the ethmoid in the orbit of the eye

Lacrimal apparatus (LAK-rih-mal ap-pah-RAT-us) The structures that produce and convey tears

Lacrimal gland (LAK-rih-mal GLAND) A glandular structure in the superior and lateral region of the orbit that produces tears

Lactase (LAK-tays) An enzyme that acts on the disaccharide lactose and breaks it into a molecule of glucose and a molecule of galactose

Lactation (lak-TAY-shun) Milk production and ejection from the mammary glands

Lacteal (lak-TEEL) Lymph capillary found in the villi of the small intestine

Lactic acid (LAK-tik AS-id) A molecule that is formed from pyruvic acid when oxygen is lacking; product of anaerobic respiration in muscles during exercise

Lactiferous duct (lak-TIFF-er-us DUKT) Duct that collects milk from the lobules of a mammary gland and carries it to the nipple

Lacuna (lah-KOO-nah) Space or cavity; space that contains bone or cartilage cells; pleural, lacunae

Lamellae (lah-MEL-ee) Concentric

rings of hard calcified matrix in bone

Lamellated corpuscle (lam-el-LAY-ted KOAR-pus-al) See Pacinian corpuscle

Laryngopharynx (lah-ring-go-FAIR-inks) Portion of the pharynx that is posterior to the larynx and extends from the level of the hyoid bone to the lower margin of the larynx

Larynx (LAIR-inks) Passageway for air between the pharynx and trachea; commonly called the voice box

Lateral (LAT-er-al) Toward the side, away from the midline; opposite of medial

Lateral sulcus (LAT-er-al SULL-kus) The deep groove between the temporal lobe below and the frontal and parietal lobes above; also called the lateral fissure or fissure of Sylvius

Left atrium (LEFT AY-tree-um) Chamber of the heart that receives oxygenated blood from the lungs through the pulmonary veins

Left ventricle (LEFT VEN-trih-kul) Chamber of the heart that pumps oxygenated blood through the aorta to systemic circulation

Leg (LEG) Portion of the lower extremity between the knee and the foot; also called the crural region

Lens (LENZ) Transparent biconvex structure that is posterior to the iris in the eye and functions in the refraction of light rays

Leukocyte (LOO-koh-syte) White blood cell

Ligament (LIG-ah-ment) Band of dense fibrous connective tissue that connects one bone to another

Ligamentum arteriosum (lig-ah-MEN-tum ahr-teer-ee-OH-sum) The fibrous remnant that results from the atrophy of the ductus arteriosus

Ligamentum venosum (lig-ah-MEN-tum veh-NO-sum) The fibrous remnant that results from the atrophy of the ductus venosus

Liminal stimulus (LIM-ih-null STIM-yoo-lus) Minimum level of stimulation that is required to start a nerve impulse or muscle contraction; also called threshold stimulus

Lipid (LIP-id) A class of organic compounds that includes oils, fats, and related substances

Lipogenesis (lip-oh-JEN-eh-sis) Series of reactions in which lipids are formed from other nutrients

Longitudinal fissure (lonj-ih-TOO-dih-null FISH-ur) Deep groove that divides the cerebrum into two halves

Lower respiratory tract (LOW-er res-PYE-rah-tor-ee TRAKT) Portion of the respiratory tract that is below the larynx, including the trachea, bronchial tree, and lungs

Lumbar region (LUM-bar REE-jun) The middle lateral portions of the abdomen, on either side of the umbilical region

Lunula (LOO-nyoo-lah) The small curved white area at the base of a nail

Luteinizing hormone (LH) (LOO-ten-eye-zing HOAR-moan) Hormone secreted by the anterior pituitary gland in both males and females; one of the gonadotropins; in males, it may be called interstitial cell–stimulating hormone

Lymph (LIMF) Fluid that is derived from interstitial fluid and found in the lymphatic vessels

Lymph capillary (LIMF KAP-ih-lair-ee) Smallest lymphatic vessel that picks up lymph from the interstitial fluid for its return to the circulating blood

Lymph node (LIMF NODE) A small, bean-shaped aggregate of lymphoid tissue along a lymphatic vessel that filters the lymph before it is returned to the blood circulation

Lymphatic (lim-FAT-ik) Relating to lymph

Lymphocyte (LIM-foh-syte) A type of white blood cell that lacks granules in the cytoplasm and has an important role in immunity

Lysosome (LYE-so-sohm) Membrane-enclosed sac of digestive enzymes within the cytoplasm

Lysozyme (LYE-soh-zyme) An enzyme found in tears, saliva, and perspiration that inhibits bacteria

Macrophage (MAK-roh-fahj) Large phagocytic connective tissue cell that functions in immune responses; name given to a monocyte after it leaves the blood and enters the tissues

Macula (MAK-yoo-lah) The structure in the utricle and saccule that detects a change in position of the head; functions in static equilibrium

Macula lutea (MAK-yoo-lah LOO-tee-ah) Yellowish spot near the center of the retina where the cones are concentrated

Malleus (MAL-lee-us) One of the tiny bones in the middle ear, adjacent to the tympanic membrane

Maltase (MAWL-tays) An enzyme that acts on the disaccharide maltose and breaks it into two molecules of glucose

Mammary (MAM-ah-ree) Pertaining to the breast

Mammary glands (MAM-ah-ree GLANDS) Organs of milk production located within the breast

Mandible (MAN-dih-bul) Bone of the lower jaw

Mandibular (man-DIB-yoo-lar) Relating to the mandible

Manubrium (mah-NOO-bree-um) Upper portion of the sternum

Mass number (MASS NUM-bur) The total number of protons and neutrons in the nucleus of an atom of an element

Mast cell (MAST SELL) A connective tissue cell that produces heparin and histamine; the name given to a basophil after it leaves the blood and enters the tissues

Mastication (mas-tih-KAY-shun) The process of chewing

Maxillae (maks-ILL-ee) Bones of the upper jaw

Meatus (mee-ATE-us) A tubelike passageway through a bone, a tunnel or canal

Mechanoreceptor (mek-ah-noh-ree-SEP-tor) A sensory receptor that responds to a bending or deformation of the cell; examples include receptors for touch, pressure, hearing, and equilibrium

Medial (MEE-dee-al) Toward the middle; opposite of lateral

Medulla (meh-DOO-lah or meh-DULL-ah) The inner portion of an organ

Medulla oblongata (meh-DOO-lah ahb-long-GAH-tah) Lowest part of the brain stem, which contains the vital cardiac center, vasomotor center, and respiratory center

Medullary cavity (MED-yoo-lair-ee KAV-ih-tee) Space in the shaft of a long bone that contains yellow marrow

Megakaryocyte (meg-ah-KAIR-ee-oh-syte) A large cell that contributes to the formation of platelets

Meiosis (my-OH-sis) Type of nuclear division in which the number of chromosomes is reduced to one half the number found in a body cell; results in the formation of an egg or sperm

Meissner's corpuscle (MYS-nerz KOAR-pus-al) A sensory receptor near the surface of the skin that detects light touch; also called corpuscle of touch

Meissner's plexus (MYS-nerz PLEK-sus) A network of autonomic nerves in the submucosa of the gastrointestinal tract; also called submucosal plexus

Melanin (MEL-ah-nin) A dark brown

or black pigment found in parts of the body, especially skin and hair

Melanocyte (meh-LAN-oh-syte) Specialized cell that produces melanin, found in the stratum basale of the epidermis

Melatonin (mell-ah-TOH-nihn) Hormone produced by the pineal body; regulates the body's internal clock and daily rhythms; responds to varying light levels; regulates onset of puberty and menstrual cycle

Membrane potential (MEM-brayn po-TEN-shall) The difference in electrical charge between inside and outside a cell membrane

Membranous labyrinth (MEM-brah-nus LAB-ih-rinth) A series of membranes located within the bony labyrinth and separated from it by perilymph; includes the cochlear duct, the utricle and saccule, and the membranous semicircular canals (ducts)

Membranous urethra (MEM-brah-nus yoo-REE-thrah) Portion of the male urethra that passes through the membranous pelvic floor

Menarche (meh-NAHR-kee) First period of menstrual bleeding at puberty

Meninges (meh-NIN-jeez) Connective tissue membranes that cover the brain and spinal cord

Meningitis (meh-nin-JYE-tis) Inflammation of the meninges

Meniscus (meh-NIS-kus) Fibrocartilaginous pads found in certain freely movable joints

Menopause (MEN-oh-pawz) Cessation of menstrual bleeding; termination of uterine cycles

Menses (MEN-seez) Periodic shedding of the stratum functionale of the uterine lining; menstruation

Menstrual cycle (MEN-stroo-al SYE-kul) Monthly cycle of events that occur in the uterus from puberty to menopause; also called the uterine cycle; occurs concurrently with the ovarian cycle

Menstruation (men-stroo-AY-shun) Periodic shedding of the stratum functionale of the uterine lining; menses

Merocrine gland (MER-oh-krin GLAND) Gland that discharges its secretions directly through the cell membrane

Mesentery (MEZ-en-tair-ee) Extensions of peritoneum that are associated with the intestine

Mesoderm (MEZ-oh-derm) The middle of the three primary germ layers, which gives rise to connective tissues, muscles, bones, and blood

Messenger RNA (mRNA) (MES-en-jer RNA) A molecule of RNA that transmits information for protein synthesis from the DNA in the nucleus to the cytoplasm

Metabolism (meh-TAB-oh-lizm) The total of all biochemical reactions that take place in the body; includes anabolism and catabolism

Metacarpals (meh-tah-KAR-pulls) Five bones that form the palm of the hand

Metacarpus (meh-tah-KAR-pus) Palm of the hand, which consists of five metacarpal bones

Metaphase (MET-ah-faze) Second stage of mitosis; stage in which visible chromosomes become aligned along the center of the cell

Metarteriole (met-ahr-TEER-ee-ohl) A microscopic vessel that directly connects an arteriole to a venule without an intervening capillary network; an arteriovenous shunt

Metatarsals (meh-tah-TAHR-sahls) Five bones that form the instep of the foot

Metatarsus (meh-tah-TAHR-sis) Instep of the foot, which consists of five metatarsal bones

Micelles (my-SELZ) Tiny droplets of monoglycerides and free fatty acids that are coated with bile salts

Microfilaments (my-kroh-FIL-ah-ments) Long, slender rods of protein within a cell

Microglia (my-kroh-GLEE-ah) Neuroglial cell that is capable of phagocytosis

Microtubules (my-kroh-TOOB-yools) Thin cylinders of protein within a cell; composed of the protein tubulin (TOOB-yoo-lin)

Microvillus (my-kroh-VIL-us) Small projection of the cell membrane that is supported by microfilaments; plural, microvilli

Micturition (mik-too-RISH-un) Act of expelling urine from the bladder; also called urination or voiding

Midbrain (MID-brayn) Region of the brain stem between the diencephalon and the pons

Middle ear (MID-dull EER) Small epithelial lined cavity in the temporal bone that contains the three auditory ossicles; also called the tympanic cavity

Midsagittal plane (mid-SAJ-ih-tal PLANE) A vertical plane that divides the body or organ into equal right and left parts; a sagittal plane that is in the midline; also called the median plane

Mineralocorticoids (min-er-al-oh-KOR-tih-koyds) A group of hormones secreted by the adrenal cortex that regulates electrolyte balance in the body; primary mineralocorticoid is aldosterone

Minerals (MIN-er-als) Inorganic substances that are needed in minute amounts in the diet to maintain growth and good health but do not supply energy

Mitochondria (my-tohe-KAHN-dree-ah) Organelles that contain the enzymes essential for producing ATP; singular, mitochondrion

Mitosis (my-TOH-sis) Process by which the nucleus of a body cell divides to form two new cells, each identical to the parent cell

Mitral valve (MY-tral VALVE) Valve between the left atrium and left ventricle; also called the bicuspid valve

Mixed nerve (MIK-st NERV) A nerve that contains both sensory and motor fibers

Mixture (MIX-chur) A combination of two or more substances that can be separated by ordinary physical means

Molecule (MAHL-eh-kyool) A particle composed of two or more atoms that are chemically bound together; smallest unit of a compound

Monocyte (MAHN-oh-syte) A type of white blood cell that lacks granules in the cytoplasm and is capable of phagocytosis

Monosaccharide (mahn-oh-SAK-ah-ride) Building block of carbohydrates; simple sugar such as glucose, fructuose, and galactose

Mons pubis (MAHNZ PYOO-bis) Rounded elevation of fat that overlies the pubic symphysis in females

Morula (MOR-yoo-lah) Solid ball of cells formed by early mitotic divisions of a zygote, usually present by the end of the third day after fertilization

Motor nerve (MOH-toar NERV) A nerve that contains primarily motor, or efferent, fibers

Motor neuron (MOH-toar NOO-ron) Nerve cell that carries impulses away from the central nervous system toward the periphery; efferent neuron

Motor unit (MOH-toar YOO-nit) A single neuron and all the muscle fibers it stimulates

Mucosa (MYOO-koh-sah) Epithelial membranes that secrete mucus and line body cavities that open directly to the exterior; also called mucous membranes

Mucous cell (MYOO-cus CELL) Cell that secretes a thick fluid called mucus

Mucous membrane (MYOO-cus MEM-brayn) Epithelial membrane that secretes mucus and lines body cavities that open directly to the exterior; also called mucosa

Multicellular (muhl-tih-SEL-yoo-lar) Consisting of many cells

Multiple motor unit summation (MUHL-tih-pul MOH-toar YOO-nit sum-MAY-shun) Type of response in which numerous motor units are stimulated simultaneously, which increases contraction strength

Multiple wave summation (MUHL-tih-pul WAYV sum-MAY-shun) Type of response in which stimuli are so rapid that the muscle is not able to relax completely between successive stimuli and sustained or more forceful contractions result

Muscle spindle (MUSS-el SPIN-dull) A receptor in skeletal muscles that is stimulated by changes in muscle length or tension; a type of proprioceptor

Muscle tone (MUSS-el TOAN) Sustained partial muscle contraction, which produces a constant tension in the muscles

Muscular (MUSS-kyoo-lar) Relating to the muscles

Myelin (MY-eh-lin) White, fatty substance that surrounds many nerve fibers

Myenteric plexus (my-en-TAIR-ik PLEK-sus) A network of autonomic nerves between the circular and longitudinal muscle layers of the gastrointestinal tract; also called Auerbach's plexus

Myocardium (my-oh-KAR-dee-um) Middle layer of the heart wall, composed of cardiac muscle tissue

Myofibrils (my-oh-FYE-brills) Threadlike structures that run longitudinally through muscle cells and are composed of actin and myosin myofilaments

Myofilaments (my-oh-FILL-ah-ments) Ultramicroscopic, threadlike structures in the myofibrils of muscle cells; composed of the contractile proteins actin and myosin

Myoglobin (my-oh-GLOH-bin) The iron-containing protein in the sarcoplasm of muscle cells that binds with oxygen and stores it; gives the red color to muscle

Myometrium (my-oh-MEE-tree-um) Thick middle layer of the uterus, which is composed of smooth muscle

Myoneural junction (my-oh-NOO-ral JUNK-shun) The area of communication between the axon terminal of a motor neuron and the sarcolemma of a muscle fiber; also called a neuromuscular junction

Myosin (MY-oh-sin) Contractile protein in the thick filaments of skeletal muscle cells

Myxedema (mik-seh-DEE-mah) Condition caused by insufficient thyroid hormone in adults

Nares (NAY-reez) Openings of the nasal cavity

Nasal conchae (NAY-zal KONG-kee) Bony ridges that project medially into the nasal cavity from the lateral walls of the nasal cavity

Nasopharynx (nay-zo-FAIR-inks) Portion of the pharynx that is posterior to the nasal cavity and extends from the base of the skull to the uvula

Natural immunity (NAT-yoor-al ih-MYOO-nih-tee) Immunity acquired through normal processes of daily living

Negative feedback (NEG-ah-tiv FEED-bak) A mechanism of response in which a stimulus initiates reactions that reduce the stimulus

Neonatal period (nee-oh-NAY-tal PEER-ee-ud) The first month after birth

Neonate (NEE-oh-nayt) Term for a baby during the neonatal period, or the first month after birth

Nephron (NEFF-rahn) Functional unit of the kidney consisting of a renal corpuscle and a renal tubule

Nerve tracts (NERV TRAKTS) Bundles of myelinated nerve fibers in the spinal cord

Nervous (NER-vus) Relating to the nerves and brain

Nervous tissue (NER-vus TISH-yoo) Specialized tissue found in nerves, brain, and spinal cord

Nervous tunic (NERV-us TOO-nik) The innermost layer of the eyeball; also called the retina

Neurilemma (noo-rih-LEM-mah) The layer of Schwann cells that surrounds a nerve fiber in the peripheral nervous system and, in some cases, produces myelin; also called Schwann's sheath

Neuroglia (noo-ROG-lee-ah) Supporting cells of nervous tissue; cells in nervous tissue that do not conduct impulses

Neurohypophysis (noo-roh-hye-PAH-fih-sis) Posterior portion of the pituitary gland

Neuromuscular junction (noo-roe-MUSK-yoo-lar JUNK-shun) The area of communication between the axon terminal of a motor neuron and the sarcolemma of a muscle fiber; also called a myoneural junction

Neuron (NOO-ron) Nerve cell, including its processes; conducting cell of nervous tissue

Neuronal pool (noo-ROH-nal POOL) Functional group of neurons within the central nervous system that receives information, processes and integrates that information, then transmits it to some other destination

Neurotransmitter (noo-roh-TRANS-mit-ter) A chemical substance that is released at the axon terminals to stimulate a muscle fiber contraction or an impulse in another neuron

Neutron (NOO-tron) An electrically neutral particle found in the nucleus of an atom

Neutrophil (NOO-troh-fill) A type of white blood cell that has granules in the cytoplasm that stain with acid and basic dyes and is capable of phagocytosis

Nociceptor (noh-see-SEP-tor) A sensory receptor that responds to tissue damage; pain receptor

Node of Ranvier (NODE OF rahn-vee-AY) Short space between two segments of myelin in a myelinated nerve fiber

Nonessential amino acids (NON-ee-sen-chul ah-MEEN-oh AS-ids) Amino acids that can be synthesized in the human body

Nonspecific resistance (non-speh-SIF-ik ree-SIS-tans) Body's ability to counteract all types of harmful agents

Noradrenalin (nor-ah-DREN-ah-lihn) A hormone secreted by the adrenal medulla that produces effects similar to epinephrine and the sympathetic nervous system; neurotransmitter released by some neurons in the sympathetic nervous system; also called norepinephrine

Norepinephrine (nor-ep-ih-NEFF-rihn) A hormone secreted by the adrenal medulla that produces effects similar to epinephrine and the sympathetic nervous system; neurotransmitter released by some neurons in the sympathetic nervous system; also called noradrenaline

Nostrils (NAHS-trils) Openings through which air enters the nasal cavity; external nares

Nucleolus (noo-KLEE-oh-lus) A dense, dark staining body within the nucleus; contains a high concentration of RNA

Nucleoplasm (NOO-klee-oh-plazm) The fluid inside the nucleus of a cell

Nucleotide (NOO-klee-oh-tide) Building block of nucleic acids; consists of a pentose sugar, an organic nitrogenous base, and a phosphate group

Nucleus (NOO-klee-us) Largest structure within the cell; contains the DNA

Nutrient (NOO-tree-ent) A chemical substance that provides energy, forms new body components, or assists in the metabolic processes of the body

Nutrient foramen (NOO-tree-ent for-A-men) Small opening in the diaphysis of bone for passage of blood vessels

Nutrition (noo-TRIH-shun) Science that studies the relationship of food to the functioning of the living organism; acquisition, assimilation, and utilization of nutrients contained in food

Occipital (ahk-SIP-ih-tal) Pertaining to the lower portion of the back of the head

Occipital bone (ahk-SIP-ih-tal BONE) Bone that forms the back of the skull and the base of the cranium

Oculomotor nerve (ahk-yoo-loh-MOH-tor NERV) Cranial nerve III; motor nerve; controls eye movements

Odontoid (oh-DON-toyd) Tooth-shaped projection on the second cervical vertebra; also called dens

Olfaction (ohl-FAK-shun) Sense of smell

Olfactory (ohl-FAK-toar-ee) Relating to the sense of smell

Olfactory bulb (ohl-FAK-toar-ee BULB) Mass of gray matter on either side of the crista galli of the ethmoid bone where olfactory neurons synapse

Olfactory cortex (ohl-FAK-toar-ee KOR-teks) Region in the temporal lobe where the sense of smell is interpreted

Olfactory epithelium (ohl-FAK-toar-ee ep-ih-THEE-lee-um) Tissue in the mucous membrane of the upper portion of the nasal cavity; contains bipolar neurons and supporting cells

Olfactory nerve (ohl-FAK-toar-ee NERV) Cranial nerve I; sensory nerve; responsible for the sense of smell

Olfactory neuron (ohl-FAK-toar-ee NOO-ron) Bipolar neuron in the upper portion of the nasal cavity that converts odors into neural signals

Olfactory tract (ohl-FAK-toar-ee TRACT) A bundle of axons that ex-

tends from the olfactory bulb to the cortex in the temporal lobe where the sense of smell is interpreted

Oligodendrocyte (ah-lee-go-DEN-droh-site) A neuroglial cell that produces myelin within the central nervous system

Oogenesis (oh-oh-JEN-eh-sis) Process of meiosis in the female in which one ovum and three polar bodies are produced from one primary oocyte

Oogonia (oh-oh-GO-nee-ah) Stem cells that give rise to ova or egg cells

Ophthalmic (off-THAL-mik) Pertaining to the eyes

Opsin (OP-sin) The protein component of the pigment in the rods

Optic chiasma (OP-tik kye-AZ-mah) Region, just anterior to the pituitary gland, where the right and left optic nerves meet and some fibers cross over to the opposite side

Optic disk (OP-tik DISK) Area in the retina where the optic nerve fibers leave the eye and there are no rods and cones; also called the blind spot

Optic nerve (OP-tik NERV) Cranial nerve II; sensory nerve; conducts visual information to the brain

Optic radiations (OP-tik ray-dee-AY-shuns) Nerve fibers in the visual pathway between the thalamus and the visual cortex in the occipital lobe

Optic tract (OP-tik TRAKT) Bundles of fibers in the visual pathway between the optic chiasma and the thalamus

Oral (OH-ral or AW-ral) Pertaining to the mouth

Organ (OR-gan) Group of tissues that work together to perform a specific function

Organ of Corti (OR-gan of KOAR-tee) The organ of hearing, consisting of supporting cells and hair cells that rest on the basilar membrane and project into the endolymph of the cochlear duct; also called spiral organ

Organelles (or-guh-NELZ) Little organs; highly organized structures suspended in the cytoplasm that are specialized to perform specific cellular activities

Organism (OR-gan-izm) A living entity

Organogenesis (or-gan-oh-JEN-eh-sis) The process of organ formation in the embryo

Origin (OR-ih-jin) The end of a muscle that is attached to a relatively immovable part; the end opposite the insertion

Oropharynx (or-oh-FAIR-inks) Portion of the pharynx that is posterior to the oral cavity and extends from the uvula to the level of the hyoid bone

Osmosis (os-MOH-sis) Diffusion of water through a selectively permeable membrane

Osseous tissue (AS-see-us TISH-yoo) Bone tissue; rigid connective tissue

Ossification (ah-sih-fih-KAY-shun) Formation of bone; also called osteogenesis

Osteoblast (AH-stee-oh-blast) Bone-forming cell

Osteoclast (AH-stee-oh-clast) Cell that destroys or resorbs bone tissue

Osteocyte (AH-stee-oh-syte) Mature bone cell

Osteogenesis (AH-stee-oh-jen-eh-sis) Formation of bone; also called ossification

Osteon (AH-stee-ahn) Structural unit of bone; haversian system

Osteonic canal (AH-stee-ahn-ik kah-NAL) Central canal in an osteon, contains blood vessels and nerves; also called haversian canal

Otic (OH-tik) Pertaining to the ears

Otoliths (OH-toh-liths) Calcium carbonate particles associated with the macula in the utricle and saccule in the inner ear; involved with static equilibrium

Oval window (OH-val WIN-dow) Small opening between the middle ear and the inner ear where the stapes fits; also called the fenestra vestibuli

Ovarian follicle (oh-VAIR-ee-an FAHL-ih-kul) An oocyte surrounded by one or more layers of cells within the ovaries

Ovarian cycle (oh-VAIR-ee-an SYE-kul) Monthly cycle of events that occur in the ovary from puberty to menopause; occurs concurrently with the uterine cycle

Ovaries (OH-vah-reez) Primary reproductive organs in the female; produce the ova or eggs

Oviducts (OH-vih-dukts) The tubes that extend laterally from the upper portion of the uterus to the region of the ovaries; also called uterine tubes or fallopian tubes

Ovulation (ah-vyoo-LAY-shun) The release of a secondary oocyte from a mature follicle at the surface of an ovary

Oxygen debt (AHKS-ee-jen DET) The amount of oxygen that must be supplied after physical exercise to convert the accumulated lactic acid into glucose

Oxyhemoglobin (ahk-see-HEE-moh-gloh-bin) Compound that is formed when oxygen binds with hemoglobin; form in which most of the oxygen is transported in the blood

Oxytocin (ahk-see-TOH-sin) Hormone produced by the hypothalamus and secreted from the posterior pituitary gland that causes uterine muscle contraction and ejection of milk from the lactating breast

P wave Deflection on an electrocardiogram that corresponds to atrial depolarization

Pacinian corpuscle (pah-SIN-ee-an KOAR-pus-al) A sensory receptor deep in the dermis of the skin that detects pressure on the surface; also called a lamellated corpuscle

Palate (PAL-at) Floor of the nasal cavity, which separates the nasal cavity from the oral cavity

Palatine (PAL-ah-tyne) Bone that forms a portion of the roof of the mouth

Palmar (PAWL-mar) Pertaining to the palm of the hand

Pancreas (PAN-kree-ahs) A glandular organ in the abdominal cavity that has both exocrine and endocrine functions; the exocrine portion consists of acinar cells, the endocrine portion is the islets of Langerhans

Pancreatic islets (pan-kree-AT-ik EYE-lets) Endocrine portion of the pancreas; consist of alpha cells that secrete glucagon and beta cells that secrete insulin

Papillary layer (PAP-ih-lair-ee LAY-er) Upper layer of the dermis

Papillary muscle (PAP-ih-lair-ee MUSS-el) Projections of cardiac muscle that extend inward from the heart wall into the chamber of the ventricle

Parasagittal plane (pair-ah-SAJ-ih-tal PLANE) A sagittal plane that is not in the midline

Parasympathetic division (pair-ah-sim-pah-THET-ik dih-VIH-shun) One of two divisions of the autonomic nervous system; primarily concerned with processes that involve the conservation and restoration of energy; sometimes referred to as the "rest and repose" division; also called the craniosacral division

Parathyroid glands (pair-ah-THIGH-royd GLANDS) A set of small glands embedded on the posterior aspect of the thyroid gland

Parathyroid hormone (PTH) (pair-ah-THIGH-royd HOAR-moan) Hormone secreted by the parathyroid glands that functions to increase blood calcium levels; also called parathormone

Paraurethral glands (pair-ah-yoo-REE-thral GLANDS) Mucus-secreting glands located on each side of the urethral orifice in the female; also called Skene's glands

Paravertebral ganglion (pair-ah-ver-TEE-brull GANG-lee-on) A chain of autonomic ganglia, the sympathetic chain, that extends longitudinally along each side of the vertebral column; a region of synapse between the two neurons in a sympathetic pathway

Parietal (pah-RYE-eh-tal) Pertains to the wall of a body cavity

Parietal bone (pah-RYE-eh-tal bone) Bone of the cranium immediately posterior to the frontal bone; forms the top of the head

Parietal cells (pah-RYE-eh-tal SELZ) Cells in the gastric mucosa that secrete hydrochloric acid and intrinsic factor

Parietal pericardium (pah-RYE-eh-tal pair-ih-KAR-dee-um) Layer of serous membrane that lines the fibrous sac around the heart

Parturition (par-too-RIH-shun) Act of giving birth to an infant

Passive immunity (PASS-iv ih-MYOO-nih-tee) Immunity that results when an individual receives the immune agents from some source other than his or her own body

Passive transport (PASS-iv TRANS-port) Membrane transport process that does not require cellular energy

Patella (pah-TELL-ah) Kneecap

Pectoral (PEK-toh-ral) Pertaining to the chest region

Pedal (PED-al) Pertaining to the foot

Pelvic (PEL-vik) Pertaining to the inferior region of the abdominopelvic cavity; lower portion of the trunk

Pelvic cavity (PEL-vik KAV-ih-tee) Inferior portion of the abdominopelvic cavity; contains the urinary bladder, part of the large intestine, and internal reproductive organs

Penile urethra (PEE-nye-al yoo-REE-thrah) Portion of the male urethra that is surrounded by corpus spongiosum and passes through the length of the penis; also called spongy urethra

Peptidase (PEP-tih-days) An enzyme that acts on protein segments called peptides

Peptide bond (PEP-tide BOND) The chemical bond that forms between two amino acids

Pericardial sac (pair-ih-KAR-dee-al SAK) Loose-fitting sac surrounding the heart that consists of fibrous connective tissue lined with a serous membrane

Pericardial cavity (pair-ih-KAR-dee-al KAV-ih-tee) Potential space between the parietal pericardium and visceral pericardium that contains a small amount of serous fluid for lubrication

Pericardium (pair-ih-KAR-dee-um) Membrane that surrounds the heart; usually refers to the pericardial sac

Perichondrium (pair-ih-KAHN-dree-um) Connective tissue covering that surrounds cartilage

Perilymph (PAIR-ih-limf) Fluid inside the bony labyrinth but outside the membranous labyrinth of the inner ear

Perimetrium (pair-ih-MEE-tree-um) Outermost layer of the uterus, which is visceral peritoneum

Perimysium (pair-ih-MY-see-um) Fibrous connective tissue that surrounds a bundle, or fasciculus, of muscle fibers (cells)

Perineal (pair-ih-NEE-al) Pertaining to the region between the anus and pubic symphysis; includes the region of the external reproductive organs

Perineurium (pair-ih-NOO-ree-um) Fibrous connective tissue that surrounds a bundle, or fasciculus, of nerve fibers

Periosteum (pair-ee-AH-stee-um) The tough, white outer membrane that covers a bone and is essential for bone growth, repair, and nutrition

Peripheral nervous system (PNS) (per-IF-er-al NER-vus SIS-tem) The portion of the nervous system that is outside of the brain and spinal cord; consists of the nerves and ganglia

Peripheral resistance (per-IF-er-al ree-SIS-tans) Opposition to blood flow caused by friction of the blood vessel walls

Perirenal fat (pair-ih-REE-nal FAT) Capsule of adipose tissue that surrounds and protects the kidney

Peristalsis (pair-ih-STALL-sis) Rhythmic contractions of the intestines that move food along the digestive tract

Peritoneum (pair-ih-toe-NEE-um) Serous membrane associated with the abdominopelvic cavity

Peritubular capillaries (pair-ih-TOOB-yoo-lar KAP-ih-lair-eez) Extensive capillary network around the tubular portions of the nephrons in the kidneys

Permanent teeth (PER-mah-nent TEETH) The teeth that replace the deciduous teeth; also called secondary teeth

Pernicious anemia (per-NISH-us ah-NEE-mee-ah) A type of anemia that is caused by a deficiency of intrinsic factor

Phagocytosis (fag-oh-sye-TOH-sis) Cell eating; a form of endocytosis in which solid particles are taken into the cell

Phalanges (fah-LAN-jeez) Bones of the fingers and toes; singular is phalanx (fah-LANKS)

Pharynx (FAIR-inks) Passageway for air and food that extends from the base of the skull to the larynx and esophagus; throat

Phospholipid (fahs-foh-LIP-id) A fat molecule that contains phosphates; an important constituent of cell membranes

Photoreceptor (foh-toh-ree-SEP-tor) A sensory receptor that detects light; located in the retina of the eye

Physiology (fiz-ee-AHL-oh-jee) Study of the functions of living organisms and their parts

Pia mater (PEE-ah MAY-ter) The innermost layer of the coverings around the brain and spinal cord; literally means "soft mother"

Pineal body (PYE-nee-al BAH-dee) A region of the epithalamus in the diencephalon that is thought to be involved with regulating the "biological clock"; also called the pineal gland because it secretes melatonin

Pineal gland See pineal body

Pinealocytes (PYE-nee-al-oh-cytes) Secretory cells of the pineal body; secrete melatonin

Pinna (PIN-nah) Visible portion of the external ear; also called the auricle

Pinocytosis (pin-oh-sye-TOH-sis) Cell drinking; a form of endocytosis in which fluid droplets are taken into the cell

Pituitary gland (pih-TOO-ih-tair-ee GLAND) Endocrine gland located in the sella turcica of the sphenoid bone, near the base of the brain; also called the hypophysis

Placenta (plah-SEN-tah) Structure that anchors the developing fetus to the uterus and provides for the exchange of gases, nutrients, and waste products between the maternal and fetal circulations

Plantar (PLAN-tar) Pertaining to the sole of the foot

Plantar flexion (PLAN-tar FLEK-shun) A movement at the ankle that increases the angle between the foot and leg; opposite of dorsiflexion

Plasma (PLAZ-mah) Liquid portion of blood

Plasma cell (PLAZ-mah SELL) A cell that develops from an activated B lymphocyte and produces antibodies

Platelet (PLATE-let) A formed element in the blood that functions in blood clotting; also called a thrombocyte

Platelet plug (PLATE-let PLUG) Accumulation of platelets at the site of blood vessel damage to prevent blood loss

Pleura (PLOO-rah) Serous membrane that surrounds the lungs; consists of a parietal layer and a visceral layer

Pleural cavity (PLOO-ral KAV-ih-tee) The small space between the parietal and visceral layers of the pleura

Plexus (PLEK-sus) A complex network of blood vessels or nerves

Plicae circulares (PLY-kee sir-kyoo-LAIR-eez) Circular folds in the mucosa and submucosa of the small intestine

Pneumotaxic center (noo-moh-TACK-sik SEN-ter) A group of neurons in the pons that affects the rate of respiration by inhibiting inspiration

Polar body (POH-lar BAH-dee) A small cell resulting from the unequal division of cytoplasm during the meiotic division of an oocyte

Polar covalent bond (POH-lar koh-VAY-lent BOND) An unequal sharing of electrons in a covalent bond

Polysaccharide (pahl-ee-SAK-ah-ride) A substance that consists of long chains of monosaccharides linked together; starch, cellulose, glycogen

Pons (PONZ) Middle portion of the brain stem, between the midbrain and the medulla oblongata

Popliteal (pop-LIT-ee-al or pop-lih-TEE-al) Pertaining to the area behind the knee

Postcentral gyrus (post-SEN-trull JYE-rus) The convolution of the brain surface immediately posterior to the central sulcus; this is the primary sensory area of the brain

Posterior (pos-TEER-ee-or) Toward the back or dorsal surface; opposite of anterior or ventral

Postganglionic fiber (post-gang-lee-AHN-ik FYE-ber) The axon that transmits impulses from a cell body in an autonomic ganglion to an effector organ

Postganglionic neuron (post-gang-lee-AHN-ik NOO-ron) A neuron that conducts impulses from an autonomic ganglion to an effector organ

Postnatal development (POST-nay-tal dee-VELL-op-ment) Development that begins with birth and lasts until death

Postsynaptic membrane (post-sih-NAP-tik MEM-brayn) The membrane that receives an impulse at a synapse

Postsynaptic neuron (post-sih-NAP-tik NOO-ron) The neuron that receives an impulse from an adjacent neuron in neuron-to-neuron communication; the neuron after the synapse

Precentral gyrus (pree-SEN-trull JYE-rus) The convolution of the brain surface immediately anterior to the central sulcus; this is the primary motor area of the brain

Preembryonic period (pree-em-bree-AHN-ik PEER-ee-ud) First 2 weeks after fertilization; period of cleavage, implantation, and formation of primary germ layers

Preganglionic fiber (pree-gang-lee-AHN-ik FYE-ber) The axon that transmits impulses from a cell body in the central nervous system to an autonomic ganglion where it synapses with a second neuron

Preganglionic neuron (pree-gang-lee-AHN-ik NOO-ron) A neuron that conducts impulses from the central nervous system to an autonomic ganglion

Pregnancy (PREG-nan-see) Presence of a developing offspring in the uterus

Prenatal development (PREE-nay-tal dee-VELL-op-ment) Development within the uterus

Prepuce (PREE-pyoos) Fold of skin that covers the distal end of the penis; also called foreskin; fold of skin that covers the clitoris in females

Presynaptic neuron (pree-sih-NAP-tik NOO-ron) The neuron that transmits an impulse to an adjacent neuron in neuron-to-neuron communication; the neuron before the synapse

Primary response (PRY-mair-ee ree-SPONS) The initial reaction of the immune system to a specific antigen

Primary teeth (PRY-mair-ee TEETH) The teeth that appear first and then are shed and replaced by permanent teeth; also called deciduous teeth

Prime mover (PRYM MOO-ver) The muscle that is mainly responsible for a particular body movement; also called agonist

Process (PRAH-sess) Any projection on a bone, often pointed and sharp

Procoagulant (pro-koh-AG-yoo-lant)

A factor in the blood that promotes blood clotting

Progesterone (proh-JESS-ter-ohn) Hormone secreted by the corpus luteum of the ovaries; prepares the uterine lining for implantation, maintains pregnancy, and prepares mammary glands for lactation

Prolactin (pro-LAK-tin) Hormone secreted by the anterior pituitary gland during pregnancy to stimulate mammary gland development for lactation

Pronation (pro-NAY-shun) Movement of the forearm that turns the palm of the hand toward the back or downward; opposite of supination

Prophase (PRO-faze) First stage of mitosis; stage of mitosis during which the chromosomes become visible

Proprioception (proh-pree-oh-SEP-shun) Sense of position, or orientation, and movement

Proprioceptor (proh-pree-oh-SEP-tor) A type of mechanoreceptor located in muscles, tendons, and joints that provides information about body position and movements

Prostaglandins (prahss-tih-GLAN-dins) A group of substances, derived from fatty acids, that are produced in small amounts and have an immediate, short-term, localized effect; sometimes called local hormones

Prostate gland (PRAHS-tayt GLAND) Accessory gland that is located below the urinary bladder in males and surrounds the proximal portion of the urethra; product is part of the seminal fluid

Prostatic urethra (prah-STAT-ik yoo-REE-thrah) Portion of the male urethra that passes through the prostate gland

Protein (PRO-teen) An organic compound that contains nitrogen and consists of chains of amino acids linked together by peptide bonds

Prothrombin (pro-THROM-bin) A protein that is produced by the liver and released into the blood where it is converted to thrombin during the process of blood clotting

Prothrombin activator (pro-THROM-bin AK-tih-vay-tor) A substance that is produced in the process of blood clotting, which functions to change prothrombin into thrombin

Proton (PRO-ton) A positively charged particle found in the nucleus of an atom

Proximal (PRAHK-sih-mal) Next or nearest; closer to a point of attachment; opposite of distal

Puberty (PYOO-ber-tee) Period during which secondary sex characteristics begin to appear and capability for sexual reproduction becomes possible

Pubis (PYOO-biss) One of the parts of the hip bone

Pudendum (pyoo-DEN-dum) Collective term for the external accessory structures of the female reproductive system; also called the vulva

Pulmonary semilunar valve (PULL-mon-air-ee seh-mee-LOO-nar VALVE) Valve between the right ventricle and pulmonary trunk that keeps blood from flowing back into the ventricle

Pulmonary trunk (PULL-mon-air-ee TRUNK) Large vessel that receives deoxygenated blood from the right ventricle

Pulmonary vessels (PULL-mon-air-ee VES-els) Blood vessels that transport blood from the heart to the lungs and then return it to the left atrium

Pulse (PULS) Expansion and recoil of arteries caused by contraction and relaxion of the heart

Pulse points (PULS POYNTZ) Where the pulse can be palpated; where an artery passes over a bone or other firm base near the surface

Pulse pressure (PULS PRESH-ur) Difference between systolic and diastolic pressures

Pupil (PYOO-pill) The hole in the center of the iris through which light enters the posterior part of the eye

Purkinje fibers (per-KIN-jee FYE-bers) Cardiac muscle cells specialized for conducting action potentials to the myocardium; part of the conduction system of the heart; also called conduction myofibers

Pyramidal tract (pih-RAM-ih-dal TRAKT) Descending, or motor, tract in the spinal cord; also called the corticospinal tract

Pyrogen (PYE-roh-jen) A chemical agent in inflammation that causes an increase in temperature

Pyruvic acid (pye-ROO-vik AS-id) A molecule with three carbons that is produced in glycolysis

QRS complex Deflection on an electrocardiogram that reflects ventricular depolarization

Radius (RAY-dee-us) Bone on the lateral side of the forearm

Ramus (RAY-mus) Vertical portion of the mandible

Reactant (ree-AK-tant) Initial substance that is changed during a chemical reaction

Reflex arc (REE-fleks ARK) Smallest unit of the nervous system that can receive a stimulus and generate a response; functional unit of the nervous system

Refraction (ree-FRAK-shun) The bending of light as it passes from one medium to another

Refractory period (ree-FRAK-toar-ee PEE-ree-od) Time during which an excitable cell cannot respond to a stimulus that is usually adequate to start an action potential

Regeneration (ree-jen-er-A-shun) Replacement of damaged tissue cells with cells that are identical to the original ones

Relative refractory period (RELL-ah-tiv ree-FRAK-toar-ee PEE-ree-od) Time during which an excitable cell can respond to a second stimulus only if the second stimulus is stronger than that normally required to start an action potential

Renal capsule (REE-nal KAP-sool) Fibrous connective tissue covering around the kidney

Renal corpuscle (REE-nal KOAR-pu-sel) Portion of the nephron where filtration occurs; consists of a glomerulus and glomerular capsule

Renal cortex (REE-nal KOAR-teks) Outer portion of the kidney that appears granular

Renal erythropoietin factor (REE-nal ee-rith-roh-poy-EE-tin FAK-tor) A substance produced by the kidneys that activates erythropoietin to stimulate the production of erythrocytes

Renal medulla (REE-nal meh-DOO-lah) Inner portion of the kidney consisting of renal pyramids

Renal papillae (REE-nal pah-PILL-ee) Pointed ends of the renal pyramids that are directed toward the center of the kidney

Renal pelvis (REE-nal PELL-vis) Large cavity in the central region of a kidney that collects the urine as it is produced

Renal pyramids (REE-nal PEER-ah-mids) Triangular-shaped regions in the kidney that appear striated

Renal sinus (REE-nal SYE-nus) Cavity within the kidney that contains the renal pelvis and branches of the renal vessels

Renal tubule (REE-nal TOOB-yool) Tubular portion of the nephron that carries the filtrate away from the glomerular capsule and where tubular reabsorption and secretion occurs

Renin (REE-nin) An enzyme secreted by the kidneys that functions in blood pressure regulation by stimulating the formation of angiotensin

Reproductive (ree-pro-DUK-tiv) Relating to reproduction

Residual volume (RV) (ree-ZID-yoo-al VAHL-yoom) Amount of air that remains in the lungs after a maximum expiration

Resistance (ree-SIS-tans) Body's ability to counteract the effects of pathogens and other harmful agents

Respiration (res-per-Ray-shun) Exchange of oxygen and carbon dioxide between the atmosphere and the body cells

Respiratory (reh-SPY-rah-tor-ee or res-per-ah-TOR-ee) Relating to respiration

Respiratory membrane (reh-SPY-rah-tor-ee MEM-brayn) Surfaces in the lungs where diffusion occurs; consists of the layers that the gases must pass through to get into or out of the alveoli

Rete testis (REE-tee TEST-is) Network of tubules on one side of the testis

Reticular layer (ree-TIK-yoo-lur layer) Lower layer of the dermis; collagenous fibers in this region provide strength to the skin

Retina (RET-ih-nah) The innermost layer of the eyeball; also called the nervous tunic; contains the photoreceptor cells for vision

Retinal (RET-ih-nal) A derivative of vitamin A that is a component of rhodopsin and is involved in reactions that trigger nerve impulses that result in vision

Rhodopsin (roh-DAHP-sin) Photosensitive pigment in the rods; also called visual purple

Ribonucleic acid (RNA) (rye-boh-noo-KLEE-ik AS-id) A nucleic acid that contains ribose sugar; functions in protein synthesis

Ribosomal RNA (rRNA) (RYE-boh-soh-mal RNA) RNA in the ribosomes in the cytoplasm; functions in protein synthesis

Ribosome (RYE-boh-sohm) Granules of RNA in the cytoplasm that function in protein synthesis

Right ventricle (RYTE VEN-trih-kul) Chamber of the heart that pumps deoxygenated blood through the pulmonary trunk to the lungs

Right lymphatic duct (ryte lim-FAT-ik DUKT) The collecting duct of the lymphatic system that collects lymph from the upper right quadrant of the body

Right atrium (RYTE AY-tree-um) Chamber of the heart that receives deoxygenated blood from coronary circulation through the coronary sinus and from systemic circulation through the superior vena cava and inferior vena cava

Rod (RAHD) A photoreceptor in the retina that is specialized for vision in dim light

Rotation (roh-TAY-shun) Movement of a part around its own axis in a pivot joint

Rough endoplasmic reticulum (RUFF end-oh-PLAZ-mik ree-TIK-yoo-lum) Endoplasmic reticulum that has ribosomes attached to it

Round window (ROWND WIN-dow) Small, membrane-covered opening between the middle ear and the inner ear, just below the oval window; also called the fenestrae cochlea

Rugae (ROO-jee) Longitudinal folds in the mucosa of the stomach

Saccule (SAK-yool) One of the divisions of the membranous labyrinth located in the vestibule of the inner ear, involved with static equilibrium

Sacral (SAY-kral) Pertaining to the posterior region between the hipbones

Sacrum (SAY-krum) Triangular structure, composed of five vertebrae fused together, that forms the base of the vertebral column

Sagittal plane (SAJ-ih-tal plane) A vertical plane that divides the body or organ into right and left portions

Saltatory conduction (SAL-tah-toar-ee kon-DUCK-shun) Process in which a nerve impulse travels along a myelinated nerve fiber by jumping from one node of Ranvier to the next

Sarcolemma (sar-koh-LEM-mah) The cell membrane of a muscle fiber (cell)

Sarcomere (SAR-koh-meer) A functional contractile unit in a skeletal muscle fiber

Sarcoplasm (SAR-koh-plazm) Cytoplasm of muscle fibers (cells)

Sarcoplasmic reticulum (sar-koh-PLAZ-mik ree-TICK-yoo-lum) Network of tubules and sacs in muscle cells; similar to endoplasmic reticulum in other cells

Satellite cell (sat-eh-LYTE SEL) Cell that binds neuron cell bodies together in peripheral ganglia

Scala tympani (SKAY-lah TIM-pah-nee) Lower portion of the cochlea, inferior to the basilar membrane, contains perilymph, and extends from the apex to the round window

Scala vestibuli (SKAY-lah ves-TIB-yoo-lee) Portion of the cochlea that is superior to the vestibular membrane, contains perilymph, and extends from the oval window to the apex

Scapula (SKAP-yoo-lah) Shoulder blade

Schwann's cells (SHVONZ SELZ) Large cells that wrap around nerve fibers in the peripheral nervous system and, in some cases, produce myelin

Sclera (SKLEE-rah) White outer coat of the posterior part of the eyeball; posterior portion of the fibrous tunic

Scrotum (SKROH-tum) A pouch of skin and subcutaneous tissue that extends below the abdomen and contains the testes

Sebaceous gland (see-BAY-shus gland) An oil gland of the skin, which produces sebum or body oil

Secondary response (SEK-on-dair-ee ree-SPONS) Rapid and intense reaction to antigens on second and subsequent exposures due to memory cells

Secondary teeth (SEK-on-dair-ee TEETH) The permanent teeth that replace the deciduous teeth; also called permanent teeth

Secretin (see-KREE-tin) A hormone that is produced in the small intestine and stimulates the pancreas to secrete a fluid with a high bicarbonate ion concentration

Selectively permeable (sel-EK-tiv-lee PER-me-ah-bul) Restricts the passage of some substances but permits the passage of other substances

Sella turcica (SELL-ah TUR-sih-kah) Depression on the superior surface of the sphenoid bone that houses the pituitary gland

Semen (SEE-men) Mixture of sperm cells and secretions from the accessory glands in the male; also called seminal fluid

Semicircular canals (seh-mee-SIR-kew-lar kah-NALS) Three curved passageways in the bony labyrinth of the inner ear, filled with perilymph and containing the membranous semicircular ducts

Semicircular ducts (seh-mee-SIR-kew-lar DUKTS) Three curved membranous channels located within the bony labyrinth of the inner ear, filled with endolymph and surrounded by perilymph; function in dynamic equilibrium

Semilunar valve (seh-mee-LOO-nar

VALVE) Valve between a ventricle of the heart and the vessel that carries blood away from the ventricle; also pertains to the valves in veins

Seminal vesicles (SEM-ih-nal VES-ih-kulz) Accessory glands located posterior to the urinary bladder in the male; secretion accounts for 60 percent of the semen volume

Seminal fluid (SEM-ih-nal FLOO-id) Mixture of sperm cells and secretions from the accessory glands in the male; also called semen

Seminiferous tubules (seh-mih-NIFF-er-us TOOB-yools) Tightly coiled structures within which sperm are produced in the testes

Senescence (seh-NESS-ens) Period of old age

Sensory nerve (SEN-soar-ee nerv) A nerve that contains primarily sensory, or afferent, fibers

Sensory neuron (SEN-soar-ee NOO-ron) Nerve cell that carries impulses toward the central nervous system from the periphery; afferent neuron

Serosa (see-ROS-ah) Epithelial membranes that secrete a serous fluid and line the closed body cavities and cover the organs within those cavities; also called serous membranes

Serotonin (sair-oh-TONE-in) One of several neurotransmitters

Serous cell (SEER-us SEL) Glandular cell that secretes a watery fluid, usually with a high enzyme content

Serous membrane (SEER-us MEM-brayn) Epithelial membrane that secretes a serous fluid and lines the closed body cavities and covers the organs within those cavities; also called serosa

Sertoli's cells (sir-TOH-leez SELZ) Cells within the seminiferous tubules that do not produce gametes but support and nourish the gamete-producing cells; also called supporting cells

Serum (SEE-rum) The fluid that remains after a blood clot has formed; plasma minus the clotting factors

Sesamoid bone (SEH-sah-moyd bone) A small bone, usually found in a tendon

Shell temperature (SHELL TEM-per-ah-chur) The temperature at or near the body surface

Simple epithelium (SIM-pul ep-ih-THEE-lee-um) Epithelial tissue that is only one layer thick

Simple series circuit (SIM-pull SEER-ees SIR-cut) The simplest conduction pathway in which a single neuron synapses with another neuron

Sinoatrial node (sye-noh-AY-tree-al NODE) Mass of specialized cardiac muscle cells that form a part of the conduction system of the heart and that are located in the right atrium near the opening for the superior vena cava; often referred to as the pacemaker of the heart

Sinus (SYE-nus) A cavity or hollow space in a bone or other body part

Skeletal muscle (SKEL-eh-tal MUS-el) Muscle that is under voluntary or willed control; also called voluntary striated muscle

Skeletal (SKEL-eh-tal) Relating to the bones of the body

Smooth muscle (SMOOTH MUS-el) Muscle tissue that is neither striated nor controlled voluntarily; also called visceral muscle

Smooth endoplasmic reticulum (SMOOTH end-o-PLAZ-mik ree-TICK-yoo-lum) Endoplasmic reticulum that does not have ribosomes attached to it and appears smooth

Soft palate (SOFT PAL-at) Posterior portion of the floor of the nasal cavity and roof of the mouth that consists of soft tissue and has no bony support

Solute (SOL-yoot) A substance that is dissolved in a solution

Solvent (SOL-vent) Fluid in which substances dissolve

Somatic nervous system (soh-MAT-ik NER-vus SIS-tem) The portion of the peripheral efferent nervous system consisting of motor neurons that control voluntary actions of skeletal muscles

Somatic sense (soh-MAT-ik sens) A general sense that is not localized but is found throughout the body; includes touch, pressure, temperature, and pain

Somatomotor cortex (soh-mat-oh-MOH-ter KOR-teks) The primary motor area of the brain, which is located in the precentral gyrus

Somatosensory cortex (soh-mat-oh-SEN-soar-ee KOR-teks) The primary sensory area of the brain, which is located in the postcentral gyrus

Somatotropic hormone (STH) (soh-mat-oh-TROH-pik HOAR-moan) A hormone secreted by the anterior pituitary gland that influences the rate of skeletal growth; also called growth hormone

Specific resistance (speh-SIF-ik ree-SIS-tans) Body's ability to counteract certain types of harmful agents; immunity

Spermatic cord (spur-MAT-ik KORD) Composite structure that contains the ductus deferens, blood vessels, nerves, lymphatic vessels, and the cremaster muscle

Spermatids (SPUR-mah-tids) Haploid cells that are the product of meiosis in the male (spermatogenesis)

Spermatogenesis (spur-mat-oh-JEN-eh-sis) Process of meiosis in the male in which four spermatids are produced from one primary spermatocyte

Spermatogonia (spur-mat-oh-GOH-nee-ah) Stem cells that give rise to sperm cells

Spermiogenesis (spur-mee-oh-JEN-eh-sis) Morphologic changes that transform a spermatid into a mature sperm

Sphenoid bone (SFEE-noyd bone) Bone that forms a portion of the cranial floor

Sphygmomanometer (sfig-moh-mah-NAHM-eh-ter) Device for measuring blood pressures

Spinal cavity (SPY-nal cavity) Part of the dorsal body cavity that contains the spinal cord

Spindle fibers (SPIN-dul FYE-burs) Microtubules that extend from the centromeres to the centrioles during cell division

Spinothalamic tract (spy-noh-thah-LAM-ik TRACT) Ascending, or sensory, tract that begins in the spinal cord and conducts impulses to the thalamus

Spirometer (spy-RAHM-eh-ter) An instrument used to measure the volume of air that moves into and out of the lungs

Spleen (SPLEEN) Large lymphoid organ that filters blood and acts as a reservoir for blood

Splenic flexure (SPLEH-nik FLEK-shur) Curve between the transverse colon and the descending colon; also called the left colonic flexure

Spongy urethra (SPUN-jee yoo-REE-thrah) Portion of the male urethra that is surrounded by corpus spongiosum and passes through the length of the penis; also called penile urethra

Squamous (SKWAY-mus) Flat, plate-like, scalelike; horizontal dimension is greater than vertical dimension

Stapes (STAY-peez) One of the tiny bones in the middle ear, adjacent to the oval window

Starch Complex polysaccharide that is the storage form of energy in plants

Starling's law of the heart Principle that the more cardiac muscle fibers are stretched, the greater the contraction strength of the heart

Static equilibrium (STAT-ik ee-kwi-LIB-ree-um) Sensing and evaluating the position of the head relative to gravity

Sternal (STIR-nal) Pertaining to the anterior midline of the thorax

Sternum (STIR-num) Breastbone

Stimulus (STIM-yoo-lus) Any agent that produces a reaction in a receptor or excitable (irritable) tissue

Straight tubule (STRAYT TOOB-yool) Single tube from each lobule of the testes that leads into the rete testis

Stratified epithelium (STRAT-ih-fyed ep-ih-THEE-lee-um) Epithelial tissue that has multiple layers of cells

Stratum basale (STRAY-tum BAY-sah-lee) Deepest layer of the epidermis, basal layer where the cells are actively mitotic; also deep layer of the endometrium that is constant and responsible for rebuilding the stratum functionale after menstruation

Stratum corium (STRAY-tum KOR-ee-um) Another name for the dermis

Stratum corneum (STRAY-tum KOR-nee-um) Outermost layer of the epidermis, consists of flattened, dead, keratinized cells

Stratum functionale (STRAY-tum FUNK-shun-al-ee) Portion of the endometrium that is sloughed off during menstruation

Stratum germinativum (STRAY-tum JER-mih-nah-tiv-um) Term used for combined stratum basale and stratum spinosum in the epidermis

Stratum granulosum (STRAY-tum gran-yoo-LOH-sum) Epidermal layer in which keratinization begins and cells appear granular; "granular layer"

Stratum lucidum (STRAY-tum LOO-sih-dum) Epidermal layer in thick skin between the stratum corneum and stratum granulosum; "clear layer"

Stratum spinosum (STRAY-tum spy-NOH-sum) Epidermal layer directly above the stratum basale; cells appear "spiny"

Striae (STRY-ee) Streaks or bands; tiny white scars that appear when elastic fibers in the dermis are stretched too much; stretch marks

Striated muscle (STRY-ate-ed MUS-el) Muscle tissue that appears to have cross-bars; voluntary striated muscle is skeletal muscle and involuntary striated muscle is cardiac muscle

Stroke volume (STROAK VAHL-yoom) The volume of blood ejected from one ventricle during one contraction; normally about 70 mL

Subarachnoid space (sub-ah-RAK-noyd SPACE) The space between the arachnoid and pia mater layers of the meninges, which contains cerebrospinal fluid

Subcutaneous layer (sub-kyoo-TAY-nee-us layer) Below the skin; a sheet of areolar connective tissue and adipose beneath the dermis of the skin; also called hypodermis or superficial fascia

Subdural space (sub-DOO-ral SPACE) The space between the dura mater and arachnoid layers of the meninges

Subliminal stimulus (sub-LIM-ih-null STIM-yoo-lus) A weak stimulus that is of insufficient intensity to start a nerve impulse or muscle contraction; also called subthreshold stimulus

Submucosal plexus (sub-myoo-KOH-sal PLEK-sus) A network of autonomic nerves in the submucosa of the gastrointestinal tract; also called Meissner's plexus

Subthreshold stimulus (sub-THRESH-hold STIM-yoo-lus) A weak stimulus that is of insufficient intensity to start a nerve impulse or muscle contraction; also called subliminal stimulus

Sucrase (SOO-krays) An enzyme that acts on the disaccharide sucrose and breaks it into a molecule of glucose and a molecule of fructose

Sudoriferous gland (soo-door-IF-er-us GLAND) A gland in the skin that produces perspiration; also called sweat gland

Sulcus (SULL-kus) A groove or furrow between parts; often refers to the grooves between the convolutions on the surface of the brain; plural, sulci (SULL-see)

Superficial (soo-per-FISH-al) On or near the body surface; opposite of deep

Superior (soo-PEER-ee-or) Higher; one part is above another; opposite of inferior

Superior colliculi (soo-PEER-ee-or koh-LIK-yoo-lye) Two upper bodies of the corpora quadrigemina on the dorsal surface of the midbrain, which function in visual reflexes

Superior vena cava (soo-PEER-ee-or VEE-nah KAY-vah) Large vein that collects blood from all parts of the body superior to the heart and returns it to the right atrium

Supination (soo-pih-NAY-shun) Movement of the forearm that turns the palm of the hand toward the front or upward; opposite of pronation

Supporting cells (suh-POR-ting SELZ) Cells within the seminiferous tubules that do not produce gametes, but support and nourish the gamete-producing cells; also called Sertoli's cells

Suprarenal gland (soo-prah-REE-null GLAND) Endocrine gland that is located on the superior pole of each kidney; divided into cortex and medulla regions; also called adrenal gland

Surfactant (sir-FAK-tant) A substance produced by certain cells in lung tissue that reduces surface tension between fluid molecules that line the respiratory membrane and helps keep the alveolus from collapsing

Susceptibility (sus-sep-tih-BILL-ih-tee) Lack of resistance to disease

Suspensory ligament (sus-PEN-soar-ee LIG-ah-ment) Stringlike structures attached to the lens of the eye that hold the lens in place and function in accommodation for near vision

Sutural bone (SOO-cher-ahl BONE) A small bone located within a suture between certain cranial bones; also called a wormian bone

Suture (SOO-cher) An immovable fibrous joint between the flat bones in the skull

Sympathetic division (sim-pah-THET-ik dih-VIH-shun) One of the two divisions of the autonomic nervous system; primarily concerned with processes that involve the expenditure of energy; sometimes referred to as the "fight or flight" division; also called the thoracolumbar division

Synapse (SIN-aps) The region of communication between two neurons

Synaptic cleft (sih-NAP-tik KLEFT) Small space between the synaptic knob of a neuron and the cell membrane of an adjacent neuron or muscle cell

Synaptic knob (sih-NAP-tik NAHB) An enlargement at the distal end of telodendria, which contains vesicles of neurotransmitters

Synarthrosis (sin-ahr-THROH-sis) An immovable joint; plural, synarthroses

Synergist (SIN-er-jist) A muscle that assists a prime mover but is not capable of producing the movement by itself

Synovial fluid (sih-NOH-vee-al FLOO-id) Fluid secreted by the synovial membrane for lubrication of freely movable joints

Synovial membrane (sih-NOH-vee-al MEM-brayn) Membrane that lines the cavity of freely movable joints and secretes synovial fluid for lubrication

System (SIS-tem) A group of organs that work together to perform complex functions

Systemic vessels (sis-TEM-ik VES-els) Blood vessels that transport blood from the heart to all parts of the body and back to the right atrium

Systole (SIS-toh-lee) Contraction phase of the cardiac cycle; opposite of diastole

Systolic pressure (sis-TAHL-ik PRESH-ur) Blood pressure in the arteries during contraction of the ventricles

T wave Deflection on an electrocardiogram that reflects ventricular repolarization

T tubules (T TOOB-yools) Invaginations of the sarcolemma that form transverse tubules in a muscle cell and permit electrical impulses to travel deeper into the cell

T lymphocytes (T LIM-foh-sytes) Cells of the immune system that differentiate in the thymus gland and are responsible for cell-mediated immunity; T cells

Talus (TAL-us) Tarsal bone that articulates with the tibia

Target tissue (TAR-get TISH-yoo) A tissue (cells) that responds to a particular hormone because it has receptor sites for that hormone

Tarsal (TAHR-sal) Pertaining to the ankle and instep of the foot

Tarsus (TAHR-sis) Ankle

Taste hair (TAYST hair) Specialized projection of the gustatory cell that extends through the taste pore and functions in the sense of taste; also called gustatory hair

Tectorial membrane (tek-TOH-ree-al MEM-brayn) A gelatinous membrane over the hair cells of the organ of Corti in the cochlear duct

Telodendria (tell-oh-DEN-dree-ah) Short branches at the distal end of an axon or axon collateral

Telophase (TELL-oh-faze) Final stage of mitosis; membrane forms around the genetic material at each end of the cell to establish two separate nuclei

Temporal bone (TEM-por-al BONE) Bone that forms the side of the cranium and surrounds the ear

Temporomandibular (tem-por-oh-man-DIB-yoo-lar) Pertaining to the temporal bone and the mandible

Tendon (TEN-dun) Band of dense fibrous connective tissue that attaches muscle to bone or another structure

Teniae coli (TEE-nee-ah KOH-lye) Bands of longitudinal muscle fibers in the large intestine

Tentorium cerebelli (ten-TOAR-ee-um sair-eh-BELL-eye) Extension of dura mater in the transverse fissure between the cerebrum and the cerebellum

Terminal ganglion (TER-mih-null GANG-lee-on) An autonomic ganglion located near, or within, the wall of the effector organ; part of the parasympathetic pathway

Testes (TEST-eez) Primary reproductive organs in the male; produce the sperm; also called testicles

Testosterone (tess-TAHS-ter-ohn) Male sex hormone produced by the interstitial cells of the testes; see androgens

Tetanus (TET-ah-nus) A smooth, sustained contraction produced by a series of very rapid stimuli to a muscle

Thalamus (THAL-ah-mus) Region of gray matter located in the diencephalon that channels sensory impulses to the appropriate regions of the cortex for discrimination, localization, and interpretation

Thermogenesis (thur-moh-JEN-eh-sis) Production of heat in response to food intake

Thermoreceptor (ther-moh-ree-SEP-tor) A sensory receptor that detects changes in temperature

Thoracic (tho-RAS-ik) Pertaining to the chest; part of the trunk inferior to the neck and superior to the diaphragm

Thoracic cavity (tho-RAS-ik KAV-ih-tee) Superior part of the ventral body cavity; contains the heart, lungs, esophagus, and trachea

Thoracic duct (tho-RAS-ik DUKT) The primary collecting duct of the lymphatic system that collects lymph from all regions of the body except the upper right quadrant

Thoracolumbar division (thoar-ah-koh-LUM-bar dih-VIH-shun) See sympathetic division

Threshold stimulus (THRESH-hold STIM-yoo-lus) Minimum level of stimulation that is required to start a nerve impulse or muscle contraction; also called liminal stimulus

Thrombin (THROM-bin) The active substance formed from prothrombin that functions to convert fibrinogen into fibrin

Thrombocyte (THROM-boh-syte) One of the formed elements of the blood, which functions in blood clotting; also called platelet

Thrombocytopenia (throm-boh-syte-oh-PEE-nee-ah) An abnormal decrease in the number of platelets in the blood

Thymosin (THYE-moh-sin) Hormone produced by the thymus; important in the development of the body's immune system

Thymus (THYE-mus) Endocrine gland and lymphoid organ located in the mediastinum; secretes thymosin; plays an important role in the body's immune system

Thyroid cartilage (THYE-royd KAR-tih-layj) Large, anterior cartilage of the larynx; commonly called Adam's apple

Thyroid gland (THYE-royd GLAND) Endocrine gland that is located anterior to the trachea at the base of the neck

Thyroid hormone (THYE-royd HOAR-moan) Hormone produced by the thyroid gland that accelerates metabolism; includes thyroxine and triiodothyronine

Thyroid-stimulating hormone (TSH) (THYE-royd STIM-yoo-lay-ting HOAR-moan) A hormone secreted by the anterior pituitary gland that stimulates the thyroid gland to produce thyroid hormone; also called thyrotropin

Thyrotropin (thye-roh-TROH-pin) See thyroid-stimulating hormone

Thyroxine (T_4) (thye-RAHK-sin) One of the thyroid hormones that stimulates cellular metabolism

Tibia (TIB-ee-ah) Large bone on the medial side of the leg

Tidal volume (TV) (TYE-dal VAHL-yoom) Amount of air that is inhaled and exhaled in a normal quiet breathing cycle

Tincture (TINK-chur) A solution that used alcohol as the solvent

Tissue (TISH-yoo) Group of similar cells specialized to perform a certain function

Tonsil (TAHN-sil) Aggregate of lymphoid tissue embedded in mucous membranes that line the nose, mouth, and throat

Total lung capacity (TLC) (TOH-tal LUNG kah-PASS-ih-tee) Amount of air in the lungs after a maximum inspiration; equals residual volume plus expiratory reserve volume plus tidal volume plus inspiratory reserve volume

Trabeculae (trah-BEK-yoo-lee) Thin plates of bone tissue, arranged in an irregular latticework, found in spongy bone

Trabeculae carneae (trah-BEK-yoo-lee KAR-nee-ee) Ridges of myocardium in the ventricles of the heart

Trachea (TRAY-kee-ah) Passageway for air that extends inferiorly from the larynx to the carina; commonly called the windpipe

Transcription (trans-KRIP-shun) Process in which a single strand of DNA acts as a template for the formation of an RNA molecule that transfers information from the nucleus to the cytoplasm

Transfer RNA (tRNA) (TRANS-fur RNA) A molecule of RNA that carries an amino acid to a ribosome during protein synthesis

Translation (trans-LAY-shun) The process of creating a new protein on the ribosome of a cell in response to messenger RNA codons

Transverse fissure (TRANS-vers FISH-ur) The deep fissure that separates the cerebrum from the cerebellum

Transverse plane (TRANS-vers PLANE) A horizontal plane that divides the body or part into superior and inferior portions

Treppe (TREP-peh) The gradual increase in the strength of muscle contraction caused by rapid, repeated stimuli of the same intensity

Tricuspid valve (trye-KUS-pid VALVE) Valve between the right atrium and right ventricle

Trigeminal nerve (trye-JEM-ih-nal NERV) Cranial nerve V; mixed nerve; responsible for chewing movements and facial sensations

Triglyceride (trye-GLIS-ser-ide) A lipid composed of glycerol and three fatty acid molecules

Trigone (TRYE-goan) Triangular area in the floor of the urinary bladder and formed by the openings for the urethra and the two ureters

Triiodothyronine (T₃) (trye-eye-oh-doh-THYE-roh-neen) One of the thyroid hormones that stimulates cellular metabolism

Trochanter (troh-KAN-tur) Large, blunt, irregularly shaped projection on a bone

Trochlear nerve (TROH-klee-ar NERV) Cranial nerve IV; motor nerve; responsible for eye movements

Trophoblast (TROH-foh-blast) Layer of cells that form the outer surface of a blastocyst; functions in the formation of the placenta

Tubercle (TOO-burr-kul) Small, rounded, knoblike projection on a bone

Tuberosity (too-burr-AHS-ih-tee) An elevation or protuberance on a bone, similar to a tubercle

Tubular reabsorption (TOOB-yoo-lar ree-ab-SORP-shun) The movement of filtrate from the renal tubules back into the blood in response to the body's needs during urine formation

Tubular secretion (TOOB-yoo-lar see-KREE-shun) The movement of substances from the blood into the renal tubules in response to the body's needs during urine formation

Tunica adventitia (TOO-nih-kah ad-ven-TISH-ah) Outermost layer of the blood vessel wall, composed of tough, fibrous connective tissue; also called tunica externa

Tunica albuginea (TOO-nih-kah al-byoo-JIN-ee-ah) Fibrous connective tissue capsule that surrounds each testis in the male; in the female, it is the layer directly under the simple cuboidal epithelium

Tunica externa (TOO-nih-kah ex-TER-nah) Outermost layer of the blood vessel wall, composed of tough, fibrous connective tissue; also called tunica adventitia

Tunica interna (TOO-nih-kah in-TER-nah) Endothelium that lines the blood vessels; also called tunica intima

Tunica intima (TOO-nih-kah IN-tih-mah) Endothelium that lines the blood vessels; also called tunica interna

Tunica media (TOO-nih-kah MEE-dee-ah) Middle layer of the blood vessel wall, primarily composed of smooth muscle

Turbinate (TURB-ih-nayte) Scroll-like bone or projection of a bone; also called concha

Tympanic cavity (tim-PAN-ik KAV-ih-tee) See middle ear

Tympanic membrane (tim-PAN-ik MEM-brayn) Membranous partition between the external ear and the middle ear; also called the eardrum

Ulna (UHL-nah) Bone on the medial side of the forearm

Umbilical (um-BIL-ih-kal) Pertaining to the navel; middle region of the abdomen

Umbilical region (um-BIL-ih-kal REE-jun) The central portion of the abdomen, where the belly button or navel is located

Unicellular (yoo-nih-SELL-yoo-lar) Consisting of one cell

Universal recipient (yoo-nih-VER-sal ree-SIP-ee-ent) An individual who has no blood type agglutinins in the plasma and thus may receive transfusions of any blood type; type AB positive

Universal donor (yoo-nih-VER-sal DOH-nor) An individual who has no blood type agglutinogens on the red blood cells and thus may donate blood to all other types; type O negative

Upper respiratory tract (UP-per res-PYE-rah-tor-ee TRACT) Portion of the respiratory tract that includes the nose, pharynx, and larynx

Ureter (yoo-REE-ter) Tubular structure that carries urine from the renal pelvis to the urinary bladder

Urethra (yoo-REE-thrah) Passageway that conveys urine from the urinary bladder to the exterior

Urinalysis (yoo-rin-AL-ih-sis) A chemical and microscopic examination of urine

Urinary (YOO-rin-air-ee) Relating to the system responsible for eliminating most fluid wastes from the body

Urinary bladder (YOO-rin-air-ee BLAD-der) Storage reservoir for urine, which is located in the pelvic cavity

Urochrome (YOO-roh-kroam) Yellow pigment, produced by the decomposition of bile pigments, that appears in the urine

Uterine tubes (YOO-ter-in TOOBS) The tubes that extend laterally from the upper portion of the uterus to the region of the ovaries; also called fallopian tubes or oviducts

Uterine cycle (YOO-ter-in SYE-kul) Monthly cycle of events that occur in the uterus from puberty to menopause; also called the menstrual cycle; occurs concurrently with the ovarian cycle

Uterus (YOO-ter-us) Hollow, muscular organ in females that is the site of menstruation, receives the developing embryo, and supports the fetus until birth

Utricle (YOO-trih-kull) One of the divisions of the membranous labyrinth located in the vestibule of the inner ear; involved with static equilibrium

Uvula (YOO-vyoo-lah) Posterior projection of the soft palate

Vaccine (vak-SEEN) A preparation of weakened or killed antigens introduced into an individual to stimulate the development of immune agents against that specific antigen

Vagina (vah-JYE-nah) Fibromuscular tube that extends from the cervix to the exterior; also called the birth canal

Vagus nerve (VAY-gus NERV) Cranial nerve X; mixed nerve; responsible for sensations and movements of the internal organs

Vasa vasorum (VAS-ah vah-SOR-um) Small blood vessels that supply nutrients to the tissues in the walls of the large blood vessels

Vascular tunic (VAS-kyoo-lar TOO-nik) Middle layer of the eyeball; also called the uvea

Vasoconstriction (vaz-oh-kon-STRIK-shun) A narrowing of blood vessels; decrease in the size of the lumen of blood vessels

Vasodilation (vaz-oh-dye-LAY-shun) An enlarging of blood vessels; increase in the size of the lumen of blood vessels

Vein (VAYN) A blood vessel that carries blood toward the heart

Ventilation (ven-tih-LAY-shun) Movement of air into and out of the lungs; breathing

Ventral (VEN-tral) Toward the front or anterior; opposite of dorsal or posterior

Ventral root (VEN-tral ROOT) Motor branch of a spinal nerve by which the nerve is attached to the spinal cord

Ventricle (VEN-trih-kull) A cavity, such as the fluid-filled cavities in the brain or in the heart

Venule (VAYN-yool) A small vessel that receives blood from a capillary and delivers it to a vein for return to the heart

Vertebrae (VER-teh-bray) Bones that make up the spinal column

Vertebral (ver-TEE-bral or VER-teh-bral) Pertaining to the spinal column; backbone

Vertebrochondral (ver-TEE-broh-kahn-dral) Pertaining to the vertebral column and the costal cartilages of the ribs

Vertebrosternal (ver-TEE-broh-stir-nal) Pertaining to the vertebral column and the sternum

Vestibular membrane (ves-TIB-yoo-lar MEM-brayn) Roof of the cochlear duct; separates the cochlear duct from the scala vestibuli; also called Reissner's membrane

Vestibule (ves-TIB-yool) A small space at the entrance to a passage; in the inner ear, the vestibule is located adjacent to the oval window, between the cochlea and the semicircular canals; in the female, the space between the two labia minora

Vestibulocochlear nerve (ves-TIB-yoo-loh-koh-klee-ar NERV) Cranial nerve VIII; sensory nerve; responsible for hearing and equilibrium

Visceral (VIS-er-al) Pertains to internal organs or the covering of the organs

Visceral muscle (VIS-er-al MUSS-el) Muscle tissue that is found in the walls of internal organs; smooth muscle

Visceral pericardium (VIS-er-al pair-ih-KAR-dee-um) Layer of serous membrane that forms the outermost layer of the heart wall; the epicardium

Vital capacity (VC) (VYE-tal kah-PASS-ih-tee) Maximum amount of air that can be exhaled after a maximum inspiration; equals tidal volume plus inspiratory reserve volume plus expiratory reserve volume

Vitamins (VYE-tah-mins) Organic compounds that are needed in minute amounts to maintain growth and good health; do not supply energy but are necessary to release energy from carbohydrates, proteins, and lipids

Vitreous humor (VIT-ree-us HYOO-mer) Jellylike substance that fills the posterior cavity of the eye, between the lens and the retina; also called vitreous body

Vomer (VOH-mer) Bone that forms the inferior part of the nasal septum

Vulva (VUL-vah) Collective term for the external accessory structures of the female reproductive system; also called the pudendum

Wormian bone (WER-mee-an BONE) A small bone located within a suture between certain cranial bones; also called sutural bone

Xiphoid (ZYE-foyd) Most inferior portion of the sternum

Yolk sac (YOHK SAK) An extraembryonic membrane that, in humans, produces the primordial germ cells and is an early source of blood cells

Zona pellucida (ZOH-nah peh-LOO-sih-dah) Glycoprotein membrane that surrounds a secondary oocyte

Zygomatic (zye-goh-MAT-ik) Triangular bone that forms the prominence of the cheek; cheek bone

Zygote (ZYE-goat) The single diploid cell that is a fertilized ovum

Index

Note: Page numbers in *italics* refer to illustrations; page numbers followed by t refer to tables.

A

A bands, 125, *125*
A blood type, 235-236, *236*, 236t
Abdominal aorta, 270, *271*, *272*, 273t, *274*
Abdominal cavity, 12, *12*
Abdominal reflex, 171, 172t
Abdominal region, 14t, *15*
Abdominal veins, *279*, 279-280
Abdominal wall, muscles of, 138t, 138-139, *139*
    veins of, *276*, *277*, 278t, 279
Abdominopelvic cavity, 12, *12*
Abdominopelvic quadrants, *12*, 13
Abdominopelvic regions, *12*, 13
Abdominopelvic veins, *276*, *277*, 278t, 279, *279*, 279-280
Abducens nerve, 172-173, *173*, 174t
Abduction, 134t
ABO blood groups, 235-236, *236*, 236t
Abruptio placentae, 420
Absolute refractory period, 160
Absorption, of fluids and electrolytes, 341, 346-347, *347*, 348t
    of nutrients, 330, 338, 339-340, 341, 346-347, *347*
Accessory nerve, 172-173, *173*, 174t
Accommodation, visual, 191, *192*
Acetabulum, 109, *110*, 110t
Acetylcholine (ACh), 126, 161, 161t, 162, 177
Acetylcholinesterase, 126
Acetyl-CoA, in glycolysis, 356, 359
    in lipid metabolism, 359, *359*, *360*
    in protein metabolism, 359, *359*, *360*
Achilles tendon, *141*, *142*, 145, 145t, 171, 172t
Acid(s), 28
    fatty, 32-33, *33*, 33t, 346, 347
        absorption of, 346, 347, *347*, 348t
        beta oxidation of, 359
        in muscle contraction, 130, *130*
        metabolism of, 343, 354, *355*, 358-359, *359*, *360*
        saturated, 33, 33t
        unsaturated, 33, 33t
    in buffer solutions, 30
    pH scale for, 29, *29*
Acid-base balance, 388-390, 391t
Acidic solutions, 29
Acidosis, 388, 389-390, 391t
    metabolic, 389-390, 391t
    respiratory, 389-390, 391t
Acinar cells, pancreatic, 344
Acinar gland, 64, *64*
Acne, 82
Acquired immunity, 299-301, *300*
Acquired immunodeficiency syndrome (AIDS), transmission of, 239
Acromegaly, 205
Acromion process, *106*, 107

Acrosome, *397*, 397-398
ACTH, 209t, *210*, 211, *214*, 215
Actin, 68, 125, *125*
Action potential, 159, *159*
    definition of, 159
    generation of, *158*, 159
    propagation of, 159-160, *160*
Active immunity, 300, *300*
Active transport, 49
Adam's apple, 309, *309*
Adaptation, sensory, 184
Addison's disease, 215-216
Adduction, 135t
Adductor brevis muscle, *141*, 143, 144t
Adductor longus muscle, *141*, 143, 144t
Adductor magnus muscle, *141*, 143, 144t
Adenocarcinoma, 64. See also *Cancer.*
Adenohypophysis, 208, *208*
    hormones of, 209t, 210-212
Adenoidectomy, 290
Adenoids, 290, 308, *309*
Adenoma, 64, 205
Adenosine diphosphate (ADP), 35
Adenosine triphosphate (ATP), 34-35, *35*
    energy storage in, 355
    in anabolism, *131*, 131-132
    in muscle contraction, 129-130, *130*
    synthesis of, 357, *357*, *358*
        aerobic respiration in, *131*, 131-132
        anaerobic respiration in, *131*, 131-132
ADH. See *Antidiuretic hormone (ADH).*
Adhesion, 60
Adipose tissue, 65t, 66, *66*, 80
Adolescence, development in, 432
ADP (adenosine diphosphate), 35
Adrenal (suprarenal) glands, *214*, 214-217
Adrenal hormones, 209t, *214*, 215-217, *216*, *217*
Adrenergic fibers, 177
Adrenocorticotropic hormone (ACTH), 209t, *210*, 211, *214*, 215
Adulthood, development in, 432
Adventitia, gastrointestinal, *330*, 331
Aerobic exercise, 146
Aerobic respiration, *131*, 131-132
Afferent arterioles, 377, *377*, 378, *378*, 379
Afferent lymphatic vessels, 289, *290*
Afferent neurons, 156, 156t
Afterbirth, 424
Age, developmental, 420
Agglutinins, ABO, 235-236, *236*, 237
    Rh, 237-238, *238*
Agglutinogens, ABO, 235-236, *236*, 237
    Rh, 237-238, *238*
Aging, blood and, 238
    circulation and, 282
    connective tissue and, 71
    digestive system and, 348
    digestive tract and, 348
    DNA damage and, 56

Aging *(Continued)*
    endocrine system and, 221
    heart and, 253-254
    immunity and, 301
    lymphatic system and, 301
    metabolism and, 369
    muscle and, 146
    nervous system and, 178
    nutrition and, 369
    reproductive system and, 413
    respiratory system and, 323
    senses and, 199-200
    skin and, 84
    urinary system and, 389
Agranulocytes, 232
AIDS, transmission of, 239
Alae, ilial, 109, *110*
Albinism, 80
Albumins, 227t, 228
Alcohol, birth defects and, 432-433
    diuresis and, 384
Aldosterone, 209t, 215, *216*
    in blood pressure regulation, 269
    in electrolyte balance, 388
    urine concentration and volume and, 384
Alimentary canal. See *Digestive system.*
Alkaline solutions, 29
Alkalis, pH scale for, 29, *29*
Alkalosis, 388, 389-390, 391t
    metabolic, 389-390, 391t
    respiratory, 389-390, 391t
Allantois, 425, *425*
Allergen, 287, 299
Allergies, 299, 301-302
    infection, 302
All-or-none principle, in muscle contraction, 127
    in nerve impulse conduction, 160-161
Alopecia, 77
Alpha globulins, 228
Alpha radiation, 36
Alveolar ducts, *310*, 311
Alveolar process, *99*, 102
Alveoli, *310*, 311
Alzheimer's disease, 178-179
Amino acid(s), 31-32, 32t, 205. See also *Protein(s).*
    absorption of, 346, *347*, 348t
    as energy source, 357
    deamination of, 357
    essential, 364
    functions of, 357
    in plasma, 228
    metabolism of, 344, 354, *355*, 357, *359*, *360*
    nonessential, 364
    production of, 364
    sequence of, 56t
Amniocentesis, 425
Amnion, 424-425, *425*, *426*

475

Amniotic cavity, 424, *424, 425*
Amniotic fluid, 425
Amniotic sac, 425
Amphiarthroses, 114
Ampulla, lactiferous, *412*, 413
  of ductus deferens, 399
  of semicircular canals, *195*, 198
Amylase, pancreatic, 345, 346t
  salivary, 334
Anabolic steroids, 147
Anabolism, 8, 354
Anaerobic exercise, 146-147
Anaerobic reactions, 355
Anaerobic respiration, 131, *131*
Anal canal, *340*, 341
Anal columns, *340*, 341
Anal sphincter, external, *340*, 341
  internal, *340*, 341
Anaphase, *50, 51*, 51t
Anaphylaxis, 287, 302
Anaplasia, 40
Anastomoses, arteriovenous, 262, *262*
Anatomical position, 11, *11*
Anatomical terms, 10-15
  for body cavities, 12, *12*
  for body directions, 11
  for body regions, *12, 13*, 13t
  for planes and sections, 11-12, *12*
Anatomy, 2, *3*
  gross human, 2
  microscopic, 2
  physiology and, 2
Androgens, 209t, 215, 218-219, *219, 402, 403*
Anemia, 226, 227
  hemolytic, 231
  pernicious, 231
Aneurysm, 261
Angina pectoris, 248
Angiography, 260
Angioplasty, 260
  excimer laser, 283
  percutaneous transluminal coronary, 283
Angiotensin, in blood pressure regulation, 269
Angiotensin II, urine concentration and volume and, 384
Angle, sternal, 105, *105*
Anions, *20*, 20-21
  formation of, 28, *28*
Ankle, 112. See also *Lower extremity.*
  muscles of, 145, 145t
Ankle-jerk reflex, 171, 172t
Anorexia nervosa, 349
Antagonists, muscle, 133
Antebrachial area, 14t, *15*
Antecubital area, 14t, *15*
Anteflexed uterus, 407
Anterior, 11
Anterior cavity, of eye, *190, 191*
Anterior crest, 112, *113*, 113t
Anterior fontanel, 102
Anterior inferior iliac spine, 109, *110*, 110t
Anterior interventricular artery, 248, *249*
Anterior median fissure, 170, *171*
Anterior superior iliac spine, 109, *110*, 110t
Anterior tibial artery, *271, 272*, 273t, 275
Anterior tibial vein, *276, 277*, 278t, 280
Anterolateral fontanel, 102
Antibodies, 297, *298*, 299t
  blood group, 235-236, *236, 237*
  in hypersensitivity, 302
Antibody-mediated immunity, 296-299, *298*
Anticoagulants, 234
Anticodons, 54, 56t

Antidiuretic hormone (ADH), 209t, *210*, 211
  urine concentration and volume and, 384
Antigens, 294-295
  blood group, 235-238, *236, 237*
    ABO, 235-236, *236*, 236t
    Rh, 236-237, *237*
  in hypersensitivity, 302
Antiserum, 300
Anuria, 375
Anus, *340*, 341
Aorta, *249*, 270, *271, 272*, 273t, *274*
  abdominal, 270, *271, 272*, 273t, *274*
  ascending, 248, *248*, 270, *271, 272*, 273t, *274*
  branches of, 270-274, *271, 272*, 273t, *274*
  descending, 270-274, *271, 272*, 273t, *274*
  thoracic, 270, *271, 272*, 273t, *274*
Aortic arch, 270, *271, 272*, 273t, *274, 275*
Aortic semilunar valve, 245, 247, *247, 248*
Apgar score, 420
Aphagia, 329
Apical foramen, 333, *333*
Apnea, sleep, 324
Apneustic area, 168
Apocrine sweat glands, *64*, 65
Aponeurosis, 124
Appendages, epiploic, *340*, *340*
Appendicitis, 341
Appendicular region, *13*, 14
Appendicular skeleton, *96*, 97, 97t, 106-113
Appendix, vermiform, *340*, *340*
Appositional growth, 96
Aqueduct, cerebral, *167*, 168, 169, *169*
Aqueous humor, *190*, 191
Arachnoid, 71, 163, *163*
Arachnoid granulations, 170
Arbor vitae, *167*, 168
Arch, aortic, 270, *271, 272*, 273t, *274, 275*
  palmar, *271, 272*, 273t, 274-275
  pubic, *110*, 110t, 111
  vertebral, 103, *103*
  zygomatic, 102
Arcuate arteries, 378, *379*
Arcuate line, 109, *110*, 110t
Arcuate veins, 378, *379*
Area(s), antebrachial, 14t, *15*
  antecubital, 14t, *15*
  apneustic, 168
  association, *164, 165*, 166t
  axillary, 14t, *15*
  brachial, 14t, *15*
  Broca's, *164*, 166t
  carpal, 14t, *15*
  celiac, 14t, *15*
  cephalic, 14t, *15*
  cervical, 14t, *15*
  costal, 14t, *15*
  cranial, 14t, *15*
  cubital, 14t, *15*
  frontal, 14t, *15*
  gluteal, 14t, *15*
  gnostic, *164*, 166t
  inguinal, 14t, *15*
  leg, 14t, *15*
  lumbar, 14t, *15*
  mammary, 14t, *15*
  motor, *164, 165*, 166t
    cerebellum as, 169
  motor speech, *164*, 166t
  occipital, 14t, *15*
  ophthalmic, 14t, *15*
  oral, 14t, *15*
  otic, 14t, *15*
  palmar, 14t, *15*

Area(s) *(Continued)*
  pectoral, 14t, *15*
  pedal, 14t, *15*
  pelvic, 14t, *15*
  perineal, 14t, *15*
  plantar, 14t, *15*
  pneumotaxic, 168
  popliteal, 14t, *15*
  sacral, 14t, *15*
  sensory, *164, 165*, 166t
  sternal, 14t, *15*
  tarsal, 14t, *15*
  thoracic, 14t, *15*
  umbilical, 14t, *15*
  vertebral, 14t, *15*
  Wernicke's, *164*, 166t
Areola, 412, *412*
Areolar connective tissue, 65t, 66, *66*
Arm, 107, *107*. See also *Upper extremity.*
  muscles of, 140t, 140-142, *141-142*
  veins of, *276, 277*, 278t, *279*
Arrector pili, 81
Arrhythmias, 250
  in myocardial infarction, 254-255
Arterectomy, 260
Arterial blood pressure, 266-269. See also *Blood pressure.*
Arteries, 260-261. See also specific arteries.
  age-related changes in, 282
  aneurysm of, 261
  function of, 260
  hardening of, 282-283
  in pulmonary circulation, *245, 248, 248, 260, 260, 271, 272*, 273t, *274, 274*
  major systemic, 270-274, *271, 272*, 273t, *274, 275*
  of head and neck, *271, 272*, 273t, *274*
  of lower extremity, *271, 272*, 273t, *275*
  of upper extremity, *271, 272*, 273t, 274-275
  origin of, 273t
  regions supplied by, 273t
  structure of, 260-261, *261*
Arterioles, 260, 261, 262, *262*
  afferent, *377, 377, 378, 378, 379*
  efferent, *377, 377, 378, 378, 379*
Arteriosclerosis, 260, 282-283
Arteriovenous anastomoses, 262, *262*
Arthritis, 91
Articular cartilage, 93, *93*, 95, 114, *115*
  age-related changes in, 116
Articulations, 114-115
Artificial immunity, 300, *300*
Artificial pacemaker, 243
Arytenoid cartilage, 309, *309*, 310
Ascending aorta, 270, *271, 272*, 273t, *274*
Ascending colon, *340*, 340-341
Ascending limb, of renal tubule, 377, *378*
Ascending tract, 171
Ascites, 329
Ascorbic acid, 366t
Aspartate aminotransferase (AST), 248
Aspiration, 307
Association areas, cortical, *164, 165*, 166t
Association neurons, 156, 156t
Asthma, 311
Astigmatism, 184
Astrocytes, 157t
Atelectasis, 307
Atheroma, 282
Atherosclerosis, 260, 282-283
Atlas, 104, *104*
Atmospheric pressure, ventilation and, 312-313, *313*

Atom(s), bonding of, 20-23
  definition of, 18, 24t
  in chemical reactions, 24-25
  structure of, 18-19, *19*
Atomic number, 10, 19
  isotopes and, 36
Atomic radiations, 36
ATP (adenosine triphosphate), 34-35, *35*
  energy storage in, 355
  in anabolism, *131*, 131-132
  in muscle contraction, 129-130, *130*
  synthesis of, 357, *357, 358*
    aerobic respiration in, *131*, 131-132
    anaerobic respiration in, *131*, 131-132
Atrial diastole, 251, *251*
Atrial natriuretic hormone, 220
  urine concentration and volume and, 384
Atrial systole, 251, *251*
Atriopeptin, 220
  urine concentration and volume and, 384
Atrioventricular bundle, *150*, 250
Atrioventricular node, 250, *250*
Atrioventricular valves, *245, 246, 247*
Atrium, left, *245, 246*
  right, *245*, 245-246, *269, 270*
Atrophy, 40
Audiometry, 184
Auditory association area, 166t
Auditory cortex, 166t
Auditory meatus, external, *98*, 101
  internal, *99, 100, 100*, 101t
Auditory ossicles, 102, *194, 195, 195, 197*
Auditory pathway, 197
Auditory sense, 194-197
Auditory tube, *194, 195*, 308, *309*
Auerbach's plexus, *330*, 331
Auricles, 195, *195*, 246
Auricular surface, 109, *110*, 110t
Auscultation, 243
Autoimmune disease, 287, 295
Autolysis, 44
Autonomic ganglion, 175, *175*
Autonomic nervous system, 155, 172, 174-177
  parasympathetic, 155, 175, *175, 176, 177*,
    177t
  sympathetic, 155, 175-176, *176*, 176t, 177
Avascular tissue, 60
Axial region, *13*, 14
Axial skeleton, *96, 97*, 97t
Axillary area, 14t, *15*
Axillary artery, *271, 272*, 273t, 274
Axillary vein, *276, 277*, 278t, 279
Axis, 104, *104*
Axon, 155, *155*, 156
Axon collaterals, *155*, 156
Azotemia, 375
Azygous vein, *276, 277*, 278t, 279

B

B blood type, 235-236, *236*, 236t
B cells, 291, 295-297, *296-298*
  memory, 297, *299*
Babinski's reflex, 171, 172t
Balance. See *Equilibrium.*
Ball-and-socket joint, 115t
Barrier defense mechanisms, 291
Barrier methods, of birth control, 414
Bartholin's glands, 408
Basal cell carcinoma, 77
Basal ganglia, 164, 165
Basal metabolic rate (BMR), 361, *361*
  age-related decline in, 369

Basement membrane, 60
Bases, 28-29
Basilar artery, *271, 272*, 273t, 274, *275*
Basilic vein, *276, 277*, 278t, 279
Basophils, 228t, 232-233
Behavioral methods, of birth control,
  414
Belly, muscle, 124
Bends, 315
Benign prostatic hyperplasia, 399
Benign tumors, 40, 57
Beta globulins, 228
Beta oxidation, of fatty acids, 359
Beta radiation, 36
Bicarbonate balance, 387-388
Bicarbonate ions, in carbon dioxide trans-
  port, 319
Biceps brachii muscle, 140t, *141*, 142-143
Biceps femoris muscle, *142*, 144t, 145
Bicuspid valve, *245, 246, 247*, 248
Bicuspids, 332, *332*, 333t
Bifid, 104
Bile, concentration and storage of, 344
  properties of, 344
  synthesis and secretion of, 343, 344
Bile canaliculi, 342, *343*
Bile pigments, 344
Bile salts, 344
  hepatic synthesis of, 343
Bilirubin, 231, 344
Binge-purge syndrome, 349
Biopsy, 60
  muscle, 123
Biotin, 366t
Birth control, 414-415
Birth control pills, 414
Birth defects, teratogens and, 432-433
Bladder, 379-380, *380*
Blastocele, *422, 423, 423*
Blastocyst, *422, 423, 423*
  implantation of, *423, 423, 424*
Blastomere, *422, 422*
Bleeding, control of, 233-235
Blepharitis, 184
Blinking, 189
Blister, 79
  fever, 331
Blood, 225-239
  age-related changes in, 238
  as connective tissue, 68, 226
  composition of, 227, 227-233
  electrolytes in, 229
  formed elements in, 226, *227*, 227-233,
    228t, 229-233
  functions of, 226-227
  gases in, 229
  nonprotein nitrogen-containing molecules
    in, 228-229
  nutrients in, 229
  osmotic pressure of, 228
  proteins in, 227t, 227-228
  solutes in, 227t, 227-228
  splenic filtering of, 290
  umbilical cord, 229
Blood cells, 65t, 68, *68*. See also *Erythro-*
  cytes; Leukocytes; Platelets.
  formation of, in bone, 92
Blood clot, formation of, 234, *234*
  lysis of, 234
Blood donor, 235
  universal, 235-236
Blood doping, 236
Blood flow. See also *Circulation.*
  cardiac, 247-249, *248*

Blood flow *(Continued)*
  pressure and, 264, *264*
  rate of, 265, *265*
  renal, 378, *379*
  resistance and, 265
Blood groups, ABO, 235-236, *236*, 236t
  Rh, 237-238, *238*
Blood pressure, 266-269
  blood flow and, 264, *264*
  blood viscosity and, 268
  blood volume and, 267-268
  cardiac output and, 267
  diastolic, 267
  measurement of, 267, *268*
  peripheral resistance and, 268
  pulse, 267
  pulse and, 266, *267, 269*
  regulation of, 253, 268-269
  systolic, 267
Blood recipient, universal, 235-236
Blood supply, 248-249, *249*. See also *Blood*
  flow; Circulation.
  myocardial, 248-249, *249*
  of muscle, 125
Blood transfusions, blood typing for, 235
  disease transmission via, 239
  universal donor in, 235-236
  universal recipient in, 235-236
Blood types, 235-238
Blood urea nitrogen (BUN), 375
Blood vessels, 259-283. See also *Arteries; Cap-*
  illaries; Circulation; Vein(s).
  age-related changes in, 282
  classification of, 260
  pulmonary, 160, 260
  structure of, 260-263, *261, 262*
  systemic, 160, 260
Blood viscosity, blood pressure and, 268
Blood volume, blood pressure and, 267-268
  cardiac output and, 267-268
Bloodborne pathogens, 239
Blood-brain barrier, 157
BMR. See *Basal metabolic rate (BMR).*
Body, ciliary, 190, *190*
  mamillary, 167
  of penis, 401, *401*
  of stomach, 335, *335*
  sternal, 105, *105*
  surface area of, rule of nines for, 85, *85*
  uterine, 407, *407*
  vertebral, 103, *103*
Body areas. See *Area(s).*
Body cavities, 12, *12*. See also *Cavity.*
Body directions, terminology for, 11
Body fat, 65t, 66, *66*, 80
  distribution of, 370
  essential, 369
  excess, 369-370
  nonessential, 369
Body heat, 8. See also *Heat; Temperature.*
Body membranes, 70-71. See also *Mem-*
  brane(s).
Body movement, 8
  types of, 134t-135t
Body organization, levels of, 2-4, *4*
  body system, 4
  cellular, 2-4
  chemical, 2
  organ, 4
  tissue, 4
  total organism, 4
Body regions, *13*, 14. See also *Region(s).*
Body systems, 4
  types of, 5

Body temperature. See *Temperature.*
Body tissues. See *Tissue.*
Bodybuilding, 147
Bonds, 20-23
  covalent, 21-22, *21-23*
    polar, 22, *23*
  hydrogen, 22-23, *23*
  intermolecular, 22-23, *23*
  intramolecular, 22
  ionic, *20,* 20-21
Bone(s), 67-68
  age-related changes in, 116
  cancellous, *92, 93*
  classification of, 93
  compact, *92, 92*
  disorders of, *118*
  endochondral, 95, *95*
  flat, 93
  growth of, 95-96
    appositional, 96
  hematopoiesis in, 92
  intramembranous, 95
  irregular, 93
  long, *93,* 93-94
  motor functions of, 91
  muscle attachment to, 124-125
  of lower extremity, *111,* 111-113, 112t, *113, 114*
  of pelvic girdle, 109-111, *110,* 110t, 111t
  of skull, 97-103, *98-100*
  of spine, *103,* 103-105, *104*
  of thoracic cage, 105, *105*
  of upper extremity, *107,* 107-109, *108,* 109t
  protective functions of, 91
  sesamoid, 97
  short, 93
  spongy, *92, 93*
  storage functions of, 92
  structure of, *92,* 92-93
  support functions of, 91
  sutural, 97
  Wormian, 97
Bone markings, 93-94, 94t
Bone marrow, blood formation in, 92
  hematopoiesis in, 229, *230*
  transplantation of, 229
Bony labyrinth, 195, *195*
Booster, vaccine, 301
Borborygmus, 329
Bowman's capsule, 377, *377*
Boyle's law, 313-314
Brachial area, 14t, *15*
Brachial artery, 271, *272,* 273t, 274
Brachial vein, *276,* 277, 278t, *279*
Brachialis muscle, 140t, *141,* 142-143
Brachiocephalic artery, *249,* 270, *271, 272,* 273t, *275*
Brachiocephalic vein, *276,* 277, *277,* 278t
Brachioradialis muscle, 140t, *141,* 142-143
Brachium, 107, *107*
Brain, 154. See also under *Cerebral.*
  structure of, *164,* 164-170, *167, 169*
Brain stem, *167,* 168
Brain testicular axis, 402
Brain tumors, 156
Breast, *412,* 412-413
  fibrocystic disease of, 413
  in lactation, 413, 428, 429-430, *431*
Breathing, 307-314. See also *Respiration; Ventilation.*
  in neonate, 429
  regulation of, 320-322, *320-322*
  voluntary control of, 321-322

Breech presentation, 429
Broad ligament, 407, *407*
Broca's area, *164,* 166t
Bronchi, *310,* 311
Bronchial tree, *310,* 311
Bronchioles, *310,* 311
Bronchogenic carcinoma, 307
Bronchopulmonary segments (lobules), 312
Bronchoscopy, 311
Brush border, 338, *339*
Buccal area, 14t, *15*
Buccinator muscle, 134, *136,* 136t, 331
Buffers, 30, 388, *389*
Bulb, olfactory, 187, *188*
  synaptic, *155,* 156
Bulbourethral glands, *396,* 400
Bulbus oculi, *190,* 190-191
Bulimia, 349
Bundle branches, *150,* 250
Bunion, 91, 113
Burns, 84-85
Bursae, 115, *115*

C

Calcaneal tendon, *141, 142,* 145, 145t
Calcaneus, 113, *114*
Calcitonin, 209t, 213, *213*
Calcium, bone storage of, 92
  dietary, 367t
  in coagulation, 234
  regulation of, calcitonin and, 213
    parathyroid hormone and, 213, *213*
Calculi, renal, 385
Callus, bony, 117
Calories, 360
Calyces, renal, 376, *376*
Canal(s), alimentary. See *Digestive system.*
  anal, *340,* 341
  carotid, *99,* 100, 101t
  central, 170
  external auditory, 195, *195*
  Haversian, 67, *68*
  hypoglossal, *100*
  inguinal, 396
  lacrimal, 189, *189*
  nasolacrimal, 100, 101t
  osteonic, 67, *68*
  root, 333, *333*
  semicircular, *195,* 198
Canaliculi, 68
  bile, 342, *343*
Cancellous bone, *92, 93*
Cancer, 57
  brain, 156
  cervical, Papanicolaou smear for, 408
  lung, 307
  metastasis in, 40, 57, 287, 289
  ovarian, 402
  prostate, 400
  skin, 77, *78*
  vaginal, Papanicolaou smear for, 408
Canines, 332, *332,* 333t
Capacitation, 420
Capillaries, function of, 261, 263-264
  lymph, *288,* 288-289
  pulmonary, *269,* 270
  structure of, *261,* 261-262, *262*
Capillary microcirculation, *263,* 263-264
Capitulum, 107, *107,* 107t
Capsule, glomerular (Bowman's), 377, *377*
  joint, 114
  lymph node, 289

Carbaminohemoglobin, 318-319
Carbohydrates, 30-32, 362t, 362-363
  classification of, 362, 362t
  digestion of, 345-346
  functions of, 362
  metabolism of, 343, 354, *355,* 355-357, *355-358, 360*
Carbon dioxide. See also *Gas(es).*
  partial pressure of, 315, 316t
  transport of, *318,* 318-320, *319*
Carbonic acid, in carbon dioxide transport, 319
Carbonic anhydrase, in carbon dioxide transport, 319
Carcinogens, 40, 57
Carcinoma, 60, 61. See also *Cancer.*
  basal cell, 77
  bronchogenic, 307
Cardiac. See also *Heart* entries.
Cardiac arrest, 243
Cardiac arrhythmias, 250
  in myocardial infarction, 254-255
Cardiac catheterization, 243
Cardiac center, 168, 253
Cardiac conduction system, 249-251, *250*
Cardiac cycle, 251, *251*
Cardiac enzymes, 248
Cardiac muscle, 68t, 69, *69,* 124t, 244, *245.*
  See also *Muscle(s); Myocardium.*
Cardiac notch, *310, 311,* 312
Cardiac output, 252, *252*
  heart rate and, *252,* 253
  stroke volume and, *252,* 252-253
Cardiac region, of stomach, 335, *335*
Cardiac sphincter, 335
Cardiac veins, 248-249, *249*
Cardiomegaly, 243
Cardiovascular system, 5, 6t. See also *Circulation; Heart.*
  age-related changes in, 253-254
  disorders of, *255*
  functional relationships of, *242*
Caries, dental, 333
Carina, *310,* 311
Carotene, 80
Carotid arteries, 271, *272,* 273t, 274
Carotid canal, *99,* 100, 101t
Carotid sinus, 274
Carpal area, 14t, *15*
Carpal bones, 108, *108*
Carpal tunnel syndrome, 91, 174
Cartilage, 65t, 67
  age-related changes in, 116
  articular, 93, *93,* 95, 114, *115*
  arytenoid, 309, 310
  bronchial, 311
  corniculate, 309
  costal, *105,* 106
  cricoid, 309, *309*
  cuneiform, 309
  elastic, 65t, 67
  fibrous, 65t, 67
  hyaline, 65t, 67, *67*
  knee, 114-115, *115*
    tear in, 115
  laryngeal, 309
  semilunar, 114-115
    tear in, 115
  thyroid, 309, *309*
  tracheal, 310, *310*
Catabolism, 354
Catalyst, 26
Cataracts, 199

Catheterization, cardiac, 243
Cations, 20, *20*
  formation of, 28, *28*
Cauda equina, 170, *170*
Caudate lobe, of liver, 342, *342*
Cavity, 12, *12*
  abdominal, 12, *12*
  abdominopelvic, 12, *12*
  amniotic, 424, *424, 425*
  anterior, of eye, 190, *191*
  cranial, 12, *12*
  dorsal, 12, *12*
  glenoid, *106*, 107
  joint, 114
  medullary, 93, *93*
  nasal, 307, *309*
  oral, *331*, 331-334, *334*
  pelvic, 12, *12*
  pericardial, 243, *245*
  pleural, *311*, 312
  posterior, of eye, 190, *191*
  pulp, 333, *333*
  spinal, 12, *12*
  thoracic, 12, *12*
  tympanic, 195
  ventral, 12, *12*
Cecum, 340, *340*
Celiac area, 14t, *15*
Celiac artery, 270, *271, 272*, 273t, *274*
Celiac disease, 354
Celiac trunk, *274, 275*
Cell(s), 2-4
  B, 291, 295-297, *296-298*
    memory, 297, *299*
  blood, 65t, 68, *68*
    formation of, in bone, 92
  chief, 336, 336t
  columnar, 61
  connective tissue, 66
  cuboidal, 61
  ependymal, 157t
  follicular, *404*, 406
  functions of, 45-56
  glial, 70, 155, 156, 157t
  goblet, 62, 64, 341
  hair, in equilibrium, 197-198, *198*
    in hearing, 196, *196*
  interstitial testicular, 396, *397*
  juxtaglomerular, 378, *378*
  Kupffer, 344
  Leydig, 396, *397*
  mast, 66, 233
    in hypersensitivity, 302
  mucous, 65
    gastric, 336, 336t
  muscle, 68, 69
  nerve. See *Neuron(s)*.
  neuroglia, 156, 157t
  pancreatic acinar, 344
  parietal, 336
  primordial germ, 396
  satellite, 157t
  Schwann, 157t
  serous, 65
  squamous, 61
  structure of, 40-45, *41*, 42t
  supporting (Sertoli's), 396, *397*
  sustentacular, 396, *397*
  T, 291, 295-296, *296-298*
    helper, 239, 296, *297*
    killer, 296, *297*
    memory, 296, *297*
    suppressor, 296, *297*
  taste (gustatory), 186

Cell division, *50*, 50-52, 51t, *52*
Cell membrane, 40-41, *42*. See also *Membrane(s)*.
  nuclear, *41*, 42t, 43
  plasma, 40-41, *42*
    selective permeability of, 40, 47
    transport across, 45-50, 46t. See also *Membrane transport*.
Cell-mediated immunity, 296, *297*
Cellular metabolism, 354
Cellular physiology, 2
Cellular respiration, 307, 354, 355
Cellulitis, 77
Cellulose, 31
Cementum, 333, *333*
Central canal, 170
Central nervous system, 154, *154*
  brain in, 164-170
    components of, 163-170
    meninges in, 163-164
    spinal cord in, 170-171
Central sulcus, 164, *164*
Central vein, 342, 343, *343*
Central venous pressure, 264
Centrioles, *41*, 42t
Centromere, in mitosis, 51
Centrosome, 45
Cephalic area, 14t, *15*
Cephalic phase, of gastric secretion, 336, *337*
Cephalic vein, *276, 277*, 278t, *279*
Cerebellar cortex, 168
Cerebellar hemispheres, 168
Cerebellum, 168-169
Cerebral aqueduct, *167*, 168, 169, *169*
Cerebral concussion, 153
Cerebral contusion, 153
Cerebral cortex, 164, 165, 166t
Cerebral hemispheres, 164, *164*
Cerebral palsy, 153
Cerebral peduncles, *167*, 168
Cerebral ventricles, 169-170
Cerebrospinal fluid, accumulation of, 169
  collection of, 170
  formation of, 170
Cerebrovascular accident (CVA), 153
Cerebrum, 164, *164*
Cerumen, 82, 194
Ceruminous glands, 82, 194
Cervical area, 14t, *15*
Cervical curvature, 103, *103*
Cervical enlargement, 170
Cervical nerves, *170*, 170-171, 173-174, 175t
Cervical vertebrae, *103*, 103-104, *104*
Cervix, 407, *407*
  cancer of, Papanicolaou smear for, 408
Cesarean section, 420
Chancre, syphilitic, 415
Chemical bonds, 20-23
  covalent, 21-22, *21-23*
    polar, 22, *23*
  hydrogen, 22-23, *23*
  intermolecular, 22-23, *23*
  intramolecular, 22
  ionic, *20*, 20-21
Chemical compounds, 23-27
  definition of, 23
  ionic, 21
  organic, 30-35
  properties of, 23-24
Chemical defense mechanisms, 291
Chemical digestion, 330, 345-346
Chemical elements, 18, 18t
Chemical equations, 24-25

Chemical equilibrium, diffusion and, 46
  reaction rate and, 27
Chemical level, of body organization, 4
Chemical reactions, 24-27
  anaerobic, 355
  catalysts in, 26
  combination, 25
  composition, 25
  decomposition, 25
  double replacement, 25
  endergonic, 26
  equilibrium in, 27
  exergonic, 25-26
  neutralization, 29-30
  rate of, 26
  reversible, 26-27
  single replacement, 25
  synthesis, 25
  types of, 25-26
Chemical symbols, 18, 18t
Chemistry, 17-36
  organic, 30
Chemoreceptors, 184, 185t
  in blood pressure regulation, 269
  in respiratory center, 321
  olfactory receptors as, 187
  taste receptors as, 186
Chiasma, optic, 193, *193*
Chief cells, 336, 336t
Childhood, development in, 431-432
Chloride, dietary, 367t
Chloride balance, 387-388
Cholecystitis, 329
Cholecystokinin, 220, 340, 344, 346t
  pancreatic secretions and, 345
Cholelithiasis, 329
Cholesterol, 33, *34*. See also *Fats; Lipids*.
  bile and, 344
  food sources of, 364t
  good vs. bad, 365
  recommended intake of, 365
Cholinergic fibers, 177
Cholinesterase, 161
Chondrin, 67
Chondrocytes, 67
Chordae tendineae, *245*, 246
Chorion, 425, *425, 426*
Chorionic villi, 425, *426*
Choroid, 190, *190*
Choroid plexus, *169*, 170
Chromatids, 51, 397, *398*
Chromatin, 42t, 43
Chromosomes, 43
Chronic obstructive pulmonary disease (COPD), 307
Chyle, 287, 347
Chylomicrons, 347
Chyme, in large intestine, 341
  in small intestine, 340
  in stomach, 336
Cigarette smoking, fetal effects of, 433
Cilia, *41*, 42t, 45, 62
Ciliary body, 190, *190*
Ciliary muscle, 189t, 190, *190*
Ciliary processes, 190, *190*
Circle of Willis, 274, *274*
Circular muscles, of iris, 189t
Circulation. See also *Arteries; Blood flow; Capillaries; Circulation; Vein(s)*.
  age-related changes in, 282
  capillary, *263*, 263-264
  fetal, *280*, 281-282, 282t, 427, 428t, 429, *430*
  physiology of, 263-269

Circulation (*Continued*)
  placental, 281
  pulmonary, 260, *260, 269,* 269-270
  renal, 378, *379*
  systemic, 260, *260,* 270
  venous, 266, *266*
Circulatory shock, 268
Circumcision, 401
Circumduction, 135t
Circumflex artery, 248, *249*
Cirrhosis, 342, 360
Cisterna chyli, 288, *289*
Citric acid cycle, 356
Clavicle, 106, *106*
Cleavage, *422,* 422-423, *423*
Cleavage lines, 79
Cleft palate, 332
Climax, female, 409
  male, 401
Clinical age, 420
Clitoris, 408, *408*
Closed fracture, 116
Clot formation, 234, *234*
Clot retraction, 234
Clubfoot, 91
Coagulation, *234,* 234-235
Coccygeal nerves, *170,* 170-171, 173-174
Coccyx, *103, 104,* 105
Cochlea, *194-197,* 195
Cochlear duct, 195, *195-197*
Cochlear implant, 200
Cochlear nerve, 196, *196,* 197
Codons, 54, 56t
Coitus interruptus, 414
Cold receptors, 186
Cold sores, 331
Collagenous fiber, 66
Collarbone, 106, *106*
Collateral ganglia, *176,* 176-177
Collecting ducts, renal, 377, *378*
Colliculi, inferior, 168
  superior, 168, *193*
Colloidal suspension, 27
Colon, *340,* 340-341
  ascending, *340,* 340-341
  descending, *340,* 341
  sigmoid, *340,* 341
  transverse, *340,* 341
Color, hair, 81
  skin, 80
Color blindness, 193
Colostomy, 329
Colostrum, 430
Column(s), anal, *340,* 341
  dorsal, 170-171, *171*
  lateral, 170-171, *171*
  renal, 376, *376*
  ventral, 170-171, *171*
Columnar cells, 61
Columnar epithelium, *60*
  pseudostratified, 61t, 62, *63*
  simple, 61t, 62, *62*
Combination reaction, 25
Combining vowel, 15
Comminuted fracture, 116
Commissural fibers, 165t
Commissure, gray, 170, *171*
Common bile duct, 342, 344
Common carotid artery, 270, *271, 272,* 273t
Common hepatic artery, *271, 272,* 273t, 275, 342, *342, 343*
Common iliac artery, *274*
Common iliac vein, *276, 277,* 278t, 280
Compensation, in acid-base balance, 390

Complement, 291-292, *294*
Complete fracture, 116
Complex polysaccharides, 31, 362, 362t. See also *Glycogen.*
Composition reaction, 25
Compound gland, 64, *64*
Compounds. See *Chemical compounds.*
Computed tomography, 153
Concentration gradient, 46
Conchae, nasal, *98, 100,* 101, 308, *309*
Concussion, cerebral, 153
Condom, 414
Conduction, heat loss via, 368
Conduction deafness, 200
Conduction myofibers, *150,* 250
Conduction system, cardiac, 249-251, *250*
Condyle, 94t
  lateral, femoral, *111,* 112, 112t
    tibial, 112, *113,* 113t
  mandibular, *98,* 102
  medial, femoral, *111,* 112, 112t
    tibial, 112, *113,* 113t
  occipital, *99, 100, 100*
Condyloid joint, 115t
Cones, 191, *192,* 192-193, 193t
Congenital malformations, teratogens and, 432-433
Conjunctiva, 188
Conjunctivitis, 189
Connective tissue, 65t, 65-68
  adipose, 65t, 66, *66*
  age-related changes in, 71
  blood as, 65t, 68, *68,* 226
  cartilage as, 65t, 67, *67*
  cell types in, 66
  collagenous fibers in, 66
  components of, 66
  dense fibrous, 65t, 67, *67*
  elastic, 66t, 67
  elastic fibers in, 66
  loose (areolar), 65t, 66, *66*
  osseous, 65t, 67-68, *68*
Contact dermatitis, 302
Continuous positive airway pressure (CPAP), 324
Contraception, 414-415
Contraction, muscle. See *Muscle contraction.*
  premature cardiac, 250
Contusion, cerebral, 153
Conus medullaris, 170, *170*
Convection, heat loss via, 368
Convergence circuit, 162, *162*
Cooper's ligaments, 412, *412*
Cor pulmonale, 243
Coracoid process, *106,* 107
Cord, spermatic, 399
Cord blood, 229
Core temperature, 367
Cornea, 190, *190*
  transplantation of, 190
Corniculate cartilage, 309
Corona radiata, 306
Coronal plane, 11
Coronal suture, *98, 100*
Coronary arteries, *245,* 248, *249,* 270, 273t, *274*
Coronary artery bypass grafting, 243, 283
Coronary veins, 248-249, *249*
Coronoid fossa, 107, *107,* 107t
Coronoid process, 108, *108,* 109t
Corpora cavernosa, 400, *401*
Corpora quadrigemina, *167,* 168
Corpus albicans, *404,* 406

Corpus luteum, *404,* 406
Corpus spongiosum, 400, *401*
Corpuscles, Meissner's, 185, *185*
  pacinian (lamellated), 185, *185*
Cortex, adrenal, 214, *214*
  auditory, 166t
  cerebellar, 168
  cerebral, *164,* 165, 166t
  gustatory, *164,* 166t
  hair, 80, *81*
  motor, *164,* 165, 166t
  olfactory, *164,* 166t, 187
  ovarian, 403, *404*
  prefrontal, 166t
  renal, 376, *376*
  sensory, *164,* 165, 166t
  somatomotor, *164,* 165, 166t
  somatosensory, *164,* 165, 166t
  visual, 166t, *193*
Corticosteroids, 205, 215-216, *216*
Cortisol, 215, *216*
Cortisone, 215
Coryza, 307
Costal area, 14t, *15*
Costal cartilage, *105,* 106
Coughing, 322, 323t
Covalent bonds, 21-22, *21-23*
Cowper's glands, *396,* 400
Coxal bones, 109, *110,* 110t
Cramps, 123, 132
Cranial area, 14t, *15*
Cranial bones, *98-100*
Cranial cavity, 12, *12*
Cranial nerves, 172-173, *173,* 174t. See also specific nerves.
Craniosacral division, 177
Creatine phosphate, in muscle contraction, 130, *130*
Creatine phosphokinase (CPK), 248
Cremaster muscle, 395
Crenation, 47
Crest, 94t
  anterior, 112, *113,* 113t
  iliac, 109, *110,* 110t
  intertrochanteric, *111,* 112, 112t
Cretinism, 205, 212
Cribriform plate, *99, 100,* 101
Cricoid cartilage, 309, *309*
Crista ampullaris, 198, *198*
Crista galli, *99, 100,* 101
Croup, 307
Crown, 333, *333*
Crying, 322, 323t
Cryptorchidism, 396
Cubital area, 14t, *15*
Cuboidal cells, 61
Cuboidal epithelium, *60,* 61, 61t, *62*
Cuneiform cartilage, 309
Cupula, 198, *198*
Cushing's syndrome, 216
Cusp, heart valve, 246, *247*
Cuspids, 332, *332,* 333t
Cutaneous membrane, 70, 77
Cutaneous region, 14t, *15*
Cuticle, *81,* 81-82
  hair, 80, *81*
Cyanocobalamin, 366t
Cyclic adenosine monophosphate (cAMP), 206
Cyclosporine, 297
Cystic duct, *342,* 344
Cystic fibrosis, 41
Cystitis, 381
Cytokinesis, 51

Cytoplasm, 41, 42t
Cytoplasmic organelles, 41, *41*, 42t, 43
Cytoskeleton, 42t

D

Dalton's law of partial pressures, 315
Dartos muscle, 395
Deafness, 199-200
Deamination, 357
Deciduous (primary) teeth, 332, *332*
Decomposition reactions, 25
Decussation, 168
Deep, 11
Deep back muscles, 137
Defecation, 330
Defense mechanism(s), barrier, 291, *292*,
    295
    chemical, 291-292, *292*, *295*
    complement in, 291-292, *295*
    inflammation as, 293, *294*, *295*
    interferon in, 292, *295*
    nonspecific, 291-293, *292*
    phagocytosis as, 292-293, *294*, *295*
    specific, 293-301. See also *Immunity*.
Defibrillation, 243
Dehydration synthesis, 26, 354, *355*
Delayed hypersensitivity, 301, *302*
Delivery, 429, *429*
    breech presentation in, 429
Deltoid muscle, 140t, 141-142, *142*
Deltoid tuberosity, 107, *107*, 107t
Dendrites, 155, *155*
Dens, 104, *104*
Dense fibrous connective tissue, 65t, 67, *67*
Dental caries, 333
Dentin, 333, *333*
Deoxyhemoglobin, 230
Deoxyribonucleic acid (DNA). See *DNA*.
Deoxyribose, 31
Depolarization, 159
Dermatitis, 77
    contact, 302
Dermis, 77, *78*
    papillary layer of, *78*, 79
    reticular layer of, *78*, 79
Descending aorta, 270-274, *271*, *272*, 273t,
    274
Descending colon, *340*, 341
Descending limb, of renal tubule, 377, *378*
Descending tract, 171
Detached retina, 191
Detrusor muscle, 380, *380*
Development, 420-433. See also *Growth*.
    embryonic, 424-426, *425*, *426*, 427t
    fertilization in, 420-422, *421*
    fetal, 426t, 427t, 427-428
    implantation in, 423, *423*, 424
    in adolescence, 432
    in adulthood, 432
    in childhood, 431-432
    in infancy, 431
    in neonatal period, 431
    organogenesis in, 426, 426t, 427t
    postnatal, 430-432
    preembryonic period of, 422-424, *422-*
        424, 427t
    prenatal, 420-430
    stages of, 427t
    teratogens and, 432-433
Developmental age, 420
Diabetes insipidus, 211

Diabetes mellitus, 221-222
    renal, 383
Dialysis, 47, 375
Diapedesis, 232
Diaphragm, contraceptive, 414
    pelvic, 138t, 139-140
    thoracic, 137, 138t, *139*, 313, *313*
    urogenital, 138t, 140
Diaphysis, 93, *93*
Diarrhea, 329
Diarthroses, 114-115
Diastole, atrial, 251, *251*
    ventricular, 251, *251*, 252
Diastolic pressure, 267. See also *Blood pres-*
    sure.
Diencephalon, 165-168, *167*
Differential count, 233
Differentiation, 8
Diffusion, capillary, 263, *263*
    facilitated, 47, *47*
    simple, *46*, 46-47
Digestion, 8
    carbohydrate, 345-346, 346t
    chemical, 330, 345-346
    deglutition in, 330
    elimination in, 330
    hydrolysis in, 345, 354, *355*
    lipid, 346, 346t
    mechanical, 330
    movements in, 330
    peristalsis in, 330
    protein, 346, 346t
    small intestine in, 339-340
    stomach in, 336t, 336-338, *337*
Digestive enzymes, 339, 344-346, 346t
Digestive system, 5, 7t, 327-350
    accessory organs of, 341-345
    age-related changes in, 348
    disorders of, *350*
    functional relationships of, *328*
    functions of, 329-330
        absorptive, 330. See also *Absorption*.
        digestive, 330. See also *Digestion*.
        ingestive, 329
    general structure of, 330-331, *331*
    histology of, 330-331, *331*
    in absorption, 346-347, 348t
    in chemical digestion, 340, 345-346
    in mechanical digestion, 330
    layers of, 330, *330*
    overview of, 329
    regions of, *331*, 331-341. See also specific
        organs.
Digitalis, 253
Dilation stage, of labor, 428, *429*
Diploë, 93
Diplopia, 184
Disaccharides, 31, 362, 362t
    absorption of, 346, *347*
Disease, autoimmune, 295
    genetic, 56
    resistance to, 291-301. See also *Immunity*.
    susceptibility to, 291-301
Disk, embryonic, 424, *424*
    intervertebral, 103, *103*
    optic, *190*, 191
Dislocation, 91
Displaced fracture, 116
Displacement reactions, 25
Dissociation, chemical, 28
Distal, 11
Distal convoluted tubule, 377, *377*, *378*
Diuresis, 375
    alcohol and, 384

Diuretics, 211, 375
Divergence circuit, 162, *162*
Dizygotic twins, 421
DNA, 33-34, *35*, 35t
    damage to, aging and, 56
    in protein synthesis, 52-53
DNA replication, 52, *53*, 53-54
Dopamine, 161, 161t
Dorsal cavity, 12, *12*
Dorsal funiculi (columns), 170-171, *171*
Dorsal horn, 170, *171*
Dorsal median sulcus, 170, *171*
Dorsal root, 173, *174*
Dorsal root ganglion, 173, *174*
Dorsalis pedis artery, *271*, *272*, 273t, *275*
Dorsalis pedis pulse, 275
Dorsiflexion, 134t
Double replacement reactions, 25
Drugs, teratogenic, 433
Dual innervation, 175
Duct(s), alveolar, *310*, 311
    cochlear, 195, *195-197*
    common bile, *342*, 344
    cystic, *342*, 344
    ejaculatory, *396*, 399
    hepatic, 342, *342*
    lacrimal, 189, *189*
    lactiferous, 412-413
    lymphatic, 288, *288*
    nasolacrimal, 189, *189*
    pancreatic, 344
    renal collecting, 377, *378*
    right lymphatic, 288, *288*
    thoracic, 288, *288*, *289*
Ductus arteriosus, *280*, 281, 281t, 428t
    closure of, 429, *430*
Ductus deferens, *396*, 399
Ductus venosus, *280*, 281, 281t, 428t, 429, *429*
Duodenum, 338-340, *339*
Dura mater, 71, 163, *163*
Dural sinuses, 163
Dysphagia, 329
Dysplasia, 40
Dystocia, 420
Dysuria, 375

E

Ear, age-related changes in, 199
    artificial, 200
    disorders of, *201*
    external, 194, *194*
    inner, 195, *195*
    middle, *194*, 195
    structure of, 194-196, *194-196*
Eating disorders, 349
Ecchymosis, 226
ECG (electrocardiogram), *250*, 250-251
    in myocardial infarction, 254-255
Echocardiography, 243
Eclampsia, 420
Ectoderm, 424, *424*
    derivatives of, 427t
Ectopic focus, 250
Ectopic pregnancy, 407
Eczema, 77
Edema, 264, 387
    pulmonary, 307
EEG (electroencephalography), 153
Effectors, 153
    in reflex arc, 162, *162*, 163t
    visceral, 176t

Efferent arterioles, 377, *377*, 378, *378*, *379*
Efferent lymphatic vessels, 289, *290*
Efferent (motor) neurons, 126, 156, 156t
  in reflex arc, 162, *162*, 163t
Ejaculation, 401
Ejaculatory duct, *396*, 399
Elastic cartilage, 65t, 67, *67*
Elastic connective tissue, 65t, 67
Elastic fibers, 66
Elastic tissue, age-related changes in, 71
Elbow, 107-108
  tennis, 107
Elderly. See *Aging.*
Electrocardiogram (ECG), *250*, 250-251
  in myocardial infarction, 254-255
Electroencephalography (EEG), 153
Electrolyte(s), 27, *28*
  absorption of, 341, 346-347, *347*, 348t
  in plasma, 229
  large intestinal absorption of, 341
Electrolyte balance, 387-388
Electromyography, 123, 128, *129*
Electrons, 19, *19*, 24t
Electron-transport chain, 356
Elements, 18, 18t
Elimination, 330
Embolus, 226
Embryo, 424
Embryonic development, 424-426, *425*, *426*, 427t
Embryonic disk, 424, *424*
Emesis, 329
Emission, 401
Emmetropia, 184
Emulsifying agents, 344, 346, 346t
Enamel, 333, *333*
Endergonic reactions, 26
Endocardium, 244-245, *245*
Endochondral bone, 95, *95*
Endochondral ossification, 95, *95*
Endocrine glands, definition of, 64
  vs. exocrine glands, 205
Endocrine system, 5, 6t, 203-223. See also
  specific glands and hormones.
  age-related changes in, 221
  disorders of, 221-222, *223*
  functional relationships of, *204*
  vs. nervous system, 205
Endocrinology, 205
Endocytosis, 49
Endoderm, 424, *424*
  derivatives of, 427t
Endolymph, 195
Endometrium, 407, *407*
Endomysium, 124, *124*
Endoneurium, 172, *172*
Endoplasmic reticulum, *41*, 42t, 44
Endorphins, 161, 161t
Endosteum, 93, *93*
Endurance exercise, 146
Energy, ATP storage of, 355
  conversion of. See *Metabolism.*
  for basal metabolism, 361, *361*
  for exercise, 361
  for thermogenesis, 361
  production of, 360. See also *Metabolism.*
  units of, 360
Energy levels, electron, 19
Enkephalins, 161, 161t
Enterokinase, 339, 346t
Enuresis, 375
Enzymes, 26
  cardiac, 248

Enzymes *(Continued)*
  digestive, 339, 344-346, 346t
  pancreatic, 344-345
Eosinophils, 228t, 232
Ependymal cells, 157t
Epicardium, 243, 244, *245*
Epicondyle, 94t, *111*, 112, 112t
  lateral, 107, *107*, 107t
  medial, 107, *107*, 107t
Epidermis, 77, *78*
Epididymis, *396*, 399
Epidural space, 170, *171*
Epigastric region, 12, *13*
Epiglottis, 309, *309*
Epimysium, 124, *124*
Epinephrine, 161, 161t, 216-217, *217*
Epineurium, 172, *172*
Epiphyseal line, 93, *93*, 96
Epiphyseal plate, 93, *93*, 95
Epiphysis, 93, *93*
Epiphysis cerebri, 219
Epiploic appendages, 340, *340*
Epithalamus, 166-167, *167*, 168
Epithelium, 60-65
  classification of, 60, 61t
  columnar, 60
    pseudostratified, 61t, 62-63, *63*
    simple, 61t, 62, *62*
  cuboidal, 60, 61, 61t, 62, *62*
  germinal (ovarian), 402-403, *404*
  glandular, 61t, *63*, 63-65, *64*, 65t. See also
    Gland(s).
  olfactory, 187, *188*
  simple, *60*, 61
  squamous, *60*
    simple, 61, *61*, 61t
    stratified, 61t, 63, *63*
  stratified, *60*, 61
  transitional, 61t, 63, *63*
Eponychium, *81*, 81-82
Equations, chemical, 24-25
Equilibrium, chemical, diffusion and, 46
  reaction rate and, 27
  positional, 197-198
    dynamic, 197, *198*
    static, 197-198
Erectile dysfunction, 401
Erection, 401
Erector spinae muscles, 137, 138t
Eructation, 329
Erythrocytes, 68, *68*, 229-231
  anucleate, 229
  characteristics of, 228t, 229
  destruction of, 231, *232*
  functions of, 228t, 230
  hemoglobin and, 230
  immature, 229
  life cycle of, 231, *232*
  production of, 230-231, *231*
  reference ranges for, 229
  shape of, 229
Erythrocytosis, 226
Erythropoietin, 230, *231*, 375
Eschar, 77
Esophagus, 335
Essential amino acids, 364
Estrogen(s), 409, *410*
  production of, by ovary, 210t, 215, 219
    by placenta, 220, 426t
Estrogen replacement therapy, 413
Ethmoid bone, *98-100*, 101
  crista galli of, *99*, *100*
Ethmoid sinus, 101, 308, *309*
Eustachian tube, *194*, 195, 308, *309*

Eutocia, 420
Evaporation, heat loss via, 368
Eversion, 135t
Exchange reactions, 25
Excimer laser angioplasty, 283
Excitatory transmission, 162
Excretion, 8
Exercise, aerobic (endurance), 146
  anaerobic (resistance), 146-147
  energy expenditure in, 361
  muscles and, 146-147
Exergonic reactions, 25-26
Exhalation, *313*, 313-314
Exocrine glands, 63-65
Exocytosis, 49-50, *50*
Exophthalmic, 205
Expiration, *313*, 313-314
Expiratory reserve volume, 314, *314*, 315t
Expulsion stage, of labor, 429, *429*
Extension, 134t
External auditory meatus, *98*, 101, 195, *195*
External carotid artery, 271, 272, 273t, 274, *275*
External ear, 194, *194*
External iliac artery, 271, 272, 273t, 275
External iliac vein, 276, *277*, 278t, 280
External intercostal muscles, 137, 138t, *139*, 313
External jugular vein, 276, *277*, *277*, 278t
External nares, 308, *309*
External oblique muscle, 138, 138t, *139*, *141*
External os, 407, *407*
External respiration, 307, 316-317, *318*
External urethral orifice, 380
External urethral sphincter, 380
Extracellular fluid, 386, *386*
Extraembryonic membranes, 424-425, *425*
Extraocular muscle, 189
Extrapyramidal tract, 171
Eye, accessory structures of, 188-189, *189*
  age-related changes in, 199
  blinking of, 189
  disorders of, *201*
  protective features of, 188
  structure of, *190*, 190-191
  vision and, *191-193*, 191-194
Eye socket, 188
Eyebrows, 188
Eyelashes, 188
Eyelids, 188

F

Facet, 94t
Facial bones, *98-100*, 102
Facial expression, muscles of, 133-137, *136*, 136t
Facial nerve, 172-173, *173*, 174t, 187
Facilitated diffusion, 47, *47*
Falciform ligament, 342, *342*
Fallopian tubes, 406-407, *407*
False labor, 428
False pelvis, 111
False ribs, *105*, 106
False vocal cords, *309*, 310
Falx cerebelli, 168
Falx cerebri, 164
Fascia, renal, 376
  superficial, 80
Fasciculus, 124, *124*, 172, *172*
Fat, perirenal, 376
  subcutaneous, 65t, 66, *66*, 80

Fat (*Continued*)
 distribution of, 370
 essential, 369
 excess, 369
 nonessential, 369
Fats, *32*, 32t, 32-33, *33*, 364-365
 digestion of, 346
 food sources of, 364t
 functions of, 364-365
 membrane, 40-42
 metabolism of, 343, 354, *355*, 358-359, *359, 360*
 recommended intake of, 365
 saturated, 365
 unsaturated, 365
Fatty acids, 32-33, *33*, 33t, 346, 347. See also *Lipids.*
 absorption of, 346, 347, *347*, 348t
 beta oxidation of, 359
 in muscle contraction, 130, *130*
 metabolism of, 343, 354, *355*, 358-359, *359, 360*
 saturated, 33, 33t
 unsaturated, 33, 33t
Fauces, 309, *331*, 334
Feces, formation and elimination of, 341
Feedback, negative, *9*, 9-10, *10*
 in hormone regulation, 206-207
 positive, 10
Feet. See *Foot.*
Femoral area, 14t, *15*
Femoral artery, 271, *272*, 273t, 275
Femoral head, *111*, 112, 112t
Femoral neck, *111*, 112, 112t
 fracture of, 112
Femoral vein, 276, *277*, 278t, 280
Femur, *111*, 111-112, 112t
Fertilization, 406, 420-422, *421*
 in vitro, 424
Fetal alcohol syndrome (FAS), 433
Fetal circulation, *280*, 281-282, 282t, 427, 428t, 429, *430*
Fetus, 427
 development of, 427, 427t
Fever, 293
Fever blisters, 331
Fiber, dietary, 362-363, 363t
Fibers, adrenergic, 177
 cholinergic, 177
 collagenous, 66
 commissural, 165t
 conduction, *150, 250*
 elastic, 66
 muscle, *124*, 125
  red, 131
  white, 131
 nerve, 155, *155*
 postganglionic, 175, *175*
 preganglionic, 175, *175*
 projection, 165t
 spindle, in mitosis, 51
Fibrillation, 243
Fibrin, 234
Fibrinogen, 227t, 228, 234
Fibrinolysis, 234
Fibroblast, 66
Fibrocartilage, 65t, 67, *67*
Fibrocartilaginous callus, 117
Fibrocystic breast disease, 413
Fibrosis, 72, *73*
Fibrous coat, of ureter, 379, *380*
Fibrous pericardium, 243, *245*
Fibrous tunic, of eye, 190, *190*
Fibula, 112, *113*, 113t

Fibular head, 112, *113*, 113t
Filamentous protein organelles, *41*, 42t, 45
Filtrate, 381
Filtration, capillary, *263*, 263-264
 membrane, 49
Filtration membrane, 381
Filtration pressure, 381
Filum terminale, 170, *170*
Fimbriae, 406, *407*
First heart sound, 251-252
First messenger, 206
First polar body, *405*, 406
First-degree burns, 84-85
Fissure(s), longitudinal, 164, *164*
 orbital, inferior, *98*, 100, 101t
  superior, *98*, 100, 101t
 osseous, 94t
  cranial, 101t
 transverse, 168
 ventral (anterior) median, 170, *171*
Flagella, 42t, 45
Flat bones, 93
Flatus, 329
Flexion, 134t
Flexure, hepatic (right colonic), *340, 341*
 splenic (left colonic), *340, 341*
Floating kidney, 376
Floating ribs, *105*, 106
Fluid, absorption of, 341, 346-347, *347*, 348t
 amniotic, 425
 cerebrospinal, accumulation of, 169
  collection of, 170
  formation of, 170
 extracellular, 386, *386*
 intake and output of, 387, *387*
 interstitial, *263*, 263, 287, 386, *386*
 intracellular, 41, 386, *386*
 intravascular, 386, *386*
 large intestinal absorption of, 341
 seminal, 400
 serous, 71
 synovial, 71, 114, *115*
Fluid balance, maintenance of, 375
 urine concentration and volume and, 384-385
Fluid compartments, 386, *386*
Fluoride, dietary, 367t
Folic acid, 366t
 in erythropoiesis, 231
Follicle, hair, 81, *81*
 ovarian, 403, *404*
  development of, *404*, 406
Follicle-stimulating hormone (FSH), 209t, *210*, 211
 in female, 409, *410*, 412
 in male, 402, *403*
Follicular cells, *404*, 406
Follicular phase, of ovarian cycle, 409, *410*
Fontanels, 102
Foot, 113, *114*. See also *Lower extremity.*
 bones of, 112, *114*
 club, 91
 muscles of, 145, 145t
Foramen (foramina), 94t
 apical, 333, *333*
 cranial, *98-100*, 100, 101t
 hypoglossal, *99*, 100, 101t
 infraorbital, *98*, 100, 101t
 intraventricular, 169, *169*
 jugular, *99*, 100, 101t
 mental, *98*, 100, 101t
 nutrient, 93, *93*
 obturator, 109, *110*, 110t
 of skull, *98-100*, 100, 101t

Foramen (foramina) (*Continued*)
 olfactory, 100, *101*, 101t
 optic, *98, 99*, 100, *101*, 101t
 stylomastoid, *99*, 100, 101t
 supraorbital, *98*, 100, *101*, 101t
 transverse, 104, *104*
 vertebral, 103, *103*
Foramen lacerum, *99*
Foramen magnum, *99*, 100, 101t
Foramen ovale, *99*, 100, 101t, *280*, 281, 281t, 428t
 closure of, 429, *430*
Foramen rotundum, *99*, 100, 101t
Forearm, 107-108, *108*, 109t. See also *Upper extremity.*
 muscles of, 140t, *141*, 142-143
Foreign bodies, tracheal, 311
Foreskin, 401, *401*
Formed elements, in blood, 226, 227, *227*, 229-233
Formula, molecular, 24
 structural, 24
Fossa(e), 94t
 coronoid, 107, *107*, 107t
 glenoid, *106*, 107
 iliac, 109, *110*, 110t
 mandibular, *98, 99*, 101
 olecranon, 107, *107*, 107t
 ovarian, 402
Fossa ovalis, 246, 429, *430*
Fourth ventricle, 169, *169*
Fovea, 94t
Fovea capitis, *111*, 112, 112t
Fovea centralis, *190*, 191
Fracture(s), 116-117
 healing of, 116-117
 of femoral neck, 112
 Pott's, 112
 reduction of, 116
 types of, 116
Fracture hematoma, 117
Free fatty acids. See *Fatty acids.*
Free nerve endings, 185, *185*
Frenulum, 332
Frontal area, 14t, *15*
Frontal bone, *98-100*, 100, 102
Frontal lobe, 164, *164*
Frontal plane, 11, *12*
Frontal sinus, 100, *101*, 308, *309*
Frontalis muscle, 133, *136*, 136t
Fructose, 31, 346, 362, 362t
 absorption of, 346, *347*
Functional residual capacity, 314, *314*, 315t
Fundus, gastric, 335, *335*
 uterine, 407, *407*
Funiculi, dorsal, 170-171, *171*
 lateral, 170-171, *171*
 ventral, 170-171, *171*

G

GABA (gamma-aminobutyric acid), 161, 161t, 162
Galactose, 31, 362, 362t
 absorption of, 341, 346, *347*, 348t
Gallbladder, *342*, 344, *345*
Gallstones, 344
Gametes, 395
Gamma globulins, 228
Gamma radiation, 36
Gamma-aminobutyric acid (GABA), 161, 161t, 162

Ganglion (ganglia), 154, 173
   autonomic, 175, *175*
   basal, 165
   collateral, *176*, 176-177
   dorsal root, 173, *174*
   paravertebral, 176
   terminal, *176*, 177
Gas(es), in plasma, 229
   partial pressure of, 315, 316t
   properties of, 315, 316t
Gas exchange, in respiration, 316, 316-317
Gas transport, in respiration, 317
Gaster, muscle, 124
Gastric arteries, *276, 277,* 278t, 280
Gastric glands, 336
Gastric juice, 336-338, *337*
Gastric mucosa, gastrin secretion by, 220
Gastric phase, of gastric secretion, 336, *337*
Gastric pits, 336
Gastric secretions, 220, 336t, 336-338, *337*
Gastrin, 220, 346t
   gastric secretion of, 336t, 336-338, *337*
Gastrocnemius muscle, *141, 142,* 145, 145t
Gastrointestinal system. See *Digestive system.*
Gavage, 329
General senses, 185-186
Genetic diseases, 56
Genetic mutations, 56
   cancer and, 57
Genital herpes, 416
Genitals, age-related changes in, 413
   female, 406-408, *407, 408*
   male, 400-401, *401*
Germ cells, primordial, 396
Germ layers, primary, formation of, 424
Germinal (ovarian) epithelium, 402-403, *404*
Gestation, 428
Gingiva, 333, *333*
Gingivitis, 333
Girdle, pectoral (shoulder), *106,* 106-107
   pelvic, 109-111, *110*
Gland(s), acinar, 64, *64*
   adrenal (suprarenal), *214,* 214-217
   apocrine, *64,* 65, 65t, 82
   Bartholin's, 408
   bulbourethral, *396,* 400
   ceruminous, 82, 194
   compound, 64, *64*
   Cowper's, *396,* 400
   endocrine, definition of, 64
     vs. exocrine glands, 205
   exocrine, 63-65
     vs. endocrine glands, 205
   gastric, 336
   greater vestibular, 408
   holocrine, *64,* 65, 65t
   intestinal, 338, *339*
   lacrimal, 189, *189*
   mammary, *412,* 412-413
   merocrine, *64,* 64-65, 65t, 80
   modes of secretion from, 65, 65t
   multicellular, 64
   parathyroid, *213,* 213-214
   paraurethral, 408
   parotid, *334,* 334
   pineal, *167,* 168, 210t, 219-220
   pituitary, 207-212, *208, 209t, 210*
   prostate, *396,* 400
   salivary, 333-334, *334*
   sebaceous, 82, 188
   simple, 64, *64*
   Skene's, 408
   sublingual, *334,* 334

Gland(s) *(Continued)*
   submandibular, *334, 334*
   sudoriferous, 82
   sweat, *64,* 64-65, 65t, 80, 82
   thyroid, *212,* 212-213
   tubular, 64
   unicellular, 64
Glandular epithelium, 61t, *63,* 63-65, *64,* 65t
Glans penis, 401, *401*
Glaucoma, 191
Glenoid cavity, *106,* 107
Glial cells, 70, 155, 156, 157t
Gliding joint, 115t
Gliomas, 156
Globins, 230, 297-298
Globulins, 227t, 228
Glomerular capsule, *377, 377*
Glomerular filtration, 381, *382, 384*
Glomerulus, *377, 377, 378*
Glossopharyngeal nerve, 172-173, *173,* 174t, 187
Glottis, *309,* 310
Glucagon, 217, *218*
Glucocorticoids, 215, *216*
Gluconeogenesis, 357
Glucose, 31, 362, 362t
   absorption of, 346, *347,* 348t
   hepatic storage of, 343
   in muscle contraction, 130, *131*
   in urine, 382
   metabolism of, 343, 354, *355,* 355-357, *355-358, 360*
   regulation of, 217-218, *218*
Glucose homeostasis, 357, *358*
   glucagon in, 217, *218*
   insulin in, 205, 217-218, *218*
Glucose tolerance test (GTT), 205
Gluteal area, 14t, *15*
Gluteal tuberosity, *111,* 112, 112t
Gluteus maximus muscle, *142,* 143, 144t
Gluteus medius muscle, *142,* 143, 144t
Gluteus minimus muscle, 143, 144t
Glycerol, 32
Glycogen, 31, 362-363
   production of, 357, *358*
   storage of, 357
Glycogenesis, 357
Glycogenolysis, 357
Glycolysis, 355-357, *357, 358*
Glycosuria, 221, 382
Gnostic area, *164,* 166t
Goblet cells, 62, 64, 341
Goiter, simple, 212
Golgi apparatus, *41,* 42t, 44, *44*
Golgi tendon organs, *185,* 186
Gonadal arteries, 270, *271, 272,* 273t, *274,* 275
Gonadocorticoids, 215-216
Gonadotropic hormones, 209t, *210,* 211
Gonadotropin-releasing hormone (GnRH), in female, 409, *410*
   in male, 401, *403*
Gonads, 395. See also *Ovary; Testis.*
   hormones of, 209t-210t, 218-219, *219*
Gonorrhea, 415
Gout, 91, 114
Gracilis muscle, *141,* 143, 144t
Graft, coronary artery bypass, 243
Granulation tissue, 72
Granulations, arachnoid, 170
Granulocytes, 232
Gray commissure, 170, *171*
Gray matter, cerebral, 164-165
   spinal, 170, *171*

Great saphenous vein, *276, 277,* 278t, 280
Greater curvature, of stomach, *335, 335*
Greater sciatic notch, 109, *110,* 110t
Greater trochanter, *111,* 112, 112t
Greater tubercle, *107, 107,* 107t
Greater vestibular glands, 408
Greater wing of sphenoid, *99,* 101
Greenstick fracture, 116
Groove, intertubercular, *107, 107,* 107t
   lacrimal, 102
Gross human anatomy, 2
Growth, 8. See also *Development.*
   appositional, 96
Growth hormone, 209t, 210, *210*
Gums, 333, *333*
Gustatory cells, 186
Gustatory cortex, *164,* 166t
Gustatory sense, 186-187, *187*
   age-related changes in, 199
   impairment of, *201*
Gyrus (gyri), *164, 164*
   postcentral, *164,* 165, 166t
   precentral, *164,* 165, 166t

H

H band, 125, *125*
H zone, 125, *125*
Hair, 80-81, *81*
   color of, 81
   lanugo, 427
   taste, 186
Hair bulb, 81, *81*
Hair cells, in equilibrium, 198, *198*
   in hearing, 196, *196*
Hair follicles, 81, *81*
Hair root, 80, *81*
Hair shaft, 80, *81*
   shape of, 81
Half-life, 36
Halitosis, 334
Hamstring muscles, *142,* 144t, 145
Hand, *108,* 108-109. See also *Upper extremity.*
   muscles of, 143
Hard palate, 308, *309,* 331, *331*
   cleft, 332
Haustra, 340, *340*
Haversian canal, 67, *68*
Haversian systems, 67, *68*
Head, femoral, *111,* 112, 112t
   fibular, 112, *113,* 113t
   humeral, *107, 107,* 107t
   osseous, 94t
   radial, 107, *108,* 109t
   ulnar, 108, *108,* 109t
Head and neck, arteries of, *271, 272,* 273t, 274
   muscles of, 133-137, *136,* 136t
   veins of, *276, 277,* 277-279, 278t
Hearing, 193, *196,* 196-197, *197*
   age-related changes in, 199
Hearing loss, 199-200
Heart, 241-255. See also *Cardiac; Cardiovascular* entries.
   age-related changes in, 253-254
   apex of, 243, *244*
   as endocrine organ, 220
   base of, 243, *244*
   blood flow in, 247-249, *248*
   chambers of, *245,* 245-246
   conduction system of, 249-251, *250*

Heart (*Continued*)
  coverings of, 243-244
  disorders of, *255*
  functional relationships of, *242*
  layers of, 244-245, *245*
  location of, 243, *244*
  muscle of, 68t, 69, *69*, 124t, 244, *245*. See
    also *Myocardium.*
  overview of, 243-244
  physiology of, 249-253
  size of, 243
  Starling's law of, 252
Heart murmurs, 252
Heart rate, 252, *253*
Heart sounds, 251-252
Heart valves, 245, 246-247, *247*
  aortic semilunar, *245*, 247, *247*, 248
  atrioventricular, 246
  cusp of, 246, *247*
  mitral (bicuspid), *245*, 246, *247*, 248
  pulmonary semilunar, *245*, 247, *247*-248
  stenosis of, 247
  tricuspid, *245*, 246, *247*, *247*
Heat, body, 8
Heat exhaustion, 354
Heat loss, 368
Heat production, 361, 368
  by muscle, 123
Heat receptors, 186
Heatstroke, 368
Helper T cells, 296, *297*
  in HIV infection, 239
Hemangioma, 260
Hematemesis, 329
Hematocrit, 227
Hematoma, fracture, 117
Hematopoiesis, 229, *230*
  in bone, 92
Heme, 230
Hemocytoblast, 229
Hemoglobin, 230
  in oxygen transport, 317, *318*
Hemolysis, 48
Hemolytic anemia, 231
Hemolytic disease of newborn, 237
Hemophilia, 226
Hemopoiesis, 229, *230*
Hemorrhoids, 260
Hemostasis, 233-235
  coagulation in, *234*, 234-235
  platelet plug formation in, 233-234, *234*
  vascular constriction in, 233, *234*
Henle's loop, 377, *377*, *378*
Henry's law, 315
Hepatic. See also *Liver.*
Hepatic artery, 342, *342*, *343*
Hepatic cirrhosis, 342, 360
Hepatic ducts, 342, *342*
Hepatic flexure, *340*, 341
Hepatic portal system, 276, *277*, 278t, 279,
    279
Hepatic portal vein, 276, *277*, 278t, 279,
    279, *342*, 342-343, *343*
Hepatic veins, 276, *277*, 278t, 279, *279*, 342,
    342, 343, *343*
Hepatitis B virus, transmission of, 239
Hepatocytes, 342
Hepatopancreatic sphincter, 344
Hering-Breuer reflex, 321
Hernia, hiatal, 336
  inguinal, 396
Herpes, genital, 416
Hiatal hernia, 336
Hiccupping, 322, 323t

High-density lipoproteins (HDLs), 365
Hilum, 2
  of kidney, 376
  of lung, 311
  of lymph node, *290*
Hinge joint, 115t
Hip girdle, 109-111, *110*
Histamine, 302
Histology, 60
HIV infection, transmission of, 239
Hives, 77
Holocrine gland, *64*, 65
Homeostasis, 9, 9-10, *10*
  negative feedback in, 9, 9-10, *10*
Horizontal plate, 102
Hormone(s), 205. See also *Endocrine system;*
    specific hormones.
  action of, control of, 206-207, *207*
    mechanisms of, 206, *206*
  adrenal, 209t, *214*, 215-217, *216*, *217*
  as proteins, 205
  as steroids, 205
  blood pressure and, 269
  characteristics of, 205-207
  definition of, 205
  hypersecretion of, 210
  hyposecretion of, 210
  in labor and delivery, 428-429
  pituitary, 209t, 210-212
  placental, 426, 426t
  receptor sites for, 205-206, *206*
  sex, female, 409-412, *410*, *411*
    male, 402, *403*
  target tissue for, 206
  thyroid, *212*, 212-213
  tropic, 207
  vs. prostaglandins, 220
Hormone replacement therapy, 413
Horn, dorsal, 170, *171*
  lateral, 170, *171*
  ventral, 170, *171*
Human chorionic gonadotropin (hCG), 220,
    423
  placental, 426t
Human immunodeficiency virus infection,
    transmission of, 239
Humerus, 107, *107*, 108t
Humoral immunity, 296-299, *298*
Hunchback, 103
Hyaline cartilage, 65t, 67, *67*
Hydrocephalus, 169
Hydrochloric acid, prostaglandins and, 221
  secretion of, 336t, 336-338, *337*
Hydrocortisone, 215, *216*
Hydrogen bond, 22-23, *23*
Hydrolysis, 25
  in chemical digestion, 345, 354, *355*
Hydrophilic, 40
Hydrophobic, 40
Hydrostatic pressure, 49
  in capillary microcirculation, 263-264
Hymen, 408
Hyoid bone, 102, *102*
Hypercortisolism, 216
Hyperextension, 134t
Hyperglycemia, in diabetes, 221
Hyperopia, 184
Hyperparathyroidism, 214
Hyperplasia, 40
Hyperplastic obesity, 369
Hyperpolarization, membrane, 162
Hypersensitivity, 299, 301-302
  delayed, 301, 302
  immediate, 301-302

Hyperthyroidism, 213
Hypertrophic obesity, 369-370
Hypertrophy, 40
Hypervitaminosis, 354
Hypochondriac region, 12, *13*
Hypocortisolism, 215-216
Hypodermis, *78*, 80
Hypogastric region, 12, *13*
Hypoglossal canal, *100*
Hypoglossal foramen, *99*, 100, 101t
Hypoglossal nerve, 172-173, *173*, 174t
Hypoglycemia, 218
Hypokalemia, 215
Hypoparathyroidism, 213-214
Hypopharynx, 334
Hypophysis, 207-212, *208*, 209t, *210*
Hypothalamus, 167, *167*, 167t
  adrenal glands and, *214*, 214-215
  pituitary and, 208, *208*, 212, *212*
  testosterone and, 219, *219*
  thyroid and, 212, *212*
Hypothermia, 354
Hypothyroidism, 212-213
Hypotonic solution, 48, *48*
Hypovolemic shock, 268

I

I bands, 125, *125*
Ileocecal junction, 340, *340*
Ileocecal sphincter, 340
Ileocecal valve, 340, *340*
Ileum, *339*, 339-340
Iliac arteries, *271*, *272*, 273t, 275
Iliac crest, 109, *110*, 110t
Iliac fossa, 109, *110*, 110t
Iliac region, 12, *13*
Iliac spine, 109, *110*, 110t
Iliac veins, 276, *277*, 278t, 280
Iliopectineal line, 109, *110*, 110t
Iliosacral joints, 109, *110*
Ilium, 109, *110*
Immediate hypersensitivity, 301-302
Immune response, primary, 297, *299*
  secondary, 297, *299*
Immunity, 291-301
  acquired, 299-301, *300*
  active, 300, *300*
  age-related changes in, 301
  antibody-mediated (humoral), 296-299,
    298
  artificial, 300, *300*
  cell-mediated, 296, *297*
  disorders of, *303*
  in hypersensitivity, 299, 301-302
  memory in, 293
  natural, 300, *300*
  passive, 299, 300, *300*
    artificial, 300
    natural, 300
  self vs. nonself in, 294-295
  specificity in, 293
Immunodeficiencies, *303*
Immunoglobulins, *298*, 299t. See also *Anti-
    bodies.*
Impetigo, 77
Implantation, 423, *423*, *424*
Impotence, 401
Incisors, 332, *332*, 333t
Inclusions, 41
Incomplete fracture, 116
Incontinence, urinary, 385

Incus, 102, *194*, 195, *195*, *197*
Infant, development in, 431
Infant respiratory distress syndrome, 314
Infarct, 254
Infection allergy, 302
Inferior, 11
Inferior cerebellar peduncle, 168
Inferior colliculi, 168
Inferior mesenteric artery, 270, *271*, *272*, 273t, 274, 275
Inferior mesenteric vein, *276*, 277, 278t, *279*, 280
Inferior oblique muscle, 189t
Inferior orbital fissure, *98*, 100, 101t
Inferior rectus muscle, 189t
Inferior vena cava, *276*, 277, 278t, *279*, *279*, 342, *342*
Inflammation, 72, 293, *294*
Infraorbital foramen, *98*, 100, 101t
Infraspinatus muscle, 140t, 141-142, *142*
Infundibulum, hypothalamic, 167, 208, *208*
  uterine tube, 406, *407*
Inguinal area, 14t, *15*
Inguinal canal, 396
Inguinal hernia, 396
Inguinal region, 12, *13*
Inhalation, 313, *313*
Inhibitory transmission, 162
Inner cell mass, *422*, 423
Inner circular layer, of digestive tract, *330*, 331
Inner ear, 195, *195*
Inner table, 93
Innominate bones, 109, *110*, 110t
Inspiration, 313, *313*
Inspiratory capacity, 314, *314*, 315t
Insula, 164, *164*
Insulin, 205, 217-218, *218*
  in diabetes, 222
Insulin-dependent diabetes, 222
Intake and output, 387, *387*
Integration, sensory, 153
Integration center, in reflex arc, 162, *162*, 163t
Integumentary system, 5, 6t. See also *Hair; Nails; Skin.*
  definition of, 77
  functional relationships of, *76*
Interatrial septal defect, 281
Interatrial septum, *245*, 246
Intercondylar notch, *111*, 112, 112t
Intercostal arteries, 270, *271*, *272*, 273t, 274
Intercostal muscles, external, 137, 138t, *139*, 313
  internal, 137, 138t, *139*, 313
Intercostal nerves, 174, 320, *320*
Interferon, 292, *294*
Interleukin-2, 297
Interleukins, 287
Interlobar arteries, 378, *379*
Interlobar veins, 378, *379*
Interlobular arteries, 378, *379*
Interlobular veins, 378, *379*
Intermolecular bonds, 22-23, *23*
Internal auditory meatus, *99*, 100, *100*, 101t
Internal carotid artery, *271*, *272*, 273t, 274, 275
Internal iliac artery, *271*, *272*, 273t, 275
Internal iliac veins, *276*, 277, 278t, 280
Internal intercostal muscles, 137, 138t, *139*, 313
Internal jugular veins, *276*, 277, *277*, 278t
Internal nares, 308, *309*
Internal oblique muscle, 138, 138t, *139*

Internal os, 407, *407*
Internal respiration, 307, 317, *318*
Internal urethral sphincter, 380
Interneurons, 156, 156t
Interphase, *50*, 50-51, 51t
Interstitial cells, testicular, 396, *397*
Interstitial cell–stimulating hormone, 209t, *210*, 211
  in female, 409
  in male, 402, *403*
Interstitial fluid, 263, *263*, 287, 386, *386*
Intertrochanteric crest, *111*, 112, 112t
Intertrochanteric line, *111*, 112, 112t
Intertubercular groove, 107, *107*, 107t
Intervertebral disks, 103, *103*
Intestinal absorption, 330
Intestinal glands, 338, *339*
Intestinal lipase, 339
Intestinal mucosa, 330, *330*, 339
Intestinal phase, of gastric secretion, 336, *337*
Intestinal villi, 287, 338, *339*
  absorption by, 341, 346-347, *347*
Intestine, large, 340-341, *341*
  small, 338-340, *339*
Intra-alveolar pressure, 312-313, *313*, 314
Intracellular fluid, 41, 386, *386*
Intramembranous bone, 95
Intramembranous ossification, 95
Intramolecular bonds, 22-23
Intrapleural pressure, 312-313, *313*
Intrauterine device, 415
Intravascular fluid, 386, *386*
Intravenous pyelogram, 375
Intraventricular foramina, 169, *169*
Intrinsic factor, 231
  gastric secretion of, 336t, 336-338, *337*
Inversion, 135t
Involuntary nervous system, I55
Iodine, dietary, 367t
  protein-bound, 213
  thyroid hormones and, 212
Ion(s), 20, 20t, 24t
  formation of, 28, *28*
Ionic bonds, 20, 20-21
Ionic compounds, 21
Iris, 190, *190*
  circular muscles of, 189t
  radial muscles of, 189t
Iron, dietary, 367t
  in erythropoiesis, 231
Irregular bones, 93
Ischial spine, *110*, 110t, 111
Ischial tuberosity, *110*, 110t, 111
Ischium, 109, *110*
Island of Reil, 164, *164*
Islets of Langerhans, 217-218, 344, *344*
Isometric contraction, 129
Isotonic contraction, 129
Isotonic solution, 47, *48*
Isotopes, radioactive, 36

J

Jejunum, *339*, 339-340
Joint(s), 114-115
  amphiarthrotic, 114
  ball-and-socket, 115t
  condyloid, 115t
  diarthrotic, 114-115
  disorders of, *118*
  gliding, 115t

Joint(s) *(Continued)*
  hinge, 115t
  pivot, 115t
  saddle, 115t
  stability of, 123
  synarthrotic, 114
  synovial, 114, *115*
Joint capsule, 114
Joint cavity, 114
Jugular foramen, *99*, 100, 101t
Jugular notch, 105, *105*
Jugular veins, *276*, 277, *277*, 278t
Juice, gastric, 336-338, *337*
  pancreatic, 344-345
Junction, ileocecal, 340, *340*
  neuromuscular, 126, *126*
Juvenile diabetes, 222
Juxtaglomerular apparatus, 378, *378*
Juxtaglomerular cells, 378, *378*

K

Keratin, 77-78
Keratinization, 77-78
Ketone bodies, 359
Ketosis, 359
Kidney(s), 375-379. See also *Renal* entries.
  age-related changes in, 389
  blood flow in, 378, *379*
  disorders of, 377, *391*
  floating, 376
  in acid-base balance, 388
  in blood pressure regulation, 269
  location of, 376, *376*
  nephrons of, 377, *377*
  polycystic disease of, 377
  stones in, 385
  structure of, 375-378, *376-378*
  urine concentration and volume and, 384
  urine formation in, 381-384
Killer T cells, 296, *297*
Kilocalories, 360
Knee, cartilage of, 114-115, *115*
  tear in, 115
  ligaments of, tears in, 115
Kneecap, *111*, 112t, 113
Knee-jerk reflex, 171, 172t
Korotkoff sounds, 267
Krebs cycle, 356
Kupffer cells, 344
Kwashiorkor, 354, 364
Kyphosis, 103

L

Labia majora, 408, *408*
Labia minora, 408, *408*
Labor, 428-429
  dilation stage of, 428, *429*
  expulsion stage of, 429, *429*
  false, 428
  placental stage of, 429, *429*
  true, 428
Labyrinth, bony, 195, *195*
  membranous, 195, *195*
Lacrimal apparatus, 189, *189*
Lacrimal bones, *98-100*, 102
Lacrimal canals, 189, *189*
Lacrimal ducts, 189, *189*
Lacrimal gland, 189, *189*
Lacrimal groove, 102

Lacrimal sac, 189, *189*
Lactase, 339, 346t
Lactate dehydrogenase (LDH), 248
Lactation, 413, 428, 429-430, *431*
Lacteals, 287, 338, *339*
Lactic acid, in glycolysis, 356
Lactiferous ducts, 412-413
Lactiferous sinus, *412*, 413
Lactogenic hormone, 209t, *210*, 211
Lactose, 31, 345-346, 362, 362t
   absorption of, 346, *347*
Lactose intolerance, 339
Lacunae, in cartilage, 67
Lambdoid suture, *98*, 100, *100*
Lamellae, 67
Lamellated corpuscles, 185, *185*
Lanugo hair, 427
Laparoscopy, 329
Large intestine, 340-341, *341*. See also *Intes-
      tinal* entries.
   functions of, 341
   structure of, *340*, 340-341
Laryngitis, 310
Laryngopharynx, 309, *309*, 334
Larynx, *309*, 309-310
Laser angioplasty, 283
Latent syphilis, 415
Lateral, 11
Lateral condyle, femoral, *111*, 112, 112t
   tibial, 112, *113*, 113t
Lateral epicondyle, 107, *107*, 107t
Lateral epicondylitis, 107
Lateral funiculi (columns), 170-171, *171*
Lateral horn, 170, *171*
Lateral malleolus, 112, *113*, 113t
Lateral meniscus, 114-115, *115*
   tear in, 115
Lateral rectus muscle, 189t
Lateral sulcus, 164, *164*
Lateral ventricles, 169, *169*
Latissimus dorsi muscle, 140t, 141, *142*
Laughing, 322, 323t
Left atrium, *245*, 246
Left bundle branch, 250, *250*
Left colonic flexure, *340*, 341
Left common carotid artery, *249*, 270, *271*,
      272, 273t, *274*, 275
Left common iliac artery, *271*, *272*, 273t,
      275
Left coronary artery, *245*, 248, *249*, 270,
      273t, *274*
Left gastric artery, *271*, *272*, 273t, 275, *276*,
      277, 278t, 280
Left hepatic ducts, 342, *342*
Left lobe, of liver, 342, *342*
Left pulmonary artery, *249*, 269, 270
Left subclavian artery, *249*, 270, *271*, *272*,
      273t, *274*, 275
Left ventricle, *245*, 246, *247*, 248
Left vertebral artery, *275*
Leg. See also *Lower extremity.*
   bones of, 112, *113*, 113t
Leg area, 14t, *15*
Lens, 190, *190*
   accommodation of, 191-192, *192*
   opacities of, 199
Lesser sciatic notch, *110*, 110t, 111
Lesser trochanter, *111*, 112, 112t
Lesser tubercle, 107, *107*, 107t
Leukocytes, 68, *68*, 228t, 232-233
   characteristics of, 228t, 232
   function of, 228t, 232
   types of, 228t, 232-233
Leukocytosis, 226

Leukopenia, 226
Levator ani muscles, 138t, 140
Levator palpebrae superioris, 188
Leydig cells, 396, *397*
LH. See *Luteinizing hormone (LH).*
Life processes, 5-8
Ligament(s), 67
   broad, 407, *407*
   falciform, 342, *342*
   of knee, tears in, 115
   periodontal, 333, *333*
   suspensory, of eye, 190, *190*, 191-192
      of uterus, 412, *412*
Ligamentum venosum, 342, *342*
Limbic system, 168
Liminal stimulus, in muscle contraction, 127
   in nerve conduction, 159
Line(s), arcuate, 109, *110*, 110t
   cleavage, 79
   epiphyseal, 93, *93*, 96
   iliopectineal, 109, *110*, 110t
   intertrochanteric, *111*, 112, 112t
   M, 125, *125*
   Z, 125, *125*
Linea alba, 138, 138t, *139*, 141
Linea aspera, *111*, 112, 112t
Linear fracture, 116
Lingual tonsils, 290, 309, *309*, 332
Lip, 331
Lipase, pancreatic, 345, 346t
   small intestinal, 339, 346t
Lipectomy, suction, 66
Lipids, *32*, 32t, 32-33, *33*, 364-365. See also
      Cholesterol; Fats.
   digestion of, 346
   functions of, 364-365
   membrane, 40-42
   metabolism of, 343, 354, *355*, 359, *359*,
      360
   restriction of, 365
Lipoproteins, high-density, 365
   low-density, 365
Lithotripsy, 375
Liver, 341-344. See also *Hepatic* entries.
   blood supply to, 342-343
   cirrhosis of, 342, 360
   functions of, 343-344
   lobes of, 342, *342*
   lobules of, 342, *343*
   structure of, 341-342, *342*, *343*
Lobar bronchi, 310, *311*
Lobe(s), frontal, 164, *164*
   liver, 342, *342*
   lung, *311*, 311-312
   mammary, 412, *412*
   parietal, 164, *164*
   temporal, 164, *164*
      in auditory pathway, 197
Lobule(s), bronchopulmonary, 312
   liver, 342, *343*
   lung, 312
   mammary, 412, *412*
   testicular, 396, *396*
Localized inflammation, 293, *294*
Long bones, 93, 93-94
Longitudinal fissure, 164, *164*
Loose connective tissue, 65t, 66, *66*
Lordosis, 103
Low-density lipoproteins (LDLs), 365
Lower extremity, arteries of, *271*, *272*, 273t,
      275
   bones of, *111*, 111-113, 112t, *113*, *114*
   muscles of, *141-142*, 143-145, 144t-145t
   veins of, 280

Lower respiratory tract, *308*, *310*, 310-312,
      311
Lumbar area, 14t, *15*
Lumbar arteries, 270, *271*, *272*, 273t, *274*,
      275
Lumbar curvatures, 103, *103*
Lumbar enlargement, 170, *170*
Lumbar nerves, *170*, 170-171, 173-174, 175t
Lumbar puncture, 170
Lumbar region, 12, *13*
Lumbar vertebrae, 103, 104, *104*
Lung(s), *311*, 311-312. See also *Pulmonary;
      Respiratory* entries.
   age-related changes in, 323
   cancer of, 307
   in neonate, 429
Lung capacities, 314, *314*, 315t
Lung volumes, 314, *314*, 315t
Lunula, 82
Luteal phase, of ovarian cycle, 409, *410*
Luteinizing hormone (LH), 209t, *210*, 211
   in female, 409, *410*, 412
   in male, 402, *403*
Lyme disease, 91
Lymph, 287
Lymph capillaries, 288, *288*
Lymph nodes, 288, *289*, 289-290, *290*
Lymph nodules, 289, *290*
Lymph sinuses, 289, *290*
Lymphadenitis, 287
Lymphangiogram, 287
Lymphatic ducts, 288, *288*
Lymphatic system, 5, 7t, 285-303
   age-related changes in, 301
   components of, 287-291
   disorders of, *303*
   functional relationships of, *286*
   functions of, 287
   organs of, *289*, 289-291, *290*
Lymphatic trunks, 288
Lymphatic vessels, *288*, 288-289
   afferent, 289, *290*
   efferent, 289, *290*
Lymphedema, 287, *288*
Lymphocytes, 228t, 233, 289
   B, 291, 295-297, *296-298*
   development of, 295-296, *296*
   differential count of, 233
   in cell-mediated immunity, 296, *297*
   splenic production of, 290
   T, 291, 295-296, *296-298*
      helper, 296, *297*
      killer, 296, *297*
      memory, 296, *297*
      suppressor, 296, *297*
Lymphoma, 287
Lysosomes, *41*, 42t, 44

M

M line, 125, *125*
Macrophages, 66, 233
   in nonspecific resistance, 292-293, *294*
   in phagocytosis, 292-293, *294*
   in specific resistance, 293-294
Macula, 197-198, *198*
Macula densa, 378, *378*
Macula lutea, 191
Magnesium, 367t
Magnetic resonance imaging, 153
Major calyx, 376, *376*
Malar bones, 102

Malignant melanoma, 77, 78
Malignant tumors, 40, 57. See also *Cancer*.
Malleolus, lateral, 113, *113*, 113t
  medial, 112, *113*, 113t
Malleus, 102, *194*, *195*, *197*
Malnutrition, 354
  kwashiorkor and, 354, 364
Maltase, 339, 346t
Maltose, 31, 345-346, 362, 362t
  absorption of, 346, *347*
  metabolism of, 354, *355*
Mamillary bodies, 167
Mammary area, 14t, *15*
Mammary glands, *412*, 412-413
Mandible, *98-100*, 102
Mandibular condyle, *98*, 102
Mandibular fossa, *98*, *99*, 101
Manubrium, 105, *105*
Marasmus, 354
Marfan's syndrome, 60
Marrow, blood formation in, 92
  hematopoiesis in, 229, *230*
  transplantation of, 229
Mass, vs. weight, 18
Mass number, 19
Masseter muscle, *136*, 136t, *137*
Mast cells, 66, 233
  in hypersensitivity, 302
Mastectomy, 288
Masticatory muscles, *136*, 136t, *137*
Mastoid fontanel, 102
Mastoid process, *98*, *99*, 101
Matrix, nail, 82
Maturity-onset diabetes, 222
Maxilla, *98-100*, 102
Maxillary sinus, 102, 308, *309*
Meatus, 94t
  external auditory, *98*, 101, *195*, 195
  internal auditory, *99*, *100*, *100*, 101t
Mechanical digestion, 330
Mechanoreceptors, 184, 185t
  in equilibrium, 197, *198*
  in hearing, 194
  in touch and pressure sense, 185, 185t
Medial, 11
Medial condyle, femoral, *111*, 112, 112t
  tibial, 112, *113*, 113t
Medial epicondyle, 107, *107*, 107t
Medial malleolus, 112, *113*, 113t
Medial meniscus, 114-115, *115*
  tear in, 115
Medial rectus muscle, 189t
Median cubital vein, *276*, *277*, 278t, *279*
Median fissure, ventral (anterior), 170, *171*
Median sulcus, dorsal (posterior), 170, *171*
Medical terminology, 10-15, *15*
Medulla, adrenal, 214, *214*
  hair, 80, *81*
  ovarian, 403, *404*
  renal, 376, *376*
Medulla oblongata, *167*, 168
  in auditory pathway, 197
Medullary cavity, 93, *93*
Megakaryocytes, 233
Meiosis, 50, *50*, 51t, 51-52, *52*
Meissner's corpuscles, 185, *185*
Meissner's plexus, *330*, 330-331
Melanin, 78, 80
Melanocytes, 78, *78*
Melanoma, 77, 78
Melatonin, 219-220
Membrane(s), basement, 60
  basilar, 195, *196*, *197*
  body, 70-71

Membrane(s) *(Continued)*
  cutaneous, 70, 77
  extraembryonic, 424-425, *425*
  filtration, 381
  mucous. See *Mucosa(e)*.
  nuclear, *41*, 42t, 43
  plasma, 40-41, *42*
    hormone receptors on, 205-206, *206*
    selective permeability of, 40, 47
    transport across, 45-50, 46t. See also
      Membrane transport.
  respiratory, 316-317, *317*
  resting, 157, *158*
  serous, 70, 70-71
    pleural, *311*, 312
  synovial, 70, 71, 114, *115*
  tectorial, 196, *196*, *197*
  tympanic, 194, *194*, *195*, *197*
  vestibular, 195, *196*, *197*
Membrane depolarization, *158*, 159
Membrane diffusion, 46
Membrane filtration, 48-49
Membrane hyperpolarization, 162
Membrane lipids, 40-42
Membrane potential, resting, 157, *158*
Membrane proteins, 40-41, *42*
Membrane repolarization, *158*, 159
Membrane transport, active, 49
  by diffusion, *46*, 46t, 46-47, *47*
  by endocytosis, 49
  by exocytosis, 49-50, *50*
  by filtration, 48-49
  by osmosis, 47, *48*
  in nutrient absorption, 346-347, *347*
Membranous labyrinth, 195, *195*
Membranous urethra, *380*, 381, *396*, 399
Memory cells, B, 297, *299*
  T, 296, *297*
Menarche, 409
Meninges, 71, *163*, 163-164
Meningitis, 164
Meniscus, 114-115, *115*
  tear in, 115
Menopause, 409, 412, 413
Menstrual cycle, 409, *410*, 410-412, *411*
Menstrual phase, of menstrual cycle, 410,
  411
Menstruation, cessation of, 412
  onset of, 409
Mental foramen, *98*, 100, 101t
Merocrine sweat glands, *64*, 64-65, 82
Mesenteric arteries, 270, *271*, *272*, 273t, *274*,
  275
Mesenteric veins, *276*, *277*, 278t, *279*, 280
Mesentery, *339*, 339-340
Mesoderm, 424, *424*
  derivatives of, 427t
Mesothelium, 70
Messenger RNA, 53-54, *54*, 206
Metabolic acidosis, 389-390, 391t
Metabolic alkalosis, 389-390, 391t
Metabolic rate, basal, 361, *361*
  age-related decline in, 369
  total, 360, *361*
Metabolism, 8, 354-361
  age-related changes in, 369
  anabolic, 354
  carbohydrate, 343, 354, *355*-357, *355*-*358*,
    360
  catabolic, 354-355
  cellular, 354
  dehydration synthesis in, 26, 354, *355*
  energy production by, 360-361
  hepatic, 343-344

Metabolism *(Continued)*
  in muscle contraction, *130-131*, 130-133
  lipid, 343-344, 354, *355*, 358-359, *359*, *360*
  protein, 344, 354, *355*, 357, *359*, *360*
Metacarpal bones, *108*, 108-109
Metacarpus, 108, *108*
Metaphase, *50*, 51, 51t
Metaplasia, 40
Metarterioles, 262, *262*
Metastasis, 40, 57, 287, 289
Metatarsal bones, 113, *114*
Metatarsus, 113, *114*
Micelles, 347
Microfilaments, 45
Microglia, 157t
Microscopic anatomy, 2
Microtubules, *41*, 45
Microvilli, 45, 62, 338, *339*
Micturition, 385
Midbrain, *167*, 168
  in auditory pathway, 197
Middle cerebellar peduncle, 168
Middle ear, *194*, 195
Middle nasal conchae, *98*, 101
Midsagittal plane, 11, *12*
Mineralocorticoids, 209t, 215, *216*
Minerals, 367, 367t
Minor calyx, 376, *376*
Miscarriage, 420
Mitochondria, *41*, 42t, 43, *43*
Mitosis, *50*, 50-52, 51t, *52*
Mitral valve, *245*, 246, *247*, 248
Mitral valve prolapse, 243
Mittelschmerz, 409
Mixtures, 27
Molars, 332, *332*, 333t
Molecular formula, 24
Molecule(s), 24, 24t
  in chemical reactions, 24-25
Monocytes, 228t, 233
  in phagocytosis, 293
Monoglycerides, absorption of, 346, 347,
  347, 348t
Mononucleosis, 287
Monosaccharides, 31, 362, 362t
  absorption of, 346, *347*
Monozygotic twins, 421
Mons pubis, 408, *408*
Morula, 422, 422-423
Motor areas, cerebellum as, 169
  cortical, *164*, 165, 166t
Motor function, 153
Motor nerves, 172, *172*
Motor neurons, 126, 156, 156t
  in reflex arc, 162, *162*, 163t
Motor output, 153
Motor speech area, *164*, 166t
Motor summation, 128
Motor unit, 126, 128
Mouth, *331*, 331-334, *334*
Movement, 8
  types of, 134t-135t
Mucosa(e), 70, *70*
  bladder, 379-380, *380*
  bronchial, 311
  gastric, 330, *330*, *331*
    gastrin secretion by, 220, 336t, 336-338,
      337
  intestinal, 330, *330*, *339*
    secretin/cholecystokinin secretion by,
      220, 340
  ureteral, 379, *380*
Mucous cells, 65
  gastric, 336, 336t

Mucous membrane. See *Mucosa(e)*.
Mucus, gastric, 336, 336t
Multipara, 420
Multiple motor unit summation, 128
Multiple myeloma, 226
Multiple sclerosis, 153
Multiple wave summation, 128
Mumps, 334
Murmurs, 252
Muscle(s), 5, 6t, 121-149. See also specific muscles.
  age-related changes in, 146
  antagonist, 133
  biopsy of, 123
  blood supply of, 125
  cardiac, 68t, 69, *69*, 124t, 244, *245*. See also *Myocardium*.
  characteristics of, 123
  contractility of, 123
  disorders of, 147
  elasticity of, 123
  excitability of, 123
  exercise and, 146-147
  extensibility of, 123
  functional relationships of, *122*
  functions of, 123
  heat production by, 123
  in joint stability, 123
  in movement, 123, 133
  in posture, 123
  names of, 133
  nerve supply of, 125, *126*
  of abdominal wall, 138t, 138-139, *139*
  of digestive tract, *330*, 331
  of eye, 188, *189*, 190, 190t
  of facial expression, 133-137, *136*, 136t
  of head and neck, 133-137, *136*, 136t
  of lower extremity, *141-142*, 143-145, 144t-145t
  of mastication, *136*, 136t, 137
  of neck, 137
  of pelvic floor, 138t, 139-140
  of trunk, 137, 138t, *139*
  of upper extremity, 140t, 140-143, *141-142*
  of vertebral column, 137
  papillary, *245*, 246
  prime mover, 133
  skeletal, 68t, 68-69, *69*, 124t, 133-145
    contraction of. See *Muscle contraction*.
    structure of, 123-126
  smooth (visceral), 124t
  striated, 68t, 69, *69*
  synergist, 133
Muscle attachments, 124-125
Muscle belly, 124
Muscle cells, 68, 69
Muscle contraction, 126-133
  all-or-none principle of, 127
  energy sources for, 129-131, *130-131*
  isometric, 129
  isotonic, 129
  muscle tone and, 129
  of whole muscle, 127-128
  oxygen debt in, 132
  sarcomere, 127
  sliding filament theory of, 127, *127*
  staircase effect in, 129, *129*
  stimulus for, 126-127
    subthreshold (subliminal), 127
    threshold (liminal), 127
  summary of, 128t
  summation in, 128
  tetany in, 128, *129*

Muscle contraction (*Continued*)
  treppe in, 129, *129*
  twitch in, 128, *129*
  venous blood flow and, 266, *266*
Muscle fibers, *124*, 125
  red, 131
  white, 131
Muscle gaster, 124
Muscle spindles, *185*, 186
Muscle tissue, 68t, 68-69
  cardiac, 68t, 69, *69*
  skeletal, 68t, 68-69, *69*
  smooth (visceral), 68t, 69, *69*
Muscle tone, 129
Muscular coat, of ureter, 379, *380*
Muscular dystrophy, 123
Muscular layer, of digestive tract, *330*, 331, 335, *335*
Muscular system, 5, 6t, 121-149
  characteristics of, 123
  functional relationships of, *122*
  functions of, 123
Muscularis layer, of bladder, 379, *380*
Mutations, 56
  cancer and, 57
Myasthenia gravis, 123
Myelin sheath, *155*, 156
Myeloma, 226
Myenteric plexus, of digestive tract, *330*, 331
Myocardial infarction, 248, 254-255
Myocardium, 244, *245*
  blood supply of, 248-249, *249*
Myofibers, conduction, *150*, 250
Myofibrils, 125, *125*
Myofilaments, 125, *125*
Myogram, 123, 128, *129*
Myometrium, 407, *407*
Myoneural junction, 126, *126*
Myopathy, 123
Myopia, 184
Myosin, 68, 125, *125*
Myositis, 123
Myxedema, 205, 212-213

N

Nails, *81*, 81-82
Nares, 308, *309*
Nasal bones, *98-100*, 102
Nasal cavity, 307, *309*
Nasal conchae, *98*, *100*, 101, 308, *309*
Nasal septum, 102, 307
Nasal turbinates, 101
Nasolacrimal canal, 100, 101t
Nasolacrimal duct, 189, *189*
Nasopharynx, 308-309, *309*, 334
Natural immunity, 300, *300*
Neck. See also under *Cervical*.
  arteries of, *271*, 272, 273t, 274
  femoral, *111*, 112, 112t
    fracture of, 112
  muscles of, *136*, 136t, 137
  of tooth, 333, *333*
  veins of, *276*, 277, 277-279, 278t
  wry, 137
Necrosis, 40
Negative feedback, 9, 9-10, *10*
  in hormone regulation, 206-207
Neonate, adjustment of, to extrauterine environment, 429, *430*
  development in, 431
  hemolytic disease of, 237

Neoplasms, 40, 57. See also *Cancer*; *Tumor(s)*.
Nephrectomy, 375
Nephritis, 375
Nephron, 377, *377*
Nephron loop, *278*, 377, *377*
Nephroptosis, 376
Nerve(s). See also specific nerves.
  age-related changes in, 178
  cranial, 172-173, *173*, 174t. See also specific nerves.
  motor, 172, *172*
  sensory, 172, *172*
  spinal, *170*, 170-171, *171*, 173-174
  stimulation of, in hormone regulation, 207
  structure of, 172, *172*
  vestibulocochlear, vestibular branch of, 198
Nerve cells. See *Neuron(s)*.
Nerve fibers, 155, *155*
  adrenergic, 177
  cholinergic, 177
  commissural, 165t
  postganglionic, 175, *175*
  preganglionic, 175, *175*
  projection, 165t
Nerve impulse conduction, 159-162, *160*
  across synapse, 161-162
  all-or-none principle of, 160-161
  excitatory transmission in, 162
  inhibitory transmission in, 162
  refractory period in, 160
  saltatory, 160, *160*
Nerve impulses, 157-163
Nerve supply, of muscle, 125, *126*
Nerve tissue, 155-157
Nervous stimulation, in hormone regulation, 207
Nervous system, 5, 6t, 151-180
  age-related changes in, 178
  autonomic, 155, 172, 174-177, *176*, 176t, 177
  central, 154, *154*
  disorders of, *179*
  functional relationships of, *152*
  functions of, 152-153
  involuntary, 155
  organization of, 154, 154-155
  parasympathetic, 155, 175, *175*, 176, 177, 177t
  peripheral, 154, *154*, 155, 171-172
  somatic, 155, 172
  sympathetic, 155, *175*, 175-176, *176*, 176t, 177
  voluntary, 155
  vs. endocrine system, 205
Nervous tissue, 69, 69-70
Nervous tunic, of eye, 191
Neurilemma, 155, *156*
Neuroglia, 70, 155, 156, 157t
Neurohypophysis, 208, *208*
  hormones of, 209t, 211
Neuromuscular junction, 126, *126*
Neuron(s), 69, 69-70, 155, 155-156
  association, 156, 156t
  conductivity of, 157
  excitability of, 157
  functional classification of, 156, 156t
  motor (efferent), 126, 156, 156t
    in reflex arc, 162, *162*, 163t
  olfactory, 187, *188*
  postsynaptic, 161, *161*
  presynaptic, 161, *161*

Neuron(s) *(Continued)*
  sensory (afferent), 156, 156t
    in reflex arc, 162, *162*, 163t
    stimulation of, 158-159
    structure of, *155*, 155-156
Neuronal pools, 162, *162*
Neurotransmitters, 161, 161t
Neutral solutions, 29
Neutralization, 29-30
Neutrons, 19, 24t
Neutrophils, 228t, 232, 292, *294*
Nevus, 77
Newborn, adjustment of, to extrauterine environment, 429, *430*
  development in, 431
  hemolytic disease of, 237
Niacin, 366t
Nipple, 412, *412*
Nitrogen, in plasma solutes, 228
Nociceptors, 184, 185t, 186
Nocturia, 375
Nodes, atrioventricular, 250, *250*
  lymph, 288, *289*, 289-290, *290*
  sinoatrial, 249, *250*
Nodes of Ranvier, *155*, 156
Nodules, lymph, 289, *290*
Nonessential amino acids, 364
Nongonococcal urethritis, 416
Non–insulin-dependent diabetes, 222
Nonrespiratory air movements, 322, 323t
Nonsteroidal anti-inflammatory drugs, 221
Norepinephrine, 161, 161t, 177, 216-217, *217*
Nose, 307, *309*. See also under *Nasal.*
Nostrils, 308
Notch, cardiac, *310*, 311, 312
  intercondylar, *111*, 112, 112t
  jugular, 105, *105*
  sciatic, greater, 109, *110*, 110t
    lesser, *110*, 110t, 111
  suprasternal, 105, *105*
  trochlear (semilunar), 107, *108*, 109t
  ulnar, 107, *108*, 109t
Nuclear membrane, *41*, 42t, 43
Nucleic acids, 33-35, *34*, *35*
Nucleolus, *41*, 42t, 43
Nucleoplasm, 43
Nucleotides, 33, *34*
Nucleus, cell, *41*, 42t, 43
Nullipara, 420
Nutrient(s), 8, 362-367. See also specific nutrients.
  absorption of, 287, 330, 338, 339-341, 346-347, *347*
  energy from, 355
  functions of, 362t
  hepatic storage of, 343
  in plasma, 229
  metabolism of, 354-361. See also *Metabolism.*
  transport of, 346-347, *347*, 348t
Nutrient foramina, 93, *93*
Nutrition, 361-368
  age-related changes in, 369
  definition of, 361
Nyctalopia, 184

O

O blood type, 235-236, *236*, 236t
Obesity, 369-370
  hyperplastic, 369
  hypertrophic, 369-370

Oblique fracture, 116
Oblique muscle, external, 138, 138t, *139*, *141*
  internal, 138, 138t, *139*
Obstructive sleep apnea, 324
Obturator foramen, 109, *110*, 110t
Occipital area, 14t, *15*
Occipital bone, *98-100*, 100, 102
Occipital condyle, *99*, 100, *100*
Oculomotor nerve, 172-173, *173*, 174t
Odontoid process, 104, *104*
Olecranon fossa, 107, *107*, 107t
Olecranon process, 107, *108*, 109t
Olfactory bulb, 187, *188*
Olfactory cortex, *164*, 166t, 187
Olfactory epithelium, 187, *188*
Olfactory foramen, 100, *101*, 101t
Olfactory nerve, 172-173, *173*, 174t
Olfactory neurons, 187, *188*
Olfactory receptors, 187-188, *188*
Olfactory sense, 187-188
  age-related changes in, 199
  impairment of, *201*
Olfactory tract, 187, *188*
Oligodendrocytes, 156, 157t
Oliguria, 375
Oocyte, 403, *404*
  primary, 404-405, *405*
  secondary, 405, *405*
    fertilization of, 406, *407*
    release of, 406
    transport of, 406-407
    sperm penetration of, 420, *421*
Oogenesis, 404-406, *405*
Oogonia, 404, *405*
Open fracture, 116
Ophthalmic area, 14t, *15*
Optic chiasma, 193, *193*
Optic disk, *190*, 191
Optic foramen, *98*, *99*, 100, *101*, 101t
Optic nerve, 172-173, *173*, 174t, *190*, 191, *193*, *193*
Optic radiations, 193, *193*
Optic tract, 193, *193*
Oral area, 14t, *15*
Oral cavity, *331*, 331-334, *334*
Oral contraceptives, 414
Orbicularis oculi muscle, 134, *136*, 136t, *188*
Orbicularis oris muscle, 133-137, *136*, 136t
Orbit, 188
Organ of Corti, 196, *196*, *197*
Organelles, 41, 42t
  cytoplasmic, *41*, 42t, 43
  filamentous protein, *41*, 42t, 45
Organic chemistry, 30
Organogenesis, 426, 426t, 427t
Organs, 4
  prenatal development of, 426, 426t, 427t
Orgasm, female, 409
  male, 401
Orifice, vaginal, 408, *408*
Oropharynx, 308-309, *334*
Osmosis, 47, *48*
  in tubular reabsorption, 383, *383*
Osmotic pressure, in capillary microcirculation, 263-264
  of blood, 228
Ossa coxae, 109, *110*, 110t
Osseous tissue, 65t, 67-68, *68*
Ossicles, auditory, 102
Ossification, endochondral, 95, *95*
  intramembranous, 95
Ossification center, primary, 95
  secondary, 95

Osteitis fibrosa cystica, 214
Osteoblasts, 94
Osteoclasts, 94
Osteocytes, 67-68, 94
Osteogenesis, 95
Osteomalacia, 91
Osteomyelitis, 91
Osteonic canal, 67, *68*
Osteons, 67, *68*
Osteoporosis, 91, 94
Osteosarcoma, 91
Otalgia, 184
Otic area, 14t, *15*
Otoliths, 198, *198*
Otosclerosis, 184, 196
Otoscopy, 184
Outer longitudinal layer, of digestive tract, *330*, 331
Outer table, 93
Oval window, *194*, 195, *195*, *197*
Ovarian cycle, 409, *410*, *411*
Ovarian epithelium, 402-403, *404*
Ovarian follicles, 403, *404*
  development of, *404*, *406*
Ovarian fossae, 402
Ovary, cancer of, 402
  hormonal control of, 409, *410*, *411*
  hormones of, 210t, 218, 219
  in oogenesis, 404-406, *405*
  structure of, 402-404, *404*
Oviducts, 406-407, *407*
Ovulation, 406
  pain of, 409
Ovulatory phase, of ovarian cycle, 409, *410*
Oxygen. See also *Gas(es).*
  blood levels of, regulation of, 321, *322*
  need for, 8
  partial pressure of, 315, 316t
Oxygen debt, in glycolysis, 356
  in muscle contraction, 132
Oxygen loading, 317, *319*
Oxygen transport, in respiration, 317, *318*, *319*
Oxygen unloading, 317, *319*
Oxyhemoglobin, 230, 317
Oxytocin, 209t, *210*, 211
  in labor, 428
  in lactation, 413, 430, *431*

P

P wave, 250, *250*
  in myocardial infarction, 254
Pacemaker, artificial, 243
  sinoatrial node as, 249, *250*
Pacinian corpuscles, 185, *185*
Packed cell volume (PCV), 227
Pain, in inflammation, 293
  ovulatory, 409
Pain receptors, 186
Palate, 308, *309*, 331
  cleft, 332
Palatine bones, *98-100*, 102
Palatine process, *99*, 102
Palatine tonsils, 290, 309, *309*, *331*, 332, 334
Palmar arches, *271*, *272*, 273t, 274-275
Palmar area, 14t, *15*
Pancreas, endocrine, 217-218
  exocrine, 344-345
  head of, 344, *345*
  islets of Langerhans of, 217-218, 344, *344*
  structure of, 344-345, *345*

Pancreas *(Continued)*
tail of, 344, *345*
Pancreatic acinar cells, 344
Pancreatic amylase, 345
Pancreatic duct, 344
Pancreatic enzymes, 344-345
Pancreatic juice, 344-345
Pancreatic lipase, 345
Pantothenic acid, 366t
Papanicolaou smear, 408
Papilla(e), 332
dermal, *78, 79*
hair bulb and, 81, *81*
renal, 376, *376*
tongue, taste buds on, 186, *187*
Papillary layer, dermal, *78, 79*
Papillary muscles, *245, 246*
Paranasal sinuses, 100, 308, *309*
Parasympathetic nervous system, 155, 175, *175, 176,* 177, 177t
Parathyroid glands, *213,* 213-214
Parathyroid hormone (PTH), 209t, *213,* 213-214
Paraurethral glands, 408
Paraverterbral ganglia, 176
Parietal, 11
Parietal bones, *98-100,* 100, 102
Parietal cells, 336
Parietal layer, *70, 70*
Parietal lobe, 164, *164*
Parietal pericardium, 243, *245*
Parietal pleura, *311,* 312
Parkinson's disease, 165
Parotid glands, 334, *334*
Partial pressure, of gases, 315, 316t
Parturition, 428
Passive immunity, 300, *300*
Patella, *111,* 113
Patellar reflex, 171, 172t
Patellar surface, *111,* 112, 112t
Pathogens, 291
bloodborne, 239
Pathology, 60
Pectoral area, 14t, *15*
Pectoral girdle, *106,* 106-107
Pectoralis major muscle, 140t, 141, *141*
Pedal area, 14t, *15*
Peduncles, cerebellar, 168
cerebral, *167,* 168
Pelvic area, 14t, *15*
Pelvic brim, 111
Pelvic cavity, 12, *12*
Pelvic diaphragm, 138t, 139-140
Pelvic floor muscles, 138t, 139-140
Pelvic girdle, 109-111, *110*
Pelvic inflammatory disease, 415
Pelvic inlet, 111
Pelvic outlet, 111
Pelvic veins, *276, 277, 278t, 279,* 279-280
Pelvimetry, 420
Pelvis, bony, male vs. female, 111t
renal, 376, *376*
Penile urethra, *380, 381, 396*
Penis, 400-401, *401*
age-related changes in, 413
erection of, 401
Pentose, 31
Pepsin, 336, 346, 346t
Pepsinogen, 336t, 336-338, *337,* 346
Peptidases, 339, 346t
Peptide bonds, 32
Peptides, 346
Percutaneous transluminal coronary angio-plasty (PTCA), 283

Pericardial cavity, 243, *245*
Pericardial sac, *70,* 71, 243, *245*
Pericarditis, 244
Pericardium, *70,* 71, 243, *245*
Perichondrium, 67
Perilymph, 195
Perimetrium, 407, *407*
Perimysium, 124, *124*
Perineal area, 14t, *15*
Perineurium, 172, *172*
Periodontal ligaments, 333, *333*
Periosteum, 93, *93*
Peripheral nervous system, 154, *154,* 155, 171-172
Peripheral vascular resistance, blood pressure and, 268
Perirenal fat, 376
Peristalsis, gastric, 338
Peritoneum, *70,* 71, *330,* 331
Peritonitis, 71
Peritubular capillaries, 378, *379*
Permanent (secondary) teeth, 332, *332*
Permeability, selective, 40, 47
Pernicious anemia, 231
Peroneal artery, *271, 272,* 273t, 275
Peroneal vein, *276, 277,* 278t, 280
Peroneus longus muscle, *142,* 145, 145t
Peroxisomes, 44
Perpendicular plate, *98,* 101
Pertussis, 307
Petechia, 226
pH, 29, *29*
blood, 388, 389, 391t
buffers and, 30
neutralization and, 29-30
regulation of, 388, 389-390
urine, 385, 385t
Phagocytes, 292, *294*
Phagocytosis, 49, *49,* 292-293, *294*
Phalanges, of foot, 113, *114*
of hand, *108,* 109
Pharyngeal tonsils, 290, 308, *309*
Pharyngitis, 309
Pharyngoplasty, 324
Pharynx, 308-309, *309,* 334-335
Phimosis, 401
Phlebitis, 260
Phlebotomy, 260
Phospholipid bilayer, 40
Phospholipids, 33
Phosphorus, dietary, 367t
Photoreceptors, 184, 185t, *192,* 192-193, 193t
Phrenic nerve, 320, *320*
Physiology, 2, *3*
anatomy and, 2
Pia mater, 71, 163, *163*
Pica, 354
Pineal gland, *167,* 168, 210t, 219-220
Pinealocytes, 219
Pinocytosis, 49
Pits, gastric, 336
Pituitary gland, 207-212, *208,* 209t, *210*
anterior, 208, *208*
hormones of, 209t, 210-212
hypothalamus and, 208, *208,* 212, *212*
posterior, 208, *208*
thyroid and, 212, *212*
Pivot joint, 115t
Placenta, 220, 424
formation of, 425-426
Placenta previa, 426
Placental circulation, 281
Placental hormones, 220, 426, 426t
Placental stage, of labor, 429, *429*

Plane(s), body, terminology for, 11
coronal, 11, *12*
frontal, 11, *12*
midsagittal, 11, *12*
sagittal, 11, *12*
transverse, 11, *12*
Plantar area, 14t, *15*
Plantar flexion, 134t
Plasma, 68, 226, *227,* 227-229, 386, *386*
electrolytes in, 229
gases in, 229
nonprotein nitrogen-containing molecules in, 228-229
nutrients in, 229
proteins in, 227t, 227-228
solutes in, 227t, 227-228
Plasma cells, 297, *299*
Plasma membrane, 40-41, *42.* See also *Membrane(s).*
hormone receptors on, 205-206, *206*
selective permeability of, 40, 47
transport across, 45-50, 46t. See also *Membrane transport.*
Plasma proteins, 227t, 227-228
synthesis of, hepatic, 343
Plate, cribriform, *99,* 100, 101
epiphyseal, 93, *93,* 95
horizontal, 102
perpendicular, *98,* 101
Platelet plug, formation of, 233-234, *234*
Platelets, 68, *68,* 228t, 233
Pleura, *70,* 71, *311,* 312
Pleural cavity, *311,* 312
Pleurisy, 312
Pleuritis, 312
Plexus, choroid, *169,* 170
myenteric (Auerbach's), *330,* 331
spinal nerve, *171,* 174, 175t
submucosal (Meissner's), *330,* 330-331
Plicae circulares, 338, *339*
Plural form, 15
Pneumoconiosis, 307
Pneumonectomy, 307
Pneumotaxic area, 168
Pneumothorax, 313
Poison ivy, 302
Polar bonds, 22, 23
Polycystic kidney disease, 377
Polycythemia, 226
Polydipsia, 221-222
Polyphagia, 222
Polysaccharides, 31
complex, 31, 362, 362t. See also *Glycogen.*
Polyuria, 375
in diabetes, 221
Popliteal area, 14t, *15*
Popliteal arteries, *271, 272,* 273t, 275
Popliteal vein, *276, 277,* 278t, 280
Pore, sweat, 82
taste, 186
Porta hepatis, 342, *342*
Portal triads, 342, *343*
Portal vein, hepatic, *342,* 342-343, *343*
Position, anatomical, 11, *11*
Position sense, *185,* 186
Positive feedback, 10
Positron emission tomography (PET), 153
Postcentral gyrus, 164, 165, 166t
Posterior cavity, of eye, *190,* 191
Posterior fontanel, 102
Posterior inferior iliac spine, 109, *110,* 110t
Posterior median sulcus, 170, *171*
Posterior superior iliac spine, 109, *110,* 110t

Posterior tibial arteries, *271, 272,* 273t, 275
Posterior tibial vein, *276, 277,* 278t, 280
Posterolateral fontanel, 102
Postganglionic fiber, 175, *175*
Postnatal development, 430-432
Postsynaptic neuron, 161, *161*
Posture, 123
Potassium, dietary, 367t
Potassium balance, 388
    aldosterone in, 215
Pott's fracture, 112
PPD test, 302
Precapillary sphincters, 262, *262,* 265
Precentral gyrus, *164,* 165, 166t
Preeclampsia, 420
Preembryonic period, 422-424, *422-424,* 427t
Prefix, 15
Prefrontal cortex, 166t
Preganglionic fiber, 175, *175*
Pregnancy, 428
    development in. See *Development.*
    drinking in, 432-433
    drugs in, 433
    ectopic, 407
    labor and delivery in, 428-429
    smoking in, 433
    teratogens in, 432-433
Premature heart contraction, 250
Premolars, 332, *332,* 333t
Prepuce, 401, *401,* 408, *408*
Presbycusis, 184, 199
Presbyopia, 184, 199
Pressure, 8
    sensation of, 185, *185*
Pressure receptors, in blood pressure regulation, 253, 268
Presynaptic neuron, 161, *161*
PRH (prolactin-releasing hormone), 430, *431*
Primary bronchi, *310,* 311
Primary follicle, ovarian, *404,* 406
Primary germ layers, formation of, 424
Primary oocyte, 404-405, *405*
Primary ossification center, 95
Primary (deciduous) teeth, 332, *332*
Prime mover, 133
Primordial germ cells, 396
Procallus, 117
Process, acromion, *106,* 107
    alveolar, *99,* 102
    bony, 94t
    ciliary, 190, *190*
    coracoid, *106,* 107
    coronoid, 108, *108,* 109t
    mastoid, *98, 99,* 101
    odontoid, 104, *104*
    olecranon, 107, *108,* 109t
    palatine, *99,* 102
    spinous, 103, *103,* 104, *104*
    styloid, *98, 99,* 101, *102,* 107, 108, *108,* 109t
    temporal, 102
    transverse, 103, *103*
    xiphoid, 105, *105*
    zygomatic, *98, 99,* 101
Procoagulants, 234
Products, reaction, 24
Progeria, 205
Progesterone, 409, *410*
    placental secretion of, 426t
    production of, by ovary, 210t, 219
        by placenta, 220
Projection fibers, 165t
Prolactin, 209t, *210, 211,* 413, 429-430, *431*

Prolactin-releasing hormone (PRH), 430, *431*
Proliferative phase, of menstrual cycle, 410-411, *411*
Pronation, 135t
Prophase, *50, 51,* 51t
Proprioception, *185,* 186
Prostaglandins, 220-221
Prostate gland, *396,* 400
    cancer of, 400
Prostatic urethra, *380, 381, 396*
Protein(s), 31-32, 32t. See also *Amino acid(s).*
    dietary, 363-364
        complete, 364
        digestion of, 346
        functions of, 363-364
        incomplete, 364
        metabolism of, 344, 354, *355, 357, 359,* 360
    hormones as, 205
    membrane, 40-41, *42*
    plasma, 227t, 227-228
        hepatic synthesis of, 343
    synthesis of, DNA in, 52-53
        messenger RNA in, 53-54, *54,* 206
        ribosomal RNA in, 54
        RNA in, 54, *55*
        transcription in, 53-54, *54*
        transfer RNA in, 54
        translation in, 54, *55*
Protein-bound iodine, 213
Prothrombin, 234
Prothrombin activator, 234
Proton, 19, 24t
Proton acceptors, 28
Proton donors, acids as, 28
Proximal, 11
Proximal convoluted tubule, 377, *377, 378*
Pruritus, 77
Pseudostratified columnar epithelium, 61t, 62-63, *63*
PTH (parathyroid hormone), 209t, 213, 213-214
Puberty, in male, 402
Pubic arch, *110,* 110t, 111
Pubic rami, *110,* 110t, 111
Pubic symphysis, *110,* 110t, 111
Pubis, 109, *110*
Pudendum, 408, *408*
Pulmonary. See also *Lung(s).*
Pulmonary arteries, *245, 248, 248, 249,* 260, *260,* 269, 270
Pulmonary capacity, 314, *314,* 315t
Pulmonary circulation, *245, 248, 248,* 260, *260, 269,* 269-270
Pulmonary edema, 307
Pulmonary semilunar valve, *245, 247,* 247-248, *269,* 270
Pulmonary trunk, *245, 248, 248, 269,* 270
Pulmonary ventilation. See *Ventilation.*
Pulmonary vessels, 260
Pulp, 333, *333*
Pulp cavity, 333, *333*
Pulsating electromagnetic fields, 117
Pulse, blood pressure and, 266, *269*
    dorsalis pedis, 275
Pulse points, 266
Pulse pressure, 267. See also *Blood pressure.*
Pupil, *190,* 190-191
Pupillary reflexes, 191
Purkinje fibers, 250, *250*
Purpura, 226
Pyloric region, 335, *335*
Pyloric sphincter, 335, *335,* 338
Pyramidal tract, 171

Pyridoxine, 366t
Pyrogens, 293
Pyruvic acid, in glycolysis, 355-356, *357,* 359
    in lipid metabolism, 359, *359, 360*
    in protein metabolism, 357, *357, 359, 359,* 360

Q

Q wave, in myocardial infarction, 254-255
QRS complex, 250, *250*
    in myocardial infarction, 254
Quadrants, abdominopelvic, *12, 13*
Quadrate lobe, of liver, 342, *342*
Quadriceps femoris muscle, *141,* 143, 144t
Quickening, 427

R

Radial artery, *271, 272,* 273t, 274-275
Radial head, 107, 108, *108,* 109t
Radial muscles, of iris, 189t
Radial notch, 108, *108,* 109t
Radial tuberosity, 107, *108,* 109t
Radial vein, *276, 277,* 278t, 279
Radiation, heat loss via, 368
Radioactive isotopes, 36
Radius, 107-108, *108,* 109t
Ramus, mandibular, *98*
    pubic, *110,* 110t, 111
Reactants, 24
Reactions, chemical, 24-27. See also *Chemical reactions.*
Receptor(s), cold, 186
    heat, 186
    hormone, 206, *206*
    in reflex arc, 162, *162,* 163t
    olfactory, 187-188, *188*
    pain, 186
    pressure, 185
        in blood pressure regulation, 253, 268
    proprioceptive, 186
    sense, 184, 185t
        in skin, 79
    stretch, pulmonary, 321
    taste, 186-187, *187*
    touch, 79, 185
Rectum, *340,* 341
Rectus abdominis muscle, 138t, *139, 139*
Red blood cells. See *Erythrocytes.*
Red fibers, 131
Red marrow, 92
Red pulp, 290
Redness, in inflammation, 293
Reflex(es), 171, 172t
    abdominal, 171, 172t
    Achilles tendon (ankle-jerk), 171, 172t
    Babinski's, 171, 172t
    Hering-Breuer, 321
    patellar (knee-jerk), 171, 172t
    pupillary, 191
    spinal, 171, 172t
Reflex arc, *162,* 162-163, 163t
Refraction, 191, *191*
Refractory period, 160
Regeneration, tissue, 72, *73*
Region(s), *12, 13, 13,* 13t, 14
    abdominal, 14t, *15*
    abdominopelvic, *12, 13*
    appendicular, *13,* 14

Region(s) (Continued)
 axial, 13, 14
 cutaneous, 14t, 15
 epigastric, 12, 13
 hypochondriac, 12, 13
 hypogastric, 12, 13
 iliac, 12, 13
 inguinal, 12, 13
 lumbar, 12, 13
 pyloric, 335, 335
 terminology of, 12, 13, 13t
 umbilical, 12, 13
Relative refractory period, 160
Remodeling, fracture, 117
Renal. See also Kidney(s).
Renal arteries, 270, 271, 272, 273t
Renal artery, 271, 272, 273t, 274, 275, 376, 376
Renal calculi, 385
Renal calyces, 376, 376
Renal columns, 376, 376
Renal cortex, 376, 376
Renal diabetes, 383
Renal erythropoietic factor, 230-231, 231
Renal fascia, 376
Renal hilum, 376
Renal medulla, 376, 376
Renal papillae, 376, 376
Renal pelvis, 376, 376
Renal pyramid, 376, 376
Renal sinus, 376
Renal threshold, 382
Renal tubule, 377, 377, 378
Renal veins, 276, 277, 278t, 279, 376, 376, 378, 379
Renin, 375, 378
 in blood pressure regulation, 269
 urine concentration and volume and, 384
Replacement reactions, 25
Replication, DNA, 52, 53, 53-54
Repolarization, 158, 159
Reproduction, 8
Reproductive organs, primary, 395
 secondary (accessory), 395
Reproductive system, 5, 7t, 393-416
 age-related changes in, 413
 disorders of, 416
 female, 402-413
  hormonal control of, 409-412
  in sexual response, 408-409
  organs of, 402-408, 404
 functional relationships of, 394
 male, 395-402
  hormonal control of, 402
  in sexual response, 401
  organs of, 395-401, 396
Residual volume, 314, 314, 315t
Resistance, disease, 291
Resistance exercise, 146-147
Respiration, 8, 307
 aerobic, 131, 131-132
 anaerobic, 131, 131-132
 carbon dioxide transport in, 318, 318-320, 319
 cellular, 307, 354, 355
 definition of, 307
 external, 307, 316-317, 318
 gas exchange in, 316, 316-317
 internal, 307, 317, 318
 overview of, 307
 oxygen transport in, 317, 318, 319
 regulation of, 320, 320-322, 321
 venous blood flow and, 266

Respiration (Continued)
 ventilation and, 307
 voluntary control of, 321-322
Respiratory acidosis, 389-390, 391t
Respiratory alkalosis, 389-390, 391t
Respiratory capacities, 314, 314-315, 315t
Respiratory center, 168, 320, 320, 321
Respiratory membrane, 316-317, 317
Respiratory rate, body temperature and, 322
 normal values for, 320
 regulation of, 320-322, 322
Respiratory system, 5, 7t, 305-325
 adjustment of, at birth, 429
 age-related changes in, 323
 disorders of, 325
 functional relationships of, 306
 functions of, 307
 in acid-base balance, 388
 lower tract, 308, 310, 310-312, 311
 upper tract, 307-312, 308, 309
Respiratory volumes, 314, 314-315, 315t
Responsiveness, 8
Resting membrane, 157, 158
Resting membrane potential, 157, 158
Rete testis, 396, 396
Reticular formation, 168
Reticular layer, dermal, 78, 79
Reticulocyte, 226, 229
Reticulocyte count, 231
Retina, 190, 191
 detached, 191
 image formation on, 191, 191-192
Reverse polarization, 158, 159
Reversible reactions, 26-27
Reye's syndrome, 153
Rh blood groups, 237-238, 238
Rhinitis, 308
Rhinoplasty, 307
Rhodopsin, 192
RhoGAM, 238
Rhythm method, 414
Riboflavin, 366t
Ribonucleic acid. See RNA.
Ribosomal RNA, 54
Ribosomes, 41, 42t, 43
Ribs, 105, 106
Rickets, 365
Right atrium, 245, 245-246, 269, 270
Right bundle branch, 250, 250
Right colonic flexure, 340, 341
Right common carotid artery, 270, 271, 272, 273t
Right common iliac artery, 271, 272, 273t, 275
Right coronary artery, 245, 248, 249, 270, 273t, 274
Right gastric artery, 276, 277, 278t, 280
Right gonadal veins, 276, 277, 278t, 279
Right hepatic ducts, 342, 342
Right hepatic flexure, 340, 341
Right lobe, of liver, 342, 342
Right lymphatic duct, 288, 288
Right pulmonary artery, 249, 269, 270
Right subclavian artery, 270, 271, 272, 273t, 274, 275
Right suprarenal vein, 276, 277, 278t, 279
Right ventricle, 245, 246, 247, 247, 269, 270
Right vertebral artery, 275
Rigor mortis, 127
RNA, 34, 35t
 in protein synthesis, 53-54, 54, 206
 messenger (mRNA), 53-54, 54, 206

RNA (Continued)
 ribosomal (rRNA), 54
 transfer (tRNA), 54
Rods, 191, 192, 192-193, 193t
Root, dorsal, 173, 174
 hair, 80, 81
 of lung, 311
 of penis, 401, 401
 of tongue, 332
 of tooth, 333, 333
 ventral, 173, 174
 word, 15
Root canal, 333, 333
Rotation, 135t
Rotator cuff muscles, 140t, 141-142, 142
Rough endoplasmic reticulum, 41, 42t, 44
Round window, 194, 195, 195, 197
Rugae, bladder, 379, 380
 gastric, 335, 355
Rule of nines, 85, 85

S

Sac, amniotic, 425
 lacrimal, 189, 189
 pericardial, 70, 71, 243, 245
 yolk, 424, 425, 425
Saccule, 195, 197
Sacral area, 14t, 15
Sacral curvature, 103, 103
Sacral nerves, 170, 170-171, 173-174
Sacroiliac joint, 105
Sacrum, 103, 104, 105
Saddle joint, 115t
Sagittal plane, 11, 12
Sagittal suture, 100
Saliva, 334
Salivary amylase, 334
Salivary glands, 333-334, 334
Saltatory conduction, 160, 160
Salts, 30
Saphenous veins, 276, 277, 278t, 280
Sarcolemma, 125
Sarcoma, 60. See also Cancer.
Sarcomere, 125
Sarcoplasm, 125
Sarcoplasmic reticulum, 125
Satellite cells, 157t
Saturated fatty acids, 33, 33t
Scala tympani, 195, 196, 197
Scala vestibuli, 195, 196, 197
Scapula, 106, 106-107
Scar formation, 72, 73
Schwann cells, 157t
Sciatic notch, greater, 109, 110, 110t
 lesser, 110, 110t, 111
Sclera, 190, 190
Scoliosis, 103
Scrotum, 395, 396
Scurvy, 60, 365
Sebaceous glands, 82, 188
Sebum, 82
Second heart sound, 251-252
Second messenger, 206
Second polar body, 405, 406
Secondary bronchi, 310, 311
Secondary follicle, ovarian, 404, 406
Secondary oocyte, 405, 405
 release of, 406
Secondary ossification center, 95
Secondary syphilis, 415
Secondary (permanent) teeth, 332, 332

Second-degree burns, 85
Secretin, 220, 340, 346t
  pancreatic secretions and, 345
Secretions, gastric, 336t, 336-338, *337*
  small intestinal, 339-340
Secretory phase, of menstrual cycle, *411,*
  411-412
Secretory vesicles, *41, 42t,* 44, *44*
Sections, body, terminology for, 11
Segmental arteries, 378, *379*
Segmental bronchi, *310,* 311
Segmental veins, 378, *379*
Segments, bronchopulmonary, 312
Selective permeability, membrane, 40, 47
Self vs. nonself, in immunity, 294-295
Sella turcica, *99, 100,* 101
Semen, 400
Semicircular canals, *195,* 198
Semilunar cartilage, 114-115
Semilunar (trochlear) notch, 107, *108,* 109t
Semilunar valves, *245, 246, 247*
Semimembranous muscle, *142,* 144t, 145
Seminal fluid, 400
Seminal vesicles, *396,* 400
Seminiferous tubules, 396, *396, 397*
Semitendinosus muscle, *142,* 144t, 145
Senescence, 432
Sense(s), age-related changes in, 199-200
  auditory, 194-197
  equilibrium, 197-198
  general (somatic), 185-186
  gustatory, 186-187, *187*
  impairment of, 199-200, *201*
  olfactory, 187-188
  special, 184, 186-198
  tactile, 185, *185*
  visual, 188-194
Sense receptors, 184, 185t
Sensitization, in hypersensitivity, 302
Sensorineural deafness, 200
Sensory adaptation, 184
Sensory areas, cortical, *164, 165,* 166t
Sensory input, 153
Sensory integration, 153
Sensory nerves, 172, *172*
Sensory neurons, 156, 156t
  in reflex arc, 162, *162,* 163t
Sensory perception, steps in, 184
Sensory reception. See *Receptor(s).*
Sensory system, 183-201
Septum (septa), interatrial, *245,* 246
  nasal, 102, 307
  testicular, *396, 396*
Serosa, *70,* 70-71
  gastrointestinal, *330, 331, 335*
Serotonin, 161, 161t, 302
Serous cells, 65
Serous fluid, 71
Serous membrane(s), *70,* 70-71
  pleural, *311,* 312
Serratus anterior muscle, 140t, 140-141, *141*
Sertoli's cells, *396, 397*
Serum, 228
Sesamoid bones, 97
Sex hormones, female, 409-412, *410, 411*
  male, 402, *403*
Sex steroids, 215-216
Sexual response, age-related changes in,
  413
  female, 408-409
  male, 401-402
Sexually transmitted diseases (STDs), 415-
  416
Shaft, penile, 401, *401*

Shell, electron, 19
Shell temperature, 368
Shingles, 153
Shock, circulatory, 268
  hypovolemic, 268
Short bones, 93
Shoulder, arteries of, *271, 272,* 273t, 274-275
  veins of, *276, 277,* 278t, 279
Shoulder blade, *106,* 106-107
Shoulder girdle, *106,* 106-107
Sighing, 322, 323t
Sigmoid colon, *340,* 341
Simple diffusion, *46,* 46-47
Simple epithelium, *60,* 61
Simple gland, 64, *64*
Simple goiter, 212
Simple series circuit, 162
Simple squamous epithelium, *60,* 61, *61,*
  61t
Single replacement reactions, 25
Sinoatrial (SA) node, 249, *250*
  heart rate and, 253
Sinus(es), carotid, 274
  dural, 163
  ethmoid, 101, 308, *309*
  frontal, 100, 308, *309*
  in bone, 94t
  lactiferous, *412,* 413
  lymph, 289, *290*
  maxillary, 102, 308, *309*
  paranasal, 100, 308, *309*
  renal, 376
  sphenoid, *100,* 101, 308, *309*
  superior sagittal, 163
Sinusoids, 342
Skeletal muscle, 68t, 68-69, *69.* See also
  Muscle(s).
Skeletal system, 5, 6t, 89-119. See also
  Bone(s); Joint(s).
  age-related changes in, 116
  disorders of, *118*
  functional relationships of, *90*
  functions of, 91-92
  structure of, 92-94
Skeleton, appendicular, *96, 97,* 97t, 106-113
  axial, *96,* 97t, 97-106
  divisions of, 97, 97t
Skene's glands, 408
Skin, accessory structures of, 80-82
  age-related changes in, 84
  burns of, 84-85
  cancer of, 77, 78
  color of, 80
  disorders of, *86*
  functions of, 82-84
  in sensory reception, 79, 83
  in temperature regulation, *83,* 83-84
  in vitamin D synthesis, 84
  protective functions of, 82-83
  structure of, 77
Skin test, tuberculin, 302
Skull, bones of, 97-103, *98-100*
  fontanels of, 102
  foramina of, *98-100,* 100, 101t
  sinuses of, 100
  sutures of, *98,* 100
Sleep apnea, 324
Sliding filament theory, 127, *127*
Small intestine, 338-340, *339.* See also *Intes-*
  tinal entries.
  secretions of, 339-340
  hormonal, 220
  structure of, 338-339, *339*
Small saphenous vein, *276, 277,* 278t, 280

Smell. See *Olfactory* entries.
Smoking, fetal effects of, 433
Smooth endoplasmic reticulum, *41, 42t,* 44
Smooth muscle, 68t, 69, *69,* 124t. See also
  Muscle(s).
Sneezing, 322, 323t
Snellen chart, 184
Sodium, dietary, 367t
  regulation of, aldosterone in, 215
Sodium balance, 387-388
Soft palate, 308, *309,* 331, *331*
Solute, 27
Solution(s), 27
  acidic, 29
  alkaline, 29
  hypertonic, 47-48, *48*
  hypotonic, 48, *48*
  isotonic, 47, *48*
  neutral, 29
Solvent, 27
  in osmosis, 47
Soma, neuronal, 155, *155*
Somatic nervous system, 155, 172
Somatic senses, 185-186
Somatomotor cortex, *164, 165,* 166t
Somatosensory association areas, *164,* 165,
  166t
Somatosensory cortex, *164, 165,* 166t
Sound, intensity of, 200
  loudness of, 197
  pitch of, 197
  transmission of, 196-197
Special senses, 184, 186-198
Sperm, capacitation of, 420
  oocyte penetration by, 420, *421*
  production of, 396-399, *398, 399*
  structure of, *397,* 397-398
Spermatic cord, 399
Spermatids, *397, 397, 398*
Spermatocytes, primary, *397, 397, 398*
  secondary, *397, 397, 398*
Spermatogenesis, 396-399, *398, 399*
Spermatogonia, 396-397, *397, 398*
Spermicides, 414
Spermiogenesis, 397-399, *398*
Sphenoid, *98-100,* 101
  greater wing of, *99,* 101
Sphenoid fontanel, 102
Sphenoid sinus, *100,* 101, 308, *309*
Sphincter(s), anal, external, *340,* 341
  internal, *340,* 341
  cardiac, 335
  hepatopancreatic, 344
  ileocecal, 340
  lower esophageal, 335
  precapillary, 262, *262,* 265
  pyloric, 335, *335,* 338
  urethral, external, 380
  internal, 380
Sphincter of Oddi, 344
Sphygmomanometer, 267, *268*
Spinal cavity, 12, *12*
Spinal cord, 154
  functions of, 171
  structure of, *170,* 170-171, *171*
Spinal curvatures, 103, *103*
Spinal nerve plexuses, 171, 174, 175t
Spinal nerves, *170,* 170-171, *171,* 173-174
Spinal reflexes, 171, 172t
Spindle fibers, in mitosis, 51
Spine, bony, 94t
  iliac, 109, *110,* 110t
  ischial, *110,* 110t, 111
  scapular, 107

Spinothalamic tract, 171
Spinous process, 103, *103*, 104, *104*
Spiral fracture, 116
Spirogram, 314, *314*
Spirometry, 314, *314*
Spleen, 290
Splenectomy, 290
Splenic artery, *271, 272*, 273t, 275
Splenic flexure, 340, *341*
Splenic vein, *276, 277*, 278t, *279*, 279-280
Spongy bone, 92, *93*
Spongy (penile) urethra, *380, 381, 396*
Sprain, 91
Squamous cells, 61
Squamous epithelium, *60*
    simple, *60, 61, 61, 61t*
    stratified, *60*, 61t, 63, *63*
Squamous suture, *98, 100*, 101
Stapes, 102, *194, 195, 195, 197*
Starch, 31, 362-363
Starling's law of the heart, 252
STDs (sexually transmitted diseases), 415-416
Stenosis, valvular, 247
Sternal angle, 105, *105*
Sternal area, 14t, *15*
Sternal body, 105, *105*
Sternocleidomastoid muscle, 137
Sternum, 105, *105*
Steroids, 33, *34*
    anabolic, 147
    hormones as, 205, 215-216, *216*
    sex, 215-216
Stethoscope, 251
Stillbirth, 420
Stomach, 335-338. See also *Gastric* entries.
    emptying of, 338
    secretions of, 336t, 336-338, *337*
    structure of, *335*, 335-336
Stones, kidney, 385
Stool, formation and elimination of, 341
Straight tubules, *396, 396*
Stratified epithelium, *60*, 61
    squamous, 61t, 63, *63*
Stratum basale, 78, *78*
    endometrial, 407, *407*
Stratum corium, 78, *79*
Stratum corneum, 78, *79*
Stratum functionale, endometrial, 407, *407*
Stratum germinativum, 78, *79*
Stratum granulosum, 78, *79*
Stratum lucidum, 78, *79*
Stratum spinosum, 78, *79*
Stress, homeostasis and, *9*, 9-10, *10*
Stressor, 9
Stretch receptors, pulmonary, 321
Striae, 79
Stroke volume, *252*, 252-253
Structural formula, 24
Stye, 188
Stylohyoid muscle, *102*
Styloid process, *98, 99*, 101, *102*, 107, *108, 108*, 109t
Stylomastoid foramen, *99, 100*, 101t
Subarachnoid space, 163, *163*
Subatomic particles, 19, *19*
Subclavian arteries, 270, *271, 272*, 273t, *274*
Subclavian vein, *276, 277*, 278t, 279
Subcutaneous fat, 65t, 66, *66*, 80
    distribution of, 370
    essential, 369
    excess, 369-370
    nonessential, 369-370
Subcutaneous layer, 77, *78*, 80

Subliminal impulse, in muscle contraction, 127
Subliminal stimulus, in nerve conduction, 159
Sublingual glands, 334, *334*
Submandibular glands, 334, *334*
Submucosa, bladder, 379, *380*
    gastrointestinal, *330*, 330-331
Submucosal plexus, *330*, 330-331
Subscapularis muscle, 140t, 141-142, *142*
Substance abuse, in pregnancy, 433
Subthreshold impulse, in muscle contraction, 127
    in nerve conduction, 159
Sucrase, 339, 345, 346t
Sucrose, 31, 345-346, 362, 362t
    absorption of, 346, *347*
Suction lipectomy, 66
Sudden infant death syndrome, maternal smoking and, 433
Sudoriferous glands, 82
Suffix, 15
Sugars, complex, 31, 362, 362t
    double, 31, 362, 362t
    metabolism of, 343, 354, 355-357, *355-358, 360*
    simple, 31, 362, 362t
        absorption of, 346, *347*
Sulcus, 164, *164*
    central, 164, *164*
    dorsal (posterior) median, 170, *171*
    lateral, 164, *164*
Summation, motor, 128
    multiple motor unit, 128
    multiple wave, 128
    wave, 128
Superficial, 11
Superficial fascia, 80
Superior, 11
Superior cerebellar peduncle, 168
Superior colliculi, 168, *193*
Superior mesenteric artery, 270, *271, 272*, 273t, *274*, 275
Superior mesenteric vein, *276, 277*, 278t, *279*, 279-280
Superior nasal conchae, 101
Superior oblique muscle, 189t
Superior orbital fissure, *98, 100*, 101t
Superior rectus muscle, 189t
Superior sagittal sinus, 163
Superior vena cava, *249, 276, 277, 277*, 278t
Supination, 135t
Supporting (Sertoli's) cells, 396, *397*
Suppressor T cells, 296, *297*
Supraorbital foramen, *98, 100, 101*, 101t
Suprarenal artery, *271, 272*, 273t, 275
Suprarenal (adrenal) glands, *214*, 214-217
    hormones of, 209t, *214*, 215-217, *216, 217*
Supraspinatus muscle, 140t, 141-142, *142*
Suprasternal notch, 105, *105*
Surface area, rule of nines for, 85, *85*
Surfactant, 314
Suspensions, 27
Suspensory ligaments, of eye, 190, *190*, 191-192
    of uterus, 412, *412*
Sustentacular cells, 396, *397*
Sutural bones, 97
Suture(s), coronal, *98, 100*
    cranial, *98, 100, 100*
    lambdoid, *98, 100, 100*
    sagittal, 100
    squamous, *98, 100*, 101
Swayback, 103

Sweat glands, 82
Swelling, in inflammation, 293
Sympathetic nervous system, 155, 175-176, *176*, 176t, 177
Symphysis pubis, 109, *110*
Synapse, components of, 161, *161*
    conduction across, 161-162
Synaptic bulb, *155*, 156
Synaptic cleft, 126
Synaptic vesicles, 161
Synarthroses, 114
Synergist muscles, 133
Synovial fluid, 71, 114, *115*
Synovial joints, 114, *115*
Synovial membranes, *70, 71*, 114, *115*
Synthesis, dehydration, 26
Synthesis reactions, 26
Syphilis, 415
Systemic circulation, 260, *260*, 270
Systemic inflammation, 293, *294*
Systole, atrial, 251, *251*
    ventricular, 251, *251*
Systolic pressure, 267. See also *Blood pressure.*

T

T cells, 291, 295-296, *296-298*
    helper, 296, *297*
        in HIV infection, 239
    killer, 296, *297*
    memory, 296, *297*
    suppressor, 296, *297*
T tubules, 125
T wave, 250, *250*
    in myocardial infarction, 254-255
Tactile sense, 179, 185, *185*
Talipes, 91
Talus, 112, 113, *113*, 113t, *114*
Tangles, in Alzheimer's disease, 179
Target tissue, 206
Tarsal area, 14t, *15*
Tarsal bones, 113, *114*
Taste, age-related changes in, 199
    impairment of, *201*
Taste blindness, 187
Taste buds, 186-187, *187*
Taste cells, 186
Taste hairs, 186
Taste pores, 186
Taste receptors, 186-187, *187*
Tears, 189
Tectorial membrane, 196, *196, 197*
Teeth, 332, 332-333, *333*
    cavities of, 333
    deciduous (primary), 332, *332*
    eruption of, 333t
    permanent (secondary), 332, *332*
    structure of, 333, *333*
Telodendria, *155*, 156
Telophase, 50, 51, 51t
Temperature, 367-368
    body heat and, 8
    core, 367
    heat loss and, 368
    heat production and, 123, 361, 368
    regulation of, 368
        skin in, 83, *83*-84
    respiratory rate and, 322
    shell, 368
Temporal bones, *98-100*, 101
Temporal lobe, 164, *164*
    in auditory pathway, 197
Temporal process, 102

Temporalis muscle, *136*, 136t, 137
Temporomandibular joint, *98*, 102
Tendon(s), 67, 124
　　Achilles, *141*, *142*, 145, 145t, 171, 172t
　　calcaneal, *141*, *142*, 145, 145t
Teniae coli, 340
Tennis elbow, 107
Tensor fasciae latae muscle, *142*, 143, 144t
Tentorium cerebelli, 168
Teratogens, 432-433
Teres minor muscle, 140t, 141-142, *142*
Terminal ganglia, *176*, 177
Terminology, anatomical, 10-14
　　medical, 15
Tertiary bronchi, *310*, 311
Tertiary syphilis, 415
Testis, 395-399, *396*, *397*
　　age-related changes in, 413
　　hormonal control of, 402, *403*
　　hormones of, 209t, 218-219, *219*
　　in spermatogenesis, 396-399, *398*, *399*
　　structure of, *396*, *396*
　　undescended, 396
Testosterone, 209t, 218-219, *219*, 402, *403*
Tetanus, 128
Tetany, 128, *129*
Thalamus, 166-167, *167*
　　in auditory pathway, 193, *193*, 197
Thermogenesis, 361, 368
Thermoreceptors, 184, 185t, 186
Thermoregulation, 368
　　skin in, *83*, 83-84
Thiamine, 366t
Thigh, 111. See also *Lower extremity*.
　　muscles of, *141-142*, 143, 144t
Third ventricle, 169, *169*
Third-degree burns, 85
Thoracic aorta, 270, *271*, *272*, 273t, *274*
Thoracic area, 14t, *15*
Thoracic cage, 105, *105*
Thoracic cavity, 12, *12*
Thoracic curvature, 103, *103*
Thoracic duct, 288, *288*, *289*
Thoracic nerves, *170*, 170-171, 173-174, 175t
Thoracic vertebrae, *103*, 104, *104*
Thoracic wall, muscles of, 137
　　veins of, *276*, *277*, 278t, *279*
Thoracocentesis, 307
Thoracolumbar division, 176
Threshold impulse, in muscle contraction, 127
　　in nerve conduction, 159
Thrombin, 234
Thrombocytes, 68, *68*, 228t, 233
Thrombocytopenia, 226
Thrombus, 226
Thymosin, 210t, 220, 291
Thymus, 210t, 220, 291
Thyroid cartilage, 309, *309*
Thyroid gland, 212, 212-213
　　hypothalamus and, 212, *212*
　　pituitary and, 212, *212*
Thyroid hormones, *212*, 212-213
Thyroid-stimulating hormone (TSH), 209t, *210*, 211
Thyroxine, 209t, *212*, 212-213
Tibia, 112, *113*, 113t
Tibial arteries, *271*, *272*, 273t, 275
Tibial tuberosity, 112, *113*, 113t
Tibial veins, *276*, *277*, 278t, 280
Tibialis anterior muscle, *141*, 145, 145t
Tics, 123
Tidal volume, 314, *314*, 315t
Tinnitus, 184

Tissue, 4, 60-70
　　adipose, 65t, 66, *66*, 80
　　age-related changes in, 71
　　avascular, 60
　　connective, 65t, 65-68. See also *Connective tissue*.
　　definition of, 60
　　epithelial, 60-65. See also *Epithelium*.
　　muscle, 68-69
　　nerve, 155-157
　　nervous, *69*, 69-70
　　organization of, 4
　　osseous, 65t, 67-68, *68*
　　regeneration of, 72, *73*
　　subcutaneous, 77, *78*, 80
　　target, 206
Tissue repair, 72, *73*
Tone, muscle, 129
Tongue, *331*, 332
Tongue tie, 332
Tonometry, 184
Tonsillectomy, 290
Tonsils, 290
　　lingual, 290, 309, *309*, *331*, 332
　　palatine, 290, 309, *309*, *331*, 332, 334
　　pharyngeal, 290, 308, *309*
Tooth. See *Teeth*.
Torso, *13*, 14
Torticollis, 137
Total lung capacity, 314, *314*, 315t
Total metabolic rate, 360, *361*
Total organism level, of body organization, 4
Touch, 179, 185, *185*
Trabeculae, *92*, 93
Trabeculae carneae, *245*, 246
Tracer, 36
Trachea, *310*, 310-311
Tracheal cartilage, 310, *310*
Tracheal foreign body, 311
Tracheotomy, 310
Tract, ascending, 171
　　descending, 171
　　extrapyramidal, 171
　　olfactory, 187, *188*
　　optic, 193
　　pyramidal, 171
　　spinothalamic, 171
Transcription, 53-54, *54*
Transfer RNA, 54
Transfusions, blood typing for, 235
　　disease transmission via, 239
　　universal donor in, 235-236
　　universal recipient in, 235-236
Transient ischemic attack (TIA), 153
Transitional epithelium, 61t, 63, *63*
Translation, 54, *55*
Transplant, bone marrow, 229
　　corneal, 190
Transverse colon, *340*, 341
Transverse fissure, 168
Transverse foramina, 104, *104*
Transverse fracture, 116
Transverse plane, 11, *12*
Transverse process, 103, *103*
Trapezius muscle, 137, 140t, 140-141, *141*, *142*
Traversus abdominis muscle, 138t, 138-139, *139*
Treppe, 129, *129*
Triceps brachii muscle, 140t, *142*, 142-143
Tricuspid valve, *245*, 246, 247, *247*, *269*, 270
Trigeminal nerve, 172-173, *173*, 174t

Triglycerides, 32, 33, *34*. See also *Lipids*.
　　absorption of, 347, *347*, 348t
　　hydrolysis of, 359
Trigone, 380, *380*
Triiodothyronine, 209t, *212*, 212-213
Trochanter, 94t
　　greater, *111*, 112, 112t
　　lesser, *111*, 112, 112t
Trochlear nerve, 172-173, *173*, 174t
Trochlear (semilunar) notch, 107, *108*, 109t
Trophoblast, *422*, 423, *424*
Tropic hormones, 207
True labor, 428
True pelvis, 111
True ribs, *105*, 106
True vocal cords, *309*, 310
Trunk(s), celiac, *274*, 275
　　lymphatic, 288
　　muscles of, 137, 138t, *139*
　　pulmonary, *245*, 248, *248*, *269*, 270
Trypsin, 345, 346
Trypsinogen, 345
TSH (thyroid-stimulating hormone), 209t, *210*, 211
Tubal ligation, 407, 414
Tube(s), auditory (eustachian), *194*, 195, 308, *309*
　　uterine (fallopian), 406-407, *407*
Tubercle, 94t
　　greater, 107, *107*, 107t
　　lesser, 107, *107*, 107t
Tuberculosis, skin test for, 302
Tuberosity, 94t
　　deltoid, 107, *107*, 107t
　　gluteal, *111*, 112, 112t
　　ischial, 110, 110t, 111
　　radial, 107, *108*, 109t
　　tibial, 112, *113*, 113t
Tubular gland, 64
Tubular reabsorption, 381-383, *383*, 384
Tubular secretion, 383-384, *384*
Tubules, seminiferous, 396, *396*, 397
　　straight, 396, *396*
　　T, 125
Tubulin, 45
Tumor(s), 57
　　benign, 40, 57
　　brain, 156
　　malignant, 40, 57. See also *Cancer*.
Tunica adventitia, 261, *261*
Tunica albuginea, 396, *396*, 403, *404*
Tunica externa, 261, *261*
Tunica interna, 260, *261*
Tunica intima, 260, *261*
Tunica media, 260, *261*
Turbinates, nasal, 101
Twins, dizygotic, 421
　　monozygotic, 421
Twitch, 128, *129*
Tympanic cavity, 195
Tympanic membrane, 194, *194*, 195, *197*
Tympanitis, 184
Type I diabetes, 222
Type II diabetes, 222

U

Ulna, 107-108, *108*, 109t
Ulnar artery, *271*, *272*, 273t, 274-275
Ulnar head, 108, *108*, 109t
Ulnar notch, 107, *108*, 109t
Ulnar vein, *276*, *277*, 278t, *279*

Umbilical area, 14t, *15*
Umbilical arteries, *280, 281,* 281t, 428t
Umbilical cord, *280, 281,* 281t
Umbilical cord blood, 229
Umbilical region, 12, *13*
Umbilical veins, *280, 281,* 281t, 428t
Undernutrition, 354
Undescended testis, 396
Universal donor, 235-236
Universal recipient, 235-236
Unsaturated fatty acids, 33, 33t
Upper extremity, arteries of, *271, 272,* 273t,
　274-275
　bones of, *107,* 107-109, *108,* 109t
　muscles of, 140t, 140-143, *141-142*
　veins of, *276, 277,* 278t, *279*
Upper respiratory tract, 307-310, *308, 309*
Urea, plasma, 228
Uremic frost, 375
Ureter, 376, *376, 379, 380*
Urethra, *380,* 380-381, *396, 399*
　membranous, *380, 381, 396, 399*
　prostatic, *380, 381, 396*
　spongy (penile), *380, 381, 396*
Urethral sphincter, 380
　external, 380
　internal, 380
Urethritis, 381
　nongonococcal, 416
Uric acid, plasma, 228
Urinary bladder. See *Bladder.*
Urinary incontinence, 385
Urinary system, 5, 7t, 373-391
　age-related changes in, 389
　components of, 375-381, *376*
　disorders of, 391
　functional relationships of, *374*
　functions of, 375
Urinary tract infection, 381
Urination, 385
Urine, abnormal constituents in, 385-386,
　386t
　characteristics of, 385t, 385-386
　chemical composition of, 385, 385t
　color of, 385, 385t
　formation of, 381-384
　　glomerular filtration in, 381, *382, 384*
　　tubular reabsorption in, 381-383, *383,*
　　384
　　tubular secretion in, 383-384, *384*
　glucose in, 221, 382
　pH of, 385, 385t
　specific gravity of, 385t
Urine concentration, regulation of, 384-385
Urine output, 387, *387*
Urine volume, 385t
　regulation of, 384-385
Urochrome, 385
Urogenital diaphragm, 138t, 140
Urolithiasis, 385
Uterine cycle, 409, *410,* 410-412, *411*
Uterine tubes, 406-407, *407*
Uterus, 407, *407*
　anteflexed, 407
Utricle, *195, 197*
Uvula, *308, 309, 331, 331*

V

Vaccination, 300, *300,* 301
Vaccine, 300, *300,* 301
Vagina, 408, *408*
　cancer of, Papanicolaou smear for, 408

Vaginal orifice, 408, *408*
Vagus nerve, 172-173, *173,* 174t
Valve(s), heart, 245, 246-247, *247.* See also
　Heart valves.
　ileocecal, 340, *340*
　venous, *261, 262*
Valvular stenosis, 247
Varicose veins, 262
Vas deferens, *396, 399*
Vasa vasorum, 261
Vascular constriction, in hemostasis, 233,
　234
Vascular tunic, of eye, 190, *190*
Vasectomy, 399, 414
Vasomotor center, 168
Vasopressin, 209t, *210,* 211
Vein(s). See also specific veins.
　age-related changes in, 282
　cardiac, 248-249, *249*
　constriction of, 266
　function of, 262
　major systemic, 275-280, *276, 277,* 278t,
　　279
　of abdominal wall, 279
　of abdominopelvic organs, *279,* 279-280
　of head and neck, *276, 277,* 277-279,
　　278t
　of lower extremity, 280
　of shoulder and arm, *276, 277,* 278t, *279*
　of thoracic wall, 279
　pulmonary, 270
　structure of, 262
　varicose, 262
Vena cava, inferior, *276, 277,* 278t, *279, 279,*
　342, 342
　superior, *249, 276, 277, 277,* 278t
Venous valves, *261, 262*
Ventilation, 307-312. See also *Respiration.*
　atmospheric pressure in, 312-313, *313*
　conducting passages in, 307-312
　expiration in, *313,* 313-314
　in neonate, 429
　inspiration in, 313, *313*
　intra-alveolar pressure in, 312-313, *313,*
　　314
　intrapleural pressure in, 312-313, *313*
　mechanics of, 312-314
　regulation of, *320-322,* 320-322
　voluntary control of, 321-322
Ventral cavity, 12, *12*
Ventral funiculi (columns), 170-171, *171*
Ventral horn, 170, *171*
Ventral median fissure, 170, *171*
Ventral root, *173, 174*
Ventricle(s), cardiac, left, *245, 246, 247,* 248
　right, *245, 246, 247, 247, 269,* 270
　cerebral, 169, *169*
Ventricular diastole, 251, *251,* 252
Ventricular systole, 251, *251*
Venules, 262, *262*
Vermiform appendix, 340, *340*
Vermis, 168
Vernix caseosa, 427
Vertebrae, *103,* 103-105, *104*
　cervical, *103,* 103-104, *104*
　lumbar, *103, 104, 104*
　sacral, *103, 104,* 105
　structure of, 103, *103*
　thoracic, *103,* 104, *104*
Vertebral arch, 103, *103*
Vertebral area, 14t, *15*
Vertebral arteries, *271, 272,* 273t, 274, *275*
Vertebral body, 103, *103*
Vertebral foramen, 103, *103*

Vertebral ribs, *105,* 106
Vertebral veins, *276, 277,* 277-279, 278t
Vertebrochondral ribs, *105,* 106
Vertebrosternal ribs, *105,* 106
Vertigo, 184
Vesicle(s), secretory, 41, 42t, 44, *44*
　seminal, *396,* 400
　synaptic, 161
Vessels. See *Blood vessels.*
Vestibular folds, *309,* 310
Vestibular membrane, 195, *196, 197*
Vestibular nerve, 198
Vestibule, of vagina, 408, *408*
　of ear, *195, 197*
Vestibulocochlear nerve, 172-173, *173,*
　174t
　cochlear branch of, 196, *196*
　vestibular branch of, 198
Villi, chorionic, 425, *426*
　intestinal, 287, 338, *339*
　　absorption by, 341, 346-347, *347*
Visceral, 11
Visceral effectors, 176t
Visceral layer, 70, *70*
Visceral muscle, 68t, 69, *69,* 124t
Visceral pericardium, 243, *245*
Visceral peritoneum, *330,* 331
Visceral pleura, *311,* 312
Vision, *191-193,* 191-194
　accommodation in, 191, *192*
　age-related changes in, 199
　photoreceptors in, *192,* 192-193, 193t
　refraction in, 191, *191*
Visual cortex, 166t, *193*
Visual pathway, *193,* 193-194
Visual sense, 188-194
Vital capacity, 314, *314,* 315t
Vitamin(s), 365-367, 366t
　deficiencies of, 365
　dietary sources of, 366t
　fat-soluble, 365, 366t
　　absorption of, 347, 348t
　functions of, 366t
　toxicity of, 366
　water-soluble, 365, 366t
　　absorption of, 347, 348t
Vitamin B$_{12}$, in erythropoiesis, 231
Vitamin D synthesis, skin in, 84
Vitamin K, in coagulation, 234
Vitreous humor, *190,* 191
Vocal cords, *309,* 310
Voiding, 385
Voluntary nervous system, 155
Volvulus, 329
Vomer, 98, *100,* 102
Vomiting, 338
Vulva, 408, *408*

W

Warm-blooded animals, 367
Warmth, in inflammation, 293
Wart, 77
Water, as compound, 23
　body, 8. See also *Fluid* entries.
　functions of, 367
　intake of, 367
Wave summation, 128
Weight, vs. mass, 18
Weightlifting, 147
Wernicke's area, *164,* 166t
White blood cells. See *Leukocytes.*
White fibers, 131

White matter, cerebral, 164-165, 165t
   spinal, 170, *171*
White pulp, 290
Wormian bones, 97
Wound repair, 72, *73*
Wrist, 108
   muscles of, 143
Wry neck, 137

X

Xiphoid process, 105, *105*

Y

Yawning, 322, 323t
Yellow marrow, 92
Yolk sac, *424*, 425, *425*

Z

Z line, 125, *125*
Zinc, dietary, 367t
Zona pellucida, *404*, 406, *422*

Zone of infarction, in myocardial infarction, 254
Zone of injury, in myocardial infarction, 254
Zone of ischemia, in myocardial infarction, 254
Zone of overlap, 125
Zygomatic arch, 102
Zygomatic bones, *98-100*, 102
Zygomatic process, *98, 99*, 101
Zygomaticus muscle, 134, *136*, 136t
Zygote, 420, *420*, 421
   cleavage of, 422, *422*

INDEX OF CLINICAL TERMS

Abruptio placentae (Ch 20)

Acromegaly (Ch 10)

Adenoma (Ch 10)

Adhesion (Ch 4)

Allergen (Ch 14)

Alopecia (Ch 5)

Amenorrhea (Ch 19)

Anaphylaxis (Ch 14)

Anaplasia (Ch 3)

Anemia (Ch 11)

Angiography (Ch 13)

Angioplasty (Ch 13)

Anuria (Ch 18)

Apgar score (Ch 20)

Aphagia (Ch 16)

Arterectomy (Ch 13)

Arteriosclerosis (Ch 13)

Arthritis (Ch 5)

Artificial pacemaker (Ch 12)

Ascites (Ch 16)

Aspiration (Ch 15)

Astigmatism (Ch 9)

Atelectasis (Ch 15)

Atherosclerosis (Ch 13)

Atrophy (Ch 3)

Audiometry (Ch 9)

Auscultation (Ch 12)

Autoimmune disease (Ch 14)

Azotemia (Ch 18)

Basal cell carcinoma (Ch 5)

Benign (Ch 3)

Biopsy (Ch 4)

Blepharitis (Ch 9)

Blood urea nitrogen (BUN) (Ch 18)

Borborygmus (Ch 16)

Bronchogenic carcinoma (Ch 15)

Bunion (Ch 6)

Carcinogen (Ch 3)

Carcinoma (Ch 4)

Cardiac arrest (Ch 12)

Cardiac catheterization (Ch 12)

Cardiomegaly (Ch 12)

Carpal tunnel syndrome (Ch 6)

Celiac disease (Ch 17)

Cellulitis (Ch 5)

Cerebral concussion (Ch 8)

Cerebral contusion (Ch 8)

Cerebral palsy (Ch 8)

Cerebrovascular accident (CVA) (Ch 8)

Cesarean section (Ch 20)

Cholecystitis (Ch 16)

Cholelithiasis (Ch 16)

Chronic obstructive pulmonary disease (COPD) (Ch 15)

Coitus (Ch 19)

Colostomy (Ch 16)

Computed tomography (CT) (Ch 8)

Cor pulmonale (Ch 12)

Coronary artery bypass grafting (CABG) (Ch 12)

Coryza (Ch 15)

Cramp (Ch 7)

Cretinism (Ch 10)

Croup (Ch 15)

Defibrillation (Ch 12)

Dermatitis (Ch 5)

Dialysis (Ch 18)

Diarrhea (Ch 16)

Diplopia (Ch 9)

Dislocation (Ch 6)

Diuresis (Ch 18)

Diuretic (Ch 18)

Dysmenorrhea (Ch 19)

Dysphagia (Ch 16)

Dysplasia (Ch 3)

Dystocia (Ch 20)

Dysuria (Ch 18)

Ecchymosis (Ch 11)

Echocardiography (Ch 12)

Eclampsia (Ch 20)

Eczema (Ch 5)

Electroencephalography (EEG) (Ch 8)

Electromyography (Ch 7)

Embolus (Ch 11)

Emesis (Ch 16)

Emmetropia (Ch 9)

Endocrinology (Ch 10)

Endometriosis (Ch 19)

Enuresis (Ch 18)

Episiotomy (Ch 19)

Eructation (Ch 16)

Erythrocytosis (Ch 11)

Eschar (Ch 5)

Eutocia (Ch 20)

Exophthalmic (Ch 10)

Fibrillation (Ch 12)

Flatus (Ch 16)

Gavage (Ch 16)

Glucose tolerance test (GTT) (Ch 10)

Gout (Ch 6)

Heat exhaustion (Ch 17)

Hemangioma (Ch 13)

Hematemesis (Ch 16)

Hemophilia (Ch 11)

Hemorrhoids (Ch 13)

Histology (Ch 4)